Pediatric *and* Adolescent Knee Surgery

Pediatric *and* Adolescent Knee Surgery

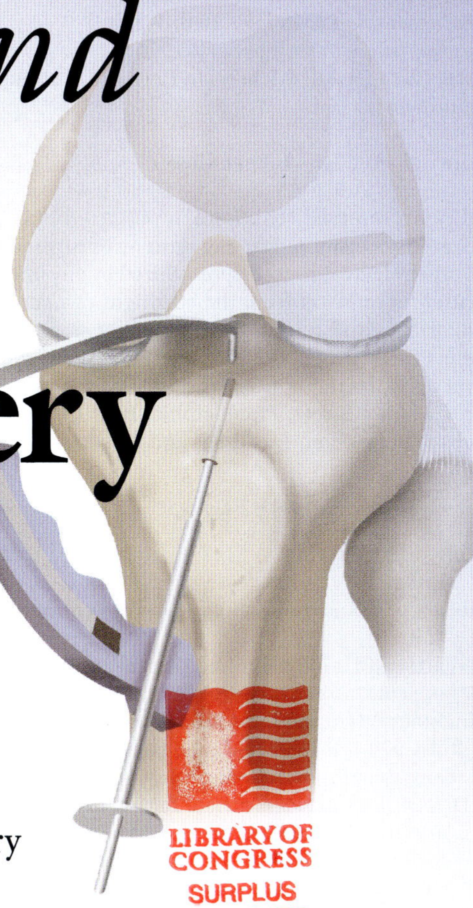

EDITORS

Frank A. Cordasco, MD, MS
Co-Medical Director
Leon Root Motion Analysis Laboratory
Attending Orthopedic Surgeon
Sports Medicine and Shoulder Service
Hospital for Special Surgery
Professor of Orthopaedic Surgery
Weill Cornell Medical College
New York, New York

Daniel W. Green, MD, MS, FAAP, FACS
Attending Orthopedic Surgeon
Pediatric Orthopedic Surgery Service
Hospital for Special Surgery
Professor of Clinical Orthopaedic Surgery
Weill Cornell Medical College
New York, New York

Wolters Kluwer

Philadelphia • Baltimore • New York • London
Buenos Aires • Hong Kong • Sydney • Tokyo

Acquisitions Editor: Brian Brown
Product Development Editor: Dave Murphy
Marketing Manager: Daniel Dressler
Production Project Manager: David Saltzberg
Design Coordinator: Steven Druding
Manufacturing Coordinator: Beth Welsh
Prepress Vendor: Absolute Service, Inc.
Cover Photo Credits: © Christian Bertrand / Shutterstock.com, © James A. Boardman / Shutterstock.com

9 8 7 6 5 4 3 2 1

Printed in China

Library of Congress Cataloging-in-Publication Data

Pediatric and adolescent knee surgery / [edited by] Frank A. Cordasco, Daniel W. Green.
p. ; cm.
Includes bibliographical references and index.
ISBN 978-1-4511-9335-0 (alk. paper)
I. Cordasco, Frank A., editor. II. Green, Daniel W., editor.
[DNLM: 1. Anterior Cruciate Ligament—surgery. 2. Knee Injuries—surgery. 3. Adolescent. 4. Anterior Cruciate Ligament Reconstruction–methods. 5. Child. 6. Knee Joint—surgery. 7. Osteochondritis Dissecans–surgery. WE 870]
RD561
617.5'82059—dc23

2015009595

LWW.com

RRS1503

To my parents, my wife Monique, my daughter Mikaela, and my son Luke

FAC

To my parents; my wife Brenda; and my daughters Kelly, Bridget, and Maggie

DWG

In addition, we would like to acknowledge our mentors and partners who have provided us with inspiration, guidance, and support. We also thank our residents and fellows who have challenged and stimulated our pursuit of knowledge throughout our careers.

FAC and DWG

Contributing Authors

Jay C. Albright, MD
Children's Hospital Colorado
Assistant Professor of Orthopedic Surgery
University of Colorado Denver
Aurora, Colorado

Allen F. Anderson, MD
Orthopedic Surgeon
Tennessee Orthopaedic Alliance
Nashville, Tennessee

Christian N. Anderson, MD
Orthopedic Surgeon
Tennessee Orthopaedic Alliance
Nashville, Tennessee

Morgan A. Anderson, MD
Internal Medicine Resident
New York University
New York, New York

Sarah M. Baker, PT, DPT
Physical Therapist
Hospital for Special Surgery
New York, New York

Davietta C. Butty, BS
Sports Medicine Research Fellow
Midwest Orthopaedics at Rush University Medical Center
Chicago, Illinois

Henry G. Chambers, MD
Professor of Clinical Orthopedic Surgery
University of California, San Diego
Rady Children's Hospital
San Diego, California

Theresa A. Chiaia, PT, DPT
Section Manager
Sports Rehabilitation and Performance Center
Department of Rehabilitation
Hospital for Special Surgery
New York, New York

Ellie Ci-En Choi, MBBS
Department of Orthopaedic Surgery
National University Hospital
Singapore

Elizabeth Cody, MD
Resident, Orthopaedic Surgery
Department of Orthopedic Surgery
Hospital for Special Surgery
New York, New York

Brian J. Cole, MD, MBA
Professor
Department of Orthopaedics
Midwest Orthopaedics at Rush University Medical Center
Chicago, Illinois

Frank A. Cordasco, MD, MS
Co-Medical Director
Leon Root Motion Analysis Laboratory
Attending Orthopedic Surgeon
Sports Medicine and Shoulder Service
Hospital for Special Surgery
Professor of Orthopaedic Surgery
Weill Cornell Medical College
New York, New York

Polly de Mille, RN, RCEP, CSCS
Clinical Supervisor, Sports Performance
Department of Rehabilitation
Hospital for Special Surgery
New York, New York

Emily R. Dodwell, MD, MPH, FRCSC
Assistant Professor, Orthopaedic Surgery
Weill Cornell Medical College
Assistant Attending Pediatric Orthopedic Surgeon
Hospital for Special Surgery
New York, New York

Shevaun M. Doyle, MD
Associate Professor of Clinical Orthopaedic Surgery
Weill Cornell Medical College
Associate Attending Orthopedic Surgeon
Hospital for Special Surgery
New York, New York

Eric W. Edmonds, MD
Director of Orthopedic Research
Co-Director, 360 Sports Medicine
Pediatric Orthopedic & Scoliosis Center
Rady Children's Hospital
Assistant Clinical Professor
Department of Orthopaedic Surgery
University of California San Diego
San Diego, California

Peter D. Fabricant, MD, MPH
Pediatric Orthopaedic Surgery Fellow
Children's Hospital of Philadelphia
Philadelphia, Pennsylvania

Donald E. Fowler III, MD
Orthopaedic Surgeon
OrthoAtlanta
Austel, Georgia

Theodore J. Ganley, MD
Director of Sports Medicine
The Children's Hospital of Philadelphia
Associate Professor of Orthopaedic Surgery
Perelman School of Medicine at the University of Pennsylvania
Philadelphia, Pennsylvania

Itai Gans, MD
Resident
Department of Orthopaedic Surgery
Johns Hopkins Hospital
Baltimore, Maryland

Matthew R. Garner, MD
Resident
Department of Orthopedics
Hospital for Special Surgery
New York, New York

Elizabeth B. Gausden, MD
Resident, Orthopaedic Surgery
Department of Orthopedic Surgery
Hospital for Special Surgery
New York, New York

Christine M. Goodbody, MD
Benjamin Fox Research Fellow
Department of Orthopaedics
The Children's Hospital of Philadelphia
Perelman School of Medicine at the University of Pennsylvania
Philadelphia, Pennsylvania

Brian Grawe, MD
Fellow Sports Medicine
Hospital for Special Surgery
New York, New York

Jessica Graziano, PT, DPT, CSCS
Physical Therapist
Sports Rehabilitation and Performance Center
Hospital for Special Surgery
New York, New York

Daniel W. Green, MD, MS, FAAP, FACS
Attending Orthopedic Surgeon
Pediatric Orthopedic Surgery Service
Hospital for Special Surgery
Professor of Clinical Orthopaedic Surgery
Weill Cornell Medical College
New York, New York

Jo A. Hannafin, MD, PhD
Professor of Orthopaedic Surgery
Weill Cornell Medical College
Orthopedic Director
Women's Sports Medicine Center
Hospital for Special Surgery
Director of Orthopedic Research
Hospital for Special Surgery
New York, New York

Jonathan D. Haskel, BS
Medical Student
Rutgers Robert Wood Johnson Medical School
New Brunswick, New Jersey

William Hennrikus, MD
Professor and Associate Dean
Penn State College of Medicine
Hershey, Pennsylvania

Benton E. Heyworth, MD
Clinical Instructor
Harvard Medical School
Attending Orthopedic Surgeon
Division of Sports Medicine
Department of Orthopedic Surgery
Boston Children's Hospital
Boston, Massachusetts

Sarah Hobart, MD
Resident
Department of Orthopaedic Surgery
Lenox Hill Hospital
New York, New York

Victor M. Ho-Fung, MD
The Children's Hospital of Philadelphia
Assistant Professor of Radiology
Perelman School of Medicine at the University of Pennsylvania
Philadelphia, Pennsylvania

James H.P. Hui, MD
Professor of Orthopaedic Surgery
Department of Orthopaedic Surgery
Yong Loo Lin School of Medicine
Clinical Director
University Orthopaedics, Hand and Reconstructive Microsurgery Cluster
Head and Senior Consultant
Division of Paediatric Orthopaedics
National University Health System
Singapore

Carl W. Imhauser, PhD
Assistant Scientist
Hospital for Special Surgery
New York, New York

Shari T. Jawetz, MD
Assistant Attending Radiologist
Hospital for Special Surgery
Assistant Professor of Radiology
Weill Cornell Medical College
New York, New York

Kristofer J. Jones, MD
Assistant Professor
Department of Orthopaedic Surgery
Division of Sports Medicine and Shoulder Surgery
University of California, Los Angeles
Los Angeles, California

Mininder S. Kocher, MD, MPH
Professor
Department of Orthopaedic Surgery
Harvard Medical School
Associate Director
Division of Sports Medicine
Boston Children's Hospital
Boston, Massachusetts

Hannah-Noemi Ladenhauf, MD
Department of Pediatric and Adolescent Surgery
University Hospital Salzburg
Salzburg, Austria

Lauren E. Lamont, MD
Orthopedic Resident
Hospital for Special Surgery
New York, New York

R. Jay Lee, MD
Assistant Professor
Department of Orthopaedic Surgery
Johns Hopkins Hospital
Baltimore, Maryland

Scott J. Luhmann, MD
Associate Professor
Department of Orthopaedic Surgery
Washington University School of Medicine
St. Louis, Missouri

Alec A. Macaulay, MD
Resident, Orthopaedic Surgery
Harvard Orthopaedics Combined Residency Program
Boston, Massachusetts

Nathan A. Mall, MD
Orthopaedic Surgeon
Regeneration Orthopedics
St. Louis Center for Cartilage Restoration and Repair
St. Louis, Missouri

Robert G. Marx, MD, MSc, FRCSC
Professor of Orthopaedic Surgery and Public Health
Weill Cornell Medical College
Hospital for Special Surgery
New York, New York

Stephanie W. Mayer, MD
Orthopaedic Surgeon
Department of Pediatric Orthopaedic Surgery
Children's Hospital Colorado
Aurora, Colorado

Moira M. McCarthy, MD
Assistant Attending Orthopaedic Surgeon
Sports Medicine and Shoulder Service
Hospital for Special Surgery
Instructor of Orthopaedic Surgery
Weill Cornell Medical College
New York, New York

Amy L. McIntosh, MD
Assistant Professor of Orthopedics
College of Medicine
Mayo Clinic
Rochester, Minnesota

Jordan D. Metzl, MD
Primary Care Sports Medicine Service
Hospital for Special Surgery
Associate Professor of Clinical Pediatrics
Weill Cornell Medical College
New York, New York

James F. Mooney III, MD
Professor
Orthopaedic Surgery
Chief
Pediatric Orthopaedic Surgery
Medical University of South Carolina
Charleston, South Carolina

Jacqueline Munch, MD
Assistant Professor of Orthopaedic Surgery
Department of Orthopaedic Surgery
Oregon Health & Science University
Portland, Oregon

Jeffrey J. Nepple, MD
Assistant Professor of Orthopaedic Surgery
Washington University in St. Louis
St. Louis, Missouri

Benedict U. Nwachukwu, MD, MBA
Resident, Orthopaedic Surgery
Department of Orthopedic Surgery
Hospital for Special Surgery
New York, New York

George A. Paletta, Jr., MD
Orthopaedic Surgeon
Regeneration Orthopedics
The Orthopedic Center of St. Louis
Chesterfield, Missouri

Gregory Pinkowsky, MD
Chief Resident
Department of Orthopaedics
Penn State College of Medicine
Hershey, Pennsylvania

John D. Polousky, MD
Orthopaedic Surgeon
Rocky Mountain Hospital for Children
Denver, Colorado

Hollis G. Potter, MD
Chairman
Department of Radiology and Imaging
Hospital for Special Surgery
The Coleman Chair in MRI Research
Attending Radiologist
Hospital for Special Surgery
Professor of Radiology
Weill Cornell Medical College
Senior Scientist
Clinical Research Section
Hospital for Special Surgery
Director of Research
Department of Radiology and Imaging
Hospital for Special Surgery
New York, New York

Ryan C. Rauck, BS
Research Assistant
The Ohio State University College of Medicine
Columbus, Ohio

Scott A. Rodeo, MD
Co-Chief Emeritus
Sports Medicine and Shoulder Service
Co-Director
Tissue Engineering, Regeneration, and Repair Program
Hospital for Special Surgery
Professor, Orthopaedic Surgery
Weill Cornell Medical College
Attending Orthopedic Surgeon
The Hospital for Special Surgery
New York, New York

Brant Sachleben, MD
Assistant Professor
Department of Orthopaedics
Arkansas Children's Hospital
Little Rock, Arkansas

Gerd Seitlinger, MD
Orthopaedic Surgeon
Department of Orthopaedic Surgery
Hospital Oberndorf
Oberndorf, Austria

Parina H. Shah, MS
Research Assistant
Department of Magnetic Resonance Imaging
Hospital for Special Surgery
New York, New York

Yong-Woon Shin, MD, PhD
Associate Professor
Department of Orthopedic Surgery
Sanggye Paik Hospital
Inje University
Seoul, Korea

Beth Shubin Stein, MD
Associate Attending Orthopedic Surgeon
Hospital for Special Surgery
Associate Professor of Orthopaedic Surgery
Weill Cornell Medical College
New York, New York

Aisling M. Toolan, PT, DPT, SCS, CSCS
Physical Therapist
Sports Physical Therapy
Sports Rehabilitation and Performance Center
Hospital for Special Surgery
New York, New York

Samir K. Trehan, MD
Orthopedic Surgery Resident
Hospital for Special Surgery
New York, New York

Tyler J. Uppstrom, BA
Research Assistant
Pediatric Orthopaedic Service
Hospital for Special Surgery
New York, New York

Curtis D. VandenBerg, MD
Pediatric Orthopaedic Surgery Fellow
Children's Hospital Colorado
Aurora, Colorado

Marcia Voigt, BA
Medical Student
Wake Forest University School of Medicine
Winston-Salem, North Carolina

Russell F. Warren, MD
Surgeon-in-Chief Emeritus
Attending Orthopedic Surgeon
Hospital for Special Surgery
Professor of Orthopaedic Surgery
Weill Cornell Medical College
New York, New York

Roger F. Widmann, MD
Chief, Division of Pediatric Orthopedic Surgery
Hospital for Special Surgery
Attending Orthopedic Surgeon
Hospital for Special Surgery
Professor of Clinical Orthopaedic Surgery
Weill Cornell Medical College
New York, New York

Keng Lin Wong, MRCS(Ed)
Resident (Clinician Scientist Track)
Department of Orthopaedic Surgery
University Orthopaedics, Hand and Reconstructive Microsurgery Cluster
National University Health System
Singapore

Adam B. Yanke, MD
Sports Medicine Fellow
Sports Medicine Division
Department of Orthopedics
Rush University Medical Center
Chicago, Illinois

Foreword

Injury to the pediatric and adolescent athlete has increasingly become an issue for the orthopedic surgeon and physical therapist. These young athletes present a series of issues that require a different approach from our adult patients. This book is beautifully organized by Dr. Dan Green and Dr. Frank Cordasco and brings to the forefront how to manage these patients throughout their years of growth.

Specifically, injuries to the anterior cruciate ligament (ACL) and the various techniques in treating this condition in young patients is well demonstrated. Patella instability and its many options are covered in detail. Epiphyseal injury and adolescent fractures about the knee are highlighted.

The authors have organized a detailed approach to the pediatric and adolescent knee that surgeons and therapists will find enlightening and enable them to provide comprehensive care to this group of patients that are increasingly seen in our orthopedic offices.

Russell F. Warren, MD

Preface

We were inspired to write this textbook by the increasing number of knee injuries in young athletes that we encounter daily in our practices. We believe that this textbook written with the support of international experts is an imperative and timely guide to the treatment of pediatric and adolescent knee injuries.

The higher volume of knee injuries in the young athlete is multifactorial and includes, but is not limited to, increased participation in sports, higher levels of competition within youth sports, increased sports specialization, and societal factors. Historically, children and adolescents with anterior cruciate ligament tears or patellofemoral instability episodes as well as other knee injuries were often treated with benign neglect. With advances in the understanding of knee anatomy, pathomechanics, and the natural history of nonoperative treatment, our therapeutic guidelines have become more focused and specific. Much of this depends on the individual athlete, his or her skeletal age, his or her sport, and the particular injury pattern.

This textbook includes 41 chapters divided into several sections with a comprehensive approach to each of the pathologic entities written by experts in their respective areas. Section 1 is composed of 13 chapters focusing on the anterior cruciate ligament. These chapters concentrate on the epidemiology, biomechanics, gender, nonoperative treatments, and a menu of five specific operative techniques followed by guidelines that offer a decision tree for selecting proper treatment as predicated by skeletal age. This section concludes with the rehabilitation, movement analysis, return to play, and prevention components necessary to complete the management of these injured athletes. Section 2 includes 6 chapters that concentrate on patellofemoral instability with an introductory chapter, 4 chapters that discuss operative technique, and a chapter on rehabilitation of these athletes. Section 3 centers on osteochondritis dissecans, with 7 chapters including an overview as well as multiple surgical techniques and ending with a chapter discussing the frontiers of cartilage restoration. Section 4 is directed toward discoid meniscus, with 3 chapters including an overview, treatment options, and meniscal transplantation. Section 5 includes 5 chapters that review the management of fractures of the tibia, femur, and patella. The textbook finishes with 6 chapters that discuss the physis, which includes imaging, anatomy, assessment of growth, the treatment of growth arrest, the applications of implant-mediated growth, and Osgood-Schlatter Disease.

Our aim is that this textbook serves as an invaluable resource to all those providers of care for our pediatric and adolescent athletes and patients including pediatric orthopedic surgeons, orthopedic sports medicine surgeons, primary care sports medicine specialists, pediatricians, fellows and residents in training, physician assistants, nurse practitioners, physical therapists, and athletic trainers. We could not have produced this work without the countless hours and contributions from the many knowledgeable colleagues who have supported this effort. We hope this resource will improve the understanding, diagnosis, and treatment of these young patients, as the function and lifespan of their knees depend on appropriate management.

Contents

SECTION 2: Patellofemoral Instability

SECTION 5: Pediatric and Adolescent Knee Fractures

SECTION 6: Physis

Videos

CHAPTER

1

Frank A. Cordasco
Daniel W. Green

Introduction

The demographic and epidemiologic changes that have occurred during the last decade have resulted in an increasing demand for specialized services regarding knee injuries in this cohort of young athletes. Sports participation is on the rise with approximately 30 to 40 million children aged 5 to 17 years participating in organized sports in the United States. Children are specializing in sport at earlier ages and training year-round. Injury rates regarding the anterior cruciate ligament (ACL), patellofemoral instability and tears of the medial patellofemoral ligament (MPFL), osteochondritis dissecans (OCD), and other articular cartilage injuries as well as discoid meniscus tears and fractures have resulted in changing injury patterns requiring the care of pediatric and adolescent sports medicine surgeons, pediatricians, primary care sports medicine specialists, physical therapists, and athletic trainers.

We have designed this textbook to review the major categories of sports injuries affecting the knee in young athletes with the express purpose to provide a guideline for the providers of care in this population. There is a technique-oriented component in each section intended to assist orthopedic surgeons with an interest in pediatric and adolescent sports medicine at the attending, fellow, and resident level. We believe these technique chapters will also help pediatricians, primary care sports medicine specialists and physical therapists, and athletic trainers who treat these young athletes to provide appropriate follow-up care and ultimately to facilitate return to play.

Section 1 includes 13 chapters from internationally renowned experts focusing on a comprehensive review of the ACL with respect to epidemiology, anatomy, gender-specific issues, historical perspectives, techniques (combined extra- and intra-articular, all-epiphyseal, partial transphyseal, and complete transphyseal), rehabilitation, return to play, and prevention.

Section 2 is a comprehensive review of patellofemoral instability beginning with epidemiology and pathomechanics, proximal and distal realignment techniques, and rehabilitation.

Section 3 focuses in the complex area of OCD from the epidemiology, etiology, and classification systems through techniques, which include transarticular and retrograde drilling, open reduction and internal fixation (ORIF), and articular cartilage restoration options.

Section 4 provides a detailed review of the discoid meniscus and covers the epidemiology, classification, patient assessment, and treatment options including saucerization, repair, and transplant.

Section 5 covers all of the primary fractures that are relevant in this cohort of pediatric and adolescent athletes.

Section 6 is the final segment and reviews the physis from imaging, anatomy, and assessment of remaining growth through the treatment of growth arrest and deformity.

Our goal is to provide a current and comprehensive review of knee injuries in the pediatric and adolescent athletes and to help all of us provide state-of-the-art care to this cohort of athletes.

SECTION

1

Anterior Cruciate Ligament Injury

Peter D. Fabricant
Emily R. Dodwell
Robert G. Marx

CHAPTER 2

Epidemiology of Pediatric and Adolescent Anterior Cruciate Ligament Injury

INTRODUCTION

There has been an increased interest in pediatric and adolescent anterior cruciate ligament (ACL) injury due to the recent spike in rates of diagnosis and treatment. With nearly 70% of children in the United States playing team sports, there has been a dramatic rise in participation in competitive athletics year-round. This, along with increased levels of competition and sports specialization in addition to improved recognition of ACL injury, has led to a significant increase in the number of ACL injuries diagnosed in skeletally immature patients.[1,2] Historically, treatment has largely been nonoperative for fear of injury to open physes. Currently, however, with improved treatment strategies, the standard of care has become reconstruction to prevent further cartilage and meniscal damage.[3,4]

Paramount to the understanding of ACL injury in children and adolescents is the recognition of the epidemiology of ACL injury in this age group as well as risk factors for ACL injury and strategies developed to prevent injury. The purpose of this chapter is to describe the epidemiology of ACL injury and reconstruction in children and adolescents as well as briefly address the risk factors for injury, which is described in greater detail throughout this section of the textbook. In addition, this chapter discusses the costs and effectiveness of ACL injury screening programs as well as ACL injury prevention programs, as these represent substantial interventions toward injury prevention in children, adolescents, and young adults.

EPIDEMIOLOGY OF ANTERIOR CRUCIATE LIGAMENT INJURY AND RECONSTRUCTION

Historically, treatment of ACL injury in the skeletally immature has largely been nonoperative for fear of injury to the physes in the growing skeleton. Currently, with improved treatment strategies, the standard of care has become reconstruction to prevent further cartilage and meniscal damage. Recent studies have shown that nonoperative management of ACL tears in the skeletally immature patient often results in poor outcomes[3,5,6] and that treatment delays increased the risk of further meniscal and cartilage damage.[3,4] Further, a recent meta-analysis reported that operatively managed ACL tears in children and adolescents have a high rate of good or excellent knee function with average Lysholm scores[7] of 96. This, coupled with improved surgical technique for ACL reconstruction in the skeletally immature, likely accounts for much of the recent increase in the rate of ACL reconstructions in this age group.

To date, there are very few large cohort and population-based studies on ACL injury in the skeletally immature athlete. A study that sampled 2,133 children aged 5 to 17 years, drawn from a cohort of nearly 140,000 patient visits treated over 9 years in a sports medicine division at a large academic pediatric medical center found that ACL tears comprised 9.4% of all presenting injuries.[8] The percentage was slightly higher in the 13- to 17-year-old age group when compared to those aged 5 to 12 years old.

The largest population-based study to date on the epidemiology of ACL reconstruction in children and adolescents was performed in New York State by Dodwell et al.[9] A billing and coding discharge database was used to identify ACL reconstructions in patients aged 3 to 20 years at the time of surgery over a 20-year period, from 1990 to 2009. The study noted that the rate of ACL reconstruction has increased steadily over the 20-year interval studied, from 17.6 to 50.9 per 100,000 population (Fig. 2.1). The authors noted that the rate of ACL reconstruction was 15% higher in boys than in girls. Although this study is the only existing population-based study to evaluate the rate of pediatric and adolescent ACL injury, its main limitation is that it quantified ACL reconstruction surgeries, which does not account for some ACL tears that are undiagnosed or treated nonoperatively. Despite this limitation, the study provides convincing evidence of the increase in rate of ACL tears in children and adolescents. As of 2009, the highest rate of ACL reconstruction was noted in 14- to 20-year-olds, with the greatest peak at age 17 years (Fig. 2.2).

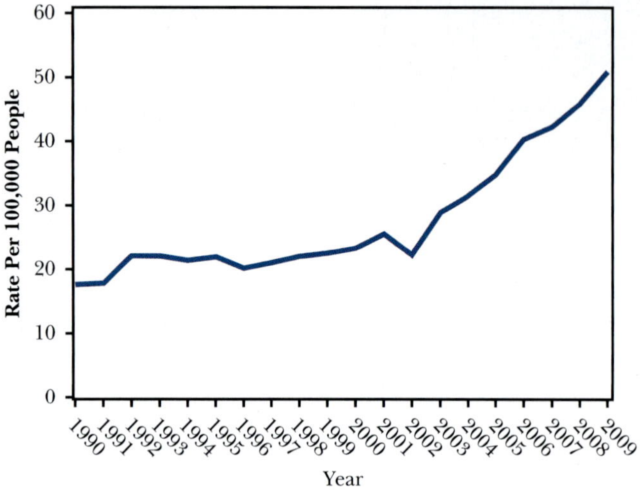

Figure 2.1. Rate of ACL reconstructions in the pediatric population (aged 3 to 20 years) in New York State from 1990 to 2009. (Adapted with permission from Dodwell ER, Lamont LE, Green DW, et al. 20 years of pediatric anterior cruciate ligament reconstruction in New York State. *Am J Sports Med.* 2014;42[3]:675–680.)

RISK FACTORS FOR ANTERIOR CRUCIATE LIGAMENT INJURY

In order to understand the risk factors for pediatric and adolescent ACL injury, one must evaluate elements that are both intrinsic to the patient as well as external factors.[10,11] Although some intrinsic risk factors are not controllable by the adolescent, many intrinsic and all extrinsic risk factors are modifiable to some extent.

Intrinsic Risk Factors

Intrinsic risk factors are variables that are inherent to the patient and include factors that are both controllable (e.g., playing style, training and preparation, skill) as well as those that are not under the athlete's control (e.g., age, previous ACL reconstruction, mechanical alignment, soft tissue laxity, hormonal differences, anatomic variation in ACL morphology and intercondylar notch geometry).[9–15] Risk for ACL injury is increased by athletic activity that requires pivoting, deceleration, and landing and can be in part related to biomechanical forces including posture, alignment, and differential muscle activation.[16] These have led to the development of strength and conditioning programs, which have been designed to mitigate these risk factors and prevent ACL injury and are discussed later in this chapter.[12,17–24]

Of the intrinsic risk factors, gender differences have drawn the most interest in the scientific literature. Clinical studies have noted increased rates of ACL tears in young female athletes when compared with males, in the order of 2 to 10 times greater.[25–29] Recent large cohort and population-based studies, however, have noted a greater frequency of ACL reconstruction surgery in males compared to females, with a rate of ACL reconstruction up to 15% higher in boys than in girls.[9,30] Although the absolute number of males with ACL reconstruction is greater than that of females, females have a higher rate of injury per athletic exposure.[1,27–29,31] On average, males experience more athletic exposures than girls, thus leading to a greater number of ACL injuries despite a lower risk per athletic exposure.[27,32–36]

The cause for females' higher rate of ACL injury per athletic exposure remains uncertain. Potential explanations include sex hormone receptors located on ACL tissue as well as "quadriceps dominant" muscle activation. Previous studies have shown associations between timing of ACL injury and phase of menstrual period, further implicating hormonal risk factors.[37–39] Anatomic risk factors placing girls at higher risk than boys include excessive femoral anteversion, increased Q angle, decreased intercondylar notch width, knee valgus, and increased posterior tibial slope.[40–42]

Higher socioeconomic status has been associated with increased rates of ACL reconstruction.[9] This may be due to differential access to "at-risk" sports or, potentially, may be related

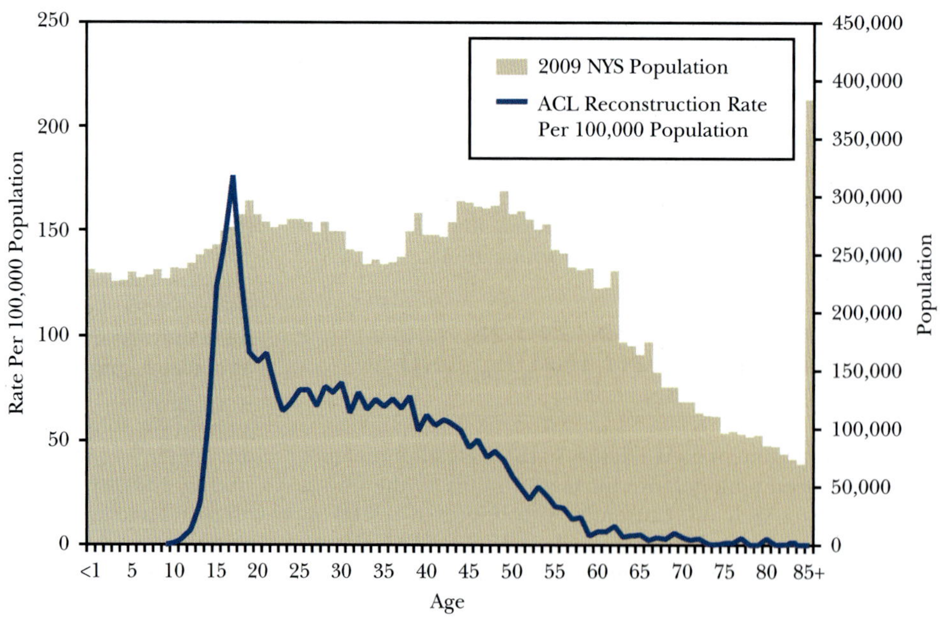

Figure 2.2. Rate of anterior cruciate ligament (*ACL*) reconstructions in 2009 compared with 2009 New York State (*NYS*) population by age. (Adapted with permission from Dodwell ER, Lamont LE, Green DW, et al. 20 years of pediatric anterior cruciate ligament reconstruction in New York State. *Am J Sports Med.* 2014;42[3]:675–680.)

to disparities in access to specialist medical care including high-technology imaging such as magnetic resonance imaging (MRI).[9] Further study is needed to elucidate specific differences in ACL injury and access to care that may be affected by socioeconomic status.

Extrinsic Risk Factors

Extrinsic risk factors are those that are external to the patient. These include weather conditions, athletic equipment, and footwear–surface interaction. Harder and dryer playing surfaces, cleat configuration, and synthetic playing surfaces can lead to increased strain on the ACL due to an increased coefficient of friction between the shoe and playing surface interface.[43,44]

Although ACL injury may occur with non–sport-related trauma, 90% of injuries occur during athletic activity.[45] Therefore, another modifiable risk factor that places the adolescent athlete at greater risk of ACL injury is participation in competitive sports year-round.[46,47] In combination with increased levels of competition and sports specialization as well as improved recognition of ACL injury, this has led to a significant increase in the number of ACL injuries diagnosed in skeletally immature patients.[1,2] Additionally, certain sports that involve cutting and pivoting (e.g., American football, wrestling, basketball, soccer) have been found to have higher rates of ACL injury than other sports (e.g., swimming, golf, baseball, softball, volleyball) and therefore patients can decrease their risk by participating in lower risk sports.[12,48]

EPIDEMIOLOGY OF ANTERIOR CRUCIATE LIGAMENT INJURY COST AND PREVENTION

ACL injury represents a large economic burden with nearly $1.4 billion spent annually on care for these patients. In addition to the financial costs, there are social and emotional hardships as well. Only 40% to 60% of patients of all ages undergoing ACL reconstruction are able to get back to asymptomatic competition, with 10% to 20% unable to return to any competitive sports activity.[49–54] Inability to participate in athletic activity can lead to both physical deconditioning as well as negative social and emotional consequences. Prevention of ACL injury may be categorized into two main approaches: screening programs[55–59] and preventive training programs.[12,17–23,59]

Recent meta-analyses evaluated the effectiveness of ACL injury prevention training programs. Those who undergo formal ACL injury prevention training experience an overall ACL injury risk reduction of 62% compared to those who do not participate.[17] When stratified by gender, the ACL injury risk reduction was 85% for males and 52% for females.[17] The cost of such prevention programs have been estimated to be approximately $1.25 per player per year.[18–24,54] Screening tests have also been developed in order to evaluate athletes and stratify them as either high or low risk of injury. Sensitivity and specificity of these tests range from 61% to 78% and 56% to 73%, respectively.[54–59] Cost of screening tests for players may be as expensive as $15 per test.[54]

In a recent cost-effectiveness analysis by Swart et al.,[54] it was noted that training all pediatric and adolescent athletes, rather than screening for those at high risk of injury and training only those athletes, was highly cost-effective. They cited the significantly large risk reduction for ACL injury with minimal cost compared to higher costs for imperfect screening tests as the driving force for this finding over such a wide range of clinical scenarios. In the interests of public health and ACL injury prevention, they argue that future resources should be geared toward universally implementing similar training programs rather than screening protocols.

ANTERIOR CRUCIATE LIGAMENT INJURY RESEARCH: POPULATION REPORTING OF YOUTH INJURY

Using ACL reconstruction as a surrogate for ACL injury has been identified as a limitation of existing research.[9] In order to continue to advance the understanding of epidemiology of pediatric and adolescent ACL injury, large injury registries are therefore needed. Recent literature comparing injury reporting methods in adolescent and high school athletes have indicated that athletic trainers may be ideally positioned to report ACL and other sports injury data into prospective registries.[60,61] In one study,[60] athletic trainers using the High School Reporting Information Online (HS-RIO) database submitted reports on 97% of high school athletic injuries, compared to only 37% reported by coaches. Athletic trainers frequently serve as medical liaisons between athletes, and medical personnel and are in frequent contact with athletes during games, at school, and around the time of practice. They therefore may notice injuries more frequently and accurately than coaches who are focused on other tasks. Because injury patterns differ by patient demographics, sport, geography, and level of competition, a simple online reporting system would allow researchers to more effectively evaluate risk factors for ACL and other sports injuries in this population.

CONCLUSION

The recent epidemic of ACL injury and surgery in pediatric and adolescent athletes is likely multifactorial, representing a combination of increased intensity and frequency of athletic competition[62] coupled with improved diagnosis and treatment.[9] Although adolescents who participate in organized sports are more likely to have a healthy self-image and less emotional distress,[63] and children with sedentary lifestyles may be at risk for obesity and other negative health outcomes, this must be balanced with the risk for overtraining and athletic injury.[62] Both intrinsic and extrinsic risk factors have been associated with an increased risk of ACL injury. Future resources designed to prevent injury should be geared toward widely implementing ACL injury prevention training programs rather than developing protocols for screening those at elevated risk of injury.[54] ACL injuries in children are an important public health concern that requires continued attention and further study in the areas of injury prevention, reporting, and treatment.[9,12]

REFERENCES

1. National Federation of State High School Associations. Participation statistics. NFHS Web site. http://www.nfhs.org/Participation/SportSearch.aspx. Accessed March 27, 2014.
2. Levey H. *Outside Class: A Historical Analysis of American Children's Competitive Activities.* Boston, MA: Pearson Allyn & Bacon; 2010.

3. Lawrence JT, Argawal N, Ganley TJ. Degeneration of the knee joint in skeletally immature patients with a diagnosis of an anterior cruciate ligament tear: is there harm in delay of treatment? *Am J Sports Med.* 2011;39(12):2582–2587.
4. Guenther ZD, Swami V, Dhillon SS, et al. Meniscal injury after adolescent anterior cruciate ligament injury: how long are patients at risk? *Clin Orthop Relat Res.* 2014;472(3):990–997.
5. Aichroth PM, Patel DV, Zorrilla P. The natural history and treatment of rupture of the anterior cruciate ligament in children and adolescents. A prospective review. *J Bone Joint Surg Br.* 2002;84(1):38–41.
6. Arbes S, Resinger C, Vecsei V, et al. The functional outcome of total tears of the anterior cruciate ligament (ACL) in the skeletally immature patient. *Int Orthop.* 2007;31(4):471–475.
7. Frosch KH, Stengel D, Brodhun T, et al. Outcomes and risks of operative treatment of rupture of the anterior cruciate ligament in children and adolescents. *Arthroscopy.* 2010;26(11):1539–1550.
8. Stracciolini A, Casciano R, Levey Friedman H, et al. Pediatric sports injuries: an age comparison of children versus adolescents. *Am J Sports Med.* 2013;41(8):1922–1929.
9. Dodwell ER, Lamont LE, Green DW, et al. 20 years of pediatric anterior cruciate ligament reconstruction in New York State. *Am J Sports Med.* 2014;42(3):675–680.
10. Fabricant PD, Jones KJ, Delos D, et al. Reconstruction of the anterior cruciate ligament in the skeletally immature athlete: a review of current concepts: AAOS exhibit selection. *J Bone Joint Surg Am.* 2013;95(5):e28.
11. Ireland ML. Anterior cruciate ligament injury in female athletes: epidemiology. *J Athl Train.* 1999;34(2):150–154.
12. Marx RG, Myklebust G, Boyle BW. *The ACL Solution: Prevention and Recovery for Sports' Most Devastating Knee Injury.* New York, NY: Demos Medical Publishing; 2012.
13. Lyman S, Koulouvaris P, Sherman S, et al. Epidemiology of anterior cruciate ligament reconstruction: trends, readmissions, and subsequent knee surgery. *J Bone Joint Surg Am.* 2009;91(10):2321–2328.
14. Wright RW, Dunn WR, Amendola A, et al. Risk of tearing the intact anterior cruciate ligament in the contralateral knee and rupturing the anterior cruciate ligament graft during the first 2 years after anterior cruciate ligament reconstruction: a prospective MOON cohort study. *Am J Sports Med.* 2007;35(7):1131–1134.
15. Flynn RK, Pedersen CL, Birmingham TB, et al. The familial predisposition toward tearing the anterior cruciate ligament: a case control study. *Am J Sports Med.* 2005;33(1):23–28.
16. Olsen OE, Myklebust G, Engebretsen L, et al. Injury mechanisms for anterior cruciate ligament injuries in team handball: a systematic video analysis. *Am J Sports Med.* 2004;32(4):1002–1012.
17. Sadoghi P, von Keudell A, Vavken P. Effectiveness of anterior cruciate ligament injury prevention training programs. *J Bone Joint Surg Am.* 2012;94(9):769–776.
18. Caraffa A, Cerulli G, Projetti M, et al. Prevention of anterior cruciate ligament injuries in soccer. A prospective controlled study of proprioceptive training. *Knee Surg Sports Traumatol Arthrosc.* 1996;4(1):19–21.
19. Gilchrist J, Mandelbaum BR, Melancon H, et al. A randomized controlled trial to prevent noncontact anterior cruciate ligament injury in female collegiate soccer players. *Am J Sports Med.* 2008;36(8):1476–1483.
20. Heidt RS Jr, Sweeterman LM, Carlonas RL, et al. Avoidance of soccer injuries with preseason conditioning. *Am J Sports Med.* 2000;28(5):659–662.
21. Hewett TE, Lindenfeld TN, Riccobene JV, et al. The effect of neuromuscular training on the incidence of knee injury in female athletes. A prospective study. *Am J Sports Med.* 1999;27(6):699–706.
22. Mandelbaum BR, Silvers HJ, Watanabe DS, et al. Effectiveness of a neuromuscular and proprioceptive training program in preventing anterior cruciate ligament injuries in female athletes: 2-year follow-up. *Am J Sports Med.* 2005;33(7):1003–1010.
23. Petersen W, Zantop T, Steensen M, et al. Prevention of lower extremity injuries in handball: initial results of the handball injuries prevention programme [in German]. *Sportverletz Sportschaden.* 2002;16(3):122–126.
24. Pfeiffer RP, Shea KG, Roberts D, et al. Lack of effect of a knee ligament injury prevention program on the incidence of noncontact anterior cruciate ligament injury. *J Bone Joint Surg Am.* 2006;88(8):1769–1774.
25. Parkkari J, Pasanen K, Mattila VM, et al. The risk for a cruciate ligament injury of the knee in adolescents and young adults: a population-based cohort study of 46,500 people with a 9 year follow-up. *Br J Sports Med.* 2008;42(6):422–426.
26. Sutton KM, Bullock JM. Anterior cruciate ligament rupture: differences between males and females. *J Am Acad Orthop Surg.* 2013;21(1):41–50.
27. Arendt E, Dick R. Knee injury patterns among men and women in collegiate basketball and soccer. NCAA data and review of literature. *Am J Sports Med.* 1995;23(6):694–701.
28. Huston LJ, Greenfield ML, Wojtys EM. Anterior cruciate ligament injuries in the female athlete. Potential risk factors. *Clin Orthop Relat Res.* 2000;(372):50–63.
29. Toth AP, Cordasco FA. Anterior cruciate ligament injuries in the female athlete. *J Gend Specif Med.* 2001;4(4):25–34.
30. Stracciolini A, Casciano R, Levey Friedman H, et al. Pediatric sports injuries: a comparison of males versus females. *Am J Sports Med.* 2014;42(4):965–972.
31. Hewett TE, Johnson DL. ACL prevention programs: fact or fiction? *Orthopedics.* 2010;33(1):36–39.
32. Bjordal JM, Arnly F, Hannestad B, et al. Epidemiology of anterior cruciate ligament injuries in soccer. *Am J Sports Med.* 1997;25(3):341–345.
33. Ferretti A, Papandrea P, Conteduca F, et al. Knee ligament injuries in volleyball players. *Am J Sports Med.* 1992;20(2):203–207.
34. Gwinn DE, Wilckens JH, McDevitt ER, et al. The relative incidence of anterior cruciate ligament injury in men and women at the United States Naval Academy. *Am J Sports Med.* 2000;28(1):98–102.
35. Lindenfeld TN, Schmitt DJ, Hendy MP, et al. Incidence of injury in indoor soccer. *Am J Sports Med.* 1994;22(3):364–371.
36. Messina DF, Farney WC, DeLee JC. The incidence of injury in Texas high school basketball. A prospective study among male and female athletes. *Am J Sports Med.* 1999;27(3):294–299.
37. Wojtys EM, Huston LJ, Boynton MD, et al. The effect of the menstrual cycle on anterior cruciate ligament injuries in women as determined by hormone levels. *Am J Sports Med.* 2002;30(2):182–188.
38. Hewett TE, Zazulak BT, Myer GD. Effects of the menstrual cycle on anterior cruciate ligament injury risk: a systematic review. *Am J Sports Med.* 2007;35(4):659–668.
39. Myklebust G, Engebretsen L, Braekken IH, et al. Prevention of anterior cruciate ligament injuries in female team handball players: a prospective intervention study over three seasons. *Clin J Sport Med.* 2003;13(2):71–78.
40. Alentorn-Geli E, Myer GD, Silvers HJ, et al. Prevention of noncontact anterior cruciate ligament injuries in soccer players. Part 1: mechanisms of injury and underlying risk factors. *Knee Surg Sports Traumatol Arthrosc.* 2009;17(7):705–729.
41. Hewett TE, Stroupe AL, Nance TA, et al. Plyometric training in female athletes. Decreased impact forces and increased hamstring torques. *Am J Sports Med.* 1996;24(6):765–773.
42. Lephart SM, Ferris CM, Riemann BL, et al. Gender differences in strength and lower extremity kinematics during landing. *Clin Orthop Relat Res.* 2002;(401):162–169.
43. Drakos MC, Hillstrom H, Voos JE, et al. The effect of the shoe-surface interface in the development of anterior cruciate ligament strain. *J Biomech Eng.* 2010;132(1):011003.
44. Taylor SA, Fabricant PD, Khair MM, et al. A review of synthetic playing surfaces, the shoe-surface interface, and lower extremity injuries in athletes. *Phys Sportsmed.* 2012;40(4):66–72.
45. Dunn WR, Spindler KP, Amendola A, et al. Which preoperative factors, including bone bruise, are associated with knee pain/symptoms at index anterior cruciate ligament reconstruction (ACLR)? A Multicenter Orthopaedic Outcomes Network (MOON) ACLR Cohort Study. *Am J Sports Med.* 2010;38(9):1778–1787.

46. McCarroll JR, Rettig AC, Shelbourne KD. Anterior cruciate ligament injuries in the young athlete with open physes. *Am J Sports Med.* 1988;16(1):44–47.
47. Souryal TO, Freeman TR. Intercondylar notch size and anterior cruciate ligament injuries in athletes. A prospective study. *Am J Sports Med.* 1993;21(4):535–539.
48. Agel J, Klossner D. Epidemiologic review of collegiate ACL injury rates across 14 sports: National Collegiate Athletic Association injury surveillance system data 2004-05 through 2011-12. *Br J Sports Med.* 2014;48(7):560.
49. Feller JA, Webster KE. A randomized comparison of patellar tendon and hamstring tendon anterior cruciate ligament reconstruction. *Am J Sports Med.* 2003;31(4):564–573.
50. Matsumoto A, Yoshiya S, Muratsu H, et al. A comparison of bone-patellar tendon-bone and bone-hamstring tendon-bone autografts for anterior cruciate ligament reconstruction. *Am J Sports Med.* 2006;34(2):213–219.
51. Marder RA, Raskind JR, Carroll M. Prospective evaluation of arthroscopically assisted anterior cruciate ligament reconstruction. Patellar tendon versus semitendinosus and gracilis tendons. *Am J Sports Med.* 1991;19(5):478–484.
52. O'Neill DB. Arthroscopically assisted reconstruction of the anterior cruciate ligament. A follow-up report. *J Bone Joint Surg Am.* 2001; 83-A(9):1329–1332.
53. Shaieb MD, Kan DM, Chang SK, et al. A prospective randomized comparison of patellar tendon versus semitendinosus and gracilis tendon autografts for anterior cruciate ligament reconstruction. *Am J Sports Med.* 2002;30(2):214–220.
54. Swart E, Redler L, Fabricant PD, et al. Prevention and screening programs for anterior cruciate ligament injuries in young athletes: a cost-effectiveness analysis. *J Bone Joint Surg Am.* 2014;96(9): 705–711.
55. Myer GD, Ford KR, Khoury J, et al. Development and validation of a clinic-based prediction tool to identify female athletes at high risk for anterior cruciate ligament injury. *Am J Sports Med.* 2010;38(10):2025–2033.
56. Myer GD, Ford KR, Hewett TE. New method to identify athletes at high risk of ACL injury using clinic-based measurements and freeware computer analysis. *Br J Sports Med.* 2011;45(4): 238–244.
57. Hewett TE, Myer GD, Ford KR, et al. Biomechanical measures of neuromuscular control and valgus loading of the knee predict anterior cruciate ligament injury risk in female athletes: a prospective study. *Am J Sports Med.* 2005;33(4):492–501.
58. Hewett TE, Ford KR, Myer GD. Anterior cruciate ligament injuries in female athletes: part 2, a meta-analysis of neuromuscular interventions aimed at injury prevention. *Am J Sports Med.* 2006;34(3): 490–498.
59. Padua DA, Marshall SW, Boling MC, et al. The Landing Error Scoring System (LESS) is a valid and reliable clinical assessment tool of jump-landing biomechanics: the JUMP-ACL study. *Am J Sports Med.* 2009;37(10):1996–2002.
60. Yard EE, Collins CL, Comstock RD. A comparison of high school sports injury surveillance data reporting by certified athletic trainers and coaches. *J Athl Train.* 2009;44(6):645–652.
61. Rechel JA, Collins CL, Comstock RD. Epidemiology of injuries requiring surgery among high school athletes in the United States, 2005 to 2010. *J Trauma.* 2011;71(4):982–989.
62. Beck NA, Patel NM, Ganley TJ. The pediatric knee: current concepts in sports medicine. *J Pediatr Orthop B.* 2014;23(1):59–66.
63. Harrison PA, Narayan G. Differences in behavior, psychological factors, and environmental factors associated with participation in school sports and other activities in adolescence. *J Sch Health.* 2003;73(3):113–120.

CHAPTER

3

Carl W. Imhauser

Functional Anatomy and Biomechanics

The knee joint allows motion in all planes based on a complicated interaction between passive constraints including bones and soft tissues and the dynamic muscle stabilizers. The structure of these constraints affords the knee large rotations in the plane of progression (flexion/extension) while allowing more subtle motions in the remaining planes.[1]

The knee joint must resist substantial multidirectional forces and moments during daily activities and sports. These loads arise from the contraction of muscles, the interaction of the foot with the ground, and the acceleration of the body. In fact, measurements from instrumented knee replacement indicate that compressive forces at the knee approach two and a half times body weight even during everyday activities such as walking.[2]

The shear forces generated between the foot and the ground are notable because they give rise to both forces and moments (i.e., torques) at the knee joint. The anterior-posterior force at the ground can be up to 20% of body weight.[3,4] Because this anterior-posterior force acts at a distance from the knee, a moment is generated about the knee that acts to flex or extend it during functional activities. The anterior-posterior forces and flexion-extension moments can be effectively countered by the cruciates and the quadriceps and hamstring muscles.

The shear forces in the mediolateral direction are also substantial during daily activities and sports. For example, at the instant in walking where the foot strikes the ground, a lateral reaction force develops that can reach 5% of body weight.[3,4] This force pushes the foot laterally, and because it acts at a distance from the knee, a moment is also generated about the knee that acts to rotate the tibia into valgus.[5] Therefore, both a medial shear force and a varus moment must be generated within the knee to counteract the effect of the lateral component of the ground reaction force (Fig. 3.1).

The varus and valgus moments generated at the knee can be even more substantial during sporting activities such as running, side-stepping, and cutting[6] and can serve as a predictor of injury risk. Elevated valgus moments during landing from a jump have been identified as a predictor of anterior cruciate ligament (ACL) injury risk in female athletes.[7]

MECHANISMS OF KNEE STABILITY

Frontal Plane Stability and the Role of Muscles

The bicondylar shape of the distal femur is well-suited to resisting the varus and valgus moments that act on the knee during daily activities and sports. When the knee compresses due to muscle contraction and/or the ground reaction force, an applied moment in the frontal plane will cause redistribution of the contact force acting on the medial and lateral condyles.[8,9] The ability of the articular surfaces to resist the applied moment is proportional to the magnitude of the contact force and its distance from the joint center. This highlights the importance of the muscles in generating contact forces that increase the ability of the articular surfaces to resist frontal plane moments.

The articular surfaces can rapidly generate resistive frontal plane moments with minimal varus or valgus angulation (≤2°) in the presence of a compressive load (Fig. 3.2). The small amounts of angulation are due to compression of the cartilage and menisci. Condylar lift-off will occur when the applied moment has exceeded the capacity of the articulating surfaces to generate an internal counteracting moment. This instant is characterized by a sudden flattening in the slope of the moment-angular displacement response (see Fig. 3.2). As the knee continues to rotate into varus or valgus, the ligaments will engage and generate forces that cause the resistive moment to once again increase (see Fig. 3.2).

Stability Provided by the Articulating Surfaces

The shapes of the articulating surfaces of the knee provide an involuntary mechanism to provide joint stability.[1] The joint will unconsciously move to a contact position that can counter the direction of an applied force within an envelope defined by the size and shape of the articular surfaces (Fig. 3.3). The bounds of this envelope can be visualized by drawing lines that are perpendicular to the articulating surfaces at the extreme ends of the joint (Fig. 3.3A).[1] The directions of these bounding lines encompass all orientations of reaction forces that can be generated by the articulating surfaces. Thus, the articular surfaces may accommodate changes in the direction of the applied

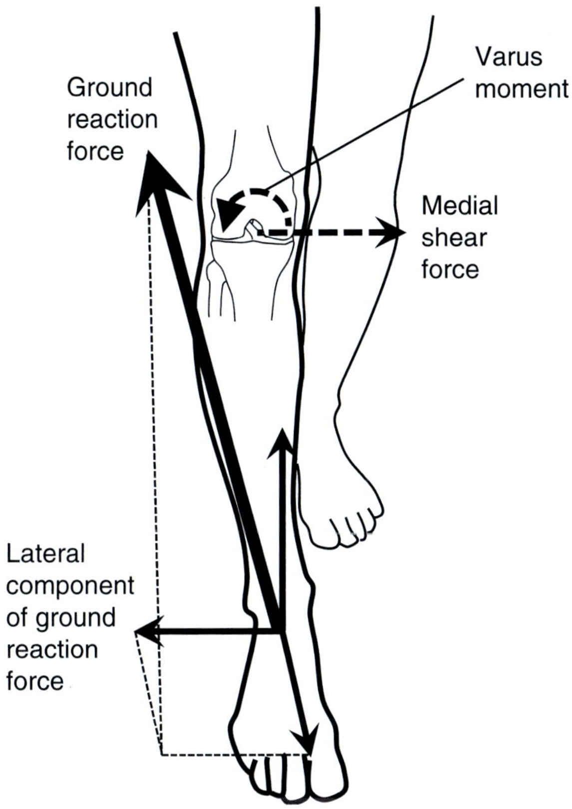

Figure 3.1. A lateral shear force is generated between the foot and the ground during the heel strike phase of the gait cycle and more so during athletic activities such as running, cutting, and jump-landing. This lateral shear force creates a valgus moment at the knee joint. The externally applied valgus moment and lateral shear force must be balanced within the knee by a medial shear force and varus moment, respectively (shown with *dashed lines*).

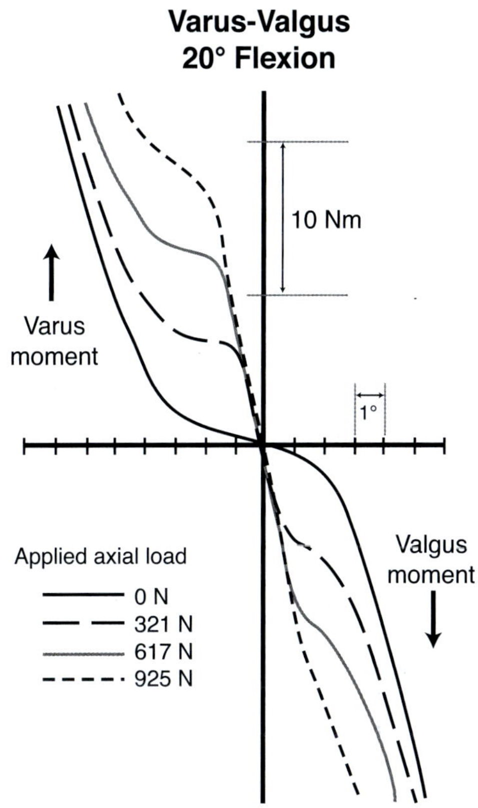

Figure 3.2. Increasing the contact force via an applied axial load increases the ability of the bicondylar articular surfaces of the knee to resist frontal plane moments. The instant of condylar lift-off is identified by a sudden decrease in the slope of the moment-angular displacement curve in varus and valgus. The torque level at which this occurs increases with increasing axial load. (Redrawn from Markolf KL, Bargar WL, Shoemaker SC, et al. The role of joint load in knee stability. *J Bone Joint Surg Am.* 1981;63[4]:570–585, with permission.)

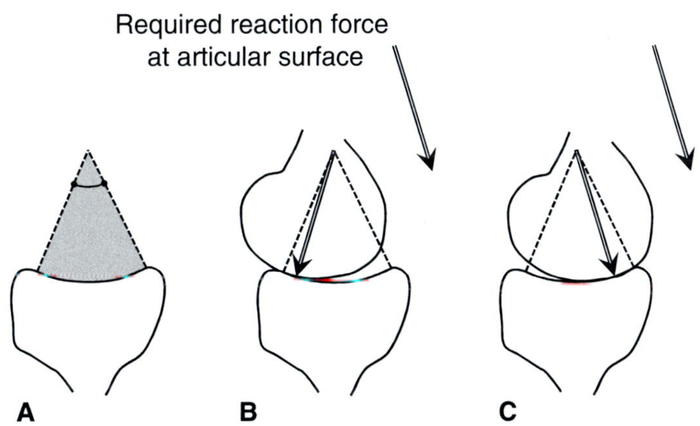

Figure 3.3. Assume that the flexion angle remains fixed. **A.** The articular surfaces are capable of generating a reaction force within the range of orientations defined by perpendiculars to the joint surface at either side of the joint (*dotted line*).[1] The sweep of achievable orientations of reaction forces that can be generated by the curvature of the articular surface is encompassed in *gray*. **B.** The reaction force that joint contact is required to generate is shown. At its current position, contact between the articular surfaces alone is unable to generate the required reaction force at the articular surface because the perpendicular to the joint surface where contact occurs is not aligned with the required reaction force. **C.** To generate the required reaction force, the femur will slide from the position shown in **B** to the position shown in **C**. Here, the perpendicular to the articulating surface aligns with the required reaction force. Therefore, no other stabilizing mechanism besides compression of the joint is needed to keep the joint stable. (Adapted from Burstein AH, Wright TM. *Fundamentals of Orthopaedic Biomechanics.* Baltimore, MD: Williams and Wilkins; 1994.)

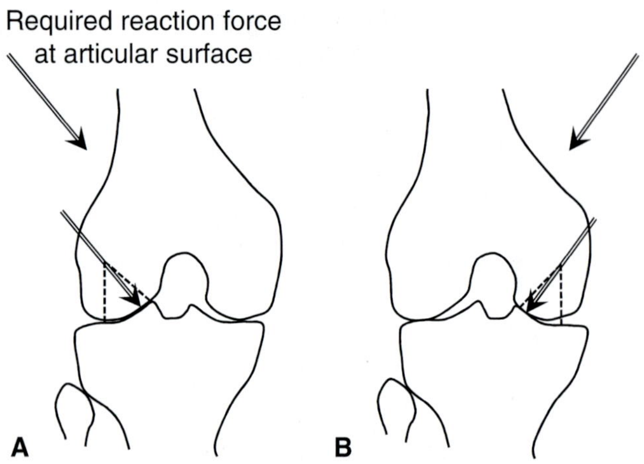

Figure 3.4. The conforming geometry of the knee joint in the frontal plane is well-suited to producing both medially and laterally directed contact forces. The required medially **(A)** and laterally **(B)** directed reaction forces are generated by a small lateral and medial shift of the tibia, respectively. The dotted lines are perpendicular to the joint surfaces. They identify the range of orientations of reaction forces that can be generated by the curvature of the articular surfaces.

loads through compression of the joint alone and by adjusting the relative position of the joint surfaces (Fig. 3.3 B,C).

Because the knee is conforming in the coronal plane, it takes only small shifts in the mediolateral position of the knee to produce mediolateral-directed contact forces (Fig. 3.4).

Similarly, the medial compartment of the knee will resist small changes in anterior-posterior–oriented forces in the sagittal plane due to its concave shape. The lateral compartment, however, based on its convex shape in the sagittal plane and lateral orientation in the frontal plane, cannot effectively resist anteriorly and medially directed external forces, respectively. Thus, it requires additional stabilizing mechanisms to accommodate these applied forces including the menisci and the ACL.

Stability Provided by Ligaments

The forces generated by ligaments also contribute to joint stability. However, when acting to restrain the joint, they must not interfere with the normal range of motion of the knee. This is accomplished because their line of action passes close to the rotation axis of the joint.[1] This makes it impossible to generate large resistive moments against flexion and extension because the distance between rotation axis and the line of action of the force generated by the ligament remains small through flexion. When this principle is not adhered to during ligament reconstruction, for example, it can lead to clinical complications including flexion contracture and overconstraint of the joint.

Ligaments must also allow some relative movement of the articular surfaces for the articular stabilizing mechanism discussed earlier to be effective.[1] Two characteristic features of ligaments facilitate this: their slack length and toe region. Slack length describes the length at which the ligament begins to carry load. The toe region refers to the initial portion of the load-displacement response of the ligament where load builds slowly as it is stretched. These two features allow the ligament to gradually generate force for the first few millimeters of relative movement of the joint surfaces. This enables the articular surfaces to move to a suitable contact point along their curvature to generate the required reaction force (Fig. 3.5).

If there is no suitable point along the curvature of the articular surfaces that can generate the required reaction force, the bones displace further apart. As the bones displace further, the ligaments will generate force more rapidly as they stiffen.[10] Thus, they will make a larger contribution to resisting loads applied to the joint.

Finally, a ligament should be oriented as closely as possible in the direction of the applied force that it must resist.[1] Thus, the collateral ligaments are appropriately oriented to resist frontal plane moments based on their mediolateral distance from the joint center and proximal-distal orientation. Similarly,

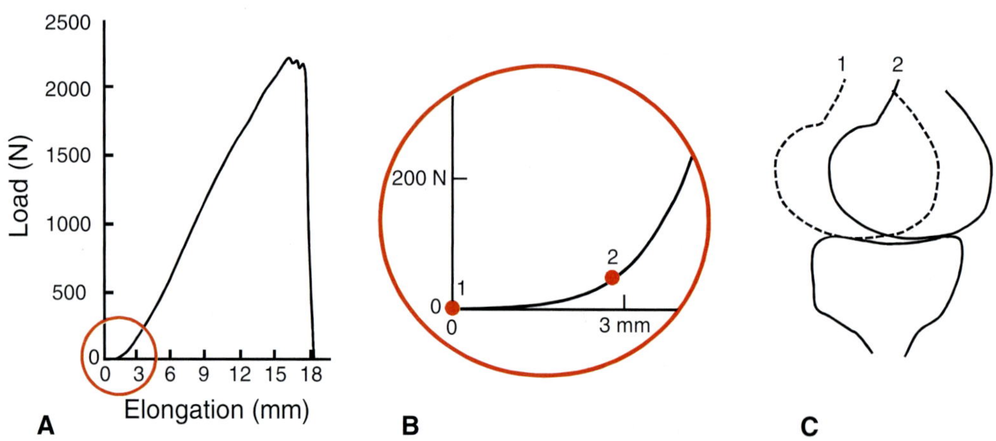

Figure 3.5. **A.** The load-displacement response of the ACL[10] includes a toe region (*circled in red*). **B.** In the toe region, the ligament gradually generates force for the first few millimeters of the load-displacement response as shown between points *1* and *2*. **C.** The toe region of the ligament allows for some relative movement of the articular surfaces between positions *1* and *2*. The toe region combined with a ligament's slack length enables motion of the contact point along the curvature of the joint. This permits the articular stabilizing mechanism to engage. (Adapted from Woo SL, Hollis JM, Adams DJ, et al. Tensile properties of the human femur-anterior cruciate ligament-tibia complex. The effects of specimen age and orientation. *Am J Sports Med.* 1991;19[3]:217–225; Burstein AH, Wright TM. *Fundamentals of Orthopaedic Biomechanics.* Baltimore, MD: Williams and Wilkins; 1994, with permission.)

the ACL has an oblique orientation with origin on the medial aspect of the lateral femoral condyle and insertion on the anterior aspect of the tibia. Thus, its orientation reveals its function in resisting forces that act to push the tibia anteriorly and medially.[11–13] Its small offset relative to the center of the joint also makes it a secondary stabilizer against varus and valgus.[13]

Knee Instability

Situations arise where the stabilizing mechanisms described earlier fail; that is, they cannot effectively counteract the magnitude and direction of the externally applied loads. This will lead to instances where the knee joint feels unstable. These instability events, or episodes where the knee gives way, compromise function and can lead to cartilage and meniscal damage.[14,15] Relief from knee instability is a primary reason why patients seek treatment for ACL injury.

Instability has been defined as large changes in the position of articular contact with small changes in applied load.[1] A stable joint is one where the articular surfaces glide smoothly relative to each other without sudden jumps or abrupt changes in their relative position. Instability can occur when a stabilizing mechanism is absent (e.g., ACL insufficiency) or when existing stabilizing mechanisms are incapable of providing an appropriate resistive force. This might happen when a movement occurs too quickly for the muscles to generate the required force such as in a quick cutting maneuver while playing sports. Stabilizing mechanisms might also fail in combination such as muscle weakness combined with a ligament injury leading to a giving-way episode in an ACL-deficient patient.

Episodes of giving way in ACL-deficient individuals have been serendipitously recorded in the gait laboratory.[16,17] This provides a unique opportunity to quantify the time sequence of loads and motions experienced by the knee over the course of this event. A moderate giving-way episode suffered by an individual while descending stairs revealed that an abnormally high applied valgus moment on the tibia preceded the instability event.[16] The instability event was associated with large and rapid anterior translation of the tibia relative to the femur and increased knee flexion compared to successfully performed trials. Another giving-way episode recorded during a cutting activity was preceded by reductions in the applied varus moment.[17] This was followed by a transition from an external rotation moment to an internal rotation moment acting on the tibia. These abnormal moments were followed by increased internal rotation of the tibia relative to the femur and increased flexion of the knee compared to successful cutting trials.

These unique data bear the hallmark signs of the clinical pivot shift, which is also generated by a complex combination of applied valgus and internal rotation moments combined with knee flexion.[14,15] This reveals the major function of the ACL as a restraint to anterolateral subluxation of the tibia against moments that tend to abduct and internally rotate the tibia.[18,19]

Interestingly, these giving-way episodes were rapid. Therefore, the restraint provided by muscle forces was likely low because the instability occurred too quickly to be resisted by a voluntary muscle response.[20] This indicates that the remaining articular and ligamentous passive stabilizers in the ACL-deficient knee were unable to maintain the position of the knee under these multiplanar loading conditions.

A closer inspection of the interaction of the articular and ligamentous stabilizers against the applied valgus and internal rotation moments provides insight into a potential cause of the instability event. This example ties together our discussion of stabilizing mechanisms of the knee focusing on the role of the ACL. First, the valgus moment acting on the tibia gives rise to a force on the convex lateral compartment that has both anterior and compressive components. Then, an internal rotation moment acts to drive the lateral compartment of the tibia anteriorly. The ACL is oriented to resist these anterior forces. However, in the ACL-deficient knee, this stabilizing mechanism is not available, and the lateral compartment of the tibia will be subject to an abrupt anterior translation relative to the femur. Only when secondary stabilizers such as the lateral meniscus engage to provide the needed posterior reaction force on the tibia will the lateral compartment cease translating anteriorly.

ANATOMY AND BIOMECHANICAL FUNCTION OF THE ANTERIOR CRUCIATE LIGAMENT

The ACL has classically been divided into two functional bundles: an anteromedial and posterolateral portion. This terminology stems from the relative location of its tibial insertion and was described initially by Abbot and colleagues[21] and later by Girgis et al.[22] This description has proven convenient in grossly demarcating function of major portions of the ACL; however, these bundles may not be easily identifiable in all individuals.[23,24] Assessment of the material properties of these bundles indicated that the elastic modulus and the maximum stress of the anteromedial bundle is about 45% greater and at least twice as high as that of the posterolateral bundle, respectively.[25] Taken to its logical extreme, the ACL could be further subdivided.[26,27] In fact, the ACL acts as a continuum of fibers[28] and has been divided into as many as 20 smaller bundles each about 1 mm in diameter.[27]

The ACL appears flat in extension and fans out about 10 to 12 mm distal to the femoral attachment,[22] thus forming a flat hourglass shape along its length.[29] This specialized shape enables the ACL to achieve an anterior and medial orientation to allow it to effectively resist loads in these directions while also accommodating the femoral notch.

Early observations by Groves[30] indicated that the bulk of the ACL was taut in extension, and this was later corroborated by Girgis et al.[22] The ACL twists on itself as the orientation of the femoral attachment changes from more vertical in extension to more horizontal in flexion.[22] The tissue inserting most proximal and anterior into the femur remains tight on visual inspection while the tissue inserting more distally into the femur slackens[22] (Fig. 3.6).

Pioneering work by Artmann and Wirth[31] quantified the relative changes in distance between the tibial insertion and various points on the femoral insertion through flexion by monitoring the change in length of cables spanning the tibial and femoral insertions. They reported that anteroproximal locations on the femur were isometric. This approach has been reproduced by others with similar results.[32] However, such studies rely on measurement of the straight-line distance between tibia and femur when in fact the individual ACL fibers wrap around one another and do not follow a linear path.[27] This was recognized

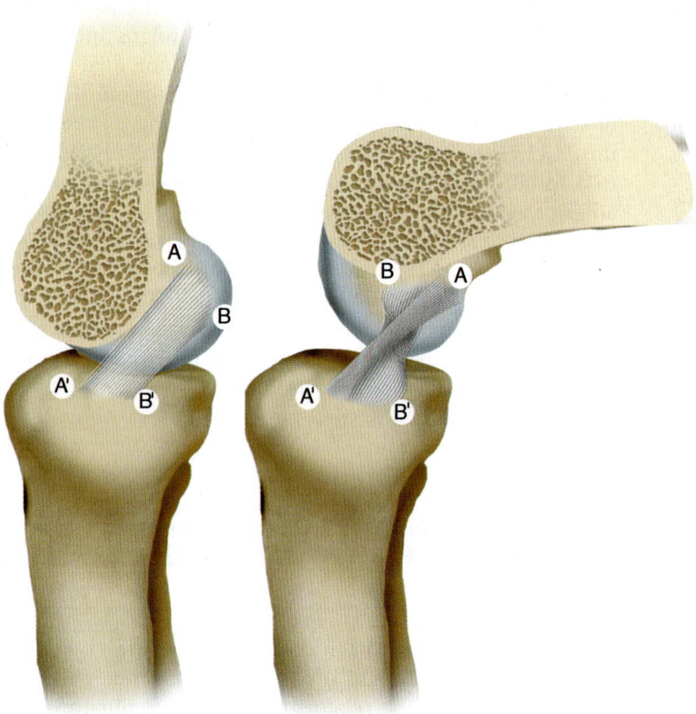

Figure 3.6. Schematic illustrating aligned ACL fibers in extension and slackened and twisted fibers in flexion. (Adapted from Girgis FG, Marshall JL, Monajem A. The cruciate ligaments of the knee joint. Anatomical, functional and experimental analysis. *Clin Orthop Relat Res.* 1975;[106]:216–231.)

and elegantly addressed by Amis and Dawkins[23] by traversing wires through the tibial insertion along fiber bundles comprising the anteromedial bundle, posterolateral bundle, and an intermediate bundle between them. The wires were fixed in the femoral insertion of each bundle. The length changes of these wires were then measured while the knee was passively flexed from full extension to 130 degrees flexion. None of the three fiber bundles was isometric through flexion[23] (Fig. 3.7). However, the anteromedial bundle did experience smaller changes in length (~3.5 mm) than the posterolateral bundle (~5 mm) from full extension to 130 degrees flexion.

Importantly, the posterolateral bundle was shown to undergo rapid shortening between full extension and 30 degrees flexion. This shortening was recognized as buckling collapse of the ligament.[33] Finally, length changes also varied up to 2 mm from specimen to specimen.[23]

These findings have implications for reconstruction of the ACL. Grafts placed at the insertion of the posterolateral bundle will be less isometric through flexion. Therefore, if fixed in flexion, they will elongate as the knee is extended. This may predispose them to high strains and elevated loads.

The high variability in length changes from specimen to specimen indicates that elongation patterns in some patients will be more sensitive to graft fixation angle. Finally, grafts cover an area of the femoral insertion, not a single point, so different regions of the graft will experience different elongation patterns based on tunnel location even if a portion of the graft encompasses an isometric point. Thus, a graft will experience varying strain patterns through its cross-section.

The anteromedial and posterolateral portions of the ACL have differential roles in resisting externally applied anterior and rotatory loads.[34] For both loading cases, the anteromedial bundle bears load throughout flexion, whereas the posterolateral bundle bears the most load near extension. In response to

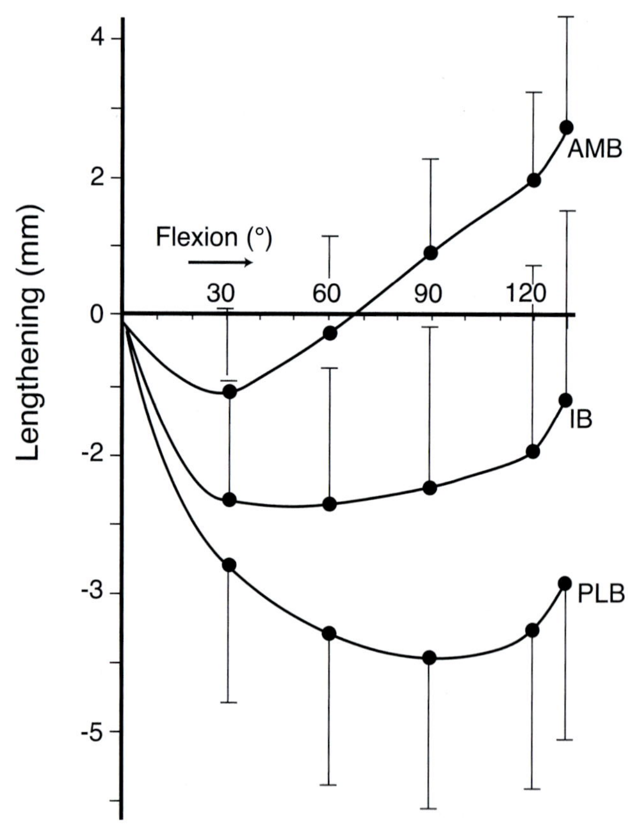

Figure 3.7. Elongation patterns of the anteromedial (*AMB*), posterolateral (*PLB*), and intermediate (*IB*) bundles of the ACL from extension to 130 degrees flexion. (Redrawn from Amis AA, Dawkins GP. Functional anatomy of the anterior cruciate ligament. Fibre bundle actions related to ligament replacements and injuries. *J Bone Joint Surg Br.* 1991;73[2]:260–267, with permission.)

an anterior applied force, the loads borne by the anteromedial portion of the ACL increased from full extension to 60 degrees flexion and then decreased. In contrast, the loads generated in the posterolateral portion of the ACL under an anterior force were highest at full extension and 15 degrees flexion but then decreased from 30 to 120 degrees flexion. At 90 degrees and greater, load in the posterolateral bundle was minimal (<10 N) in response to an anterior load. Under combined valgus and internal rotation moments, the load borne by the anterolateral and posteromedial bundles was about equal at 15 degrees flexion, whereas at 30 degrees flexion, the anteromedial bundle bore two and a half times more load than the posterolateral bundle.

Much research since the early 2000s has been devoted to evaluating ACL reconstructions that strive to recreate the differential function of the anteromedial and posterolateral bundles. Given that malposition of the femoral tunnel is a common cause of ACL graft failure, femoral tunnel placement continues to be an important consideration in ACL reconstruction.[35] This approach has evolved into an ACL reconstruction using either one or two grafts placed within the footprint of the native ACL, a so-called anatomic reconstruction.[36] In vitro biomechanical studies indicated the ability of double-bundle ACL reconstruction to better control coupled anterior translations in response to combined valgus and internal rotation moments (a so-called simulated pivot shift) than isolated reconstruction of the anteromedial bundle.[37] Furthermore, a single quadrupled hamstring tendon graft placed more posteriorly within the femoral footprint restored coupled anterior tibial translations closer to the ACL intact knee than a graft placed in a location that was more isometric[38] (Fig. 3.8).

Biomechanically, a compromise likely must be achieved between controlling coupled anterior translations (via posterior graft placement) and graft isometry. As detailed earlier, grafts placed more posteriorly on the femoral wall will be less isometric through flexion. Thus, grafts placed more posteriorly and fixed in flexion will experience larger elongations as the knee is extended and may be subject to elevated loads. This raises concern about graft failure. Indeed, posterolateral grafts fixed at 30 degrees flexion carried 67% higher loads than the native posterolateral bundle under combined rotational moments simulating the pivot shift at 15 degrees flexion.[39] Moreover, a single anteromedial bundle ACL reconstruction experienced forces that were closer to the native ACL and lower than an anatomic double-bundle reconstruction, in which the posterolateral bundle graft occasionally failed in tests near full extension.[40] Registry data reveal that anteromedial portal drilling, which is associated with posterior placement of femoral tunnels,[41] has resulted in increased rates of graft failure from 3.20% to 5.16% at 4 years when compared to transtibial drilling.[42]

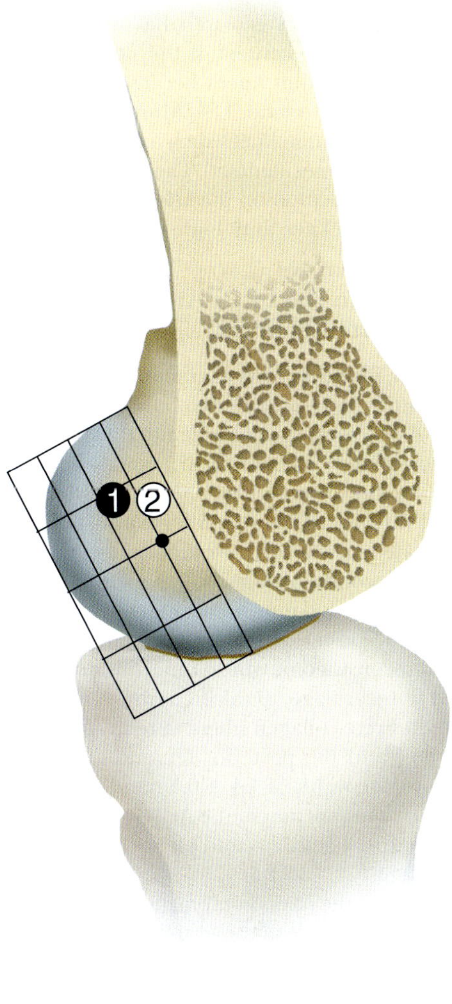

Figure 3.8. Isometric femur tunnel placement (*2*) versus so-called anatomic placement (*1*) where the tunnel is drilled more posteriorly on the medial wall of the lateral femoral condyle. (Redrawn from Musahl V, Plakseychuk A, VanScyoc A, et al. Varying femoral tunnels between the anatomical footprint and isometric positions: effect on kinematics of the anterior cruciate ligament-reconstructed knee. *Am J Sports Med.* 2005;33[5]:712–718.)

Biomechanical Comparison of Techniques for Reconstruction of the Pediatric Anterior Cruciate Ligament

The increased incidence of ACL rupture and the poor natural history of nonoperative treatment in skeletally immature patients has led to a renewed interest in surgical reconstruction of the ACL in this population.[43–46] The all-epiphyseal (AE) reconstruction, the transtibial over-the-top (OT) femoral reconstruction, and a reconstruction harvesting a portion of the iliotibial band known as the *modified McIntosh* have been developed to avoid crossing the physes.[44,47–50] Both the AE and the OT reconstruction techniques reduced high-contact stresses on the posterior aspect of the tibial plateau that arose in the ACL-deficient knee.[51,52] However, contact stress abnormalities remained in both reconstructions.[51] The AE and OT reconstructions also could not restore anterior stability to that of the native knee under an anterior load at deeper flexion angles.[51,53] The AE and OT techniques restored axial rotation to native levels at most flexion angles from 30 degrees to full extension.[51,53] However, the AE technique had the propensity to overconstrain axial rotation under combined moments.[51] Similarly, the modified McIntosh overconstrained axial rotation and varus rotation when loaded in these directions.[53] The OT technique also failed to restore loading patterns of the native

ACL at 60 and 90 degrees of flexion in response to an anterior tibial load.[54]

Cadaveric biomechanics research has limitations that are especially relevant in the context of the pediatric population. Previous studies used adult knees because of the inability to obtain juvenile donor tissue.[51–54] Morphologic differences between adult and juvenile knees such as notch size may affect stability and contact mechanics.[55] Time-zero cadaver studies also provide no information on the effects of healing, rehabilitation, and growth on knee joint biomechanics.

New Insights into the Fiber Architecture of the Anterior Cruciate Ligament

Because the ACL insertion plays a fundamental role in transmitting load from the ACL substance to bone, the architecture of the collagen fibers comprising the femoral insertion has been examined more closely. Iwahashi et al.[56] and Sasaki et al.[57] have assessed the femoral insertion of the ACL histologically and distinguished direct and indirect fiber types. The direct fiber types were located in a bony depression immediately posterior to the lateral intercondylar ridge.[57] They extended a little more than halfway (5.3 ± 1.1 mm on average) from the intercondylar ridge to the posterior femoral articular cartilage.[57] The direct insertion consisted of typical transition from ligament to noncalcified fibrocartilage, to calcified fibrocartilage, and then bone.[57] The indirect collagen fibers were located between the direct insertion and the posterior femoral articular cartilage and had an average width of 4.4 ± 0.5 mm in the anteroposterior direction.[57] This portion of the ACL was directly anchored to bone via Sharpey-like fibers and blended with the posterior articular cartilage.[57]

Macroscopically, the fibers comprising the indirect insertion have a fan-like appearance and merged with the posterior border of the cartilage on the lateral femoral condyle[58] (Fig. 3.9A).

At full extension, these fan-like fibers were nearly parallel to both the fibers inserting adjacent to the lateral intercondylar ridge and to the intercondylar roof. Interestingly, a fold developed in the femoral attachment with flexion at the demarcation between the more posterior fan-like fibers and the fibers located adjacent to the intercondylar ridge[58] (Fig. 3.9B).

Current ACL grafts do not recapitulate the complex structure of these distinct regions of the femoral insertion. Moreover, the load transmitted across these insertion regions has not been characterized. Emerging information characterizing the link between ACL structure and function may help to further guide the evolution of surgical treatment for ACL injury.

IN VIVO FUNCTION OF THE ANTERIOR CRUCIATE LIGAMENT–DEFICIENT AND RECONSTRUCTED KNEE AND IMPLICATION FOR OSTEOARTHRITIS

Abnormal mechanics may be an important contributor to osteoarthritis (OA) development following ACL injury and reconstruction. Thus, in vivo assessment of ambulatory mechanics using gait analysis tools is a common method to assess the response of the knee to functional loads. The advantage of such an approach is that knee function is measured under in vivo functional loading conditions involving the effects of muscle forces, gravity, and inertia. Although the fidelity of tracking patients performing activities in an artificial lab setting to the real-life environment has been debated, such data provide important insight into in vivo function of the knee.

Dual imaging techniques have been used to capture knee kinematics with submillimeter accuracy.[59,60] These tools have also been used to capture information about the interactions of the articulating surfaces (i.e., arthrokinematics). During a lunge activity, tibiofemoral contact points in ACL-deficient knees were found to be located more posteriorly and laterally on the medial compartment and to be located more laterally on the lateral compartment (Fig. 3.10).[61] Cartilage deformation also increased while performing a lunge activity in ACL-

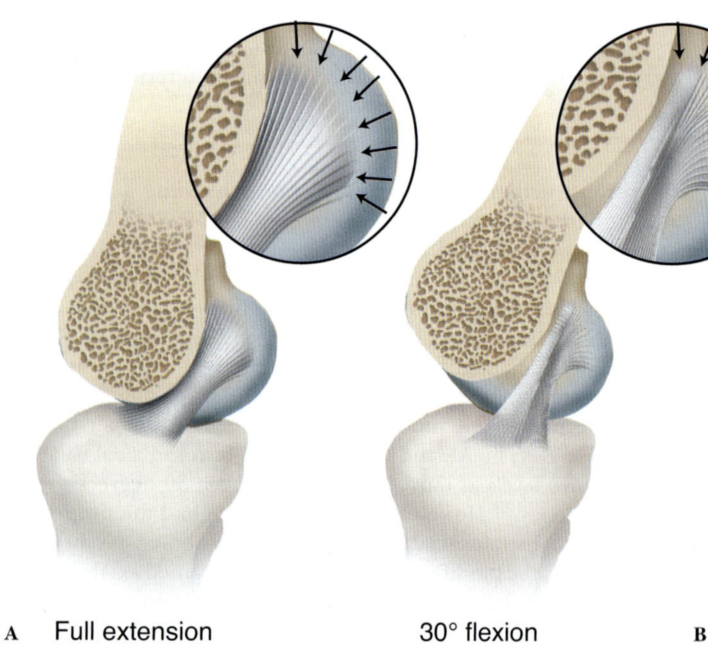

Figure 3.9. **A.** Fan-like fibers of the indirect insertion of the ACL, which insert posteriorly on the medial wall of the lateral femoral condyle. **B.** Folding of the femoral attachment with flexion, which demarcates the fan-like fibers from the remainder of the ACL. (Adapted from Mochizuki T, Fujishiro H, Nimura A, et al. Anatomic and histologic analysis of the mid-substance and fan-like extension fibres of the anterior cruciate ligament during knee motion, with special reference to the femoral attachment. *Knee Surg Sports Traumatol Arthrosc.* 2014;22[2]:336–344.)

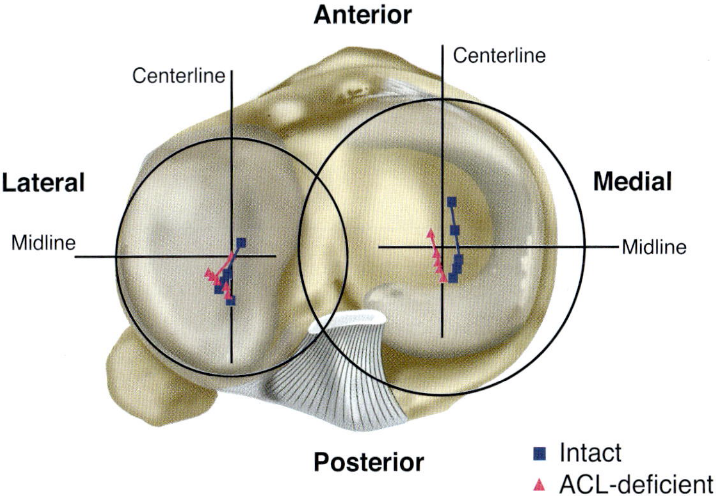

Figure 3.10. Average location of the tibiofemoral contact points projected onto the tibia during a lunge activity from 0 to 90 degrees flexion in nine people. Location of the contact points of the ACL-deficient knee are compared to the contralateral uninjured knee. Contact points were shifted posteriorly and laterally on the medial compartment of the tibia. Contact points were shifted laterally away from the tibial spine on the lateral compartment. (Adapted from Li G, Moses JM, Papannagari R, et al. Anterior cruciate ligament deficiency alters the in vivo motion of the tibiofemoral cartilage contact points in both the anteroposterior and mediolateral directions. *J Bone Joint Surg Am.* 2006;88[8]:1826–1834.)

deficient knees.[62] These data corroborate in vitro studies identifying the role of the ACL in resisting anterior and medial forces acting on the tibia.[11–13,63]

The tibia was also offset in internal rotation during gait in ACL-deficient individuals.[64] This offset was initiated during the swing phase of the gait cycle and was maintained through stance. ACL-deficient individuals also exhibited decreased peak external flexion moments during the weight acceptance portion of gait, although this was variable across individuals.[65,66] Interestingly, those individuals who adopted a gait pattern that required no increase in flexion moment had less offsets in rotation than those with higher flexion moments.[64] Thus, some people may be able to compensate for ACL deficiency by adapting their muscle activation patterns.

Knee kinematics remains abnormal following ACL reconstruction. The knees of patients receiving ACL reconstruction using either patella tendon or hamstring grafts were more adducted and more externally rotated from foot strike through midstance compared to the uninjured contralateral limb 5 months after surgery.[67] Scanlan et al.[68] corroborated these findings, showing a mean offset in external rotation through stance. Similar to the ACL-deficient knee, these small rotational offsets can lead to larger changes in the position of articular contact.[69] Interestingly, ACL-reconstructed patients with more obliquely oriented grafts were able to generate larger extension moments as would be expected in gait of uninjured individuals.[70] Changes in function continue 1 year following reconstruction including increased anterior translation of the tibia relative to the femur.[67] Altered knee function with time following reconstruction may stem from changes in graft properties, from graft slippage at the fixation site, or from neuromuscular adaptations. These remain topics for future study.

Andriacchi and colleagues have proposed that cartilage regions are attuned to their local mechanical environments[71] (Fig. 3.11). Kinematic offset after ACL injury and

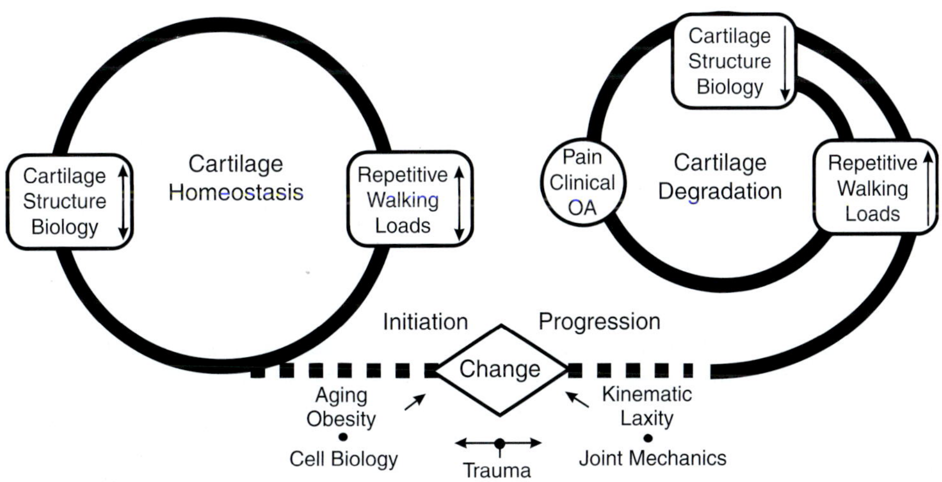

Figure 3.11. Conceptual diagram describing the role of mechanical factors in initiation and progression of osteoarthritis (OA) following traumatic injury. OA is initiated by a change, such as ACL rupture, in the homeostasis between the mechanics of walking and the biologic and/or structural status of cartilage. (From Andriacchi TP, Koo S, Scanlan SF. Gait mechanics influence healthy cartilage morphology and osteoarthritis of the knee. *J Bone Joint Surg Am.* 2009;91[suppl 1]:95–101. doi:10.2106/JBJS.H.01408, with permission.)

reconstruction could lead to degeneration if the tissue cannot adjust to the new loading regimen.[71] Animal models support the importance of altered joint motion and contact mechanics in the development of OA following ACL transection.[72]

SUMMARY

There are three mechanisms that stabilize the knee: the articulating surfaces, the ligaments, and the muscles.[1] They work in concert to allow normal function. This includes facilitating large rotations in the plane of progression while resisting forces and moments in the remaining planes. When one or more of the stabilizing mechanisms are compromised such as following ACL rupture, the knee may be susceptible to instability and suffer from large, sudden jumps in the relative position of the articulating surfaces. These giving-way episodes compromise function and can damage the cartilage and menisci.[14,15] Their elimination is a primary goal of ACL reconstruction.

The ACL is structured to resist anterior, medial, and rotational forces acting on the tibia due to its oblique orientation.[11–13,63] It also has a vital role in resisting anterolateral subluxation of the tibia in response to complex combinations of rotatory loads, described clinically as the pivot shift.[18,19,73] Its flat hourglass shape accommodates the femoral notch.[29] Classically, the ACL is divided into anteromedial and posterolateral bundles based on the location of fibers at the tibial insertion.[21,22] The anteromedial bundle resists anterior and rotatory forces throughout flexion, whereas the posterolateral bundle resists anterior and rotatory forces in extension.[34] Importantly, measures of interinsertional distance of the ACL bundles indicate that the posterolateral bundle is longest in full extension and undergoes rapid shortening from full extension to about 30 degrees flexion.[23] Therefore, close consideration should be given to the flexion angle at which a graft is fixed to avoid imposing large elongations on the graft. In practice, ACL grafts cover an area at their insertion; therefore, portions of the graft may have lengthening patterns that vary widely through its cross-section based on where the femoral tunnel is located. Although grafts placed more posteriorly toward the femoral cartilage better control anterolateral subluxation of the tibia in cadaver studies,[38] they are more anisometric through flexion. Thus, they likely experience higher loads.[39,40] Therefore, a compromise must likely be made between graft isometry through flexion and control of anterolateral subluxation of the tibia given that the fiber architecture and shape of ACL grafts do not recreate that of the native ACL.

Biomechanical evaluations of pediatric reconstruction techniques revealed the ability of over-the-top (OT) and all epiphyseal (AE) methods to reduce high posterior contact stresses generated in the ACL-deficient knee.[51,52] However, residual contact stress abnormalities remained with both methods. Although both procedures restored axial rotation, the AE approach tended to overconstrain this measure as did the modified McIntosh.[51,53] Both of these techniques failed to restore anterior stability at deeper flexion angles.[51,53] Although important for establishing proof of concept of a surgical technique, cadaver studies are limited because they account for neither anatomic differences between pediatric and adult anatomy[55] nor the effects of tissue remodeling and skeletal growth.

Recent insights into the fiber architecture of the femoral insertion based on histologic assessment may lead to future advancements in ACL reconstruction.[56,57] This includes presence of direct fibers adjacent to the intercondylar ridge and indirect fan-like fibers inserting tangentially into the bone closer to the posterior femoral cartilage.[38,60,64]

Residual differences in axial rotation during functional activities such as walking and running arise in the ACL-deficient and ACL-reconstructed knee and lead to abnormal contact mechanics.[9,33,66,68,70] Abnormal mechanics following ACL injury and reconstruction likely contribute to OA development.[20] High-resolution dynamic imaging combined with clinical outcome studies may provide insight into biomechanical factors that lead to joint degeneration over the long-term following ACL rupture and reconstruction.[74]

ACKNOWLEDGMENTS

The mentorship and guidance provided by Dr. Timothy Wright, PhD, and Professor Donald Bartel, PhD, is gratefully acknowledged. The author received funding from the following sources: grant KL2RR024997 from the Clinical and Translational Science Center at Weill Cornell Medical College, the Kirby Foundation, and the Gosnell Family.

REFERENCES

1. Burstein AH, Wright TM. *Fundamentals of Orthopaedic Biomechanics.* Baltimore, MD: Williams and Wilkins; 1994.
2. Mundermann A, Dyrby CO, D'Lima DD, et al. In vivo knee loading characteristics during activities of daily living as measured by an instrumented total knee replacement. *J Orthop Res.* 2008;26(9):1167–1172.
3. Kitaoka HB, Crevoisier XM, Hansen D, et al. Foot and ankle kinematics and ground reaction forces during ambulation. *Foot Ankle Int.* 2006;27(10):808–813.
4. Hunt AE, Smith RM, Torode M, et al. Inter-segment foot motion and ground reaction forces over the stance phase of walking. *Clin Biomech.* 2001;16(7):592–600.
5. Lewek MD, Rudolph KS, Snyder-Mackler L. Control of frontal plane knee laxity during gait in patients with medial compartment knee osteoarthritis. *Osteoarthritis Cartilage.* 2004;12(9):745–751.
6. Besier TF, Lloyd DG, Cochrane JL, et al. External loading of the knee joint during running and cutting maneuvers. *Med Sci Sport Exerc.* 2001;33(7):1168–1175.
7. Hewett TE, Myer GD, Ford KR, et al. Biomechanical measures of neuromuscular control and valgus loading of the knee predict anterior cruciate ligament injury risk in female athletes: a prospective study. *Am J Sports Med.* 2005;33(4):492–501.
8. Markolf KL, Bargar WL, Shoemaker SC, et al. The role of joint load in knee stability. *J Bone Joint Surg Am.* 1981;63(4):570–585.
9. Wang X, Malik A, Bartel DL, et al. Asymmetric varus and valgus stability of the anatomic cadaver knee and the load sharing between collateral ligaments and bearing surfaces. *J Biomech Eng.* 2014;136(8).
10. Woo SL, Hollis JM, Adams DJ, et al. Tensile properties of the human femur-anterior cruciate ligament-tibia complex. The effects of specimen age and orientation. *Am J Sports Med.* 1991;19(3):217–225.

11. Fukubayashi T, Torzilli PA, Sherman MF, et al. An in vitro biomechanical evaluation of anterior-posterior motion of the knee. Tibial displacement, rotation, and torque. *J Bone Joint Surg Am.* 1982;64(2):258–264.
12. Imhauser C, Mauro C, Choi D, et al. Abnormal tibiofemoral contact stress and its association with altered kinematics after center-center anterior cruciate ligament reconstruction: an in vitro study. *Am J Sports Med.* 2013;41(4):815–825.
13. Li G, Papannagari R, DeFrate LE, et al. The effects of ACL deficiency on mediolateral translation and varus-valgus rotation. *Acta Orthop.* 2007;78(3):355–360.
14. Galway HR, MacIntosh DL. The lateral pivot shift: a symptom and sign of anterior cruciate ligament insufficiency. *Clin Orthop Relat Res.* 1980;(147):45–50.
15. Losee RE. Concepts of the pivot shift. *Clin Orthop Relat Res.* 1983;(172):45–51.
16. Houck J, Lerner A, Gushue D, et al. Self-reported giving-way episode during a stepping-down task: case report of a subject with an ACL-deficient knee. *J Orthop Sports Phys Ther.* 2003;33(5): 273–282.
17. Houck J, Yack HJ. Giving way event during a combined stepping and crossover cutting task in an individual with anterior cruciate ligament deficiency. *J Orthop Sports Phys Ther.* 2001;31(9): 481–489.
18. Bedi A, Musahl V, Lane C, et al. Lateral compartment translation predicts the grade of pivot shift: a cadaveric and clinical analysis. *Knee Surg Sports Traumatol Arthrosc.* 2010;18(9):1269–1276.
19. Engebretsen L, Wijdicks CA, Anderson CJ, et al. Evaluation of a simulated pivot shift test: a biomechanical study. *Knee Surg Sports Traumatol Arthrosc.* 2012;20(4):698–702.
20. Di Fabio R, Graf B, Bruenig A, et al. Effect of knee joint laxity on long-loop postural reflexes: evidence for a human capsular-hamstring reflex. *Exp Brain Res.* 1992;90:189–200.
21. Abbot LC, Saunders JB, Bost FC, et al. Injuries to the ligaments of the knee joint. *J Bone Joint Surg Am.* 1944;26:503–521.
22. Girgis FG, Marshall JL, Monajem A. The cruciate ligaments of the knee joint. Anatomical, functional and experimental analysis. *Clin Orthop Relat Res.* 1975;(106):216–231.
23. Amis AA, Dawkins GP. Functional anatomy of the anterior cruciate ligament. Fibre bundle actions related to ligament replacements and injuries. *J Bone Joint Surg Br.* 1991;73(2):260–267.
24. Odensten M, Gillquist J. Functional anatomy of the anterior cruciate ligament and a rationale for reconstruction. *J Bone Joint Surg Am.* 1985;67(2):257–262.
25. Butler DL, Guan Y, Kay MD, et al. Location-dependent variations in the material properties of the anterior cruciate ligament. *J Biomech.* 1992;25(5):511–518.
26. Appel M, Gradinger R. Die architektur des kreuzbandaufbaus. *Praktische Sport-Traumatologie und Sportmedezin.* 1989;1:12–16.
27. Hara K, Mochizuki T, Sekiya I, et al. Anatomy of normal human anterior cruciate ligament attachments evaluated by divided small bundles. *Am J Sports Med.* 2009;37(12):2386–2391.
28. Arnoczky SP. Anatomy of the anterior cruciate ligament. *Clin Orthop Relat Res.* 1983;(172):19–25.
29. Triantafyllidi E, Paschos NK, Goussia A, et al. The shape and the thickness of the anterior cruciate ligament along its length in relation to the posterior cruciate ligament: a cadaveric study. *Arthroscopy.* 2013;29(12):1963–1973.
30. Groves EW. The crucial ligaments of the knee joint: their function, rupture, and the operative treatment of same. *Br J Surg.* 1920;7:505–515.
31. Artmann M, Wirth CJ. Untersuchung uber den funktionsgerechten verlauf der vorderen kreuzbandplastik. *Z Orthop.* 1974;112:160–165.
32. Hoogland T, Hillen B. Intra-articular reconstruction of the anterior cruciate ligament. An experimental study of length changes in different ligament reconstructions. *Clin Orthop Relat Res.* 1984;(185): 197–202.
33. Amis AA. The functions of the fibre bundles of the anterior cruciate ligament in anterior drawer, rotational laxity and the pivot shift. *Knee Surg Sports Traumatol Arthrosc.* 2012;20(4):613–620.
34. Gabriel MT, Wong EK, Woo SL, et al. Distribution of in situ forces in the anterior cruciate ligament in response to rotatory loads. *J Orthop Res.* 2004;22(1):85–89.
35. Morgan JA, Dahm D, Levy B, et al. Femoral tunnel malposition in ACL revision reconstruction. *J Knee Surg.* 2012;25(5):361–368.
36. Fu FH, van Eck CF, Tashman S, et al. Anatomic anterior cruciate ligament reconstruction: a changing paradigm [published online ahead of print August 3, 2014]. *Knee Surg Sports Traumatol Arthrosc.*
37. Yagi M, Wong EK, Kanamori A, et al. Biomechanical analysis of an anatomic anterior cruciate ligament reconstruction. *Am J Sports Med.* 2002;30(5):660–666.
38. Musahl V, Plakseychuk A, VanScyoc A, et al. Varying femoral tunnels between the anatomical footprint and isometric positions: effect on kinematics of the anterior cruciate ligament-reconstructed knee. *Am J Sports Med.* 2005;33(5):712–718.
39. Miura K, Woo SL, Brinkley R, et al. Effects of knee flexion angles for graft fixation on force distribution in double-bundle anterior cruciate ligament grafts. *Am J Sports Med.* 2006;34(4):577–585.
40. Markolf KL, Park S, Jackson SR, et al. Anterior-posterior and rotatory stability of single and double-bundle anterior cruciate ligament reconstructions. *J Bone Joint Surg Am.* 2009;91(1): 107–118.
41. Bowers AL, Bedi A, Lipman JD, et al. Comparison of anterior cruciate ligament tunnel position and graft obliquity with transtibial and anteromedial portal femoral tunnel reaming techniques using high-resolution magnetic resonance imaging. *Arthroscopy.* 2011;27(11):1511–1522.
42. Rahr-Wagner L, Thillemann TM, Pedersen AB, et al. Increased risk of revision after anteromedial compared with transtibial drilling of the femoral tunnel during primary anterior cruciate ligament reconstruction: results from the Danish Knee Ligament Reconstruction Register. *Arthroscopy.* 2013;29(1):98–105.
43. Fehnel DJ, Johnson R. Anterior cruciate injuries in the skeletally immature athlete: a review of treatment outcomes. *Sports Med.* 2000;29(1):51–63.
44. Guzzanti V. The natural history and treatment of rupture of the anterior cruciate ligament in children and adolescents. *J Bone Joint Surg Br.* 2003;85(4):618–619.
45. Kocher MS, Saxon HS, Hovis WD, et al. Management and complications of anterior cruciate ligament injuries in skeletally immature patients: survey of the Herodicus Society and the ACL Study Group. *J Pediatr Orthop.* 2002;22(4):452–457.
46. Mizuta H, Kubota K, Shiraishi M, et al. The conservative treatment of complete tears of the anterior cruciate ligament in skeletally immature patients. *J Bone Joint Surg Br.* 1995;77(6):890–894.
47. Andrews M, Noyes FR, Barber-Westin SD. Anterior cruciate ligament allograft reconstruction in the skeletally immature athlete. *Am J Sports Med.* 1994;22(1):48–54.
48. Lawrence JT, Bowers AL, Belding J, et al. All-epiphyseal anterior cruciate ligament reconstruction in skeletally immature patients. *Clin Orthop Relat Res.* 2010;468(7):1971–1977.
49. Lo IK, Kirkley A, Fowler PJ, et al. The outcome of operatively treated anterior cruciate ligament disruptions in the skeletally immature child. *Arthroscopy.* 1997;13(5):627–634.
50. McCarthy MM, Graziano J, Green DW, et al. All-epiphyseal, all-inside anterior cruciate ligament reconstruction technique for skeletally immature patients. *Arthrosc Tech.* 2012;1(2):e231–e239.
51. McCarthy MM, Tucker S, Nguyen JT, et al. Contact stress and kinematic analysis of all-epiphyseal and over-the-top pediatric reconstruction techniques for the anterior cruciate ligament. *Am J Sports Med.* 2013;41(6):1330–1339.
52. Stonestreet MJ, Jones KC, Kirkpatrick MS, et al. All-epiphyseal ACL reconstruction improves tibiofemoral contact: an in vitro study. *J Pediatr Orthop.* 2012;32(1):15–20.

53. Kennedy A, Coughlin DG, Metzger MF, et al. Biomechanical evaluation of pediatric anterior cruciate ligament reconstruction techniques. *Am J Sports Med.* 2011;39(5):964–971.
54. Lertwanich P, Kato Y, Martins CA, et al. A biomechanical comparison of 2 femoral fixation techniques for anterior cruciate ligament reconstruction in skeletally immature patients: over-the-top fixation versus transphyseal technique. *Arthroscopy.* 2011;27(5):672–680.
55. Kocher MS, Mandiga R, Klingele K, et al. Anterior cruciate ligament injury versus tibial spine fracture in the skeletally immature knee: a comparison of skeletal maturation and notch width index. *J Pediatr Orthop.* 2004;24(2):185–188.
56. Iwahashi T, Shino K, Nakata K, et al. Direct anterior cruciate ligament insertion to the femur assessed by histology and 3-dimensional volume-rendered computed tomography. *Arthroscopy.* 2010;26(9)(suppl):S13–S20.
57. Sasaki N, Ishibashi Y, Tsuda E, et al. The femoral insertion of the anterior cruciate ligament: discrepancy between macroscopic and histological observations. *Arthroscopy.* 2012;28(8):1135–1146.
58. Mochizuki T, Fujishiro H, Nimura A, et al. Anatomic and histologic analysis of the mid-substance and fan-like extension fibres of the anterior cruciate ligament during knee motion, with special reference to the femoral attachment. *Knee Surg Sports Traumatol Arthrosc.* 2014;22(2):336–344.
59. Li G, Wuerz TH, DeFrate LE. Feasibility of using orthogonal fluoroscopic images to measure in vivo joint kinematics. *J Biomech Eng.* 2004;126(2):314–318.
60. You BM, Siy P, Anderst W, et al. In vivo measurement of 3-D skeletal kinematics from sequences of biplane radiographs: application to knee kinematics. *IEEE Trans Med Imaging.* 2001;20(6):514–525.
61. Li G, Moses JM, Papannagari R, et al. Anterior cruciate ligament deficiency alters the in vivo motion of the tibiofemoral cartilage contact points in both the anteroposterior and mediolateral directions. *J Bone Joint Surg Am.* 2006;88(8):1826–1834.
62. Van de Velde SK, Bingham JT, Hosseini A, et al. Increased tibiofemoral cartilage contact deformation in patients with anterior cruciate ligament deficiency. *Arthritis Rheum.* 2009;60(12):3693–3702.
63. Imhauser C, Mauro C, Choi D, et al. Abnormal tibiofemoral contact stress and its association with altered kinematics after center-center anterior cruciate ligament reconstruction: an in vitro study. *Am J Sports Med.* 2013;41(4):815–825.
64. Andriacchi TP, Dyrby CO. Interactions between kinematics and loading during walking for the normal and ACL deficient knee. *J Biomech.* 2005;38(2):293–298.
65. Berchuck M, Andriacchi TP, Bach BR, et al. Gait adaptations by patients who have a deficient anterior cruciate ligament. *J Bone Joint Surg Am.* 1990;72(6):871–877.
66. Gardinier ES, Manal K, Buchanan TS, et al. Gait and neuromuscular asymmetries after acute anterior cruciate ligament rupture. *Med Sci Sports Exer.* 2012;44(8):1490–1496.
67. Tashman S, Kolowich P, Collon D, et al. Dynamic function of the ACL-reconstructed knee during running. *Clin Orthop Relat Res.* 2007;454:66–73.
68. Scanlan SF, Chaudhari AM, Dyrby CO, et al. Differences in tibial rotation during walking in ACL reconstructed and healthy contralateral knees. *J Biomech.* 2010;43(9):1817–1822.
69. Hosseini A, Van de Velde S, Gill TJ, et al. Tibiofemoral cartilage contact biomechanics in patients after reconstruction of a ruptured anterior cruciate ligament. *J Orthop Res.* 2012;30(11):1781–1788.
70. Scanlan SF, Blazek K, Chaudhari AM, et al. Graft orientation influences the knee flexion moment during walking in patients with anterior cruciate ligament reconstruction. *Am J Sports Med.* 2009;37(11):2173–2178.
71. Andriacchi TP, Koo S, Scanlan SF. Gait mechanics influence healthy cartilage morphology and osteoarthritis of the knee. *J Bone Joint Surg Am.* 2009;91[suppl 1]:95–101. doi:10.2106/JBJS.H.01408
72. Tashman S, Anderst W, Kolowich P, et al. Kinematics of the ACL-deficient canine knee during gait: serial changes over two years. *J Orthop Res.* 2004;22(5):931–941.
73. Kanamori A, Zeminski J, Rudy TW, et al. The effect of axial tibial torque on the function of the anterior cruciate ligament: a biomechanical study of a simulated pivot shift test. *Arthroscopy.* 2002;18(4):394–398.
74. Irrgang JJ, Tashman S, Moore C, et al. Challenge accepted: description of an ongoing NIH-funded randomized clinical trial to compare anatomic single-bundle versus anatomic double-bundle ACL reconstruction. *Arthroscopy.* 2012;28(6):745–747.

Moira M. McCarthy
Elizabeth Cody
Jo A. Hannafin

CHAPTER 4

Gender-Specific Issues and Anterior Cruciate Ligament

INTRODUCTION

Anterior cruciate ligament (ACL) injury is a common problem in female adolescent athletes playing cutting, pivoting, and landing sports with a greater incidence than male adolescent athletes.[1] The rise in ACL injuries in adolescents is multifactorial and may reflect widespread participation in sports at younger ages and year-round competition. The gender disparity in ACL injury incidence deserves attention secondary to potential consequences, including loss of participation in athletics, potential loss of scholarship funding and educational opportunities, and chondral and meniscal damage ultimately leading to osteoarthritis.[2,3] The intrinsic gender differences that have been proposed as risk factors are multifactorial and include anatomic, hormonal, neuromuscular, and biomechanical differences. Identification of the differences between males and females especially during the adolescent growth period is important to provide insight into design and implementation of injury prevention programs to decrease the risk of ACL injury.

GENDER DIFFERENCES IN BONE MATURITY

Females reach maturity at a younger age than males, which may affect the surgeon's decision regarding technique of ACL reconstruction. More than 25% of North American males have open physes at age 16 years, whereas 75% of females have stopped growing by age 14 years and nearly all have closed physes by age 16 years.[4]

There are also significant differences in the characteristics of female bone compared to male bone, which begin to appear during puberty. Several imaging modalities have been used to study the changes that occur in female and male bone from childhood to adulthood. Macdonald et al.[5] used peripheral quantitative computed tomography (pQCT) to assess total bone cross-sectional area and cortical area in the tibial midshaft of 128 females and males during various stages of puberty. They found no gender differences in these variables in prepubertal children. However, during puberty, males had significantly greater increases in both total cross-sectional area and cortical area as compared to females.

Hogler et al.[6] found similar results: They performed magnetic resonance imaging (MRI) and dual-energy x-ray absorptiometry (DEXA) studies on the femurs of 145 males and females ranging in age from 6 to 25 years. They found that in prepubertal children, there was no gender difference in bone mineral content, cortical bone mineral density, cross-sectional bone geometry, and muscle area in the proximal third of the femur. After puberty, males had a greater total and cortical bone area, bone diameter, and muscle area than their female counterparts, even when adjusted for femur length and weight. However, relative to muscle area, postpubertal females had greater total and cortical bone area than men.

Neu et al.[7] assessed volumetric bone density in addition to total and cortical cross-sectional bone area. They used pQCT to analyze the radial diaphysis of 469 subjects ranging in age from 6 to 40 years. From childhood to adulthood, females increased their total cross-sectional area by 50%, compared to 116% in males, with similar increases in cortical area. Bone mineral content increased by 111% in females and 140% in males; however, volumetric bone mineral content increased by 48% in females, more than double the 23% increase seen in males. Kontulainen et al.[8] also used pQCT of the tibial mid-diaphysis to show that during puberty, females increase the density of their cortical bone to a greater extent than males. By adulthood, females have a smaller volume of bone than males, but it is more dense bone. Some authors have hypothesized that this additional bone mineral content in women functions as a reservoir of calcium and other minerals needed for reproduction.[9,10]

The amount and strength of bone that women have also appears to be modifiable by physical activity. Ward et al.[11] used pQCT and DEXA studies to compare 86 prepubertal gymnasts with age-matched controls. The gymnasts had 5% greater cortical area and 6% greater cortical thickness than controls, corresponding to about a 5% greater bone strength. In the distal radius and tibia, sites of primarily trabecular bone, volumetric bone density was up to 17% greater in the gymnasts than in controls.[11]

Kontulainen et al.[12] studied 64 female tennis and squash players compared to age-matched controls using pQCT and DEXA. Their findings were similar to those of Ward et al.[11] in that the athletes had greater cortical bone area, higher bone mineral content, and higher volumetric trabecular bone density. Interestingly, they also compared the athletes who began playing their sport before or after menarche. Early starters, who began the sport before menarche, had higher bone mineral content, total cross-sectional area, cortical area, cortical thickness, and torsional bone strength index than the older starters. Their findings suggest that physical activity has an even greater effect on bone mineral content and bone architecture if started prior to puberty.[12]

Females who engage in more physical activity before puberty may increase their bone mineral content and bone size to an extent greater than that seen in males. Hasselstrom et al.[13] evaluated 135 males and 108 females aged 6 to 8 years who participated in a program in which the time spent in physical education classes was doubled to 3 hours per week. DEXA evaluation after 3 years showed that the females had a 12.5% increase in distal forearm bone mineral content and a 13.2% increase in distal forearm scanned area compared to controls who participated in the standard curriculum. Among the males, however, there was no difference between the intervention group and the control group.

It is important to note for the young female athlete that bone age may be affected by sport participation. The most common example may be gymnastics. Markou et al.[14] studied 169 female elite artistic gymnasts. In this group, bone age was delayed by 2 years compared to chronologic age.

Overall, major changes occur in the architecture and composition of bone in both females and males during puberty. Compared to males, females reach adulthood with less bone volume and less cortical thickness but with higher density of bone. The bone variables are more likely to be modifiable by increased activity. The young female athlete sees primarily increases in thickness at cortical bone sites and in bone density at trabecular bone sites. With high intensity of exercise, however, bone age may be delayed. The surgeon should be aware of these factors when treating an adolescent female athlete with an ACL injury.

EPIDEMIOLOGY OF ANTERIOR CRUCIATE LIGAMENT INJURIES

ACL injuries are most common in patients in their late teens and early 20s, with soccer being the most common sport implicated.[15] Approximately 70% of ACL injuries occur by a noncontact mechanism. The characteristic mechanism described is at foot strike when landing or decelerating, with a valgus stress on the knee, the tibia in internal rotation, and the knee in slight flexion.[16]

Females have been reported to have higher rates of ACL injury than males, with some estimating up to an eight times greater incidence of ACL tears in women than in men.[16] Prodromos et al.[17] conducted a meta-analysis of all studies which reported ACL tear incidence in an effort to clarify the roles of gender, sport, and knee injury reduction regimens. Most significantly, they found that the gender difference varies by sport. The female-to-male ACL tear incidence ratio was highest in basketball at 3.5, decreasing to 2.67 in soccer, 1.18 in lacrosse, and 1.0 in alpine skiing. From their data, the authors deduced that women playing high-level soccer or basketball have a 5% risk each year for ACL injury. Women playing handball, rugby, and wrestling also had increased risk relative to men, although due to the low number of exposures reported, these findings were less reliable.[17]

Age may also play a role in the gender difference in ACL incidence. In the meta-analysis, Prodromos[17] noted that in basketball, the overall incidence of ACL tears was significantly higher in collegiate female athletes than in high school female athletes (0.29 tears per 1,000 exposures vs. 0.09). However, the female-to-male incidence ratio was higher in the high school athletes (4.5 vs. 3.63).[17]

These findings correlate with the observation that increased risk in females appears to arise at puberty.[18] ACL injury in children younger than the age of 10 years is extremely rare; incidence increases throughout adolescence to a peak incidence at age 17 years. The incidence of ACL injury in the pediatric population has been increasing, possibly due to increased sports participation at increasingly younger ages.[19] Caine et al.[20] conducted a review of studies reporting incidence rates of sports injuries in children. Females younger than the age of 18 years who play basketball were found to have approximately doubled the risk of sustaining any knee injury and up to nine times the risk of sustaining an ACL injury.[20]

Parkkari et al.[21] reported on ACL tear incidence among 46,000 Finnish adolescent athletes aged 14 to 18 years over a period of 9 years. In this population, the incidence of ACL injury was 60.9 per 100,000 person-years. The incidence in male subjects was more than three times the incidence in female subjects. However, the risk of ACL injury was greatest in females who participated in organized sports at least four times per week; this risk was double that seen by males.[21]

Dodwell et al.[19] examined New York State database records over 20 years, from 1990 to 2009, to identify the rate of ACL reconstruction per 100,000 person-years in the population aged 3 to 20 years. In this population, the rate of ACL reconstruction increased from 17.6 in 1990 to 50.9 in 2009. The youngest patient to undergo ACL reconstruction was age 9 years. At the peak age of 17 years, the rate was 176.7. Males had a 15% higher rate of ACL reconstruction compared to females. Although the rate of ACL tears is almost certainly higher than the rate of ACL reconstruction, the data still highlights the fact that ACL injury in children and adolescents is likely on the rise.[19]

ACL injuries are frequently associated with other injuries, including injuries to the menisci, articular cartilage, medial collateral ligament (MCL), and posterior cruciate ligament (PCL). These injuries tend to vary by mechanism: Compared to ACL injuries sustained from soccer, skiing injuries are more often associated with PCL, MCL, and multiligamentous injuries, and basketball injuries are more frequently associated with meniscus and cartilage injuries.[22]

Reported rates of meniscal injury in patients with ACL tears range from about 40% to 60%.[15,23] Isolated injury to the medial meniscus is most common, followed by injury to the lateral meniscus. Females have a lower rate of injury to the menisci, suggesting that a less forceful mechanism may be required to cause an ACL tear in females.[23–25]

REASONS FOR INCREASED FEMALE ANTERIOR CRUCIATE LIGAMENT INJURY RATE—RISK FACTOR ANALYSIS

Females are more likely than males to sustain an ACL injury. Differences between the anatomy and biomechanics of males and females exist only after puberty, which corresponds with the developmental time period when the gender differences in ACL injury rates occur.[26–28]

Anatomic, hormonal, neuromuscular, and biomechanical risk factors in female athletes have been investigated in numerous sports, including soccer, basketball, volleyball, and handball. Specific risk factors that are often discussed and widely studied are body mass index (BMI), generalized and specific knee joint laxity, Q angle and other anatomic considerations, intercondylar notch width, ACL size and strength, pelvic anatomy, posterior tibial slope, and foot pronation.[29] In addition, neuromuscular and biomechanical gender differences exist, and, together, these form the basis for ACL injury prevention programs.[30]

Anatomic Gender-Based Risk Factors

Anatomic risk factors such as tibia length and thigh length and height have been minimally studied because the ability to modify these factors is low. Beynnon et al.[31] suggested that an increased thigh length in female skiers was related to an increased injury rate. However, these static anthropometric differences have not correlated well with dynamic injury mechanisms.[32]

Females have a higher BMI than males. A prospective study of cadets at the U.S. Military Academy demonstrated that a higher BMI in females was associated with an increased injury risk.[33] Uhorchak et al.[33] reported that females with a BMI 1 standard deviation (SD) above the mean had a 3.2 to 3.5 times greater risk of ACL injury than those with normal or below normal BMI. Height and weight were also shown to be predictors of injury in adolescent females in a longitudinal study of adolescent soccer players.[34] In prepubescent athletes, there was no gender difference in knee injury, but females aged older than 11 years had an increased risk of knee injury.[34] In females older than age 8 years, higher BMI was also correlated with an increase in knee injury risk.[34] The authors estimated that females began to have a higher risk of knee injury at age 12 years, which correlated with the timing of increased BMI in females related to pubertal development.[34] Brown et al.[35] noted in college-aged recreational athletes that an increase in BMI resulted in a more extended position of the lower extremity with a decreased knee flexion velocity on landing, which was postulated to lead to an increase in ACL injury. Knapik et al.[36] prospectively evaluated males and females in basic combat training and noted no increased risk of female cadets with higher BMIs. Ostenberg and Roos[37] also found no correlation with BMI and injury in female soccer players. Thus, although BMI has not been shown in the literature to have a profound impact on increasing ACL injury risk, there are other risk factors associated, such as improper lower extremity positioning during landing, which may play a more prominent role in ACL injury.

Pubertal development and maturation is a distinct point when females become more at risk for ACL injuries than males. There is no evidence for a gender discrepancy in ACL injury rates in prepubescent athletes.[34,38,39] Knee injuries do occur in pediatrics, and the percentage of those presenting as ACL injuries may be rising. And although ACL injuries are on the rise in both male and female pubescent athletes, females have a higher rate of ACL injuries immediately after their growth spurt.[40] The growth of the tibia and femur is rapid around puberty in both genders.[41] As these two bones grow rapidly, the knee is subject to greater torques.[42] Males and females show differing neuromuscular activation patterns during and following puberty[42] with females showing decreased adaptation after puberty.[28] Males increase power, strength, and coordination with age and maturational stage which allows increased dynamic lower extremity control. Females do not follow the same postpubertal course. Thus, the growth and development during and following puberty related to neuromuscular, biomechanical, and hormonal factors are likely responsible for the differences in ACL injury risk based on age and gender.

Another widely studied risk factor for female ACL injury relates to the increased Q angle of females. The Q angle is formed by a line from the anterior superior iliac spine (ASIS) to the middle of the patella and then another line from the middle of the patella to the tibial tubercle. Some authors have reported that a higher Q angle may alter lower limb mechanics and place the knee at risk for higher static and dynamic valgus stresses.[43,44] Shambaugh et al.[45] reported a higher incidence of knee injuries in female basketball players with higher Q angles. Other authors, however, have suggested that a static measurement of the Q angle is not predictive of either knee valgus angles, neuromuscular patterns, or ACL injury risk during movement.[32,46] Soderman et al.[47] studied Q angle effect on leg injuries in female soccer players and noted no increase in leg injuries. Pantano et al.[48] showed that peak knee valgus in a single-leg squat was not significantly greater in collegiate athletes with high or low Q angles. Pantano et al.[48] also noted that a better ratio to predict valgus knee was pelvic width to femoral length ratio. This ratio was related to both static and dynamic knee valgus. Overall, static measurements such as Q angle do not appear to be entirely predictive of knee valgus or ACL risk, but this leaves the door open for evaluation and emphasis on dynamic neuromuscular factors and the role of muscle activation and control in the landing, pivoting, and cutting maneuvers known to induce ACL injury.[32,46]

Females have increased joint laxity and flexibility compared to males.[47,49] Uhorchak et al.[33] reported that females with generalized joint laxity had a 2.7 times greater risk of ACL injury than those without joint laxity. Generalized joint laxity and hyperextension were found to increase the risk of injury in female soccer players.[47] Joint laxity is defined not only in the sagittal plane as hyperextension but also in the coronal plane as valgus which both can lead to strain in the ACL and possibly an increased risk of ACL injury.[28,33,49–51]

Notch width differences between males and females have been proposed as a risk factor for ACL injury. Uhorchak et al.[33] reported a 16.8 times greater risk ratio for women with a smaller intercondylar notch (<13 mm) than those with a larger notch. Emerson[52] hypothesized that a narrower notch width was a predisposing factor for ACL injury because it resulted in a smaller, weaker ligament. Shelbourne et al.[53] agreed that notch width was indicative of a smaller ACL and that more females than males had smaller, narrower notches. Dienst et al.[54] reported an in vivo MRI study that there was a correlation with smaller ACL cross-sectional area with smaller notch surface area and postulated an increase in ACL injury with smaller notches because of impingement of the ACL in the notch with tibial external rotation and abduction. Although many have accepted this theory regarding notch size as a risk factor for ACL injury, others refute that there is an association between notch width and ACL injury or that there are smaller notches in females compared to males when the notch width is normalized to bone width in both genders.[1,28,55,56]

Hamstring flexibility has been postulated as an additional risk factor for the increased ACL rates in females. Hamstring muscles were significantly more lax in ACL-injured athletes than matched controls.[49] Hamstring flexibility is a marker for overall flexibility, with males and females showing divergent flexibility patterns after puberty. Males show decreased flexibility with age and maturation, whereas females have increased flexibility with puberty.[57] After the pubertal growth spurt with significant changes in height and weight, males have decreased flexibility, whereas females do not,[58] coincident with the time that ACL injury rates increase in females.

Increased hamstring flexibility in females may be responsible for the decreased dynamic control of the knee in adolescent female athletes.[59,60] A potential mechanism is that lax hamstrings may lead to a delay in hamstring muscle activation. During early foot strike, hamstring and quadriceps cocontraction is required. It is postulated that with increased hamstring flexibility and laxity, hamstring activation may be delayed or absent, resulting in abnormalities in gait at foot strike.[61] Further study is required to assess hamstring flexibility and laxity patterns during cutting and pivoting maneuvers in adolescent females; however, the disparity in female hamstring flexibility may be a potential risk factor for increased ACL injury in adolescent females.

The primary restraint to anterior translation of the tibia on the femur is the ACL.[51] Uhorchak et al.[33] in the study on female cadets reported that females with a 1 SD above the mean increase in anterior tibial translation, or anterior–posterior laxity of the knee, had a 2.7 times greater risk of ACL injury than those without laxity. Rosene and Fogarty[62] reported that females had increased anterior tibial translation and hypothesized that the natural laxity in female ligaments allowed the tibia to shift anteriorly before dynamic muscle control could take over. However, tibial translation is modifiable by hamstring and quadriceps muscle activation and control.[63] Cutting, jumping, pivoting, and landing sports involve repetitive acceleration but, more importantly, deceleration that may result in anterior tibial translation and stress the ACL. When dynamic muscle control is impacted and ligamentous laxity occurs, this may be a prime situation for an increased rate of ACL injury.

In addition to generalized joint laxity, ligamentous laxity in the foot may also play a role in increased ACL injury in females.[64,65] Trimble et al.[65] reported that navicular drop occurs in females, resulting in anterior shift of the tibia placing increased strain on the ACL. Loudon et al.[64] reported an association with subtalar joint overpronation and noncontact ACL injuries and reported that females with ligamentous laxity are prone to overpronation. Beckett et al.[66] established a direct relationship between subtalar joint hyperpronation and ACL injury. They noted that with excessive pronation of the subtalar joint, the tibia remains internally rotated, placing the preloaded ACL at a greater stress, which may increase risk of ACL injury.

Hormonal Gender-Based Risk Factors

As the rate of ACL injuries between males and females diverges at the onset of puberty, it has been hypothesized that there is a hormonal influence on injury rates. Wojtys et al.[67] showed a trend toward an increase in noncontact ACL injuries during ovulation and a decrease during the follicular phase, whereas Slauterbeck et al.[68] and Möller Nielsen and Hammar[69] reported increased rates during the luteal phase. In female recreational skiers, Ruedl et al.[70] showed that ACL injury rates were higher in the preovulatory phase coincident with an estrogen spike.

The evidence regarding oral contraceptive use and ACL injury prevention is controversial. Ruedl et al.[70] reported that oral contraceptive use did not result in any protective effect on ACL injury in alpine skiing. Martineau et al.[71] noted that oral contraceptive use decreased the ligamentous laxity in female soccer players. Arendt and Dick[1] and Wojtys et al.[72] studies provide evidence in support of a protective effect of contraceptives on ACL injury. There is insufficient evidence at this time to recommend the use of oral contraceptives to decrease the rate of ACL injury.

The data on the effect of estrogen on the strength of the ACL is unclear. Estrogen at physiologic concentrations has been shown to decrease ligament strength.[73] However, there were no reported differences in force, stiffness, or energy to failure of ACLs from sheep with or without estrogen.[74] There are other conflicting reports about whether there is increased ligament laxity during the menstrual cycle and whether that has an effect on the mechanical properties of the ACL. The effects of the menstrual cycle on neuromuscular function are complex with significant differences in isokinetic strength, anaerobic capacity, aerobic capacity, and high-intensity endurance during different phases of the menstrual cycle.[75] Hormonal factors are likely not the only risk factor, but they may contribute to alterations in neuromuscular control.

Neuromuscular Gender-Based Risk Factors

Several neuromuscular mechanisms have been proposed to explain the increased risk of ACL injury in female athletes. Wojtys et al.[76] reported that females have greater maximal rotation of the tibia in relaxed and active muscle states and that women exhibit less muscular protection of the knee ligaments under internal rotation loading than males. When decelerating from landing, males demonstrated threefold higher knee flexor moments than females, and females had decreased hamstring-to-quadriceps peak torque ratios and increased knee abduction (valgus) moments compared to males.[59] Hewett et al.[59] also suggested that the imbalance in the hamstring-to-quadriceps strength and recruitment in female athletes could affect the ability to decelerate from a landing and to control dynamic valgus and anterior tibial translation and rotation, resulting in an increased risk of ACL injury. Females also have a decreased ability to balance muscular recruitment in positions of high joint loading, thereby increasing the risk of ACL injury.[28] Additionally, disproportionate activation of quadriceps contraction may lead to anterior shear forces during dynamic exercise resulting from imbalances between hamstring and quadriceps activation, leading to stress on the ACL.[50,77]

Huston and Wojtys[60] reported that female athletes have a slower response to activation of hamstrings in response to a stress on the ACL, suggesting that muscle activation response time may be a gender-based risk factor. Cowling and Steele[78] reported that female hamstring activation before landing activities occurred before males but in a pattern that suggested the male activation response was more in synchrony with landing, resulting in better control of joint loading during landing. Zazulak et al.[79] showed that females activated the rectus femoris in the precontact phase of landing, resulting in potential increases for ACL injury. Imbalance in activation of the quadriceps and hamstring would contribute to lowered energy absorption and increased ground reaction forces associated with ACL injury.

In response to torque and elongation of the ACL, the agonist musculature about the knee fires.[80] The stretch reflex responds through hamstring activation, which is lower and possibly delayed in females.[63]

Fatigue is another risk factor that has generated interest in the study of female athletes and ACL injury risk. Nyland et al.[81] showed that in crossover cutting in female athletes, fatigue of the quadriceps produced early gastrocnemius and delayed rectus femoris activation. Wojtys et al.[76] studied the effects of fatigue on anterior tibial translation and found that fatigue altered the neuromuscular response to anterior tibial translation but did not affect the dynamic stability of the knee.

Biomechanical Gender-Based Risk Factors

The most common position associated with a noncontact ACL injury is tibial external rotation, the knee close to full extension, and the foot planted during a deceleration when the leg collapses into valgus.[49] There are conflicting studies which report that females land with less knee flexion than their male counterparts, whereas others report that females land with more knee flexion. Thus, there is no consensus in the literature with regard to gender differences in landing knee flexion. Hewett et al.[28] reported that peak external hip flexion moments were greater in females who sustained an ACL injury versus those who did not sustain an injury. Decker et al.[82] reported that females had higher ground reaction forces during landing because of decreased use of hip musculature to absorb the forces. Zazulak et al.[79] reported that females had decreased gluteus maximus activity compared to males during single leg landings. Hip control and biomechanics may play an important role in the gender disparity of ACL injury.

Hewett et al.[28] showed that knee abduction moments (valgus torques) were significant predictors of ACL injury. Ford et al.[61] reported that females had greater knee abduction angles when preparing for a cutting maneuver compared to males. These gender differences suggest a role of altered dynamic neuromuscular activation and indicate different patterns of contraction of the adductors and abductors in females.[28] Additionally, females have greater hip adduction moments during landing which could lead to dynamic valgus position of the knee and higher risk of ACL injury.[32,59,83]

Female athletes may be less adept at handling unanticipated situations and high-risk movements such as cutting and pivoting or landing from a jump. Ford et al.[61] reported that females had greater lower extremity valgus during unanticipated cutting than males. This dynamic valgus, as described earlier, may be a cause of increased ACL injuries in female athletes.

ANTERIOR CRUCIATE LIGAMENT INJURY PREVENTION PROGRAMS FOR FEMALES

Due to the increased incidence in ACL injuries in female athletes, multiple prevention programs have been developed with the goal of assessing and modifying the risk factors and ultimately lowering the incidence of ACL injuries in males and females.

Ettlinger et al.[84] published the first study on ACL prevention training programs and demonstrated a decreased incidence of knee injuries in alpine skiers following a training program as compared with controls. This set the stage for evaluation of potential training programs to decrease the rate of ACL injuries in total, whereas a subset of risk factor analyses led to training programs specifically designed to decrease the rate of ACL injury in female athletes.

Stevenson et al.[85] provided a recent systematic review on the effectiveness of neuromuscular training programs in reducing the incidence of ACL injuries in female athletes. They found that most studies showed either a trend toward improvement or a significant improvement in ACL injury rates and that the most effective programs included plyometric exercises and a preseason component.[85] Noyes and Barber-Westin [86] published a more recent systematic review of neuromuscular retraining intervention programs on ACL injury rates in adolescent female athletes. They found wide variability in the programs in terms of frequency, duration, timing, control or supervision, the specific components of the training program, noncontact ACL injury incidence rates, and compliance with training. The authors concluded that the three ACL intervention programs successfully reduced noncontact ACL injury rates in adolescent female athletes. The overall relative risk reduction ranged from 75% to 100% and the number of athletes needed to treat to prevent one noncontact ACL injury ranged from 70 to 98 athletes.

A recent meta-analysis by Myer et al.[87] reported that female athletes enrolled in a preventive neuromuscular training program had significantly decreased knee injury rates than the control group. The preventive group was more effective in the mid-teen (age 14 to 18 years) group than the late-teen (age 18 to 20 years) or the early adult (age older than 20 years) groups, although all groups treated with the preventive training had decreased rates of injury compared to controls.[87]

Prevention programs, as shown earlier, can be beneficial to some female athletes when compliance is complete, but there is a cost to these programs. The cost of these programs is financial but, more importantly, time-intensive for the athlete and trainer to ensure compliance. However, with the most recent estimate of the cost of an ACL injury[88] at $38,121, cost of a prevention program pales in comparison and can be seen as an investment.

GRAFT CHOICE

One of the prime topics of controversy surrounding ACL reconstruction is graft choice. In male versus female patients who are skeletally immature, soft tissue grafts are the preferred treatment option. The purpose of the soft tissue grafts in patients with open physes is to avoid creation of a bone bridge across the physis that may result in growth abnormalities including angular and rotational deformities. Several authors have reported on the role of gender in surgical outcome comparing the most common grafts: hamstring and bone-patellar tendon-bone autografts. Allografts are not recommended in adolescent patients due to the higher rates of failure.[89]

Ma et al.[90] reported that females had smaller diameter hamstring grafts than males (7.5 mm vs. 8.1 mm, respectively) and that preoperative screening of height and weight were not predictive of tendon size. Xie et al.[91] found that females had smaller diameter and shorter length hamstring tendons than males but that height and weight could predict graft size intraoperatively. Laboute et al.[92] recently reported on the outcomes for hamstring tendon autograft versus patellar tendon autograft and found that age and gender did not influence the reinjury rate. Despite this conclusion, in females, there were no reinjuries in the patellar tendon group (26 females), whereas there were five reinjuries in the hamstring autograft group (38 females). Ahldén et al.[93] evaluated clinical outcomes in patients undergoing ACL reconstruction and found no gender differences after 2 years following hamstring autograft reconstruction.

There are no specific studies designed to determine the appropriate graft choice for young, active females, which demonstrate any difference in failure rates as compared to males. Biomechanical data has shown that smaller grafts experience larger strain[94] and that soft tissue grafts smaller than 8 mm in diameter have a higher failure rate in both genders.[95]

Female patients treated with autogenous hamstring tendon grafts in particular may be at risk for an inferior outcome. Several authors have found increased laxity and worse outcomes on follow-up in female patients treated with autogenous hamstring tendon grafts.[96–98] Noojin et al.[97] reported on 39 female and 26 male patients who underwent quadruple-looped hamstring autograft anterior cruciate ligament reconstruction (ACLR). At an average of about 40 months follow-up, the clinical failure rate was 23% for women and 4% for men. There was a trend toward increased laxity in the female patients. Women also reported more pain and were less likely to return to their preinjury level of activity. The authors believed that the women may have had a higher failure rate due to having smaller tendons than the men and also potentially from a higher frequency of greater ligamentous laxity.[97]

OUTCOMES OF ANTERIOR CRUCIATE LIGAMENT INJURIES IN FEMALES

In the short term, ACL injuries result in impaired joint stability and biomechanics and can lead to further injury to the joint in the form of meniscus and cartilage damage. In the long term, 10 to 20 years after injury, 50% of patients have pain and limited function related to osteoarthritis.[98]

Among patients who do not undergo surgery, females may be more likely than males to lack dynamic knee stability, impairing their return to activity. Hurd et al.[99] reported on 340 patients with ACL insufficiency, all of whom were very active prior to injury. Their ability to cope with conservative management was assessed based on functional exam, questionnaires, and residual giving-way episodes. Sixty-four percent of the females in the study were deemed non-copers, compared to 54% of males. Females who had a noncontact mechanism of injury were more likely to be classified as non-copers than those whose injury was contact-related.[99]

A number of studies have found that surgical intervention within 6 to 12 months of injury decreases the incidence of further injury to the joint in the form of meniscus tears and/or chondral injury.[25,100–103] Long-term follow-up (>10 years) of patients who received ACLR compared to patients treated nonoperatively has shown that ACLR decreases the need for additional surgery (12.4% vs. 24.9%). Patients treated with ACLR also preserve their activity level better than patients treated nonoperatively, as measured by the Tegner score.[104]

Following ACLR, several authors have reported no differences between males and females in terms of complications or failure rate.[105,106] However, when other objective and subjective outcomes are assessed, females may have worse outcomes from ACLR than males. Data from the Swedish National Knee Ligament Register[107] demonstrated that males were more likely than females to achieve functional recovery by 2 years after ACLR. Using the same registry, Ageberg et al.[24] found that at 1 and 2 years after ACLR, females reported significantly worse outcomes than males on the Knee injury and Osteoarthritis Outcome Score (KOOS), despite having a lower rate of meniscal and cartilage injuries than men. The score difference was most marked on the sport/recreation section of the KOOS, and although women made significant gains from postoperative year 1 to year 2, men made more gains so that the gender difference increased from postoperative year 1 to year 2.[24]

Females may also be at higher risk for reinjury and/or contralateral injury. Paterno et al.[108] studied the rate of recurrent ACL injury (ipsilateral or contralateral) following ACLR in athletes. The incidence of recurrent injury was 15 times greater than that of new ACL injury in controls. Female athletes were four times more likely than men to reinjure their ipsilateral ACL and six times more likely to sustain a contralateral ACL tear. However, the sample size was relatively small (63 subjects and 39 controls), limiting the use of this observation.[108]

Shelbourne et al.[109] followed 1,415 patients for 5 years after ACLR and found that women were significantly more likely to injure the contralateral ACL (7.8% vs. 3.7%) but were not more likely to reinjure the reconstructed knee (4.3% vs. 4.1%). Among the 528 patients younger than 18 years of age at the time of initial injury, the risk of subsequent injury was even higher, with a combined 17.4% incidence of reinjury and contralateral injury over the study period. Females were significantly more likely to injure the contralateral knee (11.6% vs. 4.6%), whereas males were significantly more likely to sustain an ACL graft tear (10.6% vs. 4.6%). The incidence of subsequent injury to either knee was lowest in patients older than 25 years of age at the time of injury, at less than 4%.[109]

Gobbi et al.[96] reviewed 80 athletes who underwent patellar tendon or hamstring grafting. Among the patellar tendon patients, there was no significant difference in subjective or objective outcomes between men and women. However, women in the hamstring group had significantly greater laxity and worse results on isokinetic testing at 1 year.[96] Aldrian et al.[110] found that female patients who underwent computer-navigated double-bundle ACLR had significantly worse clinical outcome scores on the International Knee Documentation Committee (IKDC) scale, Lysholm scale, and Tegner score than male counterparts.[110]

Laboute et al.[92] reported on reinjury rates after ACLR at a 3- to 4-year follow-up. Although they did not find a gender difference in rate of reinjury, there was a higher reinjury rate among patients who received hamstring tendon grafts compared to patellar tendon grafts. Reinjury rates were 12.7% for hamstring tendon autograft recipients and 6.1% for patellar tendon autograft recipients. The major risk factor for reinjury that was identified was early return to competition: Patients who returned to competition within 7 months of surgery had an at least doubled risk of reinjury compared to those who returned after 7 months.[92]

CONCLUSION

ACL injuries are an increasingly common injury sustained by adolescents due to increased participation in sporting activities. Gender-based differences that may account for the increased ACL injury risk in female as compared to male athletes include anatomic, biomechanical, neuromuscular, and hormonal differences. Injury prevention programs have shown some success in decreasing the injury risk in the adolescent female athlete.

REFERENCES

1. Arendt E, Dick R. Knee injury patterns among men and women in collegiate basketball and soccer. NCAA data and review of literature. *Am J Sports Med.* 1995;23(6):694–701.
2. Freedman KB, Glasgow MT, Glasgow SG, et al. Anterior cruciate ligament injury and reconstruction among university students. *Clin Orthop Relat Res.* 1998;(356):208–212.
3. Ruiz AL, Kelly M, Nutton RW. Arthroscopic ACL reconstruction: a 5-9 year follow-up. *Knee.* 2002;9(3):197–200.
4. Tanner J, Oshman D, Bahhage F, et al. Tanner-Whitehouse bone age reference values for North American children. *J Pediatr.* 1997;131(1, pt 1):34–40.
5. Macdonald HM, Kontulainen SA, Mackelvie-O'Brien KJ, et al. Maturity- and sex-related changes in tibial bone geometry, strength and bone-muscle strength indices during growth: a 20-month pQCT study. *Bone.* 2005;36(6):1003–1011.
6. Hogler W, Blimkie CJ, Cowell CT, et al. Sex-specific developmental changes in muscle size and bone geometry at the femoral shaft. *Bone.* 2008;42(5):982–989.
7. Neu CM, Rauch F, Manz F, et al. Modeling of cross-sectional bone size, mass and geometry at the proximal radius: a study of normal bone development using peripheral quantitative computed tomography. *Osteoporosis Int.* 2001;12(7):538–547.
8. Kontulainen SA, Macdonald HM, McKay HA. Change in cortical bone density and its distribution differs between boys and girls during puberty. *J Clin Endocrinol Metab.* 2006;91(7):2555–2561.
9. Frisancho AR, Garn SM, Ascoli W. Subperiosteal and endosteal bone apposition during adolescence. *Hum Biol.* 1970;42(4): 639–664.
10. Schoenau E, Neu CM, Rauch F, et al. Gender-specific pubertal changes in volumetric cortical bone mineral density at the proximal radius. *Bone.* 2002;31(1):110–113.
11. Ward KA, Roberts SA, Adams JE, et al. Bone geometry and density in the skeleton of pre-pubertal gymnasts and school children. *Bone.* 2005;36(6):1012–1018.
12. Kontulainen S, Sievänen H, Kannus P, et al. Effect of long-term impact-loading on mass, size, and estimated strength of humerus and radius of female racquet-sports players: a peripheral quantitative computed tomography study between young and old starters and controls. *J Bone Miner Res.* 2002;17(12):2281–2289.
13. Hasselstrom HA, Karlsson MK, Hansen SE, et al. A 3-year physical activity intervention program increases the gain in bone mineral and bone width in prepubertal girls but not boys: the prospective Copenhagen school child interventions study (CoSCIS). *Calcif Tissue Int.* 2008;83(4):243–250.
14. Markou KB, Mylonas P, Theodoropoulou A, et al. The influence of intensive physical exercise on bone acquisition in adolescent elite female and male artistic gymnasts. *J Clin Endocrinol Metab.* 2004;89(9):4383–4387.
15. Maletis GB, Granan LP, Inacio MC, et al. Comparison of community-based ACL reconstruction registries in the U.S. and Norway. *J Bone Joint Surg Am.* 2011;93(suppl 3):31–36.
16. Hewett TE, Myer GD, Ford KR. Anterior cruciate ligament injuries in female athletes: part 1, mechanisms and risk factors. *Am J Sports Med.* 2006;34(2):299–311.
17. Prodromos CC, Han Y, Rogowski J, et al. A meta-analysis of the incidence of anterior cruciate ligament tears as a function of gender, sport, and a knee injury-reduction regimen. *Arthroscopy.* 2007;23(12):1320.e6–1325.e6.
18. Ford KR, Shapiro R, Myer GD, et al. Longitudinal sex differences during landing in knee abduction in young athletes. *Med Sci Sports Exerc.* 2010;42(10):1923–1931.
19. Dodwell ER, Lamont LE, Green DW, et al. 20 years of pediatric anterior cruciate ligament reconstruction in New York State. *Am J Sports Med.* 2014;42(3):675–680.
20. Caine D, Maffulli N, Caine C. Epidemiology of injury in child and adolescent sports: injury rates, risk factors, and prevention. *Clin Sports Med.* 2008;27(1):19–50.
21. Parkkari J, Pasanen K, Mattila VM, et al. The risk for a cruciate ligament injury of the knee in adolescents and young adults: a population-based cohort study of 46 500 people with a 9 year follow-up. *Br J Sports Med.* 2008;42(6):422–426.
22. Granan L, Inacio MCS, Maletis GB, et al. Sport-specific injury pattern recorded during anterior cruciate ligament reconstruction. *Am J Sports Med.* 2013;41(12):2814–2818.
23. Kilcoyne KG, Dickens JF, Haniuk E, et al. Epidemiology of meniscal injury associated with ACL tears in young athletes. *Orthopedics.* 2012;35(3):208–212.
24. Ageberg E, Forssblad M, Herbertsson P, et al. Sex differences in patient-reported outcomes after anterior cruciate ligament reconstruction: data from the Swedish Knee Ligament Register. *Am J Sports Med.* 2010;38(7):1334–1342.
25. Sri-Ram K, Salmon LJ, Pinczewski LA, et al. The incidence of secondary pathology after anterior cruciate ligament rupture in 5086 patients requiring ligament reconstruction. *Bone Joint J.* 2013;95-B(1):59–64.
26. Griffin LY, Albohm MJ, Arendt EA, et al. Understanding and preventing noncontact anterior cruciate ligament injuries: a review of the Hunt Valley II meeting, January 2005. *Am J Sports Med.* 2006;34(9):1512–1532.
27. Hewett TE, Lindenfeld TN, Riccobene JV, et al. The effect of neuromuscular training on the incidence of knee injury in female athletes. A prospective study. *Am J Sports Med.* 1999;27(6):699–706.
28. Hewett TE, Myer GD, Ford KR, et al. Biomechanical measures of neuromuscular control and valgus loading of the knee predict anterior cruciate ligament injury risk in female athletes: a prospective study. *Am J Sports Med.* 2005;33(4):492–501.
29. Alentorn-Geli E, Myer GD, Silvers HJ, et al. Prevention of non-contact anterior cruciate ligament injuries in soccer players. Part 1: mechanisms of injury and underlying risk factors. *Knee Surg Sports Traumatol Arthrosc.* 2009;17(7):705–729.
30. Toth AP, Cordasco FA. ACL injuries in the female athlete. *J Gend Specif Med.* 2001; 4(4):25–34.
31. Beynnon B, Slauterbeck J, Padua D, et al. Update on ACL risk factors and prevention strategies in the female athlete. In: *National Athletic Trainers Association Annual Meeting and Clinical Symposia.* Los Angeles, CA: Human Kinetics; 2001:15–18.
32. Myer GD, Ford KR, Hewett TE. The effects of gender on quadriceps muscle activation strategies during a maneuver that mimics a high ACL injury risk position. *J Electromyogr Kinesiol.* 2005;15(2):181–189.
33. Uhorchak JM, Scoville CR, Williams GN, et al. Risk factors associated with noncontact injury of the anterior cruciate ligament: a prospective four-year evaluation of 859 West Point cadets. *Am J Sports Med.* 2003;31(6):831–842.
34. Buehler-Yund C. A longitudinal study of injury rates and risk factors in 5 to 12 year old soccer players. In: *Environmental Health.* Cincinnati, OH: University of Cincinnati; 1999:161.

35. Brown CN, Yu B, Kirkendall DT, et al. Effects of increased body mass index on lower extremity motion patterns in a stop-jump task: National Athletic Trainers Association Annual Meeting. *J Athl Train.* 2005;404(suppl):5.
36. Knapik JJ, Sharp MA, Canham-Chervak M, et al. Risk factors for training-related injuries among men and women in basic combat training. *Med Sci Sports Exerc.* 2001;33(6):946–954.
37. Ostenberg A, Roos H. Injury risk factors in female European football. A prospective study of 123 players during one season. *Scand J Med Sci Sports.* 2000;10(5):279–285.
38. Andrish JT. Anterior cruciate ligament injuries in the skeletally immature patient. *Am J Orthop (Belle Mead NJ).* 2001;30(2):103–110.
39. McCarroll JR, Rettig AC, Shelbourne KD. Anterior cruciate ligament injuries in the young athlete with open physes. *Am J Sports Med.* 1988;16(1):44–47.
40. Tursz A, Crost M. Sports-related injuries in children. A study of their characteristics, frequency, and severity, with comparison to other types of accidental injuries. *Am J Sports Med.* 1986;14(4):294–299.
41. Tanner JM, Davies PS. Clinical longitudinal standards for height and height velocity for North American children. *J Pediatr.* 1985;107(3):317–329.
42. Hewett TE, Myer GD, Ford KR. Decrease in neuromuscular control about the knee with maturation in female athletes. *J Bone Joint Surg Am.* 2004;86-A(8):1601–1608.
43. Heiderscheit BC, Hamill J, Caldwell GE. Influence of Q-angle on lower-extremity running kinematics. *J Orthop Sports Phys Ther.* 2000;30(5):271–278.
44. Mizuno Y, Kumagai M, Mattessich SM, et al. Q-angle influences tibiofemoral and patellofemoral kinematics. *J Orthop Res.* 2001;19(5):834–840.
45. Shambaugh JP, Klein A, Herbert JH. Structural measures as predictors of injury basketball players. *Med Sci Sports Exerc.* 1991;23(5): 522–527.
46. Gray J, Taunton JE, McKenzie DC, et al. A survey of injuries to the anterior cruciate ligament of the knee in female basketball players. *Int J Sports Med.* 1985;6(6):314–316.
47. Soderman K, Alfredson H, Pietilä T, et al. Risk factors for leg injuries in female soccer players: a prospective investigation during one out-door season. *Knee Surg Sports Traumatol Arthrosc.* 2001;9(5): 313–321.
48. Pantano KJ, White SC, Gilchrist LA, et al. Differences in peak knee valgus angles between individuals with high and low Q-angles during a single limb squat. *Clin Biomech (Bristol, Avon).* 2005;20(9): 966–972.
49. Boden BP, Dean GS, Feagin JA Jr, et al. Mechanisms of anterior cruciate ligament injury. *Orthopedics.* 2000;23(6):573–578.
50. Markolf KL, Burchfield DM, Shapiro MM, et al. Combined knee loading states that generate high anterior cruciate ligament forces. *J Orthop Res.* 1995;13(6):930–935.
51. Markolf KL, Graff-Radford A, Amstutz HC. In vivo knee stability. A quantitative assessment using an instrumented clinical testing apparatus. *J Bone Joint Surg Am.* 1978;60(5):664–674.
52. Emerson RJ. Basketball knee injuries and the anterior cruciate ligament. *Clin Sports Med.* 1993;12(2):317–328.
53. Shelbourne KD, Davis TJ, Klootwyk TE. The relationship between intercondylar notch width of the femur and the incidence of anterior cruciate ligament tears. A prospective study. *Am J Sports Med.* 1998;26(3):402–408.
54. Dienst M, Schneider G, Altmeyer K, et al. Correlation of intercondylar notch cross sections to the ACL size: a high resolution MR tomographic in vivo analysis. *Arch Orthop Trauma Surg.* 2007;127(4): 253–260.
55. Hutchinson MR, Ireland ML. Knee injuries in female athletes. *Sports Med.* 1995;19(4):288–302.
56. LaPrade RF, Burnett QM II. Femoral intercondylar notch stenosis and correlation to anterior cruciate ligament injuries. A prospective study. *Am J Sports Med.* 1994;22(2):198–202; discussion 203.
57. Malina RM, Bouchard C. Timing and sequence of changes in growth, maturation, and performance during adolescence. In: Malina RM, Bouchard C, eds. *Growth, Maturation, and Physical Activity.* Champaign, IL: Human Kinetics; 1991:267–272.
58. Beunen GP, Malina RM, Renson R, et al. Physical activity and growth, maturation and performance: a longitudinal study. *Med Sci Sports Exerc.* 1992;24(5):576–585.
59. Hewett TE, Stroupe AL, Nance TA, et al. Plyometric training in female athletes. Decreased impact forces and increased hamstring torques. *Am J Sports Med.* 1996;24(6):765–773.
60. Huston LJ, Wojtys EM. Neuromuscular performance characteristics in elite female athletes. *Am J Sports Med.* 1996;24(4):427–436.
61. Ford KR, Myer GD, Toms HE, et al. Gender differences in the kinematics of unanticipated cutting in young athletes. *Med Sci Sports Exerc.* 2005;37(1):124–129.
62. Rosene JM, Fogarty TD. Anterior tibial translation in collegiate athletes with normal anterior cruciate ligament integrity. *J Athl Train.* 1999;34(2):93–98.
63. Solomonow M, Baratta R, Zhou BH, et al. The synergistic action of the anterior cruciate ligament and thigh muscles in maintaining joint stability. *Am J Sports Med.* 1987;15(3):207–213.
64. Loudon JK, Jenkins W, Loudon KL. The relationship between static posture and ACL injury in female athletes. *J Orthop Sports Phys Ther.* 1996;24(2):91–97.
65. Trimble MH, Bishop MD, Buckley BD, et al. The relationship between clinical measurements of lower extremity posture and tibial translation. *Clin Biomech (Bristol, Avon).* 2002;17(4):286–290.
66. Beckett ME, Massie DL, Bowers KD, et al. Incidence of hyperpronation in the acl injured knee: a clinical perspective. *J Athl Train.* 1992;27(1):58–62.
67. Wojtys EM, Huston LJ, Lindenfeld TN, et al. Association between the menstrual cycle and anterior cruciate ligament injuries in female athletes. *Am J Sports Med.* 1998;26(5):614–619.
68. Slauterbeck JR, Fuzie SF, Smith MP, et al. The menstrual cycle, sex hormones, and anterior cruciate ligament injury. *J Athl Train.* 2002;37(3):275–278.
69. Möller Nielsen J, Hammar M. Sports injuries and oral contraceptive use. Is there a relationship? *Sports Med.* 1991;12(3):152–160.
70. Ruedl G, Ploner P, Linortner I, et al. Are oral contraceptive use and menstrual cycle phase related to anterior cruciate ligament injury risk in female recreational skiers? *Knee Surg Sports Traumatol Arthrosc.* 2009;17(9):1065–1069.
71. Martineau PA, Al-Jassir F, Lenczner E, et al. Effect of the oral contraceptive pill on ligamentous laxity. *Clin J Sport Med.* 2004;14(5):281–286.
72. Wojtys EM, Huston LJ, Boynton MD, et al. The effect of the menstrual cycle on anterior cruciate ligament injuries in women as determined by hormone levels. *Am J Sports Med.* 2002;30(2):182–188.
73. Booth FW, Tipton CM. Ligamentous strength measurements in prepubescent and pubescent rats. *Growth.* 1970;34(2):177–185.
74. Strickland SM, Belknap TW, Turner SA, et al. Lack of hormonal influences on mechanical properties of sheep knee ligaments. *Am J Sports Med.* 2003;31(2):210–215.
75. Lebrun CM. The effect of the phase of the menstrual cycle and the birth control pill on athletic performance. *Clin Sports Med.* 1994;13(2):419–441.
76. Wojtys EM, Huston LJ, Schock HJ, et al. Gender differences in muscular protection of the knee in torsion in size-matched athletes. *J Bone Joint Surg Am.* 2003;85-A(5):782–789.
77. Sell TC, Ferris CM, Abt JP, et al. Predictors of proximal tibia anterior shear force during a vertical stop-jump. *J Orthop Res.* 2007;25(12):1589–1597.
78. Cowling EJ, Steele JR. Is lower limb muscle synchrony during landing affected by gender? Implications for variations in ACL injury rates. *J Electromyogr Kinesiol.* 2001;11(4):263–268.
79. Zazulak BT, Ponce PL, Straub SJ, et al. Gender comparison of hip muscle activity during single-leg landing. *J Orthop Sports Phys Ther.* 2005;35(5):292–299.

80. Nichols TR. The contributions of muscles and reflexes to the regulation of joint and limb mechanics. *Clin Orthop Relat Res.* 2002;(403)(suppl):S43–S50.
81. Nyland JA, Caborn DN, Shapiro R, et al. Fatigue after eccentric quadriceps femoris work produces earlier gastrocnemius and delayed quadriceps femoris activation during crossover cutting among normal athletic women. *Knee Surg Sports Traumatol Arthrosc.* 1997;5(3):162–167.
82. Decker MJ, Torry MR, Wyland DJ, et al. Gender differences in lower extremity kinematics, kinetics and energy absorption during landing. *Clin Biomech (Bristol, Avon).* 2003;18(7):662–669.
83. Ford KR, Myer GD, Hewett TE. Valgus knee motion during landing in high school female and male basketball players. *Med Sci Sports Exerc.* 2003;35(10):1745–1750.
84. Ettlinger CF, Johnson RJ, Shealy JE. A method to help reduce the risk of serious knee sprains incurred in alpine skiing. *Am J Sports Med.* 1995;23(5):531–537.
85. Stevenson JH, Beattie CS, Schwartz JB, et al. Assessing the effectiveness of neuromuscular training programs in reducing the incidence of anterior cruciate ligament injuries in female athletes: a systematic review [published online ahead of print February 25, 2014]. *Am J Sports Med.*
86. Noyes FR, Barber-Westin SD. Neuromuscular retraining intervention programs: do they reduce noncontact anterior cruciate ligament injury rates in adolescent female athletes? *Arthroscopy.* 2014;30(2):245–255.
87. Myer GD, Sugimoto D, Thomas S, et al. The influence of age on the effectiveness of neuromuscular training to reduce anterior cruciate ligament injury in female athletes: a meta-analysis. *Am J Sports Med.* 2013;41(1):203–215.
88. Mather RC III, Koenig L, Kocher MS, et al. Societal and economic impact of anterior cruciate ligament tears. *J Bone Joint Surg Am.* 2013;95(19):1751–1759.
89. Lamblin CJ, Waterman BR, Lubowitz JH. Anterior cruciate ligament reconstruction with autografts compared with non-irradiated, non-chemically treated allografts. *Arthroscopy.* 2013;29(6):1113–1122.
90. Ma CB, Keifa E, Dunn W, et al. Can pre-operative measures predict quadruple hamstring graft diameter? *Knee.* 2010;17(1):81–83.
91. Xie G, Huangfu X, Zhao J. Prediction of the graft size of 4-stranded semitendinosus tendon and 4-stranded gracilis tendon for anterior cruciate ligament reconstruction: a Chinese Han patient study. *Am J Sports Med.* 2012;40(5):1161–1166.
92. Laboute E, Savalli L, Puig P, et al. Analysis of return to competition and repeat rupture for 298 anterior cruciate ligament reconstructions with patellar or hamstring tendon autograft in sportspeople. *Ann Phys Rehabil Med.* 2010;53(10):598–614.
93. Ahldén M, Sernert N, Karlsson J, et al. Outcome of anterior cruciate ligament reconstruction with emphasis on sex-related differences. *Scand J Med Sci Sports.* 2012;22(5):618–626.
94. Lipps DB, Oh YK, Ashton-Miller JA, et al. Morphologic characteristics help explain the gender difference in peak anterior cruciate ligament strain during a simulated pivot landing. *Am J Sports Med.* 2012;40(1):32–40.
95. Mariscalco MW, Flanigan DC, Mitchell J, et al. The influence of hamstring autograft size on patient-reported outcomes and risk of revision after anterior cruciate ligament reconstruction: a Multicenter Orthopaedic Outcomes Network (MOON) Cohort Study. *Arthroscopy.* 2013;29(12):1948–1953.
96. Gobbi A, Domzalski M, Pascual J. Comparison of anterior cruciate ligament reconstruction in male and female athletes using the patellar tendon and hamstring autografts. *Knee Surg Sports Traumatol Arthrosc.* 2004;12(6):534–539.
97. Noojin FK, Barrett GR, Hartzog CW, et al. Clinical comparison of intraarticular anterior cruciate ligament reconstruction using autogenous semitendinosus and gracilis tendons in men versus women. *Am J Sports Med.* 2000;28(6):783–789.
98. Lohmander LS, Englund PM, Dahl LL, et al. The long-term consequence of anterior cruciate ligament and meniscus injuries: osteoarthritis. *Am J Sports Med.* 2007;35(10):1756–1769.
98. Pinczewski LA, Deehan DJ, Salmon LJ, et al. A five-year comparison of patellar tendon versus four-strand hamstring tendon autograft for arthroscopic reconstruction of the anterior cruciate ligament. *Am J Sports Med.* 2002;30(4):523–536.
99. Hurd WJ, Axe MJ, Snyder-Mackler L. Influence of age, gender, and injury mechanism on the development of dynamic knee stability after acute ACL rupture. *J Orthop Sports Phys Ther.* 2008;38(2):36–41.
100. Anstey DE, Heyworth BE, Price MD, et al. Effect of timing of ACL reconstruction in surgery and development of meniscal and chondral lesions. *Phys Sportsmed.* 2012;40(1):36–40.
101. Fanelli GC, Orcutt DR, Edson CJ. The multiple-ligament injured knee: evaluation, treatment, and results. *Arthroscopy.* 2005;21(4):471–486.
102. Fok AW, Yau WP. Delay in ACL reconstruction is associated with more severe and painful meniscal and chondral injuries. *Knee Surg Sports Traumatol Arthrosc.* 2013;21(4):928–933.
103. Michalitsis S, Vlychou M, Malizos K, et al. Meniscal and articular cartilage lesions in the anterior cruciate ligament-deficient knee: correlation between time from injury and knee scores. *Knee Surg Sports Traumatol Arthrosc.* 2015;23(1):232–239.
104. Chalmers PN, Mall NA, Moric M, et al. Does ACL reconstruction alter natural history?: a systematic literature review of long-term outcomes. *J Bone Joint Surg Am.* 2014;96(4):292–300.
105. Barber-Westin SD, Noyes FR, Andrews M. A rigorous comparison between the sexes of results and complications after anterior cruciate ligament reconstruction. *Am J Sports Med.* 1997;25(4):514–526.
106. Ferrari JD, Bach BR Jr, Bush-Joseph CA, et al. Anterior cruciate ligament reconstruction in men and women: an outcome analysis comparing gender. *Arthroscopy.* 2001;17(6):588–596.
107. Barenius B, Forssblad M, Engstrom B, et al. Functional recovery after anterior cruciate ligament reconstruction, a study of health-related quality of life based on the Swedish National Knee Ligament Register. *Knee Surg Sports Traumatol Arthrosc.* 2013;21(4):914–927.
108. Paterno MV, Rauh MJ, Schmitt LC, et al. Incidence of contralateral and ipsilateral anterior cruciate ligament (ACL) injury after primary ACL reconstruction and return to sport. *Clin J Sport Med.* 2012;22(2):116–121.
109. Shelbourne KD, Gray T, Haro M. Incidence of subsequent injury to either knee within 5 years after anterior cruciate ligament reconstruction with patellar tendon autograft. *Am J Sports Med.* 2009;37(2):246–251.
110. Aldrian S, Valentin P, Wondrasch B, et al. Gender differences following computer-navigated single- and double-bundle anterior cruciate ligament reconstruction. *Knee Surg Sports Traumatol Arthrosc.* 2014;22(9):2145–2152.

CHAPTER

5

Morgan A. Anderson
Jordan D. Metzl

Historical Approach: Nonoperative

INTRODUCTION

Injuries to the anterior cruciate ligament (ACL) in the pediatric population are predominantly in the form of tibial spine avulsion fractures and ACL tears. Tibial spine avulsion fractures are one of the most common knee injuries in children, usually resulting in avulsions of the anterior intercondylar eminence from the pull of ACL, with posterior intercondylar eminence avulsions being much less common. ACL tears are classified as partial- or full-thickness tears, depending on the degree of disruption to the ligament. Tibial spine avulsion fractures and partial ACL tears constitute a greater percentage of ACL injuries in preadolescents when compared to complete tears due to the ability of the immature skeleton to absorb force. As children mature, the risk of a complete ACL tear increases secondary to increased skeletal rigidity.[1] The two basic treatment options available for ACL injuries are conservative nonoperative management and surgical reconstruction. The management of ACL injuries in the pediatric population continues to be controversial, as there is low methodologic quality of published studies on the outcomes of each treatment.[2] Regardless of the modality, treatment is directed at restoring the stability of the knee in order to maintain the integrity and long-term durability of the remaining knee structures. The degree of skeletal maturity is an important factor in deciding which treatment modality is most appropriate. The skeletally immature patient is one in whom the growth plates are open and significant axial growth is expected. Historically, a tibial spine avulsion fracture and a midsubstance injury to the ACL in a patient with significant growth remaining were treated with a nonoperative regimen aimed at restoring stability through bracing, active rehabilitation, and modification of activity. As time has progressed, there has been a shift toward reconstructive surgery of the ACL in the pediatric population, particularly in adolescents who have reached skeletal maturity.[3] This chapter discusses the nonoperative approach to treating an injury to the ACL in the preadolescent and adolescent patient and the indications for doing so.

The management of an ACL injury in patients with open growth plates presents a challenge as physicians and patients must weigh the risks of nonoperative treatment with the risks of early surgical treatment. In addition, there is the option of delaying surgical reconstruction in a skeletally immature child until the physes have fused. The management remains controversial as nonoperative and operative treatment both have the potential for serious risks. Nonoperative treatment can result in increased meniscal and articular cartilage damage from chronic instability, leading to a greater risk of early degenerative disease. Early surgical intervention on an immature skeleton carries the risk of growth arrest and angular deformities from disruption of the tibial and femoral growth plates. The chief concern in this growing population is the potential for iatrogenic injury to the physes, as the distal femoral physes and proximal tibial physes contribute 70% and 55% to the growth of their respective bones.[4] Damage to the physis can result in limb length inequality and angular joint deformity. Due to the potential for long-term complications resulting from either of the available treatment options, it is essential to determine which patients are potential candidates for nonoperative management and which patients are better suited for surgical reconstruction.

The nonoperative treatment algorithm involves a structured and supervised rehabilitation program, usually broken into three distinct phases. The patient must progress through the phases based on specific functional milestones before returning to their preferred activities. Discussion of the first phase includes modes of decreasing swelling, the use of a custom-fit knee brace, the use of crutches, and the duration of activity modification and limitation. The second phase details the specifics of the rehabilitation program, including strength, balance, and plyometric exercises. The final phase is a secondary prevention program composed of neuromuscular and functional muscle strengthening exercises that should be continued indefinitely to maintain strength and stability of the knee joint.[5] All three phases are integral components of the nonoperative treatment approach. Historically, some individuals who have been managed nonoperatively have required subsequent reconstructive surgery after reaching skeletal maturity. The indications for adolescent ACL reconstruction in a patient who has maximized nonoperative care are also discussed in this chapter.

INDICATIONS FOR NONOPERATIVE TREATMENT

The treatment approach for a skeletally immature or mature pediatric patient with an ACL injury is different for each patient, depending on their unique traits and the specifics of their injury. Regardless of how the ACL is torn, an experienced physician will work with each patient to determine a personalized course of treatment. It is important to recognize which young patients are potential candidates for nonoperative treatment. The initial assessment, obtained through the history, physical examination, and a magnetic resonance imaging (MRI), should include sexual maturity, skeletal age, associated injuries, location and extent of the ACL injury, and the predicted level of compliance of the child.

Although chronologic age can provide a rough estimate of the patient's maturity, it is important to determine their physiologic and skeletal age, which can vary significantly from the chronologic age of the child. The maturity assessment allows patients to be classified as either prepubescent or pubescent. Tanner staging of sexual maturity is the most commonly used method of assessing physiologic maturity[6] (Table 5.1). Tanner staging takes into account the secondary sex characteristics in both males and females and the menarche history in females. Skeletal age, another measure of determining maturity, can be evaluated by a variety of different methods. The Hospital for Special Surgery (HSS) shorthand bone age assessment tool facilitates evaluation of the bone age without the use of an atlas (Table 5.2). This tool has been validated and shown to be equally as accurate as the Greulich and Pyle method used at other institutions.[7] The prepubescent child has physiologic characteristics defined by Tanner stages 1 and 2 and a skeletal age of less than 12 years in boys and less than 11 years in girls. The pubescent child has physiologic characteristics defined by Tanner stages 3 and 4 and a bone age of 13 to 16 years in boys and 12 to 14 years in girls. The management of a tibial spine avulsion fracture is not dependent on the sexual and skeletal maturity of the patient. Conversely, physiologic and skeletal maturity, in combination with the features discussed in the following text, play a large role in which patients are candidates for nonoperative management of a torn ACL.

The extent of the ACL injury is an important determinant of which children can be considered for nonoperative management. In a tibial spine avulsion injury, the fracture of the intercondylar eminence is classified by severity of the displacement and angulation, which guides management. A nondisplaced or minimally displaced tibial spine avulsion injury can be treated nonoperatively with positive results, whereas more severely displaced and angulated avulsion injuries require arthroscopic reduction and internal fixation regardless of the child's age or skeletal maturity.[8] Similarly, the location of the ACL tear and the amount of ligament torn play a large role in differentiating which patients are candidates for nonoperative therapy. Patients with partial tears of the ACL, particularly those compromising less than 50% of the diameter of the ligament, have been shown to be promising candidates for nonsurgical management. Kocher et al.[9] performed a prospective cohort study on 45 skeletally mature and immature patients 17 years of age or younger to assess the functional outcome after partial ACL tears in children and adolescents treated nonoperatively. Of the 45 patients treated with a nonoperative structured rehabilitation program and followed for at least 2 years, only 14 of the patients (31%) underwent subsequent reconstruction due to symptoms of instability or episodes of reinjury. The study found that the need for reconstruction after initial nonoperative treatment was significantly associated with tears greater than 50% of the thickness of the ligament, tears that were predominantly posterolateral in location, and patients older in chronologic and skeletal age. Therefore, the research advocates for consideration of nonoperative management for ACL tears in children and adolescents 14 years of skeletal age or less with less than 50% tear of the ligament.[9] While assessing the degree of the ACL tear through the physical examination and MRI studies, it is important to evaluate the knee joint as a whole to determine if there has been damage to any other structures. Many studies have evaluated skeletally immature patients with ACL tears and concomitant tears to the meniscus and have found poor outcomes with nonoperative treatment.[10] Therefore, the nonoperative approach is best suited for those with isolated injuries to the ACL with no other ligamentous or cartilage involvement.

Compliance with both the rehabilitation program and willingness to modify activity is essential for a patient to be successful with nonoperative treatment. Many children and adolescents with ACL injuries are competitive athletes who desire to pursue sports that involve cutting and pivoting movements for a lifetime. The modification and limitation of certain activities is temporary, with the hope that proper rehabilitation can nurture the patient back into their desired activities without hindrance. However, every patient should know that both nonoperative and operative treatment carry the risk of not returning to high-risk activities, such as cutting and pivoting sports. The benefit of each treatment far outweighs the risk, as the patient would be unable to engage in such activities without one treatment or the other. A prospective cohort study by Moksnes et al.[11] investigated changes in functional performance following a nonoperative treatment algorithm for ACL injuries in skeletally immature children 12 years and younger. A majority (78%) of the 36 children treated nonoperatively remained ACL deficient with adequate knee function.

TABLE 5.1 Tanner Stages of Maturity

Tanner Stage	*Male Specific (Genitals)*	*Female Specific (Breasts)*	*Both Genders (Pubic Hair)*
1	Small	No glandular tissue	None
2	Slight enlargement of scrotum; penis length unchanged	Breast bud forms	Small amount and fine
3	Further enlargement of scrotum and penis	Enlargement of breast and areola	Coarse and curly extending laterally
4	Further enlargement of scrotum and penis	Projection of areola and papilla to form secondary mound	Adultlike hair that crosses pubis
5	Adult size and shape	Adult size and shape	Adult hair extending to medial thigh

TABLE 5.2 The Hospital for Special Surgery Shorthand Bone Age Assessment Tool

Girls Age (y)	*Boys Age (y)*	*Hand Radiograph Finding*
10	12.5	Appearance of hook of hamate
11	13	Appearance of MP sesamoid of thumb
NA	13.5	Proximal radial aspect of radial epiphysis has met maximum width of distal radial metaphysis; no capping
12	14	Capping of distal radial epiphysis
13	15	Closure of thumb distal phalanx physis
13.5	15.5	Closure of index finger distal phalanx physis
14	16	Closure of index finger proximal phalanx physis

MP, metacarpophalangeal; NA, not available; closure, bridging by more than 50% bone across physis.

Ninety-one percent of the ACL-deficient children reported consistent participation in pivoting sports and/or physical education classes in school.[11] These patients did also report changing their primary sport to one that does not pose a risk to the ACL, which can be attributed to apprehension of reinjury.

The nonsurgical approach is most effective in a highly compliant patient with a partial ACL tear and no additional intra-articular injury who is willing and able to decrease their activity level during a given period of time. Despite these generalizations, every young patient should be well informed about the nonoperative treatment option and the pros and cons of this management program if faced with an ACL injury.

INDICATIONS FOR ADOLESCENT ANTERIOR CRUCIATE LIGAMENT RECONSTRUCTION AFTER NONOPERATIVE MANAGEMENT

Adolescent ACL reconstruction may be advised if there is persistent knee instability, multiple giving-way episodes, a secondary injury, or an unacceptable lowering of the patient's activity level after nonoperative management has been maximized. Patients who experience repeated instability episodes during a course of nonoperative treatment have demonstrated an increased risk of accelerated joint disease secondary to the instability.[12]

CONTRAINDICATIONS TO NONOPERATIVE MANAGEMENT

Tears involving more than 50% of the diameter of the ACL have demonstrated unsatisfactory outcomes with conservative management, and some of these tears have progressed to a complete tear when initial reconstruction was not performed.[13] Full-thickness tears of the ACL treated with nonoperative management carry the risk of increased intra-articular damage in the form of meniscal tears and damage to the cartilage. Although animal studies have shown that there is increased healing potential of an injured ACL in the skeletally immature compared with adults,[14] nonoperative management of complete tears generally has a poor prognosis when compared to the surgical reconstruction options available today.

As discussed earlier, many children who have sustained an ACL injury will also have coexistent meniscal damage, which is a relative contraindication to nonoperative management. In addition, a patient who is poorly compliant will not succeed with nonoperative treatment, as it requires complete dedication and discipline. Poor compliance will put the young individual at significant risk of further meniscal injury or articular cartilage damage.

A functionally unstable knee, as evidenced by multiple episodes of giving out, has been shown to have poor results with nonoperative treatment. Children approaching skeletal maturity and with little growth remaining should go straight to reconstruction without delay if they are experiencing instability symptoms.

AUTHORS' PREFERRED NONOPERATIVE TREATMENT

After initial injury to the ACL, rehabilitation is divided into three subsequent phases. The initial phase is directed at resolving knee impairments related to swelling and range-of-motion (ROM) deficits. The second phase aims to restore muscle strength and adequate neuromuscular responses. The goal of the third phase is to equip patients with a series of exercises and stretches that can be continued indefinitely as preventive medicine. Active rehabilitation will not be entirely the same for every child or adolescent with an ACL injury, but there are fundamental principles that will be consistent throughout the treatment.

Phase 1: Control Swelling, Restore Range of Motion, Normalize Gait

Phase 1 aims to control pain and swelling, restore ROM to the knee joint, improve flexibility, normalize gait mechanics, and establish good quadriceps activation. The patient should elevate and apply ice immediately after injury with an elastic wrap to control the initial swelling. Ice can be applied for 20-minute periods multiple times throughout the day. Always maintain one layer between the ice and the skin, such as a cloth or paper towel, to prevent damage to the skin. If the entire leg is swollen, elevating the leg and using elastic stockings can help to decrease the general swelling. Anti-inflammatory medications are also very beneficial immediately after injury, and the physician will prescribe their medication of choice if they see fit. The primary goal immediately after the injury is to decrease the swelling so that the patient can work toward regaining full ROM. During the early period of immobilization, it is crucial to avoid any pivoting or twisting motions of the knee that might lead to instability and giving out. It is important to alert the physician if the child has any episodes of knee buckling. The knee is extremely unstable immediately after injury and the thigh muscles can become very weak. It may be difficult to support the weight of the body when walking during the first few days, which is why most children and adolescents require crutches to avoid full weight bearing. The knee can also be protected with the use of a knee brace to aid in immobilization. Although the knee brace is a useful aid, it is not sufficient when used without intentional restriction of activities. A study by Graf et al.[10] showed that bracing alone does not prevent meniscal tears in the absence of activity modification, making it imperative that the patient does not try to return to weight bearing or activity too soon. The experienced physician will monitor progression and determine when the patient can wean from two crutches to one crutch, and then from one crutch to walking without aid. The single crutch is always held on the opposite side of the injured knee. Patients may progress to walking without aid when they are able to walk without a limp and with no pain. If the patient cannot demonstrate pain-free normal walking mechanics, they cannot walk without crutches. Every pediatric or adolescent with an injury to the ACL will progress at their own rate, as swelling can remain anywhere from days to weeks, so there is no exact time frame that one can expect to follow during this phase. Once the swelling has diminished and the pain subsides, a stretching and strengthening program is of utmost importance in regaining the full motion and strength of the knee joint. Rehabilitation with an experienced physical therapist is important in ensuring that the pediatric or adolescent patient is performing the exercises and stretches properly and with enough frequency.

During phase 1, there are ROM and strength exercises that can be gradually introduced as the swelling decreases to initiate the return to full strength. The swelling and ROM deficits must be resolved before progressing to phase 2. An adolescent patient can use an exercise bike machine daily at a very low effort level for 10 minutes to increase blood flow and aid in ROM recovery. The focus of this acute phase is on maintaining muscle tone in the quadriceps muscle, which will help straighten the knee, as quadriceps muscle weakness has been associated with ACL injury. Many studies have demonstrated that if an adequately designed rehabilitation program is not performed soon after the injury, strength in the quadriceps muscle group is difficult to recover.[15] In another study, Zebis et al.[16] emphasized the importance of the hamstring muscles in stabilizing the knee in order to restore full knee flexion after an injury to the ACL. The Nordic hamstring exercise described in phase 2 will increase eccentric hamstring muscle strength, which is important as the hamstrings help the ACL during stopping and jumping.

Strength Exercises during Phase 1: Perform These Exercises Once Daily during the Acute Phase

Quad Sets: Quad sets will help build and maintain strength in the muscles on top of the thigh. Sit on the floor with the injured leg straight out in front of the body. Tighten the muscles on top of the thigh by pressing the back of the knee flat down to the floor. Hold for about 6 seconds, then rest for up to 10 seconds. Perform 1 set of 8 to 12 repetitions, increasing to 2 sets as the phase progresses. If there is any discomfort under the knee, place a small towel beneath the knee during the exercise (Fig. 5.1).

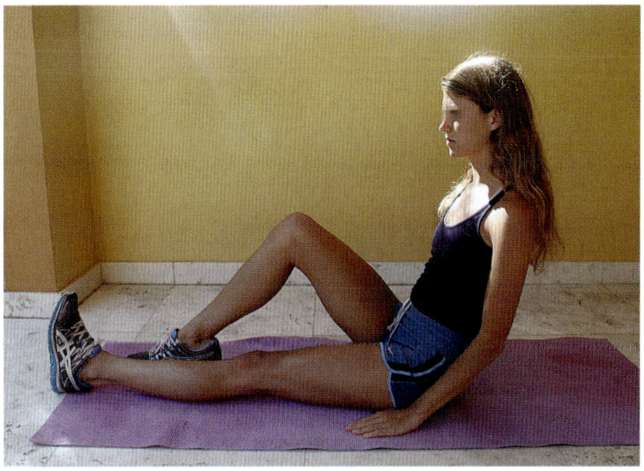

Figure 5.1. Quad sets.

Straight-Leg Raise to the Front: These straight-leg raises will strengthen both the muscles on top of the thigh and the muscles around the hip. Lie on the back with the good knee bent so that the foot rests flat on the floor. The injured leg should be straight to start. Tighten the thigh muscles in the injured leg by pressing the back of the knee flat down to the floor. Hold the knee straight, and lift the injured leg up so that the heel is about 1 foot off the floor. Hold for 5 seconds then lower slowly. Do 8 to 12 repetitions (Fig. 5.2).

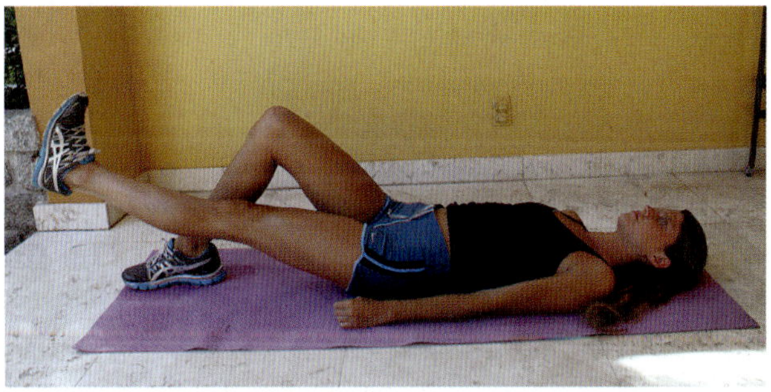

Figure 5.2. Straight-leg raise to the front.

Heel Raise: Using a table for stabilization, gently raise the heel off the floor and balance on the balls of the feet, holding for 6 seconds before easing slowly back down. Perform 2 sets of 10 repetitions daily.

Hip Abduction/Adduction: Lie on the back with the legs straight out on the floor, keeping the toes pointed toward the ceiling throughout the exercise. Move one leg outward as far as possible. Slowly return to the starting position with a straight leg. Perform 2 sets of 10 repetitions.

Clam Shells: Lying on one side of the body with your knees bent at 90 degrees, slowly raise the knee of the upper leg while keeping the feet sealed together. Slowly return to the closed position. Perform 2 sets of 15 repetitions on each leg (Fig. 5.3).

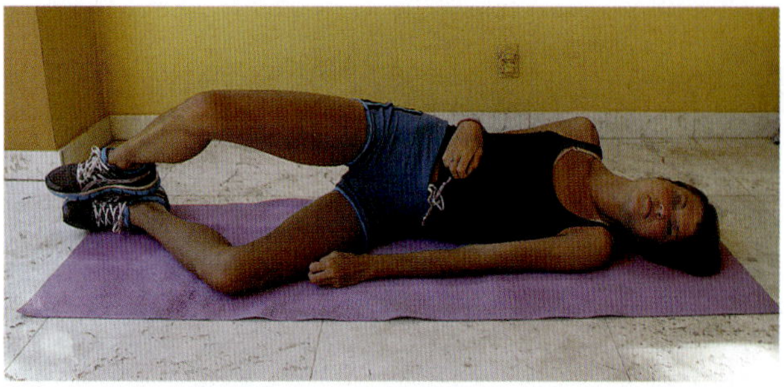

Figure 5.3. Clam shells.

Range-of-Motion Exercises in Phase 1: Perform These Exercises Three to Five Times a Day

Patella Mobilization: Repeat each position 10 times (Fig. 5.4).

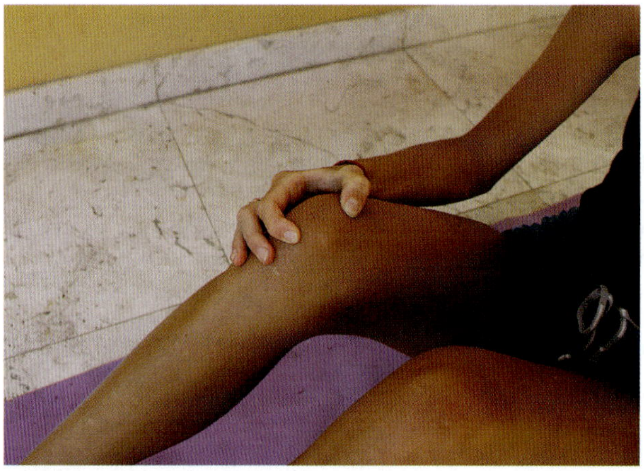

Figure 5.4. Patella mobilization.

Inferior Glide: With thumbs on the upper border of the kneecap, gently push the kneecap toward the foot, holding for 5 seconds.

Superior Glide: With thumbs on lower border of the kneecap, gently pull the kneecap toward the body, holding for 5 seconds.

Medial/Lateral Glide: Using a pincer grip, grab the inside and outside edges of the kneecap and gently push the kneecap in toward your other leg, holding for 5 seconds before gently pushing the kneecap out, holding for another 5 seconds.

Towel Stretch (Calf/Hamstring): While lying on the back, which allows the muscles to relax, place your foot in the center of a towel while holding the ends. Pull the involved leg straight up in the air until a stretch is felt along the back of the thigh. Hold the stretch for 30 seconds, and repeat three times (Fig. 5.5).

Heel Slides: While seated on a chair, use a towel and place the foot on the ACL-injured side in the middle of the towel, holding one end of the towel in each hand. Slowly pull the towel while bending the knee to feel a stretch, holding for 10 seconds before releasing. Repeat 10 times.

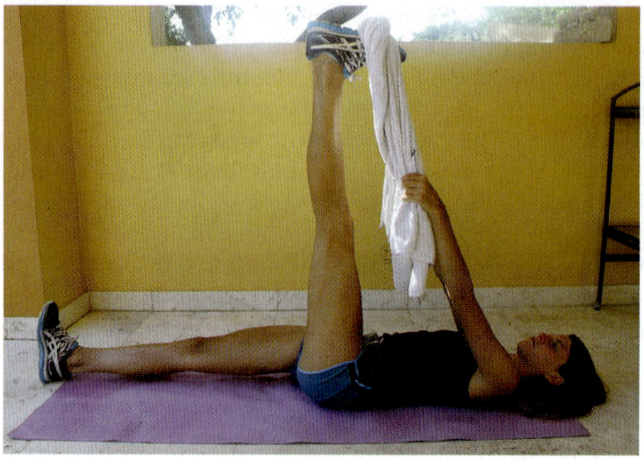

Figure 5.5. Towel stretch of calf and hamstring.

Prone Hamstring Stretch: Lie on the stomach on a flat surface that is raised from the ground, with one foot hanging off. Place a pillow under the knee for comfort. Keep the leg straight, avoiding the temptation to roll the hip in or out, and be sure to relax the muscles of the leg and keep the hips down. Stay in this prone hang for a couple of minutes. Once ROM improves, use an ankle weight to increase knee extension and stretch the quadriceps muscles.

Stationary Bike with Minimal Resistance: Cycle for 10 minutes daily if there is no pain. If it is too painful to make a full circle, raise the bike seat. As time progresses and ROM improves, the bike seat can be lowered and the length of time on the bike can be gradually increased.

Phase 2: Strength, Balance, and Plyometrics

Phase 2 of the nonoperative treatment of an ACL injury aims to restore muscle strength, maintain ROM and flexibility, and improve neuromuscular control, all the while avoiding patella femoral pain. Phase 2 depends on a structured rehabilitation program containing a variety of exercises that focus on strength, balance, and plyometrics while simultaneously continuing the ROM exercises that were initiated in phase 1. The combination of these three elements is essential for achieving success with the nonoperative approach and forms the foundation for phase 3 of treatment, the ACL injury prevention program. Training for young individuals must be enjoyable, safe, and effective in order to keep them motivated and moving forward. Although many adults can understand the importance of strength training because they are able to see the physical benefits as their muscles become stronger and more defined, gains in muscle strength in children are believed to be facilitated primarily through neural adaptive mechanisms, as opposed to the hypertrophy that is more commonly seen in adults.[17] Therefore, the rehabilitation should be directed toward neuromuscular knee-stabilizing exercises and plyometric exercises in order to facilitate increased motor unit activation and changes in motor unit coordination, recruitment, and firing.

Proprioception is defined as the sense of the relative position of neighboring parts of the body and strength of effort being employed in movement. Proprioceptive training increases the patient's awareness of the relative position of his or her body parts, which translates to a greater sense of balance. Most patients engage in exercises and activities that develop their proprioception and thus improve their ability to balance without realizing that they are doing so. For example, when performing an athletic motion for the first time, an athlete must consciously focus on the task at hand. After a certain number of repetitions, the body develops a neuromuscular pattern that enables the athlete to perform the motion effortlessly. Improving proprioception in a prepubescent child during the rehabilitation of an ACL injury can develop neuromuscular pathways that will support the injured ACL currently and protect both knees for a lifetime. Therefore, there are a variety of exercises detailed here to increase core stability and proprioception through balance training, resulting in a greater sense of coordination. It is essential to pay close attention to the position of the knees during these exercises, as any exercise performed in the wrong position can be detrimental to the knees. In order to keep the knee flexed at the correct angle, the patient should aim to keep the knee over the toe. In addition, individuals recovering from an ACL injury with decreased strength surrounding the knee joint may be inclined to let their knees cave inward. It is essential to avoid this dangerous valgus position, more commonly known as a *knock-kneed position.* With this in mind, the exercises detailed here can be incorporated into the nonoperative rehabilitation program of a young patient with an ACL injury. While focusing on strength, balance, and plyometrics, a rehabilitation program must provide enough variation and progression among the three elements to keep young patients engaged and interested in the recovery process. The patient should begin with the simplest form of the exercise, progressing as the physician and physical therapist see fit.

Range-of-Motion Exercises during Phase 2

Continue ROM exercises from phase 1.

Strength Exercises during Phase 2

The Plank: Place the elbows directly underneath the shoulders with hands on the ground and toes gripping the ground and lift the entire body up, supporting the weight on the forearms and toes. Pull in the navel so that there is neither an arch nor a caving in of the back. Hold this position for 30 seconds and progress by adding 5 seconds each time the exercise is performed (Fig. 5.6).

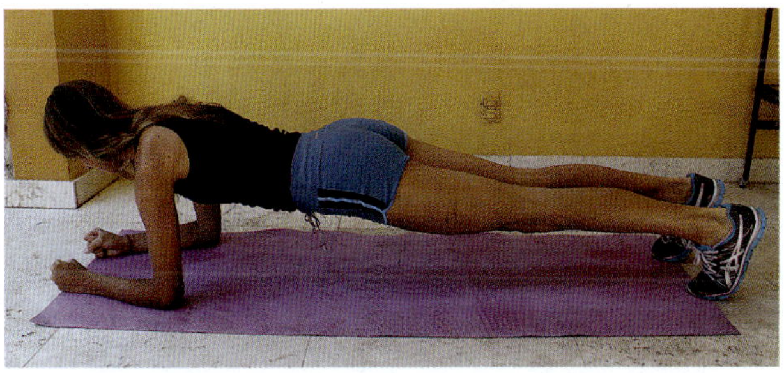

Figure 5.6. The plank.

Side Plank: Lying on one side of the body, lift the entire body with one side facing the ground as one foot and one forearm hold the body above ground. The outstretched arm should be positioned at 90 degrees to the upper arm with the elbow directly below the shoulder. Hold this position for 30 seconds and progress by adding 5 seconds each time the exercise is performed (Fig. 5.7).

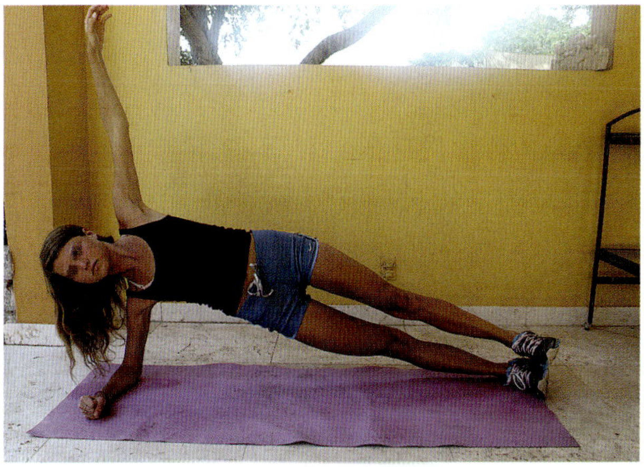

Figure 5.7. Side plank.

Nordic Hamstrings: Kneeling on a flat surface, have a partner hold both ankles firmly. Keeping the body perfectly straight from the shoulders to the knees, use the muscles in the buttocks and the back of the thighs to support the body as the torso leans forward in a smooth, controlled manner. After leaning forward as far as possible, hold the position for as long as possible, after which the hands can aid in lowering the body down, gradually accepting all body weight on the hands and ending in a push-up position (Fig. 5.8).

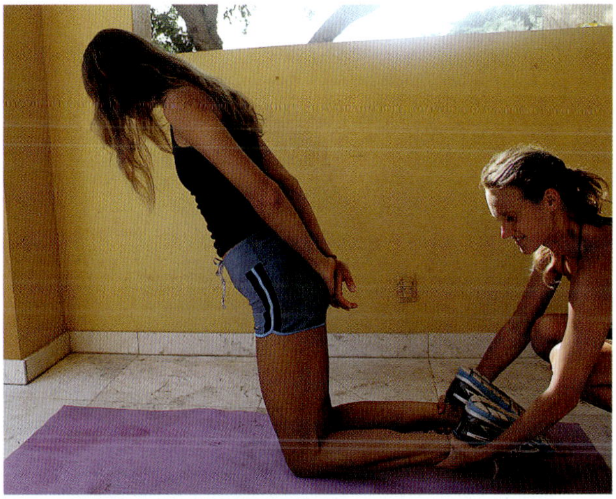

Figure 5.8. Nordic hamstrings.

Balance during Phase 2

Single-Leg Balance: Progress from level 1 to level 3 throughout phase 2.

Level 1: Hold the ball.

Stand on one leg while holding a ball outstretched in front. Rest the weight of the body in the middle of the foot, flexing the knee slightly between 15 and 20 degrees, but do not let the knee cave inward. Hold the position for 30 seconds before switching to the opposite leg (Fig. 5.9).

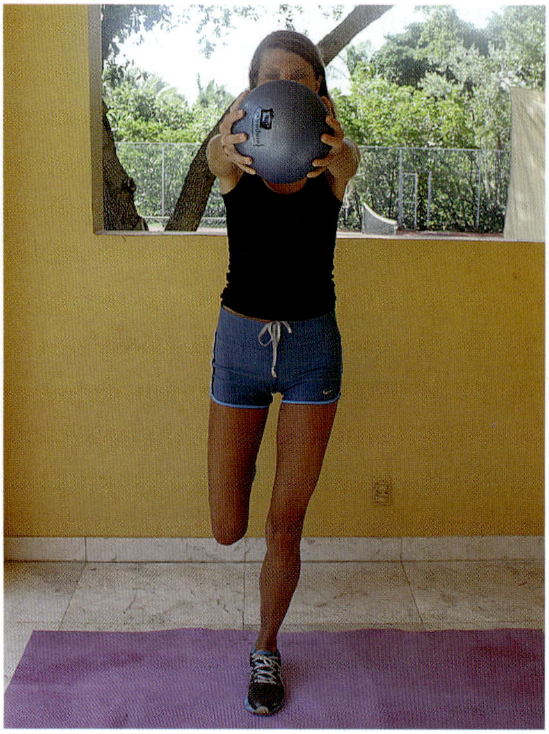

Figure 5.9. Hold the ball with knee bent.

Level 2: Throwing the ball with a partner

Stand 2 to 3 yd from a partner, each balancing on one leg with the supporting leg slightly flexed as in level 1. Throw a ball back and forth to one another while remaining balanced and avoiding the knock-kneed position (Fig. 5.10).

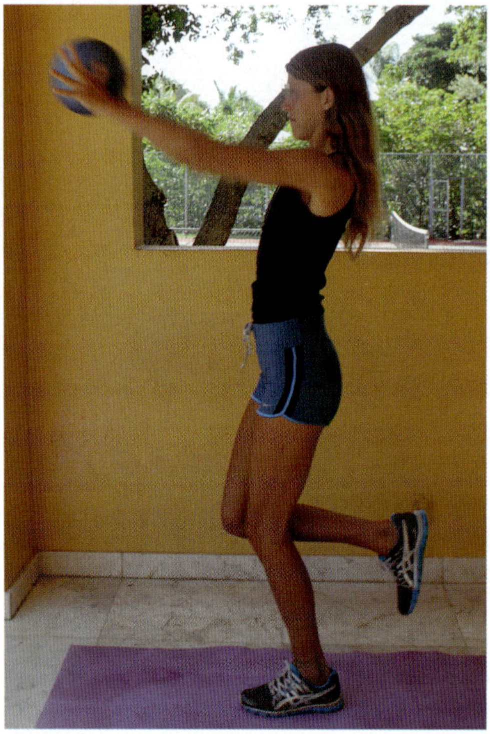

Figure 5.10. Throwing the ball with a partner.

Level 3: Throwing the ball with partner on a wobble board

This exercise is similar to level 2, but this time, each partner stands on one leg on a wobble board as the ball is passed back and forth.

Plyometrics during Phase 2

Squats: Progress from level 1 to level 5 throughout phase 2.

Level 1: Squats with toe raise

Stand with the feet hip-width apart, and slowly bend both the hips and knees to 90 degrees. Quickly straighten the body completely, continuing upward to stand on the toes. Repeat for 30 seconds. Be careful not to let the knees cave inward. Increase by 5 seconds each time the exercise is performed (Fig. 5.11).

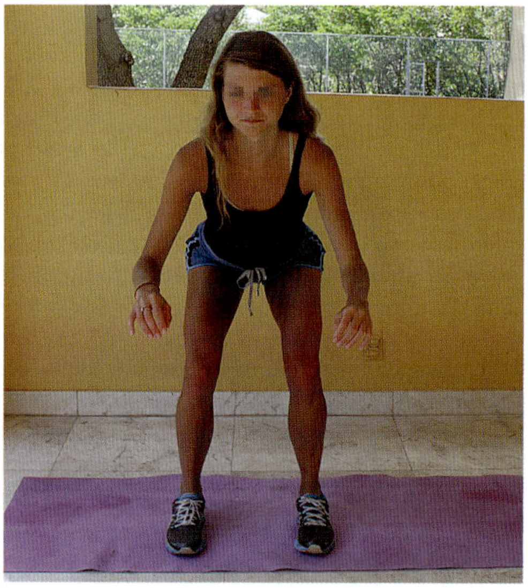

Figure 5.11. Squats with toe raise.

Level 2: Walking lunges

With the feet separated a hip-width apart, lunge forward until the hips and knees are bent to 90 degrees. Continue to lunge across the room at a brisk pace for 30 seconds, increasing by 5 seconds each time the exercise is performed (Fig. 5.12).

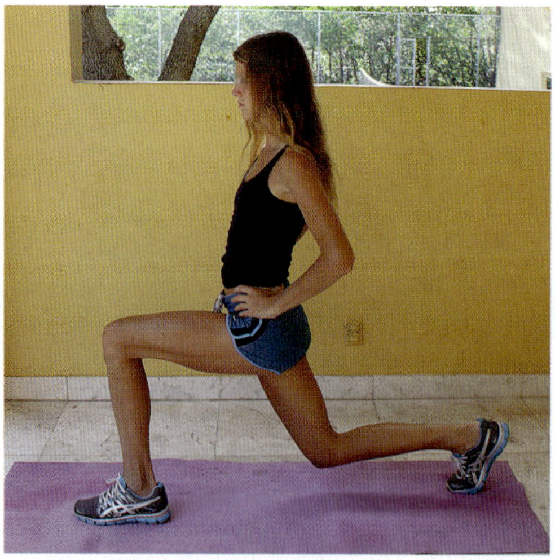

Figure 5.12. Walking lunges.

Level 3: One-leg squats

Standing on one leg, slowly bend the supporting knee as far as you can without losing balance. In a faster motion, straighten the knee and raise the body back to the start, keeping the knee over the toes at all times. Repeat 10 times before switching legs.

Level 4: Squats with toe raise on a wobble board

Squat while standing on both legs on top of the wobble board. Quickly raise and lower the body for 20 seconds, progressing by 5 seconds each time the exercise is performed until you are able to do squats for 1 minute.

Level 5: One-leg squats on a wobble board

Balance on one leg on the wobble board, performing squats for 20 seconds, progressing by 5 seconds each time the exercise is performed until you are able to do squats for 1 minute.

Phase 3: Anterior Cruciate Ligament Injury Prevention Program

Phase 3 is very similar to the advanced stages of phase 2. The combination of strength, balance, and plyometric exercises discussed in phase 2 should be continued indefinitely in order to prevent a repeat injury to the affected ACL or a new injury to the patient's other ACL. In addition, jumping and running exercises will be incorporated during this phase. It is important to remember that a young individual is more likely to comply with a prevention program when it is efficient, enjoyable, and productive. The running exercises incorporated at this stage of recovery will also influence the neuromuscular pathways of young athletes. Running and jumping exercises will improve athletic performance, build strength, and give young individuals a base of skills to move and land that will preserve their ACL for the long term.[18]

Ultimately, return to activity, especially those including cutting and pivoting, depends on how the child has progressed in therapy and whether or not they continue to have episodes of instability, such as buckling and giving out.

RECOGNIZING IF THE NONOPERATIVE APPROACH HAS FAILED

Although many young patients have success with the three phases of nonoperative rehabilitation, it is important to recognize when a patient who has maximized nonoperative care is not reaching a desirable end point. Giving-way episodes at the knee during functional activity are examples of instability. Giving-way is defined as buckling, or subluxation, of the tibiofemoral joint. These episodes can result in pain and an effusion of the joint. Any patient experiencing repeated episodes of instability after maximizing this nonoperative approach should be evaluated, as they will likely require physeal-sparing ACL reconstructive surgery.[19] Reconstructive surgery should be considered in these patients because recurrent episodes of giving-way have been associated with an increased incidence of irreparable meniscus tears and articular cartilage damage.[20–23]

CONCLUSION

The management of an ACL injury in adolescents presents a challenge as physicians and patients must weigh the risks of nonoperative treatment with the risks of early surgical treatment, which poses a risk to open growth plates. The skeletal maturity of the patient, the degree and location of injury to the ACL, and the compliance of the patient will all play a role in which patients can be managed nonoperatively. A patient who is dedicated to the stretching, strengthening, and plyometric exercises detailed in this chapter have the highest rates of return to baseline activity without episodes of instability. Adolescent patients who have experienced an injury to the ACL are encouraged to continue the ACL injury prevention program indefinitely to protect their knees from further damage.

REFERENCES

1. Alharby SW. Anterior cruciate ligament injuries in growing skeleton. *Int J Health Sci (Qassim).* 2010;4(1):71–79.
2. Moksnes H, Engebretsen L, Risberg MA. The current evidence for treatment of ACL injuries in children is low: a systematic review. *J Bone Joint Surg Am.* 2012;94:1112–1119.
3. Micheli LJ, Metzl JD, Di Canzio J, et al. Anterior cruciate ligament reconstructive surgery in adolescent soccer and basketball players. *Clin J Sports Med.* 1999;9:138–141.
4. Ogden J. Radiologic aspects. In: Ogden J, ed. *Skeletal Injury in the Child.* 2nd ed. Philadelphia, PA: Saunders;1990:65–96.
5. Moksnes H, Engebretsen L, Eitzen I, et al. Functional outcomes following a non-operative treatment algorithm for anterior cruciate ligament injuries in skeletally immature children 12 years and younger. A prospective cohort with 2 years follow-up. *Br J Sports Med.* 2013;47(8):488–494.
6. Tanner JM. The development of the reproductive system. In: Tanner JM, ed. *Growth at Adolescence.* 2nd ed. Oxford, United Kingdom: Blackwell Scientific;1962:28–39.
7. Heyworth BE, Osei DA, Fabricant PD, et al. The shorthand bone age assessment: a simpler alternative to current methods. *J Pediatr Orthop.* 2013;33(5):569–574.
8. Wheeless CR. Intercondylar eminence fracture. Wheeless' Textbook of Orthopaedics Web site. http://www.wheelessonline.com/ortho/intercondylar_eminence_fracture. Updated July 3, 2012. Accessed March 25, 2014.
9. Kocher MS, Micheli LJ, Zurakowski D, et al. Partial tears of the anterior cruciate ligament in children and adolescents. *Am J Sports Med.* 2002;30(5):697–703.
10. Graf BK, Lange RH, Fujisaki CK, et al. Anterior cruciate ligament tear in skeletally immature patients: meniscal pathology at presentation and after attempted conservative treatment. *Arthroscopy.* 1992;8:229–233.
11. Moksnes H, Engebretsen L, Eitzen I, et al. Functional outcomes following a non-operative treatment algorithm for anterior cruciate ligament injuries in skeletally immature children 12 years and younger. A prospective cohort with 2 years follow-up. *Br J Sports Med.* 2013;47:488–494.
12. Mizuta H, Kubota K, Shiraishi M, et al. The conservative treatment of complete tears of the anterior cruciate ligament in skeletally immature patients. *J Bone Joint Surg Br.* 1995;77:890–894.
13. Kocher MS, Micheli LJ, Zurakowski D, et al. Partial tears of the anterior cruciate ligament in children and adolescents. *Am J Sports Med.* 2002;30(5):697–703.
14. Murray MM, Magarian EM, Harrison SL, et al. The effect of skeletal maturity on functional healing of the anterior cruciate ligament. *J Bone Joint Surg Am.* 2010;92:2039–2049.
15. Eitzen I, Moksnes H, Snyder-Mackler L, et al. A progressive 5-week exercise therapy program leads to significant improvement in knee

function early after anterior cruciate ligament injury. *J Orthop Sports Phys Ther.* 2010;40:705–721.

16. Zebis MK, Bencke J, Andersen LL, et al. Acute fatigue impairs neuromuscular activity of anterior cruciate ligament-agonist muscles in female team handball players. *Scand J Med Sci Sports.* 2011; 21:833–840.
17. Faigenbaum AD, Kraemer WJ, Blimkie CJ, et al. Youth resistance training: updated position statement paper from the national strength and conditioning association. *J Strength Cond Res.* 2009;23:S60–S79.
18. Marx RG, Myklebust G, Boyle BW. *The ACL Solution: Prevention and Recovery for Sports' Most Devastating Knee Injury.* New York, NY: Demos Medical Publishing; 2012.
19. McCarthy MM, Graziano J, Green DW, et al. All-epiphyseal, all-inside anterior cruciate ligament reconstruction technique for skeletally immature patients. *Arthrosc Tech.* 2012;1(2):e231–e239.
20. Fabricant PD, Jones KJ, Delos D, et al. Reconstruction of the anterior cruciate ligament in the skeletally immature athlete: a review of current concepts: AAOS exhibit selection. *J Bone Joint Surg Am.* 2013;95(5):e28.
21. Fitzgerald GK, Axe MJ, Snyder-Mackler L. A decision-making scheme for returning patients to high-level activity with nonoperative treatment after anterior cruciate ligament rupture. *Knee Surg Sports Traumatol Arthrosc.* 2000;8:76–82.
22. Lawrence JT, Agrawal N, Ganley TJ. Degeneration of the knee joint in skeletally immature patients with a diagnosis of an anterior cruciate ligament tear: is there harm in delay of treatment? *Am J Sports Med.* 2011;39(12):2582–2587.
23. Millett PJ, Willis AA, Warren RF. Associated injuries in pediatric and adolescent anterior cruciate ligament tears: does a delay in treatment increase the risk of meniscal tear? *Arthroscopy.* 2002; 18:955–959.

Brant Sachleben
Mininder S. Kocher

CHAPTER

6

Technique: Modified McIntosh

INTRODUCTION

Injuries to the anterior cruciate ligament (ACL) were once thought to be rare occurrences among skeletally immature patients. Tibial eminence fractures were considered the pediatric equivalent to ACL injuries and thought to occur much more frequently.[1–4] However, a 10% to 65% incidence of ACL tears in the setting of acute hemarthrosis has been reported in pediatric patients in recent years.[5–11] The increase in ACL ruptures in the growing athlete has led to a reevaluation of treatment options for the immature patient. Historically, treatment of ACL injuries has been largely nonsurgical consisting of physical therapy, activity modification, and bracing until skeletal maturity due to the fear of physeal injury. At maturity, these patients would receive a standard ACL reconstruction; however, high rates of instability and subsequent meniscal and articular cartilage injuries have been the hallmark of this approach.[12–25] Aichroth et al.[21] conducted a prospective natural history study of 33 patients for 10 years: 10 of these patients could not tolerate nonsurgical treatment and opted for surgical intervention and 23 patients remained in the study. At the time of injury, the mean age was 12.5 years (range, 11 to 15 years), and the mean follow-up was 72 months (range, 36 to 144 months). The mean Lysholm score decreased from 78.6 (range, 54 to 93) at the time of injury to 52.4 (range, 30 to 83) at final follow-up; the mean Tegner score decreased from 6.7 (range, 4 to 9) at the time of injury to 4.2 (range, 2 to 6) at final follow-up. At the time of injury, 14 meniscal tears (8 medial, 6 lateral) and 3 osteochondral fractures were reported, all of which underwent surgical intervention. At final follow-up, an additional 7 meniscal tears were reported and 10 patients had degenerative radiographic changes.

In a more recent study, Lawrence et al.[25] reviewed the results of delayed versus acute treatment in 70 patients (mean age, 12.9 years; range, 10 to 14 years). Of these, 29 (41%) underwent at least 12 weeks of nonsurgical treatment and 41 underwent acute ACL reconstruction. Logistic regression analysis exhibited that time from injury to surgery greater than 12 weeks was independently associated with an increased rate of meniscal tears and chondral injuries at the time of surgery. Survivorship analysis showed that patients without meniscal tears or high-grade chondral defects (Outerbridge grades II to IV) underwent surgery at a median of 9 weeks. This implies causality of the presence of these lesions to the timing of surgery. The authors also noted that rates of irreparable meniscal tears were over three times more frequent (24% vs. 7%) among patients who were treated nonoperatively for more than 12 weeks versus those patients who underwent acute surgery. The authors also reported that 45% of patients who underwent surgery more than 12 weeks from the time of injury had Outerbridge grade II, III, or IV chondral lesions of the lateral femoral condyle versus 10% of patients in the early treatment group. Among the patients who underwent delayed surgery, 7% sustained grade IV lesions versus none in the acute surgery group. Within the last decade, other studies have reported similar findings.[22–24]

TREATMENT (BRIEF LITERATURE REVIEW)

Indications/Contraindications

Although nonoperative management of ACL injuries has led to poorer outcomes, ACL reconstruction is not emergency surgery and nonsurgical treatment remains an option for patients irrespective of skeletal maturity. It involves rehabilitation aimed at maximizing quadriceps and hamstring strength, bracing, and avoiding cutting and pivoting sports. Adherence to this protocol can be exceedingly difficult for pediatric and adolescent patients.[18,21,26–29] This decision should be made on an individual basis and should involve the family, patient, and physician. For partial ACL ruptures in patients younger than the age of 14 years involving less than 50% of the ligament, we continue to recommend nonoperative management.

Surgical treatment can restore knee stability, theoretically minimizing the risk of future meniscal and chondral injury and providing greater potential for return to cutting and pivoting sports.[29–31] Several methods of ACL reconstruction are considered physeal respecting, including all-epiphyseal tunnels, transtibial over-the-top with soft tissue graft, and combined intra-articular/extra-articular reconstruction using the iliotibial band.[17,32–64] This chapter principally concerns the combined intra-articular/extra-articular reconstruction using the iliotibial band. Indications for intra-articular/extra-articular reconstruction using the iliotibial band in Tanner 1 or 2 patients include complete ACL tear with functional instability, partial ACL tear that has failed nonoperative treatment, and ACL injury with associated repairable meniscal or chondral injury (Diagram 1). Surgery is typically delayed 3 weeks from the time of injury or until adequate range of motion has been achieved.

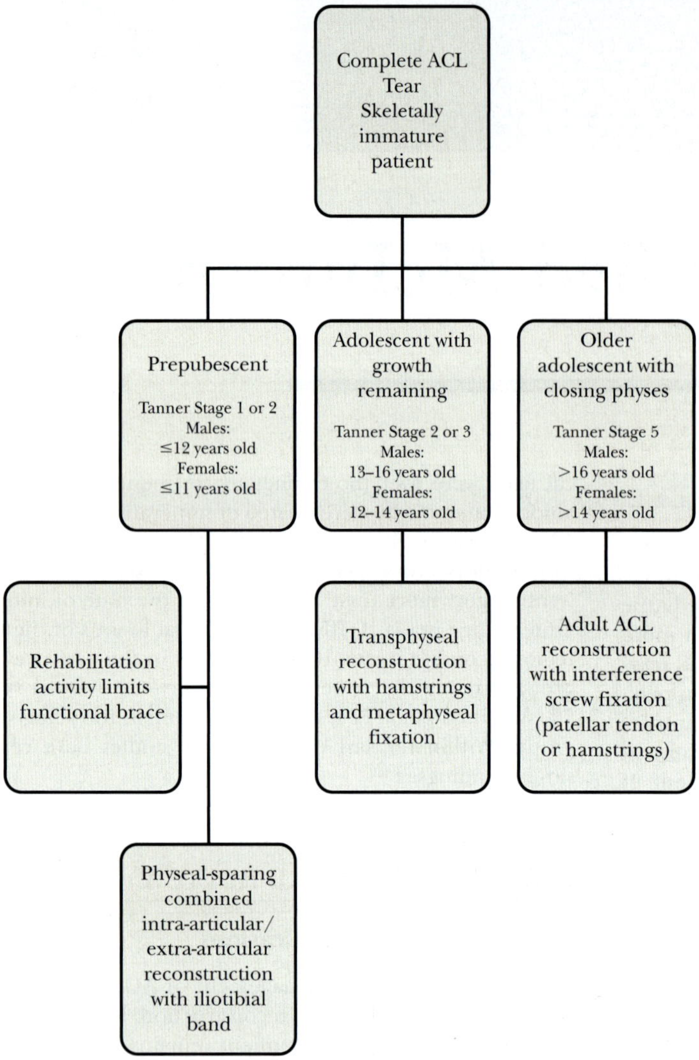

Diagram 6.1. Algorithm for surgical decision making.

Contraindications include active knee infection, no functional instability with activity, lack of acceptable knee range of motion, or an inability to comply with the postoperative protocol for rehabilitation.

AUTHORS' PREFERRED TREATMENT

Our approach to ACL reconstruction in the skeletally immature patient is based on physiologic and skeletal age using the Tanner staging system and the Greulich and Pyle wrist atlas for each respective age. In prepubescent patients (Tanner 1 or 2), the author of this chapter prefer the combined intra-articular/extra-articular reconstruction with autogenous iliotibial band graft due to personal experience, technical ease, and recent biomechanical evidence exhibiting more closely restored anterior posterior and rotatory stability using this technique compared with other physeal-respecting reconstruction options (Fig. 6.1A–D). Kocher et al.[37] reported on 44 prepubescent patients (mean age, 10.3 years; range, 3.6 to 14.0 years) who underwent a combined extra-articular/intra-articular reconstruction using autogenous iliotibial band. The mean skeletal age was 10.1 years (range, 3.5 to 14.0 years). Of the 44 patients,

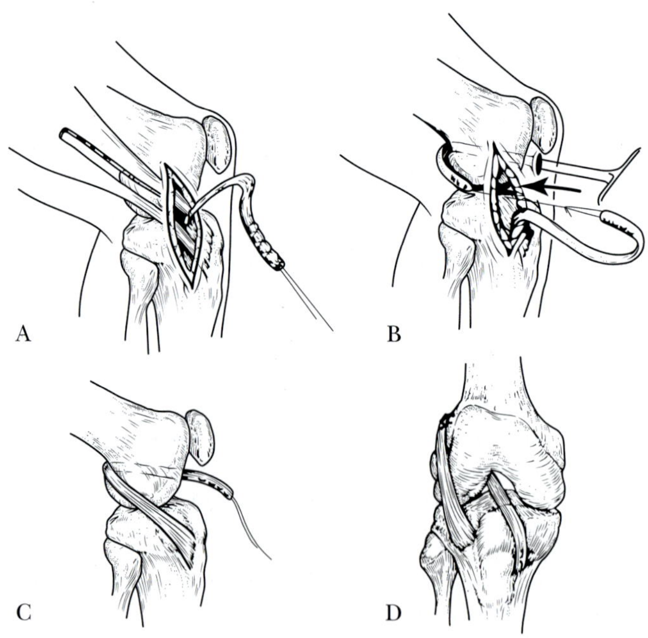

Figure 6.1. **A–D.** Visual outline of steps.

31 were Tanner stage 1 and 13 were Tanner stage 2. There were two traumatic reruptures (4.5%): one at 4.7 years and one at 8.3 years postoperatively, no growth disturbances, and mean (± SD) International Knee Documentation Committee (IKDC)[65] score of 96.7 ± 6 and mean (± SD) Lysholm[66] score of 95.7 ± 6.7 in the remaining patients. The mean follow-up was 5.3 years (range, 2.0 to 15.1 years), and the mean total height gained after surgery was 21.5 cm (range, 9.5 to 118.5 cm).

Although it is true that this reconstruction is not anatomic, a recent study by Kennedy et al.[67] examined the kinematics of the combined intra-articular/extra-articular reconstruction with autogenous iliotibial band versus an all-epiphyseal reconstruction and a transtibial over-the-top reconstruction in a cadaver model. Their findings concluded that the iliotibial band reconstruction technique most closely restore native ACL kinematics. There was, however, a tendency for the technique to overconstrain the knee to varus rotational forces at certain angles of knee flexion. As is noted in the following texts, we have modified a portion of the technique from the original publication to prevent this occurrence. There is no explanation offered by the authors as to why this reconstruction technique was better able to restore native ACL kinematics. Anecdotally, we believe that the extra-articular tenodesis eliminates the rotatory instability, whereas the intra-articular reconstruction from other techniques principally eliminates only the anterior to posterior translational instability.

Surgical Technique Step by Step

For this procedure, the child is placed in the supine position on a standard flat-top operating room (OR) table. A pneumatic tourniquet is placed as far proximally as possible on the thigh but is not routinely inflated during harvest to prevent iliotibial band tethering. The tourniquet is routinely inflated after harvest at the commencement of arthroscopy. Alternatively, a sterile tourniquet can be applied after harvest. An oblique 6-cm incision is made from the midlateral joint line to the anterior border of the iliotibial band (Fig. 6.2A). Subcutaneous fat should be dissected off the iliotibial band with a Cobb elevator. The anterior and posterior borders of the iliotibial band should be identified and incised; the incisions are carried proximally under the skin with a curved meniscotome. The iliotibial band is detached proximally with a curved meniscotome or an open tendon stripper. Alternatively, an additional proximal incision can be made to detach the tendon. Distal dissection of the tendon off the joint capsule and lateral patellar retinaculum is performed, but the tendon is left attached to the Gerdy tubercle (Fig. 6.2B). The free end is tubularized with a no. 5 nonabsorbable braided suture using a whipstitch technique. The graft is typically 10 cm relative to the lateral incision at this point. The graft is placed back in the wound, the tourniquet is inflated, and diagnostic arthroscopy is performed via standard

A

B

C

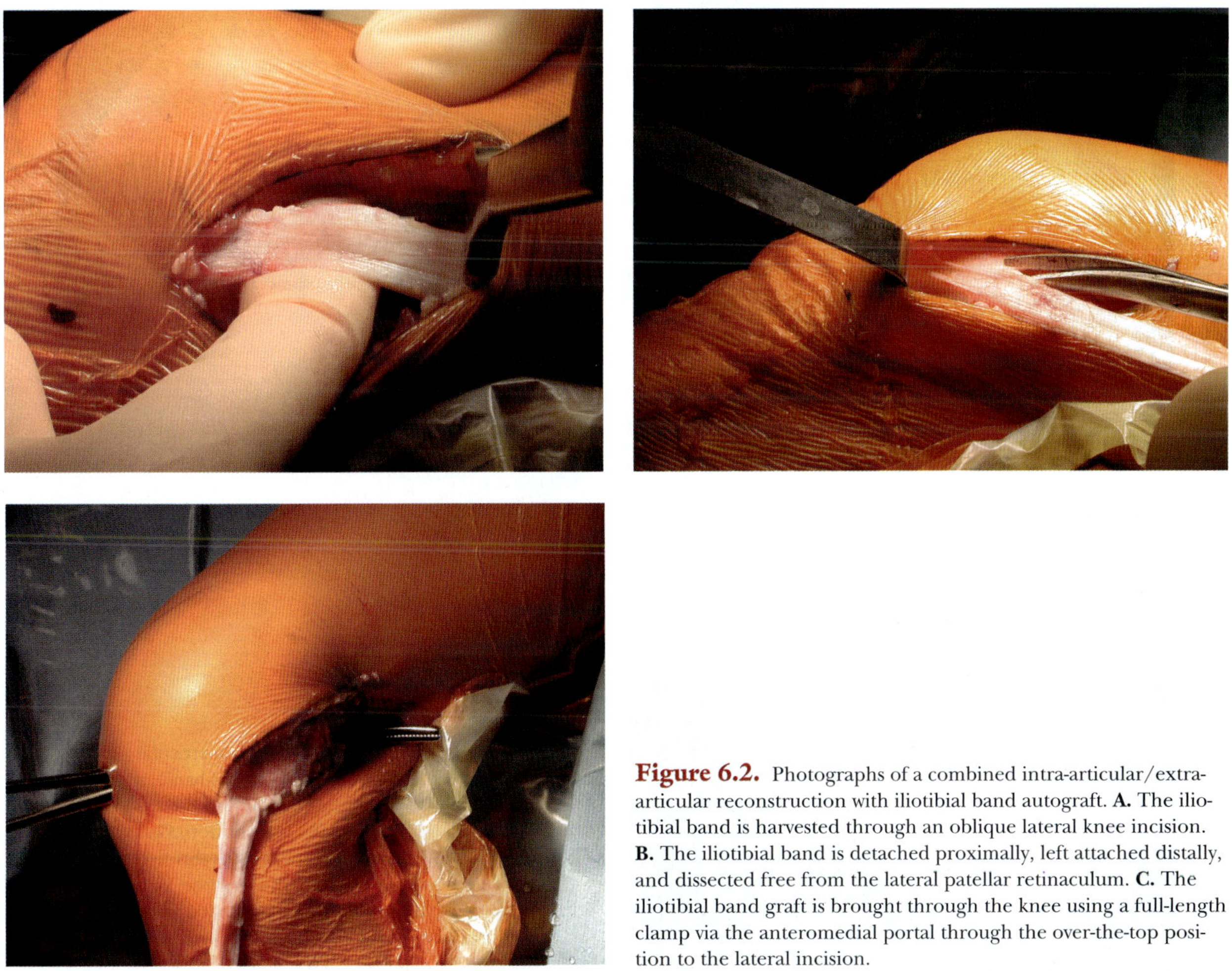

Figure 6.2. Photographs of a combined intra-articular/extra-articular reconstruction with iliotibial band autograft. **A.** The iliotibial band is harvested through an oblique lateral knee incision. **B.** The iliotibial band is detached proximally, left attached distally, and dissected free from the lateral patellar retinaculum. **C.** The iliotibial band graft is brought through the knee using a full-length clamp via the anteromedial portal through the over-the-top position to the lateral incision.

anterolateral and anteromedial portals. The ACL remnant is excised and any intra-articular pathology can be treated at this point. The over-the-top position on the femur and the over-the-front position under the intermeniscal ligament on the tibia are identified. At most, a minimal notchplasty should be performed to avoid injury to the perichondral ring of the distal femoral physis.[68] A curved clamp is passed through the anteromedial portal and bluntly through the capsule, out through the posterolateral compartment of the knee, and into the lateral incision (Fig. 6.2C). It is important to maintain the clamp on the posterolateral femur during dissection to avoid neurovascular injury. The free end of the graft is passed through the knee in the over-the-top position and the sutures are passed out via the anteromedial portal (Fig. 6.3A,B). A two-incision rear-entry guide can also be used. A second incision is made on the anterior tibia near the pes anserinus, and the dissection

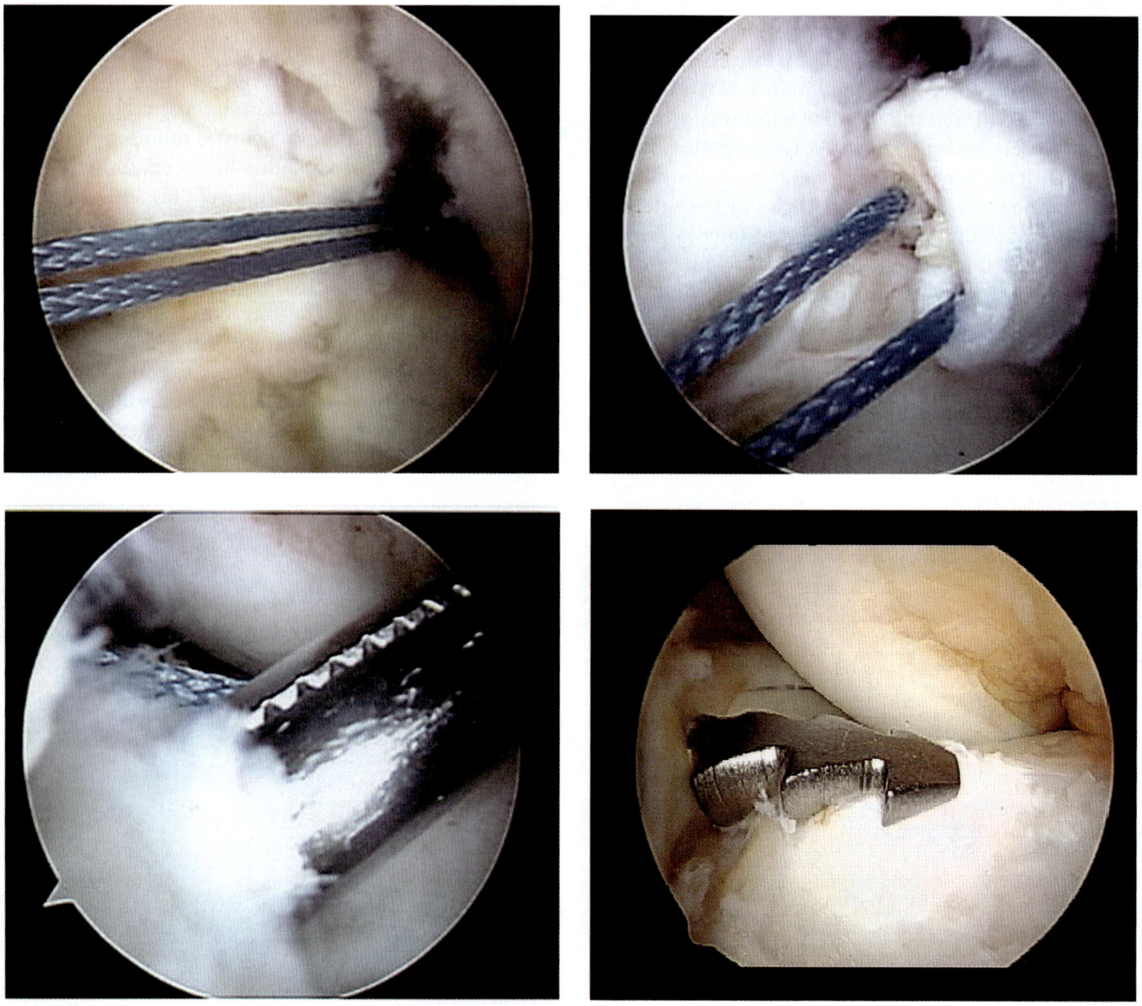

A B C D

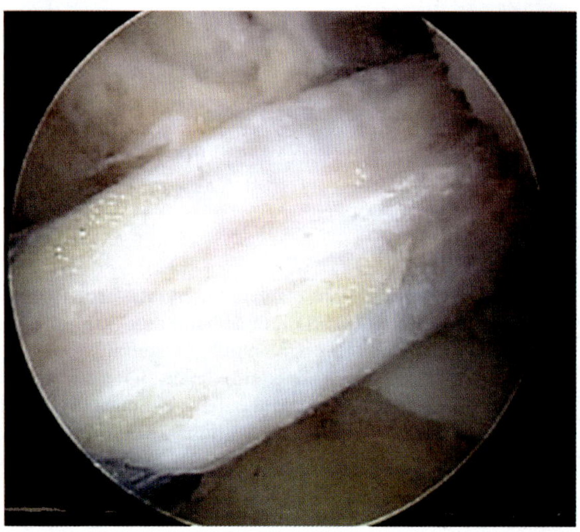

E

Figure 6.3. Images of a combined intra-articular/extra-articular reconstruction with iliotibial band autograft. Arthroscopic views show the sutures **(A)** and the graft **(B)** brought through the over-the-top position. **C.** A clamp is placed under the intermeniscal ligament through a proximal medial tibial incision. **D.** Illustration shows a curved rasp used to create a groove in the proximal tibial epiphysis under the intermeniscal ligament. **E.** Arthroscopic view shows the graft brought through the knee in the over-the-top position and under the intermeniscal ligament.

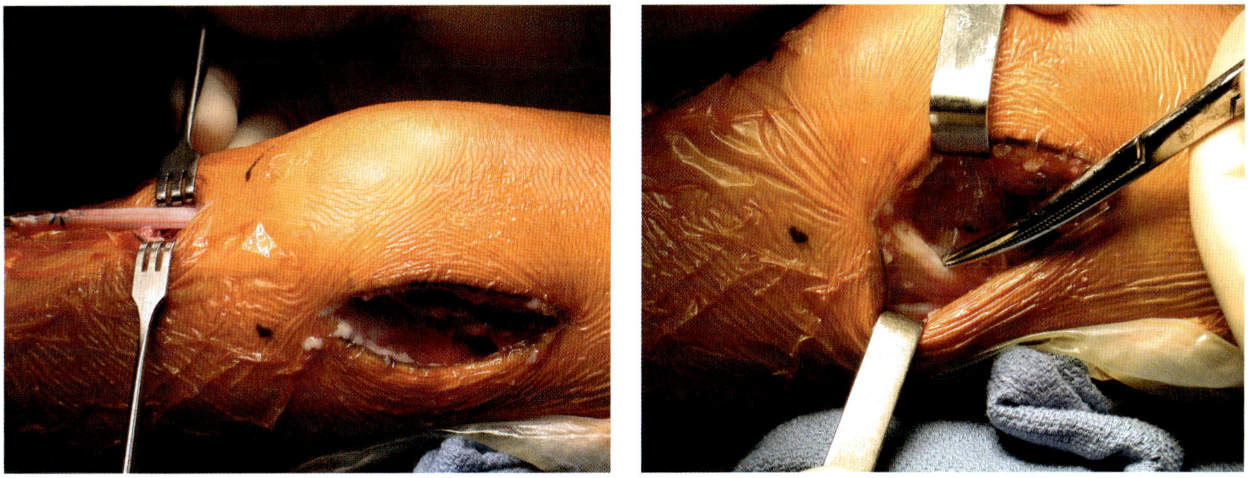

A B

Figure 6.4. Photographs of graft placement during a combined intra-articular/extra-articular reconstruction with iliotibial band autograft. **A.** The graft is brought out through the proximal medial tibial incision. **B.** On the femoral side, the graft is sutured to the intermuscular septum and the periosteum of the lateral femoral condyle.

is carried down 4.5 cm to the periosteum to ensure that the proximal tibial physis and tibial tubercle apophysis are not in the area of dissection. A curved clamp is used to tunnel up to and through the joint capsule under the intermeniscal ligament (Fig. 6.3C). The clamp is replaced with a rasp, which is used to create a groove for passage of the graft (Fig. 6.3D). The clamp is reintroduced via the tibial incision to grasp the sutures attached to the graft, and the graft is passed under the intermeniscal ligament (Fig. 6.3E), out of the knee joint, and into the tibial incision (Fig. 6.4A). The extra-articular portion of the reconstruction procedure is performed by securing the graft to the lateral femoral condyle at the insertion of the intermuscular septum with mattress sutures with the knee placed in 90 degrees of flexion (Fig. 6.4B). The author of this chapter have modified this portion of the procedure and no longer externally rotate the knee 15 degrees at this point to prevent overconstraint.[67] Tibial fixation is subsequently accomplished by elevating two small flaps of periosteum in the anterior tibial incision and creating a shallow bony trough in the tibia with a motorized burr. Fluoroscopy can be used to confirm that the physis has not been violated. With the knee in 20 degrees of flexion and appropriate tension on the graft, the graft is secured to the periosteum in the bony trough with mattress sutures. With the knee in 20 to 30 degrees of flexion, distal tension is applied to the graft. No. 2 FiberWire sutures are thrown from proximal to distal then tied after all are placed. We use mattress sutures from superficial to deep through the medial periosteum, medial to lateral through graft, then deep to superficial through lateral periosteum, angling the stitches proximally to increase graft tension when tied. At least three sutures should be placed proximally in the femur and distally in the tibia. Tibial fixation may be supplemented with a post if necessary.

Patients are typically admitted overnight for pain control and therapy on postoperative day 1 to ensure safety with crutches or a walker if the child is very young.

List of Equipment

- Standard arthroscopy equipment (30-degree scope, shaver, etc.)
- Long right-angle retractor (Fig. 5)
- Rat-tail rasp (Fig. 5)
- Full-length clamp (Fig. 5)
- Curved and straight meniscotomes (Fig. 5)
- No. 2 FiberWire or similar suture

Rehabilitation

Postoperative management consists of touchdown weight bearing with the knee locked in full extension for initial 6 weeks when upright and range of motion from 0 to 30 degrees for the initial 2 weeks. Continuous passive motion (CPM) from 0 to 30 degrees is used during this time, mainly to overcome the child's fear and anxiety about knee motion. After 2 weeks, CPM is discontinued and range of motion from 0 to 90 degrees in the hinged knee brace is permitted until 6 weeks postoperative.

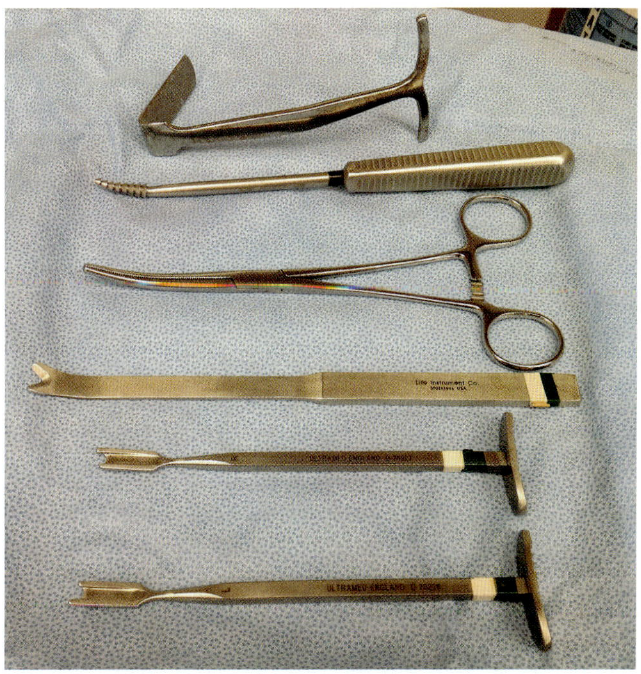

Figure 6.5. Photograph of long right-angle retractor, rat-tail rasp, full-length clamp, and curved and straight meniscotomes.

Use of the postoperative brace is discontinued at 6 weeks, with full weight bearing and unrestricted range of motion permitted thereafter in a simple hinge brace. More formal strengthening also commences at this time. Straight-ahead jogging is allowed at 3 months, and return to sport is usually allowed at approximately 6 months. A custom-made ACL brace is worn during high-risk activities for 2 years after return to sport. Clinical follow-up with assessment for leg length discrepancy or angular deformity is done yearly for at least 2 years. Additional radiographs are obtained as indicated by clinical exam.

Complications/Pearls on Avoiding

- Failure to adequately asses the stage of growth and development of the patient
- Harvesting too short of an iliotibial band graft
  - This can be minimized by using a longer incision or by making a second incision proximally.
  - If the graft is too short, it can be augmented with allograft.
- Avoid detachment of the iliotibial band from Gerdy tubercle.
- Avoid vigorous notchplasty or dissection of the over-the-top position. It can lead to perichondral ring injury.
- A sling of tissue at the inferior portion of the lateral femoral condyle typically exists. Avoid taking this down. It aids in keeping the graft in the correct position.
- Failure to bring the graft under the intermeniscal ligament
- We no longer tension the extra-articular portion in external rotation to avoid overconstraint.
- Given that the procedure incises the lateral iliotibial band, it is important to warn patients of a possible lateral muscular bulge.
- Avoid making the posterior capsulotomy too large with Kelley or graft will slide down the wall into joint.
  - If the graft slides too distal in between the femur and tibia, it can be fixed in the over-the-top position using a suture anchor.
- Ensure adequate tibial fixation.
- Avoid prolonged immobilization because it can lead to postoperative stiffness.

REFERENCES

1. Rang M. *Children's Fractures.* 2nd ed. Philadelphia, PA: Lippincott; 1983: xviii, 365.
2. Kocher MS, Foreman ES, Micheli LJ. Laxity and functional outcome after arthroscopic reduction and internal fixation of displaced tibial spine fractures in children. *Arthroscopy.* 2003;19(10):1085–1090.
3. Kocher MS, Micheli LJ, Gerbino P, et al. Tibial eminence fractures in children: prevalence of meniscal entrapment. *Am J Sports Med.* 2003;31(3):404–407.
4. Kocher MS, Mandiga R, Klingele K, et al. Anterior cruciate ligament injury versus tibial spine fracture in the skeletally immature knee: a comparison of skeletal maturation and notch width index. *J Pediatr Orthop.* 2004;24(2):185–188.
5. Eiskjaer S, Larsen ST, Schmidt MB. The significance of hemarthrosis of the knee in children. *Arch Orthop Trauma Surg.* 1988;107(2): 96–98.
6. Kloeppel-Wirth S, Koltai JL, Dittmer H. Significance of arthroscopy in children with knee joint injuries. *Eur J Pediatr Surg.* 1992;2(3): 169–172.
7. Luhmann SJ. Acute traumatic knee effusions in children and adolescents. *J Pediatr Orthop.* 2003;23(2):199–202.
8. Stanitski CL, Harvell JC, Fu F. Observations on acute knee hemarthrosis in children and adolescents. *J Pediatr Orthop.* 1993;13(4): 506–510.
9. Vähäsarja V, Kinnuen P, Serlo W. Arthroscopy of the acute traumatic knee in children: prospective study of 138 cases. *Acta Orthop Scand.* 1993;64(5):580–582.
10. Matelic TM, Aronsson DD, Boyd DW Jr, et al. Acute hemarthrosis of the knee in children. *Am J Sports Med.* 1995;23(6):668–671.
11. Sullivan JA. Ligamentous injuries of the knee in children. *Clin Orthop Relat Res.* 1990;(255):44–50.
12. Kannus P, Järvinen M. Knee ligament injuries in adolescents: eight year follow-up of conservative management. *J Bone Joint Surg Br.* 1988;70(5):772–776.
13. McCarroll JR, Rettig AC, Shelbourne KD. Anterior cruciate ligament injuries in the young athlete with open physes. *Am J Sports Med.* 1988;16(1):44–47.
14. Angel KR, Hall DJ. Anterior cruciate ligament injury in children and adolescents. *Arthroscopy.* 1989;5(3):197–200.
15. Graf BK, Lange RH, Fujisaki CK, et al. Anterior cruciate ligament tears in skeletally immature patients: meniscal pathology at presentation and after attempted conservative treatment. *Arthroscopy.* 1992;8(2):229–233.
16. Drongowski RA, Coran AG, Wojtys EM. Predictive value of meniscal and chondral injuries in conservatively treated anterior cruciate ligament injuries. *Arthroscopy.* 1994;10(1):97–102.
17. McCarroll JR, Shelbourne KD, Porter DA, et al. Patellar tendon graft reconstruction for midsubstance anterior cruciate ligament rupture in junior high school athletes: an algorithm for management. *Am J Sports Med.* 1994;22(4):478–484.
18. Mizuta H, Kubota K, Shiraishi M, et al. The conservative treatment of complete tears of the anterior cruciate ligament in skeletally immature patients. *J Bone Joint Surg Br.* 1995;77(6):890–894.
19. Janarv PM, Nyström A, Werner S, et al. Anterior cruciate ligament injuries in skeletally immature patients. *J Pediatr Orthop.* 1996; 16(5):673–677.
20. Pressman AE, Letts RM, Jarvis JG. Anterior cruciate ligament tears in children: an analysis of operative versus nonoperative treatment. *J Pediatr Orthop.* 1997;17(4):505–511.
21. Aichroth PM, Patel DV, Zorrilla P. The natural history and treatment of rupture of the anterior cruciate ligament in children and adolescents: a prospective review. *J Bone Joint Surg Br.* 2002;84(1): 38–41.
22. Millett PJ, Willis AA, Warren RF. Associated injuries in pediatric and adolescent anterior cruciate ligament tears: does a delay in treatment increase the risk of meniscal tear? *Arthroscopy.* 2002;18(9): 955–959.
23. Arbes S, Resinger C, Vécsei V, et al. The functional outcome of total tears of the anterior cruciate ligament (ACL) in the skeletally immature patient. *Int Orthop.* 2007;31(4):471–475.
24. Henry J, Chotel F, Chouteau J, et al. Rupture of the anterior cruciate ligament in children: early reconstruction with open physes or delayed reconstruction to skeletal maturity? *Knee Surg Sports Traumatol Arthrosc.* 2009;17(7):748–755.
25. Lawrence JT, Argawal N, Ganley TJ. Degeneration of the knee joint in skeletally immature patients with a diagnosis of an anterior cruciate ligament tear: is there harm in delay of treatment? *Am J Sports Med.* 2011;39(12):2582–2587.
26. Shelbourne KD, Patel DV, McCarroll JR. Management of anterior cruciate ligament injuries in skeletally immature adolescents. *Knee Surg Sports Traumatol Arthrosc.* 1996;4(2):68–74.
27. Fehnel DJ, Johnson R. Anterior cruciate injuries in the skeletally immature athlete: a review of treatment outcomes. *Sports Med.* 2000;29(1):51–63.
28. Schachter AK, Rokito AS. ACL injuries in the skeletally immature patient. *Orthopedics.* 2007;30(5):365–372.
29. Vavken P, Murray MM. Treating anterior cruciate ligament tears in skeletally immature patients. *Arthroscopy.* 2011;27(5):704–716.

30. McConkey MO, Bonasia DE, Amendola A. Pediatric anterior cruciate ligament reconstruction. *Curr Rev Musculoskelet Med.* 2011; 4(2):37–44.
31. Finlayson CJ, Nasreddine A, Kocher MS. Current concepts of diagnosis and management of ACL injuries in skeletally immature athletes. *Phys Sportsmed.* 2010;38(2):90–101.
32. Anderson AF. Transepiphyseal replacement of the anterior cruciate ligament in skeletally immature patients: a preliminary report. *J Bone Joint Surg Am.* 2003;85-A(7):1255–1263.
33. Guzzanti V, Falciglia F, Stanitski CL. Physeal-sparing intraarticular anterior cruciate ligament reconstruction in preadolescents. *Am J Sports Med.* 2003;31(6):949–953.
34. Anderson AF. Transepiphyseal replacement of the anterior cruciate ligament using quadruple hamstring grafts in skeletally immature patients. *J Bone Joint Surg Am.* 2004;86-A(pt 2, suppl 1):201–209.
35. Lawrence JT, Bowers AL, Belding J, et al. All-epiphyseal anterior cruciate ligament reconstruction in skeletally immature patients. *Clin Orthop Relat Res.* 2010;468(7):1971–1977.
36. Micheli LJ, Rask B, Gerberg L. Anterior cruciate ligament reconstruction in patients who are prepubescent. *Clin Orthop Relat Res.* 1999;(364):40–47.
37. Kocher MS, Garg S, Micheli LJ. Physeal sparing reconstruction of the anterior cruciate ligament in skeletally immature prepubescent children and adolescents. *J Bone Joint Surg Am.* 2005;87(11): 2371–2379.
38. Lipscomb AB, Anderson AF. Tears of the anterior cruciate ligament in adolescents. *J Bone Joint Surg Am.* 1986;68(1):19–28.
39. Andrews M, Noyes FR, Barber-Westin SD. Anterior cruciate ligament allograft reconstruction in the skeletally immature athlete. *Am J Sports Med.* 1994;22(1):48–54.
40. Bisson LJ, Wickiewicz T, Levinson M, et al. ACL reconstruction in children with open physes. *Orthopedics.* 1998;21(6):659–663.
41. Kim SH, Ha KI, Ahn JH, et al. Anterior cruciate ligament reconstruction in the young patient without violation of the epiphyseal plate. *Arthroscopy.* 1999;15(7):792–795.
42. Guzzanti V, Falciglia F, Stanitski CL. Preoperative evaluation and anterior cruciate ligament reconstruction technique for skeletally immature patients in Tanner stages 2 and 3. *Am J Sports Med.* 2003; 31(6):941–948.
43. Brief LP. Anterior cruciate ligament reconstruction without drill holes. *Arthroscopy.* 1991;7(4):350–357.
44. Parker AW, Drez D Jr, Cooper JL. Anterior cruciate ligament injuries in patients with open physes. *Am J Sports Med.* 1994;22(1):44–47.
45. Robert H, Bonnard C. The possibilities of using the patellar tendon in the treatment of anterior cruciate ligament tears in children. *Arthroscopy.* 1999;15(1):73–76.
46. Steadman JR, Cameron-Donaldson ML, Briggs KK, et al. A minimally invasive technique ("healing response") to treat proximal ACL injuries in skeletally immature athletes. *J Knee Surg.* 2006;19(1):8–13.
47. Bonnard C, Fournier J, Babusiaux D, et al. Physeal-sparing reconstruction of anterior cruciate ligament tears in children: results of 57 cases using patellar tendon. *J Bone Joint Surg Br.* 2011;93(4): 542–547.
48. Lo IK, Kirkley A, Fowler PJ, et al. The outcome of operatively treated anterior cruciate ligament disruptions in the skeletally immature child. *Arthroscopy.* 1997;13(5):627–634.
49. Matava MJ, Siegel MG. Arthroscopic reconstruction of the ACL with semitendinosus-gracilis autograft in skeletally immature adolescent patients. *Am J Knee Surg.* 1997;10(2):60–69.
50. Aronowitz ER, Ganley TJ, Goode JR, et al. Anterior cruciate ligament reconstruction in adolescents with open physes. *Am J Sports Med.* 2000;28(2):168–175.
51. Edwards PH, Grana WA. Anterior cruciate ligament reconstruction in the immature athlete: long-term results of intra-articular reconstruction. *Am J Knee Surg.* 2001;14(4):232–237.
52. Fuchs R, Wheatley W, Uribe JW, et al. Intra-articular anterior cruciate ligament reconstruction using patellar tendon allograft in the skeletally immature patient. *Arthroscopy.* 2002;18(8):824–828.
53. Volpi P, Galli M, Bait C, et al. Surgical treatment of anterior cruciate ligament injuries in adolescents using double-looped semitendinosus and gracilis tendons: supraepiphysary femoral and tibial fixation. *Arthroscopy.* 2004;20(4):447–449.
54. Gebhard F, Ellermann A, Hoffmann F, et al. Multicenter-study of operative treatment of intraligamentous tears of the anterior cruciate ligament in children and adolescents: comparison of four different techniques. *Knee Surg Sports Traumatol Arthrosc.* 2006;14(9): 797–803.
55. McIntosh AL, Dahm DL, Stuart MJ. Anterior cruciate ligament reconstruction in the skeletally immature patient. *Arthroscopy.* 2006; 22(12):1325–1330.
56. Sankar WN, Wells L, Sennett BJ, et al. Combined anterior cruciate ligament and medial collateral ligament injuries in adolescents. *J Pediatr Orthop.* 2006;26(6):733–736.
57. Thompson M, Flynn J, Wells L, et al. Single incision arthroscopic ACL reconstruction in skeletally immature patients with direct visualization of the femoral and tibial physes. *Orthopedics.* 2006; 29(6):488–492.
58. Kocher MS, Smith JT, Zoric BJ, et al. Transphyseal anterior cruciate ligament reconstruction in skeletally immature pubescent adolescents. *J Bone Joint Surg Am.* 2007;89(12):2632–2639.
59. Schneider FJ, Kraus T, Linhart WE. Anterior cruciate ligament reconstruction with semitendinosus tendon in children. *Oper Orthop Traumatol.* 2008;20(4–5):409–422.
60. Salzmann GM, Spang JT, Imhoff AB. Double-bundle anterior cruciate ligament reconstruction in a skeletally immature adolescent athlete. *Arthroscopy.* 2009;25(3):321–324.
61. Cho Y, Jang SJ, Son JH. Transphyseal anterior cruciate ligament reconstruction in a skeletally immature knee using anterior tibialis allograft. *Orthopedics.* 2011;34(5):397.
62. Courvoisier A, Grimaldi M, Plaweski S. Good surgical outcome of transphyseal ACL reconstruction in skeletally immature patients using four-strand hamstring graft. *Knee Surg Sports Traumatol Arthrosc.* 2011;19(4):588–591.
63. Nikolaou P, Kalliakmanis A, Bousgas D, et al. Intraarticular stabilization following anterior cruciate ligament injury in children and adolescents. *Knee Surg Sports Traumatol Arthrosc.* 2011;19(5): 801–805.
64. Shelbourne KD, Gray T, Wiley BV. Results of transphyseal anterior cruciate ligament reconstruction using patellar tendon autograft in Tanner stage 3 or 4 adolescents with clearly open growth plates. *Am J Sports Med.* 2004;32(5):1218–1222.
65. Irrgang JJ, Anderson AF, Boland AL, et al. Development and validation of the international knee documentation committee subjective knee form. *Am J Sports Med.* 2001;29(5):600–613.
66. Lysholm J, Gillquist J. Evaluation of knee ligament surgery results with special emphasis on use of a scoring scale. *Am J Sports Med.* 1982; 10(3):150–154.
67. Kennedy A, Coughlin DG, Metzger MF, et al. Biomechanical evaluation of pediatric anterior cruciate ligament reconstruction techniques. *Am J Sports Med.* 2011;39(5):964–971.
68. Behr CT, Potter HG, Paletta GA Jr. The relationship of the femoral origin of the anterior cruciate ligament and the distal femoral physeal plate in the skeletally immature knee: an anatomic study. *Am J Sports Med.* 2001;29(6):781–787.

CHAPTER

7

Allen F. Anderson
Christian N. Anderson

Technique: Anderson Technique

INTRODUCTION

Intrasubstance tears of the anterior cruciate ligament (ACL) have been recently reported with increasing frequency in skeletally immature patients. Epidemiologic data from a large integrated health care system demonstrates an incidence of 0.11 per 10,000 at 8 years of age that gradually increases to 2.42 per 10,000 by 14 years of age.[1] Although ACL injuries in children and adolescents are relatively rare, an increased rate of ACL reconstructions in this population has been observed over the last 20 years.[2] This increase in pediatric ACL surgery is thought to be commensurate with increasing injury incidence[2]; however, this phenomenon may also represent a change in management preferences from nonoperative to operative because of improved surgical techniques[3–12] and increased awareness that meniscal and chondral pathology may be associated with nonoperative[13–19] or delayed surgical treatment.[20–25]

Pediatric knee injuries, including ACL tears, present a public health problem because of the detrimental effects they can have on the health and well-being of young athletes.[26] ACL reconstruction in skeletally immature patients has been shown to be effective at restoring normal knee function and stability.[4,27] Surgical reconstruction techniques can be categorized into three groups: transphyseal, physeal-sparing, and hybrid techniques. The type of surgical treatment should be determined by the patient's physiologic and skeletal age at the time of injury. Appropriate treatment is paramount in avoiding iatrogenic growth disturbance and for return to sports participation and overall quality of life.

TREATMENT

Nonoperative Treatment or Delayed Surgical Management

Nonoperative treatment of ACL injuries in pediatric patients typically involves a regimen of functional bracing, physical therapy, and activity modification. Studies evaluating the efficacy of conservative treatment generally demonstrate poor and "unacceptable" outcomes, including high rates of recurrent instability, meniscal damage, early arthritis, and sports-related disability.[13–19] Both noncompliance[21] and significantly higher activity levels observed in children[28] have been cited as contributing factors for these poor results. Delayed surgical reconstruction until skeletal maturity in an effort to avoid risking iatrogenic growth disturbance has also been associated with recurrent instability and an increased incidence of associated knee pathology.[20–25]

In contrast to the growing body of literature demonstrating poor outcomes with conservative or delayed treatment, relatively few studies support the use of nonoperative treatment algorithms in skeletally immature patients.[29–32] Even so, a recent meta-analysis overwhelmingly favored early surgical stabilization over conservative treatment or delayed reconstruction.[24] In this study, the aggregate data of nonoperative or delayed treatment was associated with a 34-fold increase in knee instability.[24] Furthermore, patients treated nonoperatively had a 12-fold increase in the rate of medial meniscus tears and none were able to return to their preinjury level of play.[24] Given the increasing evidence of poor outcomes with nonoperative and delayed surgical treatment, our current recommendation is early reconstruction to avoid recurrent instability and associated knee pathology.

Surgical Treatment Options

The first step in surgical treatment of ACL injuries in pediatric individuals is determining the skeletal maturity and growth potential of the patient. The most common method for assessing skeletal maturity is comparing hand and wrist radiographs to the Greulich and Pyle atlas.[33] In determining the skeletal age, the relative risk and potential consequences of iatrogenic physeal injury can be estimated. Subsequently, the appropriate surgical technique can be selected to minimize the chance of limb length discrepancy (LLD) or angular deformity.

Surgical reconstruction options include transphyseal, physeal-sparing, and hybrid techniques. Transphyseal and hybrid techniques involve drilling through one or both of the growth plates. Favorable results have been achieved using these techniques, with good subjective outcome scores, objective measures, and low complication rates.[34–38] However, both basic science[39–45] and clinical research studies[34,35,46–50] indicate a risk of iatrogenic LLD or angular deformity with transphyseal drilling. To decrease physeal damage and risk of growth deformity, advocates of transphyseal ACL reconstruction recommend minimizing drill tunnel diameter and drilling femoral tunnels using a transtibial technique or as vertically as possible.[34–38] However, vertical femoral tunnel placement results in a nonanatomic ACL graft position[51] that does not restore the normal kinematics of the knee.[52]

Physeal-sparing techniques can be described as extraphyseal,[6,12] transepiphyseal,[4,5] or all-epiphyseal.[7,9–11] The advantage of these techniques is a theoretical decrease in the risk of growth disturbance by avoiding damage to the physis. Micheli et al.[12] described a modification of the McIntosh and Darby intra-articular and extra-articular ACL reconstruction, whereby the iliotibial band is rerouted to an over-the-top femoral position and through the knee. Although clinical results for this procedure are favorable,[6,12] almost 30 years ago, Odensten and Gillquist[53] noted this technique lacked isometry and resulted in 10 mm of graft elongation with knee extension.

In 2003, Anderson[4] described a transepiphyseal reconstruction that followed the generally accepted principles of ACL reconstruction in adults but relied on anatomic tunnels drilled completely within the epiphysis, thereby theoretically minimizing the chance of growth disturbance by not transgressing either the tibial or femoral physis. Compared to the Micheli technique, the Anderson technique has been shown to be more effective at restoring native knee kinematics with dynamic pivot shift loading.[27] The Anderson technique relies on graft fixation distal to the physis on the tibial side (Fig. 7.4), whereas the Micheli technique uses extraphyseal fixation on both the femoral and tibial sides. Fixation of the graft outside of the epiphysis theoretically risks soft tissue tethering on the growth plate; however, the clinical results of these techniques in patients with substantial postoperative growth have not demonstrated growth deformity.[4,6,12]

We have subsequently modified our approach by using all-epiphyseal graft fixation (Figs. 7.5 to 7.8) (OrthoPediatrics, Warsaw, IN), thereby theoretically eliminating the potential of soft tissue tethering of the growth plate. The modified Anderson technique uses suspensory fixation on the tibial side and shielded screw fixation on the femoral side that prevents the physis from being damaged by the interference screw.

Our algorithm for determining the appropriate surgical technique involves risk stratifying patients based on skeletal maturity—a direct indicator of the amount of knee growth remaining.[54] Males with bone age less than 13 years and females less than 12 years are placed in a high-risk category because they have significant knee growth remaining[54] and the effects of growth arrest would be severe.[55] Males with bone age from 13 to 15 years and females from 12 to 13 years have at least 1 to 2 cm of knee growth remaining[54] and are consequently placed in an intermediate-risk category. Males with bone age greater than 15 years and females greater than 13 years are placed in a low-risk category because they have 1 cm or less of knee growth remaining[54] and iatrogenic physeal damage would likely result in no significant growth disturbance.

Patients categorized as high risk undergo an all-epiphyseal reconstruction with suspensory fixation on the tibial side and shielded screw fixation on the femoral side. Younger patients in the intermediate group may be treated with transepiphyseal or all-epiphyseal reconstruction (males with bone age 13 to 14 years and females 12 years). Older patients in the intermediate risk category (males with bone age 14 to 15 years and females 13 years) may be treated with transphyseal reconstruction using quadruple hamstring grafts and a modified vertical femoral tunnel. Patients classified as low risk undergo adult-type reconstruction with quadrupled hamstring autografts and anatomic femoral tunnel drilling through the anteromedial portal.

SURGICAL TECHNIQUE

Anderson Technique—Transepiphyseal Anterior Cruciate Ligament Reconstruction

Place the injured leg in an arthroscopic leg holder, and flex the hip to 20 degrees to facilitate visualization of the knee in the lateral plane using fluoroscopy. Position the C-arm on the side of the table opposite the injured leg, and place the monitor at the head of the table on the same side as the injured knee. Before the leg is prepared and draped, visualize the tibial and femoral physes in both anteroposterior and lateral planes. Then, rotate the C-arm 30 degrees externally to visualize the extension of the tibial physis into the tibial tubercle on the lateral view of the tibia.

Make an oblique incision 3 to 4 cm long; dissect the semitendinosus and gracilis tendons free. Then, transect the tendons at the musculotendinous junction using a standard tendon stripper and detach them distally. Next, double the tendons and place a no. 2 FiberWire suture (Arthrex, Naples, FL) in the tendon ends using a locking whipstitch. Place the doubled tendons on the back table under 4.5 kg of tension using the Graft Master device (Acufex, Smith & Nephew, Andover, MA). Insert the arthroscope into the anterolateral portal, and insert the probe through the anteromedial portal. Perform an intra-articular examination in a standard manner. Remove the debris from the intercondylar notch so the anatomic footprint of the ACL on the femur can be visualized. At this point in the procedure, repair any tears of the menisci.

Place an arthroscope in the anteromedial portal and the ACL drill guide in the anterolateral portal. Place the tip of the guide at the center of the anterior footprint of the ACL on the femur. Elevate the handle of the guide 30 degrees anteriorly so the drill hole does not damage the lateral collateral ligament or popliteus tendon attachment. At this point, visualize the position of the drill guide and guide wire with the C-arm in the anteroposterior plane and then advance the guide wire across the femoral epiphysis. Using the arthroscope, visualize entry of the guide wire into the intercondylar notch (Fig. 7.1). The proper entry point is at the center of the anatomic footprint of the ACL on the femur. With the femoral guide wire in place, insert a second guide wire into the anteromedial aspect of the tibia, passing through the epiphysis, with the aid of the drill guide. From a direct lateral position, externally rotate the C-arm approximately 30 degrees to reveal the physis extending into the tibial tubercle. Lift the handle of the drill guide so the pin clears the anterior portion of the tibial physis. Then, drill the guide wire into the tibial epiphysis using real-time fluoroscopic imaging. Ensure the pin enters the joint just anterior to the free edge of the lateral meniscus and in the footprint of the ACL on the tibia (Fig. 7.2).

Before proceeding, confirm that both guide wires are in the correct position. Measure the diameter of the quadruple hamstring graft using tendon sizers; these grafts typically range from 6 to 8 mm in diameter. Because a tight fit is essential, use the smallest reamer possible to ream over the guide wires. Chamfer the edge of the femoral hole intra-articularly, and measure the width of the lateral femoral condyle. Choose an EndoButton continuous loop (Acufex, Smith & Nephew, Memphis, TN; 2 to 3 cm) that allows 1.5 to 2 cm of the quadruple hamstring graft to remain within the lateral femoral condyle. Pass the

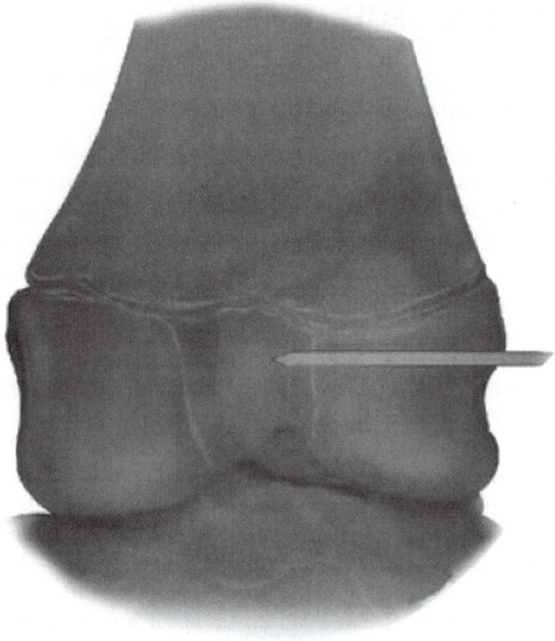

Figure 7.1. Anteroposterior view demonstrating the position of the guide wire in the femoral epiphysis. (From Anderson AF, Anderson CN. Anterior cruciate ligament reconstruction in skeletally immature patients. In: Prodromos C, Brown C, Fu FH, et al, eds. *The Anterior Cruciate Ligament: Reconstruction and Basic Science.* Philadelphia, PA: Saunders; 2008:464, with permission.)

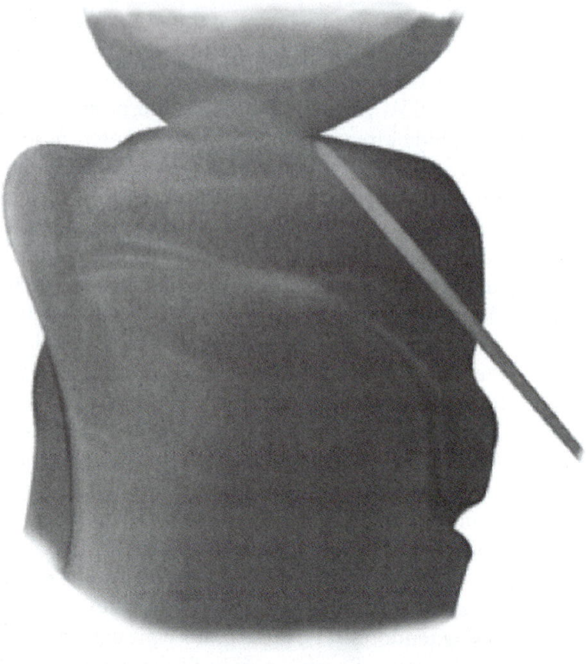

Figure 7.2. Lateral view of the tibia demonstrating the position of the tibial guide wire. Although the guide wire appears to enter the tibial tubercle in this view, it actually enters the epiphysis medial to the tibial tubercle. (From Anderson AF, Anderson CN. Anterior cruciate ligament reconstruction in skeletally immature patients. In: Prodromos C, Brown C, Fu FH, et al, eds. *The Anterior Cruciate Ligament: Reconstruction and Basic Science.* Philadelphia, PA: Saunders; 2008:464, with permission.)

EndoButton continuous loop around the middle of the double tendons, and loop it inside itself to secure the tendons. This will shorten the length of the EndoButton continuous loop substantially. An alternative method is to place the tendons through the continuous loop before suturing the tendons together. This method requires drilling and measuring the length of the femoral hole to determine the appropriate length of the EndoButton continuous loop before the graft is prepared.

In one end of the EndoButton, place a no. 2 FiberWire suture. Pass the suture from anterior to posterior through the tibia and out the lateral femoral condyle using a suture passer. Then pull the EndoButton and tendons up through the tibia and out the femoral hole using the suture (Fig. 7.3). Place an AO washer that is 3 to 4 mm larger than the femoral hole over the EndoButton. Apply tension to the tendons distally and pull both the EndoButton and the washer to the surface of the lateral femoral condyle. The washer anchors the graft proximally, so the EndoButton does not get pulled through the hole in the lateral femoral condyle. Place the graft under tension and extend the knee to arthroscopically ensure that the graft is not impinging on the intercondylar notch. It is usually unnecessary to perform an anterior notchplasty when performing transepiphyseal ACL reconstruction; however, a small area of the anterior intercondylar notch may be removed if it comes in contact with the graft in terminal extension. Place the knee in 20 degrees of flexion and secure the quadruple hamstring graft distally by tying the no. 2 FiberWire sutures over a 4.5- × 25-mm long cancellous screw and post (Smith & Nephew) located medial to the tibial tubercle apophysis and distal to the proximal tibial physis (Fig. 7.4). Close the subcutaneous tissue and skin using standard technique.

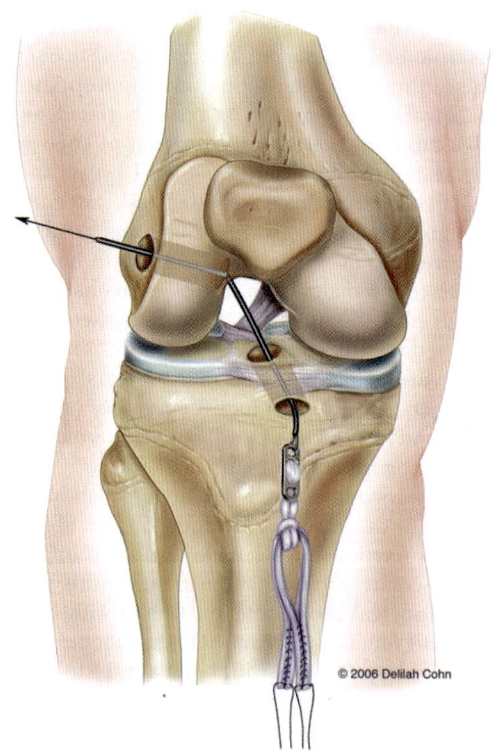

Figure 7.3. The semitendinosus and gracilis tendons are pulled up through the tibia and out the lateral femoral condyle with use of the no. 2 suture in the EndoButton. (With permission from Delilah Cohn.)

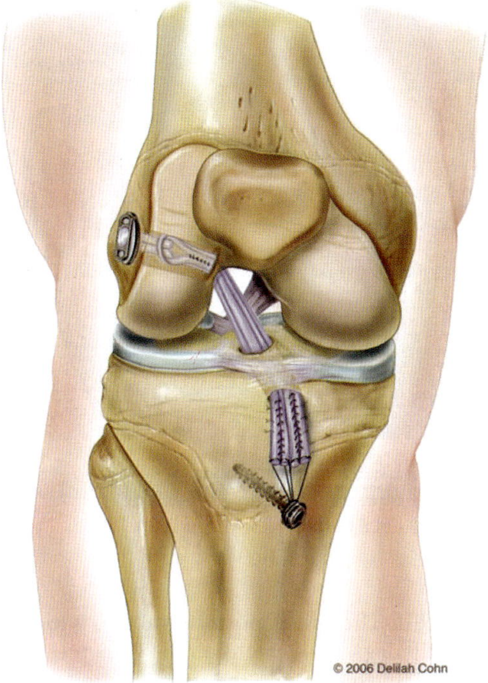

Figure 7.4. The EndoButton washer is placed over the EndoButton, and the washer is pulled back to the surface of the lateral femoral condyle. The quadruple hamstring grafts are secured distally by tying the no. 2 FiberWire sutures over the screw and post. (With permission from Delilah Cohn.)

Modified Anderson Technique—All-Epiphyseal Anterior Cruciate Ligament Reconstruction

The setup of the room, diagnostic arthroscopy, harvesting and preparing the grafts, insertion of the guide wires, and drilling the holes in the tibial and femoral epiphyses is performed just as described in the transepiphyseal technique. However, the OrthoPediatrics set has all of the necessary instrumentation to perform each step. After drilling the tibial and femoral holes, it is necessary to insert the ShieldLoc sleeve into the femoral hole. Insert the counter bore reamer into the femoral hole until it bottoms out on the lateral femoral cortex. During this step, the counter bore is inserted to a depth of 8 mm and increases the diameter of the femoral hole by 2 mm. The small amount of bone removal occurs rapidly. Retract the iliotibial band and carefully remove the soft tissue immediately around the hole to allow for clear placement of the ShieldLoc. The appropriately sized ShieldLoc sleeve is screwed on to the insertion device (Fig. 7.5A) and then gently tapped into the femoral tunnel (Fig. 7.5B). The fluted fins on the outside of the ShieldLoc sleeve prevent the device from backing out of the femoral tunnel while removing the insertion device. The ShieldLoc sleeve is designed to protect the physis from radial pressure caused by the insertion of the interference screw. After the ShieldLoc sleeve has been inserted, place the Graft Passer from the Disposable Kit through the femoral tunnel and with an arthroscopic grasper; pull the Graft Passer loop out of the tibial tunnel. Place one end of each graft through the Graft Passer loop on the femoral side. Then pull the tibial end of the Graft Passer, bringing the graft through the femoral tunnel into the tibial tunnel. Gently pull 1 to 2 cm of the graft loop outside of the anterior tibial cortex to allow installation of the ArmorLink implant. With the use of hemostat, pass the ArmorLink around the tendons (Fig. 7.6A). Pull on the free strands of the graft coming out of the femoral tunnel in order to seat the ArmorLink on the tibial cortex (Fig. 7.6B). The ArmorLink may be positioned in any orientation. Observe the ShieldLoc when pulling the free strands of the graft to make sure the ShieldLoc sleeve does not catch on the sutures in the free ends of the graft and become displaced. If the ShieldLoc sleeve moves when pulling the tendons through, then stabilize the ShieldLoc sleeve with a hemostat to prevent displacement. With the knee in approximately 20 to 30 degrees of flexion,

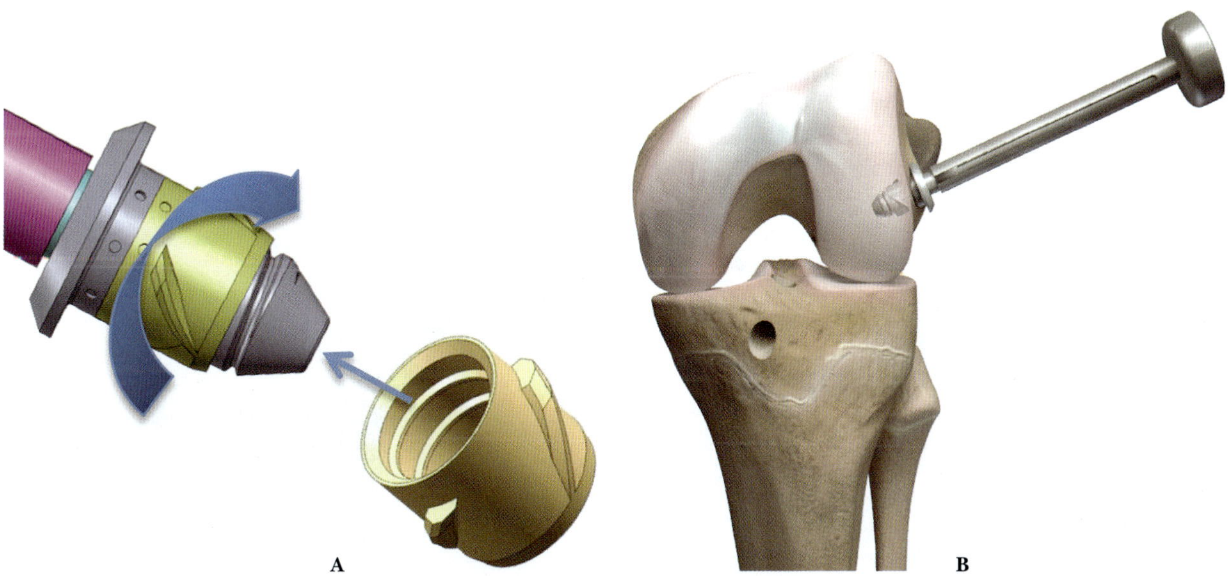

Figure 7.5. **A.** The appropriately sized ShieldLoc is screwed onto the ShieldLoc insertion device. **B.** The ShieldLoc is then inserted into the femoral tunnel by gently tapping on the insertion device until it is fully seated. The insertion device is removed by unscrewing it from the ShieldLoc. (Copyright 2013 OrthoPediatrics Corp., with permission.)

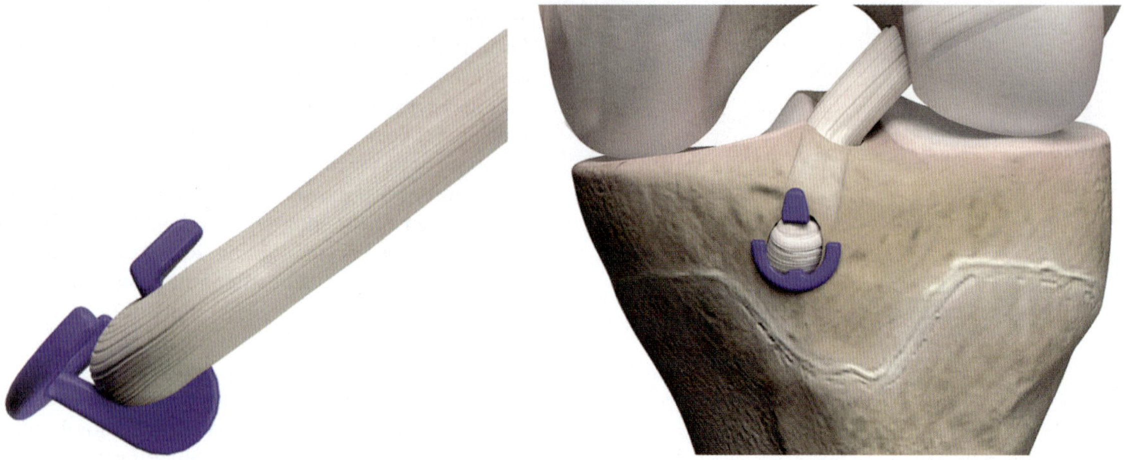

Figure 7.6. **A.** The ArmorLink device is grasped with a hemostat and passed around the loops formed from doubling over both the semitendinosus and gracilis tendons. **B.** The free strands of the graft exiting the femoral tunnel are then pulled laterally to seat the ArmorLink on the tibial cortex. (Copyright 2013 OrthoPediatrics Corp., with permission.)

apply tension with the graft tensioner and insert the screw of the ShieldLoc (Fig. 7.7). Evaluate the graft for intercondylar notch impingement and then close the wound in a standard fashion (Fig. 7.8). The postoperative rehabilitation is the same with this technique as for the transepiphyseal technique.

Postoperative Rehabilitation for Transepiphyseal or All-Epiphyseal Anterior Cruciate Ligament Reconstruction

Postoperative rehabilitation following the transepiphyseal ACL reconstruction procedure has three phases. Phase I begins when the patient awakens from surgery. Encourage the patient to perform straight-leg raises and to contract the quadriceps muscles. Use cryotherapy for 5 to 10 minutes each hour. The day after surgery, the patient performs range-of-motion exercises and hamstring stretches in a prone position. Patients without meniscal repairs may ambulate with crutches and partial weight bearing for 4 weeks. For patients who required meniscal repair, only toe-touch weight bearing is allowed for the first 6 weeks. The 1-week postsurgical goal is to have a range of motion of 0 degrees of extension to 90 degrees of flexion.

Phase II of rehabilitation is the strengthening phase that may last from 2 to 11 weeks. During this phase, patients perform active range-of-motion exercises and patellar mobilization and undergo electrical muscle stimulation. Patients should work at a comfortable pace. At postsurgical week 2, the patient is fitted with a functional knee brace and is encouraged to bear weight. Exercises should be introduced in order of increasing difficulty, including hamstring stretches, quadriceps muscle stretches and strengthening, proprioception exercises, and functional strengthening. Finally, strengthening exercises may be

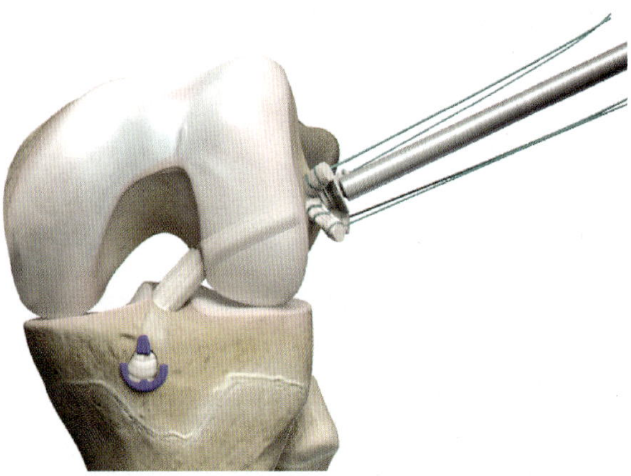

Figure 7.7. The graft is then tensioned with the knee at 20 to 30 degrees of flexion and the interference screw is then inserted into the ShieldLoc. (Copyright 2013 OrthoPediatrics Corp., with permission.)

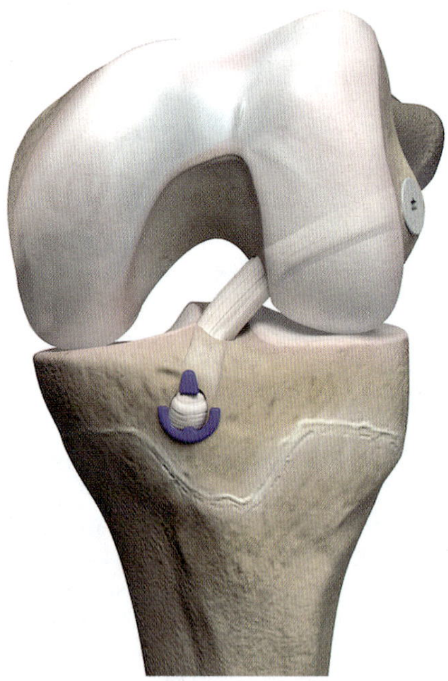

Figure 7.8. The knee is then extended and the graft is evaluated for impingement in the intercondylar notch. The free ends of the semitendinosus and gracilis are trimmed after satisfactory stability is confirmed. (Copyright 2013 OrthoPediatrics Corp., with permission.)

performed in a pool. The goal is for the operative knee to have the same range of motion as the normal knee by postsurgical week 6.

The goal of the final rehabilitation phase is to regain full function of the knee. This phase lasts from 12 to 20 weeks. Rehabilitation activities during this phase include functional strengthening exercises, straight line jogging, plyometric exercises, sport cord exercises for jogging, lateral movement, and foot agility exercises. Between postsurgical weeks 16 and 20, patients may resume functional activities (full speed running) while wearing the brace. At postsurgical week 32, patients may return to full participation in sports.

REFERENCES

1. Funahashi KM, Moksnes H, Maletis GB, et al. Anterior cruciate ligament injuries in adolescents with open physis: effect of recurrent injury and surgical delay on meniscal and cartilage injuries. *Am J Sports Med.* 2014;42(5):1068–1073.
2. Dodwell ER, LaMont LE, Green DW, et al. 20 years of pediatric anterior cruciate ligament reconstruction in New York State. *Am J Sports Med.* 2014;42(3):675–680.
3. Kim SH, Ha KI, Ahn JH, et al. Anterior cruciate ligament reconstruction in the young patient without violation of the epiphyseal plate. *Arthroscopy.* 1999;15(7):792–795.
4. Anderson AF. Transepiphyseal replacement of the anterior cruciate ligament in skeletally immature patients a preliminary report. *J Bone Joint Surg Am.* 2003;85(7):1255–1263.
5. Guzzanti V, Falciglia F, Stanitski CL. Physeal-sparing intraarticular anterior cruciate ligament reconstruction in preadolescents. *Am J Sports Med.* 2003;31(6):949–953.
6. Kocher MS, Garg S, Micheli LJ. Physeal sparing reconstruction of the anterior cruciate ligament in skeletally immature prepubescent children and adolescents. *J Bone Joint Surg Am.* 2005;87(11):2371–2379.
7. Lawrence JT, Bowers AL, Belding J, et al. All-epiphyseal anterior cruciate ligament reconstruction in skeletally immature patients. *Clin Orthop Relat Res.* 2010;468(7):1971 1977.
8. Bonnard C, Fournier J, Babusiaux D, et al. Physeal-sparing reconstruction of anterior cruciate ligament tears in children: results of 57 cases using patellar tendon. *J Bone Joint Surg Br.* 2011;93(4):542.
9. Lykissas MG, Nathan ST, Wall EJ. All-epiphyseal anterior cruciate ligament reconstruction in skeletally immature patients: a surgical technique using a split tibial tunnel. *Arthrosc Tech.* 2012;1(1): e133–e139.
10. McCarthy MM, Graziano J, Green DW, et al. All-epiphyseal, all-inside anterior cruciate ligament reconstruction technique for skeletally immature patients. *Arthrosc Tech.* 2012;1(2):e231–e239.
11. Makani A, Franklin CC, Kanj WW, et al. All-epiphyseal anterior cruciate ligament reconstruction using fluoroscopic imaging. *J Pediatr Orthop B.* 2013;22(5):445–449.
12. Micheli LJ, Rask B, Gerberg L. Anterior cruciate ligament reconstruction in patients who are prepubescent. *Clin Orthop Relat Res.* 1999;(364):40–47.
13. Angel KR, Hall DJ. Anterior cruciate ligament injury in children and adolescents. *Arthroscopy.* 1989;5(3):197–200.
14. Streich NA, Barié A, Gotterbarm T, et al. Transphyseal reconstruction of the anterior cruciate ligament in prepubescent athletes. *Knee Surg Sports Traumatol Arthrosc.* 2010;18(11):1481–1486.
15. Aichroth PM, Patel DV, Zorrilla P. The natural history and treatment of rupture of the anterior cruciate ligament in children and adolescents. A prospective review. *J Bone Joint Surg Br.* 2002;84(1):38–41.
16. Graf BK, Lange RH, Fujisaki CK, et al. Anterior cruciate ligament tears in skeletally immature patients: meniscal pathology at presentation and after attempted conservative treatment. *Arthroscopy.* 1992;8(2): 229–233.
17. Mizuta H, Kubota K, Shiraishi M, et al. The conservative treatment of complete tears of the anterior cruciate ligament in skeletally immature patients. *J Bone Joint Surg Br.* 1995;77(6):890–894.
18. McCarroll JR, Rettig AC, Shelbourne KD. Anterior cruciate ligament injuries in the young athlete with open physes. *Am J Sports Med.* 1988;16(1):44–47.
19. Kannus P, Järvinen M. Knee ligament injuries in adolescents. Eight year follow-up of conservative management. *J Bone Joint Surg Br.* 1988;70(5):772.
20. Millett PJ, Willis AA, Warren RF. Associated injuries in pediatric and adolescent anterior cruciate ligament tears: does a delay in treatment increase the risk of meniscal tear? *Arthroscopy.* 2002;18(9): 955–959.
21. Lawrence JT, Argawal N, Ganley TJ. Degeneration of the knee joint in skeletally immature patients with a diagnosis of an anterior cruciate ligament tear: is there harm in delay of treatment? *Am J Sports Med.* 2011;39(12):2582–2587.
22. Dumont GD, Hogue GD, Padalecki JR, et al. Meniscal and chondral injuries associated with pediatric anterior cruciate ligament tears: relationship of treatment time and patient-specific factors. *Am J Sports Med.* 2012;40(9):2128–2133.
23. McCarroll JR, Shelbourne KD, Porter DA, et al. Patellar tendon graft reconstruction for midsubstance anterior cruciate ligament rupture in junior high school athletes. An algorithm for management. *Am J Sports Med.* 1994;22(4):478–484.
24. Ramski DE, Kanj WW, Franklin CC, et al. Anterior cruciate ligament tears in children and adolescents: a meta-analysis of nonoperative versus operative treatment. *Am J Sports Med.* 2014;42(11):2769–2776.
25. Henry J, Chotel F, Chouteau J, et al. Rupture of the anterior cruciate ligament in children: early reconstruction with open physes or delayed reconstruction to skeletal maturity? *Knee Surg Sports Traumatol Arthrosc.* 2009;17(7):748–755.
26. Yang J, Marshall SW, Bowling JM, et al. Use of discretionary protective equipment and rate of lower extremity injury in high school athletes. *Am J Epidemiol.* 2005;161(6):511–519.
27. Sena M, Chen J, Dellamaggioria R, et al. Dynamic evaluation of pivot-shift kinematics in physeal-sparing pediatric anterior cruciate ligament reconstruction techniques. *Am J Sports Med.* 2013;41(4):826–834.
28. Wall EJ, Myer GD, May MM. Anterior cruciate ligament reconstruction timing in children with open growth plates: new surgical techniques including all-epiphyseal. *Clin Sports Med.* 2011;30(4): 789–800.
29. Woods GW. Delayed anterior cruciate ligament reconstruction in adolescents with open physes. *Am J Sports Med.* 2004;32(1):201–210.
30. Moksnes H, Engebretsen L, Eitzen I, et al. Functional outcomes following a non-operative treatment algorithm for anterior cruciate ligament injuries in skeletally immature children 12 years and younger. A prospective cohort with 2 years follow-up. *Br J Sports Med.* 2013;47(8):488–494.
31. Moksnes H, Engebretsen L, Risberg MA. Prevalence and incidence of new meniscus and cartilage injuries after a nonoperative treatment algorithm for ACL tears in skeletally immature children: a prospective MRI study. *Am J Sports Med.* 2013;41(8): 1771–1779.
32. Moksnes H, Engebretsen L, Risberg MA. Performance-based functional outcome for children 12 years or younger following anterior cruciate ligament injury: a two to nine-year follow-up study. *Knee Surg Sports Traumatol Arthrosc.* 2007;16(3):214–223.
33. Pyle SI, Greulich WW. *Radiographic Atlas of Skeletal Development of the Hand and Wrist.* Stanford, CA: Stanford University Press; 1959.
34. Kohl S, Stutz C, Decker S, et al. Mid-term results of transphyseal anterior cruciate ligament reconstruction in children and adolescents. *Knee.* 2014;21(1):80–85.
35. Kumar S, Ahearne D, Hunt DM. Transphyseal anterior cruciate ligament reconstruction in the skeletally immature. *J Bone Joint Surg Am.* 2013;95(1):e1.

36. Goddard M, Bowman N, Salmon LJ, et al. Endoscopic anterior cruciate ligament reconstruction in children using living donor hamstring tendon allografts. *Am J Sports Med.* 2013;41(3): 567–574.
37. Redler LH, Brafman RT, Trentacosta N, et al. Anterior cruciate ligament reconstruction in skeletally immature patients with transphyseal tunnels. *Arthroscopy.* 2012;28(11):1710–1717.
38. Hui C, Roe J, Ferguson D, et al. Outcome of anatomic transphyseal anterior cruciate ligament reconstruction in Tanner stage 1 and 2 patients with open physes. *Am J Sports Med.* 2012;40(5):1093–1098.
39. Guzzanti V, Falciglia F, Gigante A, et al. The effect of intra-articular ACL reconstruction on the growth plates of rabbits. *J Bone Joint Surg Br.* 1994;76(6):960–963.
40. Houle JB, Letts M, Yang J. Effects of a tensioned tendon graft in a bone tunnel across the rabbit physis. *Clin Orthop Relat Res.* 2001;391:275.
41. Mäkelä EA, Vainionpää S, Vihtonen K, et al. The effect of trauma to the lower femoral epiphyseal plate. An experimental study in rabbits. *J Bone Joint Surg Br.* 1988;70(2):187–191.
42. Janarv PM, Wikström B, Hirsch G. The influence of transphyseal drilling and tendon grafting on bone growth: an experimental study in the rabbit. *J Pediatr Orthop.* 1998;18(2):149–154.
43. Chudik S, Beasley L, Potter H, et al. The influence of femoral technique for graft placement on anterior cruciate ligament reconstruction using a skeletally immature canine model with a rapidly growing physis. *Arthroscopy.* 2007;23(12):1309–1319.
44. Edwards TB, Greene CC, Baratta RV, et al. The effect of placing a tensioned graft across open growth plates a gross and histologic analysis. *J Bone Joint Surg Am.* 2001;83(5):725–734.
45. Babb JR, Ahn JI, Azar FM, et al. Transphyseal anterior cruciate ligament reconstruction using mesenchymal stem cells. *Am J Sports Med.* 2008;36(6):1164–1170.
46. Yoo WJ, Kocher MS, Micheli LJ. Growth plate disturbance after transphyseal reconstruction of the anterior cruciate ligament in skeletally immature adolescent patients: an MR imaging study. *J Pediatr Orthop.* 2011;31(6):691.
47. McIntosh AL, Dahm DL, Stuart MJ. Anterior cruciate ligament reconstruction in the skeletally immature patient. *Arthroscopy.* 2006;22(12):1325–1330.
48. Higuchi T, Hara K, Tsuji Y, et al. Transepiphyseal reconstruction of the anterior cruciate ligament in skeletally immature athletes: an MRI evaluation for epiphyseal narrowing. *J Pediatr Orthop B.* 2009;18(6):330–334.
49. Chotel F, Henry J, Seil R, et al. Growth disturbances without growth arrest after ACL reconstruction in children. *Knee Surg Sports Traumatol Arthrosc.* 2010;18(11):1496–1500.
50. Kocher MS, Saxon HS, Hovis WD, et al. Management and complications of anterior cruciate ligament injuries in skeletally immature patients: survey of the Herodicus Society and the ACL Study Group. *J Pediatr Orthop.* 2002;22(4):452–457.
51. Strauss EJ, Barker JU, McGill K, et al. Can anatomic femoral tunnel placement be achieved using a transtibial technique for hamstring anterior cruciate ligament reconstruction? *Am J Sports Med.* 2011;39(6):1263–1269.
52. Wang H, Fleischli JE, Zheng N. Transtibial versus anteromedial portal technique in single-bundle anterior cruciate ligament reconstruction: outcomes of knee joint kinematics during walking. *Am J Sports Med.* 2013;41(8):1847–1856.
53. Odensten M, Gillquist J. Functional anatomy of the anterior cruciate ligament and a rationale for reconstruction. *J Bone Joint Surg Am.* 1985;67(2):257–262.
54. Green WT, Anderson M. Experiences with epiphyseal arrest in correcting discrepancies in length of the lower extremities in infantile paralysis; a method of predicting the effect. *J Bone Joint Surg Am.* 1947;29(3):659–678.
55. Wester W, Canale ST, Dutkowsky JP, et al. Prediction of angular deformity and leg-length discrepancy after anterior cruciate ligament reconstruction in skeletally immature patients. *J Pediatr Orthop.* 1994;14(4):516–521.

CHAPTER

8

Elizabeth B. Gausden
Daniel W. Green
Frank A. Cordasco

Technique: Anterior Cruciate Ligament Reconstruction: All-Epiphyseal Sockets

INTRODUCTION

Although previously considered uncommon in skeletally immature patients, given the strength of the cruciate ligaments over physeal integrity, current literature suggests an increase in incidence of anterior cruciate ligament (ACL) injury in pediatric patients.[1,2] Dodwell et al.[3] reported that the rate of ACL reconstruction per 100,000 population aged 3 to 20 years in New York State has increased from 17.6 in 1990 to 50.9 in 2009. In a Scandinavian database study, the incidence of ACL reconstruction was 76 in 100,000 girls and 47 per 100,000 boys between the ages of 10 and 19 years.[4,5]

Nonoperative management of ACL injuries in the skeletally immature population is associated with poor outcomes, including cartilage and meniscal damage as well as instability.[6] Children with ACL tears treated nonoperatively have a 50% sport dropout rate because of recurrent instability.[6] As standard adult ACL reconstruction involves drill holes that traverse physes, there is a risk of physeal damage and potentially leg length discrepancy over time. Orthopedic surgeons and researchers have not been able to fully quantify the risk of angular deformities and growth disturbances resulting from standard ACL reconstruction with transphyseal tunnels. Part of the difficulty in assessing risk is that the injury creating an ACL tear may independently cause a growth disturbance.[7]

One meta-analysis of 55 studies found a rate of growth disturbance following ACL reconstruction in the skeletally immature patient of 2%.[8] Similarly, Kocher et al.[9] found that 11% of knee surgeons reported a growth disturbance in skeletally immature patients following ACL reconstruction. A study that assessed physeal injury with magnetic resonance imaging (MRI) found that the graft diameter was the most critical variable affecting the volume of physeal injury, whereas increased drill angle was associated with less physeal injury.[10]

In the past, delaying ACL reconstruction until patients reached skeletal maturity was a more common approach. However, studies indicate that delaying ACL reconstruction can predispose the young athlete to chondral injury and meniscal tears as a result of recurrent knee instability. Furthermore, fewer patients and parents are willing to accept bracing and activity restriction required for nonoperative management or delayed surgical management.

Both the increasing incidence of ACL injuries in juvenile populations as well as consistently poor results with nonoperative treatment have stimulated interest in developing ACL reconstruction techniques suitable for the pediatric population.[9,11,12] Therefore, we recommend pediatric ACL reconstruction for the majority of our young active pediatric and adolescent athletes with a complete tear. Although various techniques for pediatric ACL reconstruction have been published in the literature, there is currently a lack of high-level research to suggest that one technique is superior to the others at this time.

TECHNIQUES DESCRIBED IN LITERATURE

As described in the previous and subsequent chapters, there are a variety of surgical techniques used to reconstruct the ACL in a skeletally immature patient. These techniques can be classified into three broad categories: extraphyseal reconstruction, transphyseal reconstruction, and the all-epiphyseal reconstruction. The most popular "over-the-top" reconstruction uses a pedicled iliotibial band and is known as the *modified McIntosh reconstruction*, which is an extraphyseal reconstruction using a combined extra- and intra-articular approach.[13]

The disadvantage of extraphyseal reconstructions is that they do not accurately recreate the anatomy of the ACL and may tend to overconstrain the knee, but the clinical consequence of this has yet to be fully elucidated.[31] There are numerous transphyseal or partial transphyseal techniques that involve transphyseal stabilization of an ACL graft on either the femoral or tibial side, or both.[14] Finally, a number of all-epiphyseal techniques, or techniques that involve graft fixation within the epiphysis without crossing the physes, have been popularized recently.[15–19]

The remainder of this chapter focuses on the all-epiphyseal technique developed by the co-editors of this textbook (F.A.C. & D.W.G).[16]

One of the unique aspects of this technique is that, in addition to socket positioning that is all-epiphyseal, the sockets are created from the inside out, leaving a cortical bone bridge on the lateral femoral condyle and medial proximal tibia. These sockets may allow for improved graft to bone healing.[19a] Furthermore, our technique uses suture tensioning buttons across the bone rather than tenodesis screws within the softer noncortical epiphyseal bone to achieve graft fixation.

OUR PREOPERATIVE PLANNING

Our preferred all-inside, all-epiphyseal ACL reconstruction technique is intended for skeletally immature patients with more than 3 years of growth remaining. The specific algorithm we use for addressing ACL injuries in pediatric patients is discussed in a later chapter.[20]

In preparation for ACL reconstruction in a skeletally immature patient, we routinely obtain a posteroanterior (PA) radiograph of the patient's left hand to assess skeletal age as well as standing radiographs to evaluate leg length and overall alignment. An MRI of the affected knee including physeal-specific sequences (frequency-selective fat suppressed 3D spoiled gradient recalled echo [SPGFR]) is a routine component of the workup. After the acute injury phase, patients are enrolled in a strengthening program prior to surgery, depending on their age.

Once in the operating room (OR), a thorough exam under anesthesia is performed. The landmarks are identified, including the tibial tubercle, the distal femoral physis laterally along with the popliteus tendon insertion, the joint line, the inferior pole of the patella, and the anteromedial and anterolateral arthroscopic portals (Fig. 8.1).

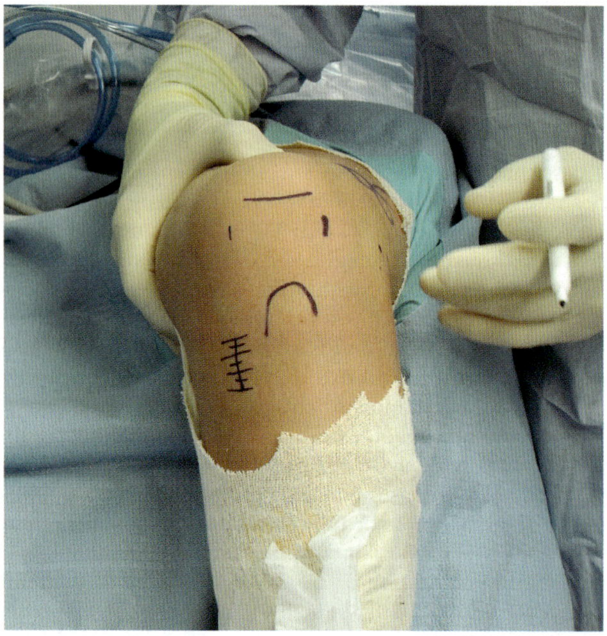

Figure 8.1. Prior to incision, the landmarks are identified including the borders of the patella, tibial tubercle, the incision for hamstring harvest, the popliteus tendon insertion, and the femoral condyles.

Step 1: Graft Harvest

Hamstring autograft is the graft choice in this skeletally immature population. A 2-cm vertical incision over the distal insertion of the hamstring tendon is the preferred approach. The vertical incision allows evaluation of the tibial physis and will be used later for placement of the tibial guide (see Step 5).

Layer one of the medial structures of the knee, the sartorius fascia, is incised.[21] The gracilis and semitendinosus tendons, which lie between the first and second layers of the knee, are identified. In general, both tendons are harvested unless the semitendinosus is large enough to provide a diameter of 9 mm or more. The semitendinosus and gracilis are left attached distally to facilitate the graftlink preparation. A native graft length of 27 cm will provide enough tissue to allow for an appropriate length for the final graftlink autograft (between 55 and 65 mm for the all-epiphyseal construct). If the combined tendons do not allow for a final diameter of at least 8.5 mm, we consider adding an allograft semitendinosus to the construct. This is discussed as a routine part of the consent preoperatively with the patient and family. Although it is clear from the literature that allograft alone is not an appropriate choice in this population of young athletes,[22,23] we have not found that adding allograft to autograft tissue when the diameter is less than 8.5 mm has been a clinical problem and we are not comfortable using a graft less than 8.5 mm in diameter given the evidence in the literature.[24–27] An alternative is to harvest the contralateral semitendinosus in this setting. Given the incidence of contralateral injury in this population of young athletes, we prefer to supplement with allograft than to harvest contralateral autograft.

Step 2: Graft Preparation

A graft preparation table is used to construct the tendon graft and to secure the surgical fixation on the femoral end (Fig. 8.2). The tendons are looped together on this table to increase the graft's diameter. The result is a shorter and thicker graft, which is biomechanically stiffer (Fig. 8.3). A TightRope RT suture (Arthrex, Naples, FL) is used on the femoral end of the graft, and a free TightRope Attachable Button System (ABS) is used for fixation on the tibial end.

Our preference is to secure the graft on both the tibial and femoral side using suspensory fixation in the form of a reverse tensioning (RT) button (TightRope RT device) and a free tensioning button (ABS device) on the tibial side using the GraftLink technique. We modified the original technique of using TightRope RT buttons on both sides, as we found that passing the tibial button through the anteromedial portal and through the tibial socket was unnecessary. The length of the graft is generally 55 to 65 mm (Fig. 8.4). If the length of the graft is too long, it will "bottom out" in one of the sockets; but if it is too short, it may compromise biologic fixation within the socket. The diameter of the graft is assessed through the same sizing block.

We also bundle the graft using four separate Ethibond sutures through and around the graft to form a more compact and denser graft. This stitch is started by passing the needle through the inner graft limb to the outer graft limb, then wrapping the suture around the graft and finally passing the needle through the outer limb back to the inner limb. This results in

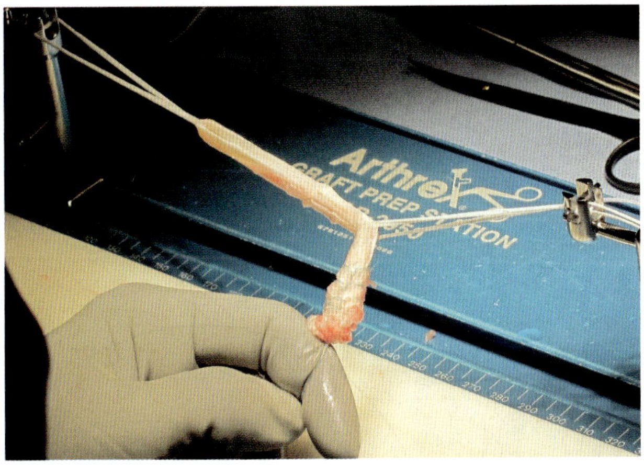

Figure 8.2. Graft is secured on the preparation station with suspensory sutures. Here, the graft has been doubled and the free ends sutured together with a FiberLoop (Arthrex) in a whipstitch. The free ends of the FiberLoop are then wrapped around the post of the tensioner to hold the graft in place. Additionally, the free ends of the graft have FiberLoop sutures that have been brought out through the free ends and are passed through the tibial aspect of the graft. These will be used for backup fixation on the ABS button and can facilitate docking the tibial end of the graft within the tibial socket.

a buried knot tucked inside the graft. This is repeated three more times to create two stitches at 15 and 20 mm from each end of the graft for four stitches total (see Fig. 8.4).

The graft is generally symmetrical throughout in diameter, approximately 9 to 11 mm. However, if one end of the graft has a greater diameter than the other, we can adjust the size of our femoral or tibial socket accordingly. While we move on to the diagnostic knee arthroscopy, the graft is pretensioned to 20 lb for 5 minutes on the back table. Following tensioning, the graft is wrapped in moist gauze and stored in a sealed plastic bag.

Step 3: Diagnostic Knee Arthroscopy and Site Preparation

Standard diagnostic knee arthroscopy is performed via anteromedial and anterolateral portals. At this time, any meniscal or chondral pathology is addressed appropriately. The ACL tear is visualized and confirmed, and the footprints are débrided. We use the anterolateral portal with a 70-degree lens to visualize the femoral footprint. We identify both footprints, débride the stumps, and leave intact portions of the ligament that do not interfere with the procedure for the theoretical benefit

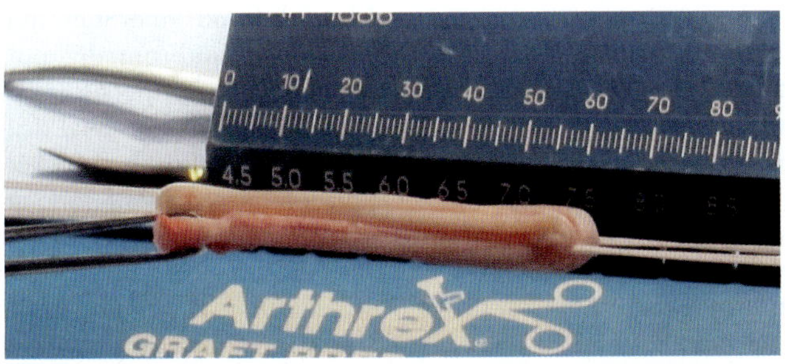

Figure 8.3. Graft length once quadrupled prior to placement of tibial and femoral suspensory sutures.

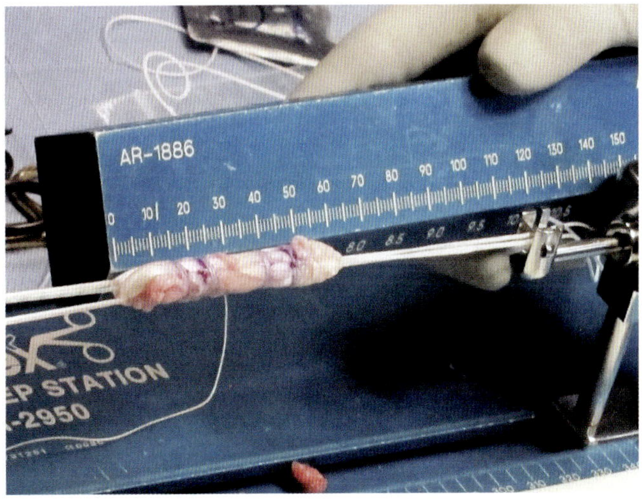

Figure 8.4. Appearance of the hamstring graft once prepared. Generally, it is between 55 and 65 mm in length prior to fixation.

of facilitating proprioception by leaving behind Pacinian corpuscles, Golgi apparatus, etc. Rubberized flexible cannulas (PassPort, Arthrex Inc., Naples, FL) are used to facilitate suture management and graft passage.

Step 4: Femoral Socket Preparation

We prepare the femoral socket first and, at this time, switch the arthroscope from the 70-degree lens in the anterolateral portal to a 30-degree lens in the anteromedial portal. We start by first placing the side-specific small-angle femoral marking hook (Arthrex) through the anterolateral portal. We have found that the optimal angle for the guide is between 90 and 95 degrees, onto the center of the femoral footprint, approximately 2 to 3 mm from the back wall. Once we have established the guide's correct intra-articular position within the ACL's femoral footprint, we need to align the trajectory of the tunnel correctly. To do this, we carefully palpate the posterolateral femoral condyle with respect to the marks we made on the distal femoral physis. The insertion of the popliteus tendon can be a useful landmark for placement of the guide pin.[28] A less than 1-cm incision is made just anterior to the lateral epicondyle, and the guide is seated onto the lateral cortex of the lateral femoral condyle.

Then, we insert a small guide pin under fluoroscopic guidance to assess its position relative to the physis and articular surfaces. After the guide pin position is verified fluoroscopically, a FlipCutter (Arthrex) of the appropriate diameter based on measurements of the graft on the back table is drilled through the stepped drill sleeve to reach the ACL footprint in the notch. Again, the position of the FlipCutter is confirmed by fluoroscopy (Fig. 8.5).

The stepped drill sleeve is then gently placed through the lateral cortex using a mallet to ensure a bone bridge of at least 7 mm between the end of the tunnel and the lateral cortex of the lateral femoral condyle. Next, the FlipCutter is deployed and the femoral socket is reamed retrograde to approximately 25 mm. The intraosseous length of the socket is noted at this time and used to mark the femoral side of the GraftLink construct to facilitate arthroscope visualization during the graft

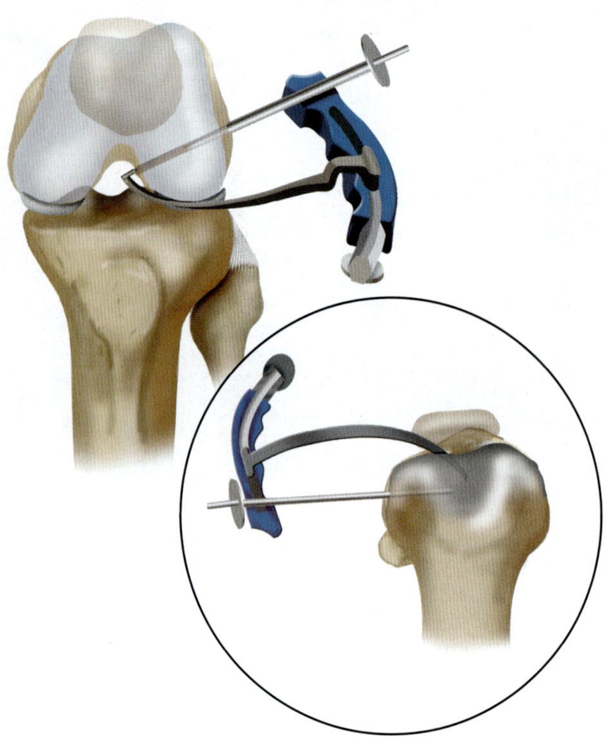

Figure 8.5. Illustration of the pediatric-specific femoral marking hook and drill sleeve. The position of the FlipCutter is confirmed prior to reverse drilling of the femoral socket.

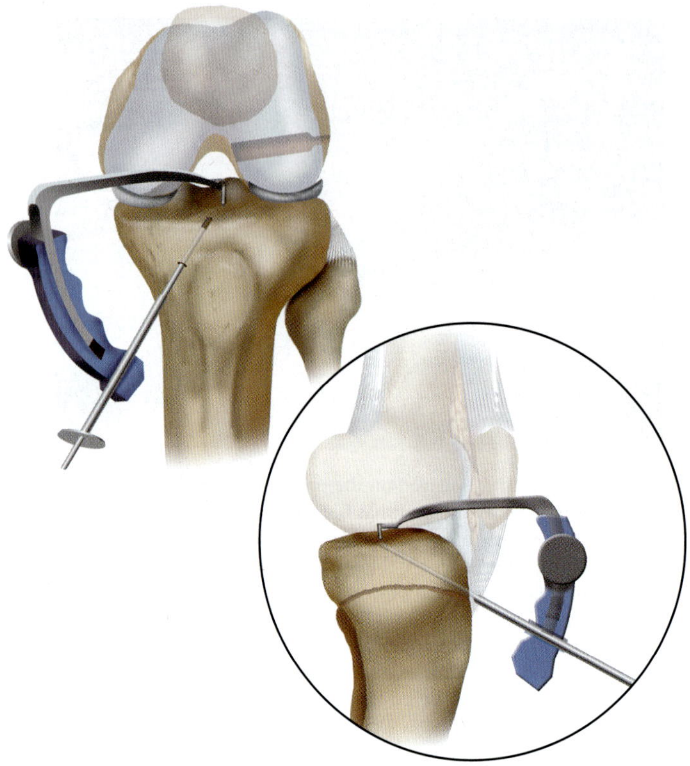

Figure 8.6. Illustration of the pediatric-specific tibial marking hook and drill sleeve. The position of the FlipCutter is confirmed prior to reverse drilling of the tibial socket.

passage step (see the following texts). Then, the FlipCutter is removed, and a FiberStick (Arthrex) is inserted through the drill sleeve and exits via the anteromedial portal for later graft passage.

Step 5: Tibial Socket Preparation

At this time, the arthroscope is returned to the anterolateral portal, and again, a 70-degree lens is used. Using a radiofrequency probe, the ACL's tibial footprint is prepared. The pediatric-specific tibial ACL guide, which is set to approximately 30 to 40 degrees, is inserted through the anteromedial portal. The correct intra-articular position of the guide on the tibial footprint of the ACL is confirmed via arthroscopic visualization. The extra-articular point of the guide is just proximal to the proximal tibial physis. Correct placement is aided by palpation of the physis through the vertical incision made for graft harvest.

The small-angle tibial marking hook (Arthrex), which is attached to the stepped drill sleeve, is inserted and placed onto the tibial footprint. This positioning is directly visualized with the arthroscope. A guide pin is generally placed and evaluated fluoroscopically to confirm correct placement within the epiphysis. The stepped drill sleeve is then gently placed through the tibial cortex using a mallet. Then the appropriate-sized FlipCutter is drilled through the guide and exits through the tibial footprint, visualized fluoroscopically and via the arthroscope in the anterolateral portal. If positioned correctly, the FlipCutter is deployed and reamed retrograde to a predetermined depth, but typically between 15 and 20 mm and a bone bridge of at least 7 mm (Fig. 8.6). A FiberStick is advanced through the guide, traversing the socket and retrieved intra-articularly to exit through the anterolateral portal for later graft passage.

Step 6: Graft Passage

The graft is passed through the anteromedial portal into the femoral socket. The intraosseous length markings on the femoral side sutures are visualized arthroscopically while docking the graft in the femoral socket to help avoid passing the RT button through the skin on the lateral side of the distal femur. The RT button is passed through the lateral femoral epiphyseal cortex, flipped, and secured onto the lateral epiphyseal cortex. Once secured, the slack is removed from the suture and it is partially tensioned. Pulling back on the graft will provide tactile feedback that the RT button is secured on the cortical bone. The strands should be pulled one at a time in 2-mm increments to advance the graft.

The tibial aspect of the graft is brought in through the anteromedial portal using the previously placed FiberStick that has been shuttled from the anterolateral to anteromedial portals. Then the TightRope suture is shuttled into the suture in the FiberStick, and that stitch is pulled through the tibial drill hole, pulling the tibial end of the graft into the tibial socket. Then a TightRope ABS button is placed onto the ABS loop attached to the tibial end of the graft. Any soft tissue blocking the path of the button to the bone needs to be cleared so the RT button can lie flush on the periosteum. Once the button abuts the medial tibial cortex, the ABS button is partially tensioned onto the medial proximal epiphyseal cortex of the tibia. Then the whipstitch sutures are loaded onto the button and secured for backup fixation.

Step 7: Graft Tensioning

Markings were placed on the graft at the 15- and 20-mm level on both the femoral and tibial side to help assess how much graft is docked into both the femoral and tibial socket. The graft is tensioned with the knee in 20 degrees of flexion, first on the femoral side and then on the tibial side. The knee is then cycled through flexion and extension 50 times and then final tensioning is performed. We recommend backing up the RT and ABS buttons by tying knots over the buttons once final tensioning has been accomplished. The graft is evaluated throughout a full range of motion under direct visualization arthroscopically. The pivot shift and Lachman tests are performed and compared to the patient's preoperative assessment. We then tie knots over the self-tensioning suspensory fixation devices. Prior to wound closure, the position of the tensioning buttons is confirmed fluoroscopically. The incisions are thoroughly irrigated and closed. A hinged knee brace locked in extension is placed in the OR.

REHABILITATION

In general, we have admitted this cohort of young athletes for one night following ACL reconstruction. Cryotherapy is applied in the postanesthesia care unit. Physical therapy begins in the hospital on postoperative day 1. Patients are weight bearing as tolerated unless they have concomitant injuries that dictate otherwise. The postoperative program is extensive and outlined in a later chapter of this textbook.

OUTCOMES

Despite the dramatic surge in ACL reconstruction surgery in pediatric patients over the past 20 years, there is still no consensus on the best technique. Historically, the physeal-sparing technique used most commonly has been the modified McIntosh, popularized by Micheli.[29,30] Although some authors have reported good outcomes with this extraepiphyseal ACL reconstruction technique,[29] recent biomechanical evidence has found that this technique may overconstrain the knee.[31,32] We have reported favorable kinematic and contact stress results in a biomechanical study of the all-epiphyseal technique.[33] Our group has also reported that the AE technique is safe with the absence of growth disturbance in a cohort of athletes following physeal-sparing techniques using SPGR MRI analysis.[33a]

When an ACL-deficient knee sustains an anterior load, increased contact pressures are noted at the posterior aspect of the tibial plateau, which may lead to degenerative changes to the meniscus and the articular cartilage.[34]

Colleagues at our institution compared the all-epiphyseal femoral technique to over-the-top and transphyseal techniques in a canine model, finding less angular deformity and better position of the femoral graft origin after growth in the all-epiphyseal model.[7] We have compared this all-epiphyseal technique to the complete transphyseal (CT) technique biomechanically and have found that the all-epiphyseal technique is superior to the CT technique, which uses vertical tunnels to avoid physeal compromise.[35]

The clinical outcomes of our all-epiphyseal ACL reconstruction technique begin with a routine imaging assessment of standing radiographs and MRI at the 6-month, 1-year, and 2-year postoperative time frames to check for growth disturbances, injury to the physis, and graft incorporation.[33a] These athletes begin standard objective testing including KT-1000, isokinetic testing and a movement assessment and return to play evaluations. Symmetry, alignment control and the ability to decelerate are assessed during progressively challenging movement patterns encountered in sport. This is indicated in preparation for return to play clearance by our multidisciplinary team.[36] The athlete and his or her parents are prepared for this process pre-operatively with the understanding that at the 6 month stage the rate-limiting step is less about the knee and more about how the body moves in space around both the ipsilateral and contralateral knees in an attempt to minimize the potential for injury to either knee.

Our group has reported on the 2 year follow-up of a group of 23 athletes following all-inside, all-epiphyseal ACL reconstructions using the technique described in this chapter.[37] There were 6 females and 17 males. The average chronologic age was 11.8 and the average skeletal age using the HSS Shorthand Bone Age method was 12.1. The majority sustained a non-contact injury during sports participation. These athletes were injured playing a number of sports and Lacrosse (38%) and Soccer (31%) were the two most common. Lachman and Pivot Shift testing were negative in all patients at final follow-up. The KT-1000 arthrometry demonstrated no significant differences between the injured and contralateral knees. Isokinetic testing revealed deficits at both 180 and 300 degrees per second to be acceptable at less than 10% deficits in those athletes cleared for return to play. Two of the 23 (8.6%) skeletally immature athletes in this study required a second surgery. One athlete sustained an ipsilateral graft rupture 10 months post-op and the second athlete required a partial medial meniscectomy 18 months post-operatively for an incompletely healed medial meniscus repair that had been performed at the index operation. The average time for return to unrestricted competitive activity after successful completion of the Movement Assessment and Return to Play process was 12.5 +/− 1.25 months from the time of surgery.

While awaiting long term clinical outcomes, the theoretical benefit of the all-inside, all-epiphyseal technique is clear. The technique fulfills both the requirements of creating an ACL reconstruction that has demonstrated favorable kinematics and contact stress results while avoiding physeal injury. Studies to date have reported in vitro biomechanical results comparing different physeal-sparing and physeal-traversing techniques and results in animal models. Long-term outcomes in pediatric patients comparing various techniques will be the most useful in determining a superior technique.

CASE

The patient is an 11-year-old male with no other medical history who presented with a left knee effusion after a twisting injury during a soccer game. His exam was notable for a moderate knee effusion and a grade IIB Lachman and 2+ pivot shift test. His preoperative standing radiographs demonstrate equal leg lengths (Fig. 8.7). On MRI, he had a complete midsubstance ACL tear (Fig. 8.8). His bone age was 11 years and 6 months by the Greulich and Pyle system. Given his growth remaining, he was indicated for an all-epiphyseal ACL reconstruction. His postoperative images demonstrate placement of the tensioning buttons (Fig. 8.9).

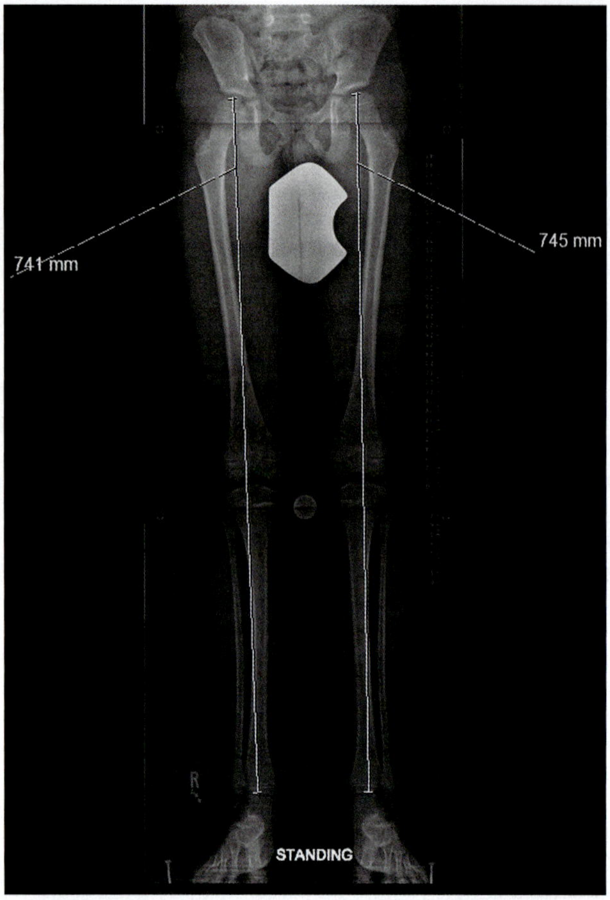

Figure 8.7. Preoperative standing radiograph demonstrating equal leg lengths.

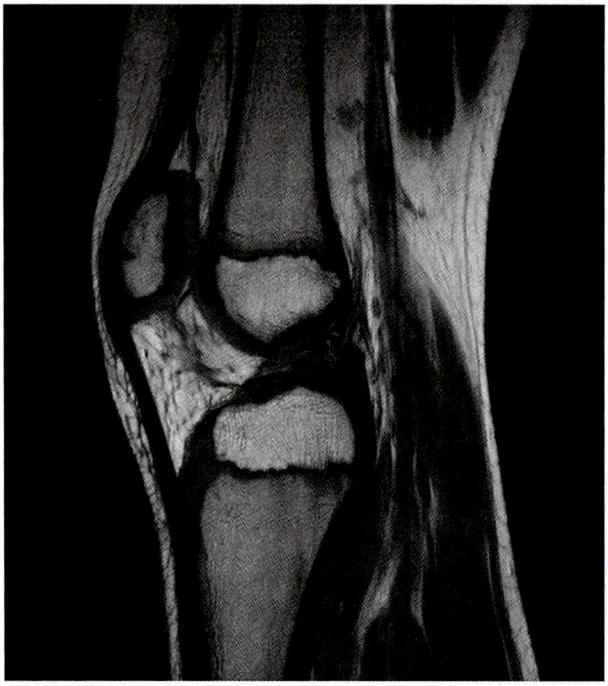

Figure 8.8. Cartilage-sensitive sagittal image of the left knee demonstrating the ACL tear in this patient.

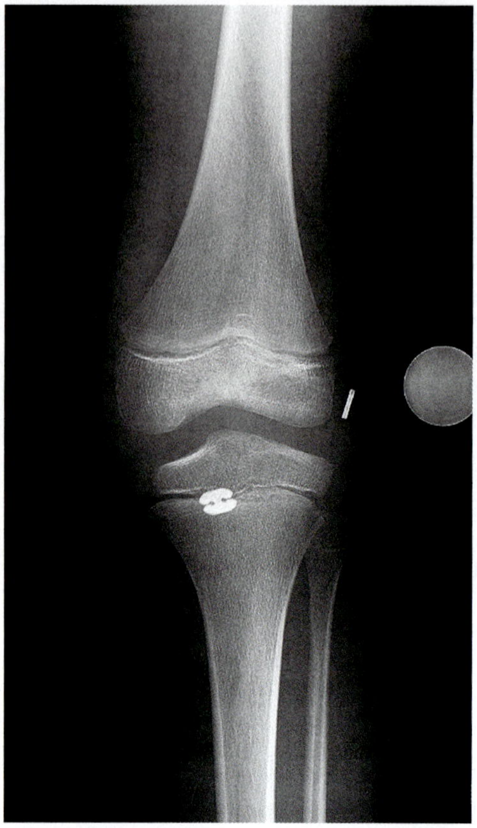

Figure 8.9. Postoperative radiograph demonstrating the location of the RT and ABS buttons on the anteroposterior (AP) view.

At his 6-month follow-up appointment, his KT-1000 was 1 mm of side-to-side difference at 30 degrees and 30 psi. Postoperative standing radiographs reveal no evidence of growth disturbance (Fig. 8.10), and MRI demonstrates no evidence of physeal compromise with excellent graft incorporation (Fig. 8.11). After completing a return to play program, he returned to sports activity at 13 months postoperative without recurrent episodes of knee instability.

Implants Used

Implants

ACL TightRope RT (AR-1588RT)
TightRope ABS (AR-1588TN)
TightRope ABS Button (AR-1588TB)

Instruments

RetroConstruction Drill Guide Set (AR-1510S)
Pin Tip Tibial Marking Hook ACL Guide, small angle
Footprint Femoral ACL Guide, small angle (R and L)
FlipCutter II (6 to 13 mm)
Drill Sleeve for RetroConstruction Drill Guide (AR 1510D)
PassPort, Arthrex Inc., Naples, FL

Suture

0 FiberWire, 38 in (blue) with Tapered Needle, 22.2 mm ½ circle
FiberStick no. 2 FiberWire, 50 in (blue) (one end stiffened)

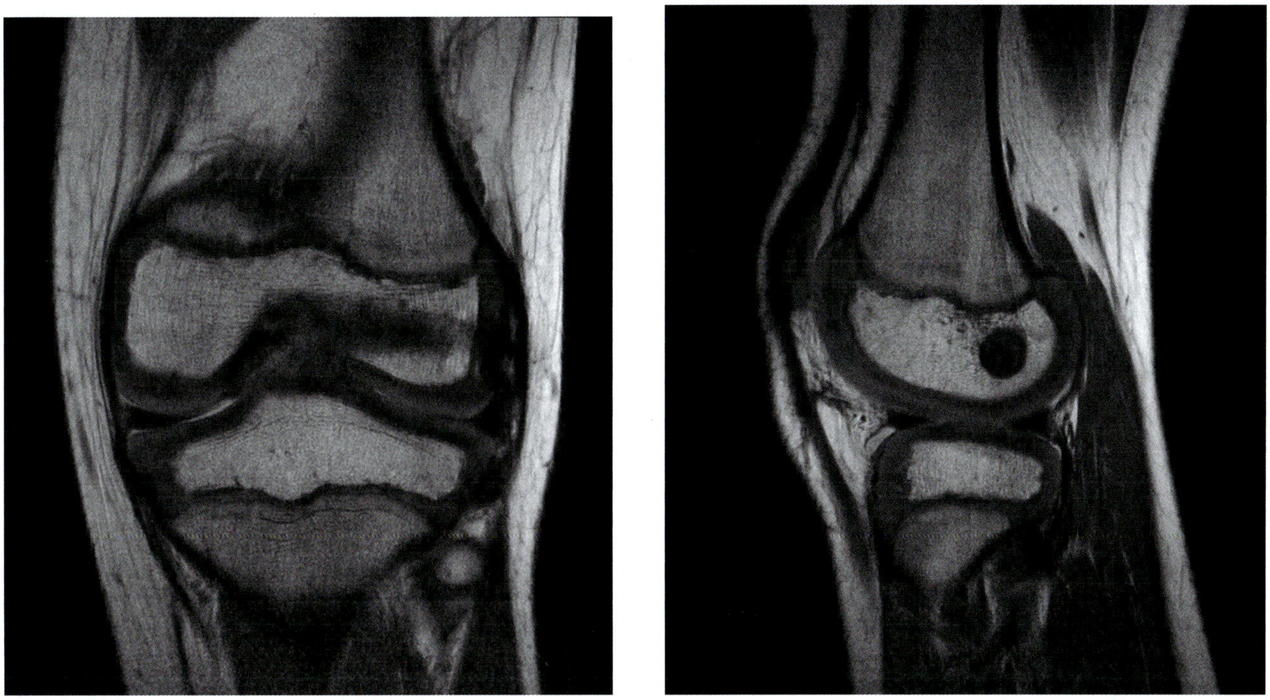

A B

Figure 8.10. Cartilage-sensitive coronal **(A)** and sagittal **(B)** images demonstrating the all-epiphyseal placement of the hamstring graft.

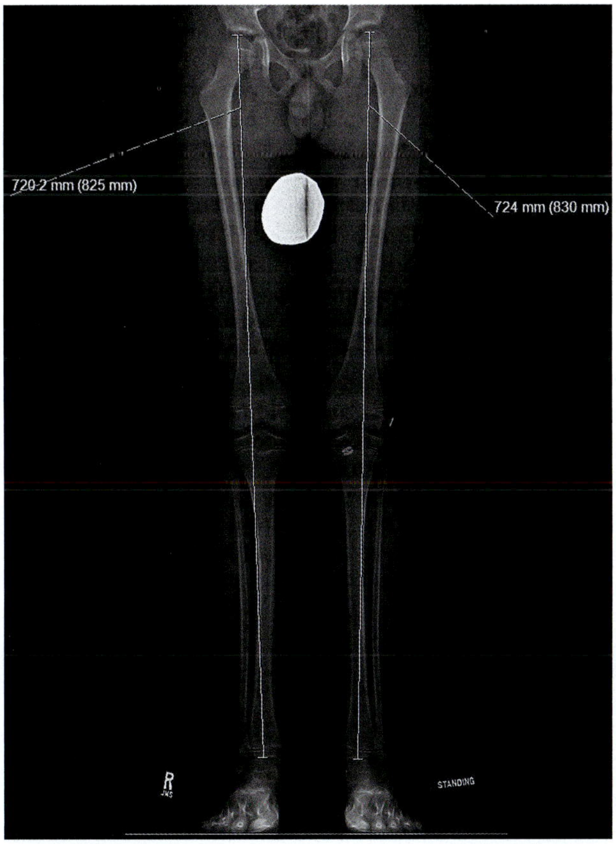

Figure 8.11. Postoperative standing radiograph demonstrating no significant leg length discrepancy.

REFERENCES

1. Lyman S, Koulouvaris P, Sherman S, et al. Epidemiology of anterior cruciate ligament reconstruction: trends, readmissions, and subsequent knee surgery. *J Bone Joint Surg Am.* 2009;91(10):2321–2328.
2. Bollen SR, Scott BW. Rupture of the anterior cruciate ligament—a quiet epidemic? *Injury.* 1996;27(6):407–409.
3. Dodwell ER, Lamont LE, Green DW, et al. 20 years of pediatric anterior cruciate ligament reconstruction in New York State. *Am J Sports Med.* 2014;42(3):675–680.
4. Granan LP, Forssblad M, Lind M, et al. The Scandinavian ACL registries 2004-2007: baseline epidemiology. *Acta Orthop.* 2009;80(5):563–567.
5. Dumont GD, Hogue GD, Padalecki JR, et al. Meniscal and chondral injuries associated with pediatric anterior cruciate ligament tears: relationship of treatment time and patient-specific factors. *Am J Sports Med.* 2012;40(9):2128–2133.
6. McCarroll JR, Rettig AC, Shelbourne KD. Anterior cruciate ligament injuries in the young athlete with open physes. *Am J Sports Med.* 1988;16(1):44–47.
7. Chudik S, Beasley L, Potter H, et al. The influence of femoral technique for graft placement on anterior cruciate ligament reconstruction using a skeletally immature canine model with a rapidly growing physis. *Arthroscopy.* 2007;23(12):1309.e1–1319.e1.
8. Frosch KH, Stengel D, Brodhun T, et al. Outcomes and risks of operative treatment of rupture of the anterior cruciate ligament in children and adolescents. *Arthroscopy.* 2010;26(11):1539–1550.
9. Kocher MS, Saxon HS, Hovis WD, et al. Management and complications of anterior cruciate ligament injuries in skeletally immature patients: survey of the Herodicus society and the ACL study group. *J Pediatr Orthop.* 2002;22(4):452–457.
10. Kercher J, Xerogeanes J, Tannenbaum A, et al. Anterior cruciate ligament reconstruction in the skeletally immature: an anatomical study utilizing 3-dimensional magnetic resonance imaging reconstructions. *J Pediatr Orthop.* 2009;29(2):124–129.

11. Guzzanti V. The natural history and treatment of rupture of the anterior cruciate ligament in children and adolescents. *J Bone Joint Surg Br.* 2003;85(4):618–619; author reply 619.
12. Lawrence JT, Argawal N, Ganley TJ. Degeneration of the knee joint in skeletally immature patients with a diagnosis of an anterior cruciate ligament tear: is there harm in delay of treatment? *Am J Sports Med.* 2011;39(12):2582–2587.
13. Kocher MS, Garg S, Micheli LJ. Physeal sparing reconstruction of the anterior cruciate ligament in skeletally immature prepubescent children and adolescents. *J Bone Joint Surg Am.* 2005;87(11): 2371–2379.
14. Hui C, Roe J, Ferguson D, et al. Outcome of anatomic transphyseal anterior cruciate ligament reconstruction in Tanner stage 1 and 2 patients with open physes. *Am J Sports Med.* 2012;40(5): 1093–1098.
15. Anderson AF. Transepiphyseal replacement of the anterior cruciate ligament using quadruple hamstring grafts in skeletally immature patients. *J Bone Joint Surg Am.* 2004;86-A(suppl 1, pt 2): 201–209.
16. McCarthy MM, Graziano J, Green DW, et al. All-epiphyseal, all-inside anterior cruciate ligament reconstruction technique for skeletally immature patients. *Arthrosc Tech.* 2012;1(2):e231–e239.
17. Lemos SE, Keating PM, Scott TP, et al. Physeal-sparing technique for femoral tunnel drilling in pediatric anterior cruciate ligament reconstruction using a posteromedial portal. *Arthrosc Tech.* 2013;2(4):e483–e490.
18. Lawrence JT, Bowers AL, Belding J, et al. All-epiphyseal anterior cruciate ligament reconstruction in skeletally immature patients. *Clin Orthop Relat Res.* 2010;468(7):1971–1977.
19. Lykissas MG, Nathan ST, Wall EJ. All-epiphyseal anterior cruciate ligament reconstruction in skeletally immature patients: a surgical technique using a split tibial tunnel. *Arthrosc Tech.* 2012; 1(1):e133–e1339.

19a. Smith P, Cook JL, Stannard J, Pfeiffer F, Kuroki K. Suspensory versus interference screw fixation for arthroscopic ACL reconstruction in a novel canine model. 2014 ACL Study group meeting; February 4, 2014; Cape Town, South Africa.

20. Fabricant PD, Jones KJ, Delos D, et al. Reconstruction of the anterior cruciate ligament in the skeletally immature athlete: a review of current concepts: AAOS exhibit selection. *J Bone Joint Surg Am.* 2013;95(5):e28.
21. Warren LF, Marshall JL. The supporting structures and layers on the medial side of the knee: an anatomical analysis. *J Bone Joint Surg Am.* 1979;61(1):56–62.
22. Pallis M, Svoboda SJ, Cameron KL, et al. Survival comparison of allograft and autograft anterior cruciate ligament reconstruction at the united states military academy. *Am J Sports Med.* 2012; 40(6):1242–1246.
23. Kaeding CC, Aros B, Pedroza A, et al. Allograft versus autograft anterior cruciate ligament reconstruction: predictors of failure from a MOON prospective longitudinal cohort. *Sports Health.* 2011;3(1):73–81.
24. Park SY, Oh H, Park S, et al. Factors predicting hamstring tendon autograft diameters and resulting failure rates after anterior cruciate ligament reconstruction. *Knee Surg Sports Traumatol Arthrosc.* 2013;21(5):1111–1118.
25. Magnussen RA, Lawrence JT, West RL, et al. Graft size and patient age are predictors of early revision after anterior cruciate ligament reconstruction with hamstring autograft. *Arthroscopy.* 2012;28(4):526–531.
26. Kamien PM, Hydrick JM, Replogle WH, et al. Age, graft size, and Tegner activity level as predictors of failure in anterior cruciate ligament reconstruction with hamstring autograft. *Am J Sports Med.* 2013;41(8):1808–1812.
27. Mariscalco MW, Flanigan DC, Mitchell J, et al. The influence of hamstring autograft size on patient-reported outcomes and risk of revision after anterior cruciate ligament reconstruction: a multicenter orthopaedic outcomes network (MOON) cohort study. *Arthroscopy.* 2013;29(12):1948–1953.
28. Xerogeanes JW, Hammond KE, Todd DC. Anatomic landmarks utilized for physeal-sparing, anatomic anterior cruciate ligament reconstruction: an MRI-based study. *J Bone Joint Surg Am.* 2012; 94(3):268–276.
29. Kocher MS, Garg S, Micheli LJ. Physeal sparing reconstruction of the anterior cruciate ligament in skeletally immature prepubescent children and adolescents. surgical technique. *J Bone Joint Surg Am.* 2006;88(suppl 1, pt 2):283–293.
30. Micheli LJ, Rask B, Gerberg L. Anterior cruciate ligament reconstruction in patients who are prepubescent. *Clin Orthop Relat Res.* 1999;(364):40–47.
31. Kennedy A, Coughlin DG, Metzger MF, et al. Biomechanical evaluation of pediatric anterior cruciate ligament reconstruction techniques. *Am J Sports Med.* 2011;39(5):964–971.
32. Sena M, Chen J, Dellamaggioria R, et al. Dynamic evaluation of pivot-shift kinematics in physeal-sparing pediatric anterior cruciate ligament reconstruction techniques. *Am J Sports Med.* 2013; 41(4):826–834.
33. McCarthy MM, Tucker S, Nguyen JT, et al. Contact stress and kinematic analysis of all-epiphyseal and over-the-top pediatric reconstruction techniques for the anterior cruciate ligament. *Am J Sports Med.* 2013;41(6):1330–1339.

33a. Nawabi DH, Jones KJ, Lurie B, et al. All-inside, physeal-sparing anterior cruciate ligament reconstruction does not significantly compromise the physis in skeletally immature athletes: a post-operative physeal magnetic resonance imaging analysis. *Am J Sports Med.* 2014;42:2933–2940.

34. Scarvell JM, Smith PN, Refshauge KM, et al. Comparison of kinematics in the healthy and ACL injured knee using MRI. *J Biomech.* 2005;38(2):255–262.
35. McCarthy MM, Jagander H, Fabricant PD, et al. Kinematics and contact stress analysis of pediatric anterior cruciate ligament reconstructions: do the all-epiphyseal and complete transphyseal reconstructions restore anterior and rotational stability? *Orthop J Sports Med.* 2014;2(suppl 2).
36. Nawabi D, McCarthy MM, Graziano J, et al. Return to play and clinical outcomes after all-inside anterior cruciate ligament reconstruction in skeletally immature athletes. *Orthop J Sports Med.* 2014; 2(2 suppl).
37. Cordasco FA, Mayer S, Graziano J, et al. All-inside, all-epiphyseal ACL reconstruction in skeletally immature athletes: return to play, incidence of second surgery and two year clinical outcomes. *2015 AANA Annual Meeting.* April 23, 2015; Los Angeles, California.

CHAPTER

9

Kristofer J. Jones

Technique: Partial Transphyseal (Hybrid)

INTRODUCTION

Anterior cruciate ligament (ACL) tears were once considered an uncommon injury in the skeletally immature population. The low incidence of ACL injury was largely attributed to the notion that the native ligament was stronger than the developing bone and physis, resulting in tibial eminence fractures (the pediatric equivalent of the ACL tear) instead of intrasubstance tears.[1] Current literature suggests a significant rise in the rate of pediatric ACL injuries.[2,3] A population-based study demonstrated the rate of ACL reconstruction per 100,000 patients aged 3 to 20 years has steadily increased over the last two decades from 17.6% in 1990 to 50.9% in 2009.[3] The peak age for ACL reconstruction was 17 years in 2009, and the overall rate of surgery was 15% higher in boys relative to girls.[3] Ultimately, this new epidemic of sports-related injuries can be largely attributed to several factors, including year-round participation, increased concentration on a single sport, and increased intensity with sport-specific training.

Treatment strategies for ACL tears in skeletally immature patients have evolved; however, there are no definitive guidelines to direct management of these injuries. In general, a nonoperative approach was historically favored in this population due to the perceived risk of physeal damage with the use of conventional ACL reconstruction techniques. However, current literature suggests nonoperative management of complete ACL tears generally leads to poor clinical outcomes and a low rate of return to athletic activity in this population.[4] Similar treatment for partial ACL tears has also demonstrated a low return to athletic activity, as Kocher et al.[5] found that approximately 33% of children (mean age, 13.7 years) in a single cohort required surgical reconstruction due to persistent instability. Ultimately, progressive instability with activity is a cause for significant concern, as recent studies demonstrate high rates (up to 61%) of progressive meniscal and articular cartilage damage in pediatric patients that are treated with nonoperative management.

Poor clinical outcomes following nonoperative management have resulted in earlier consideration for surgical intervention. There has been a considerable amount of controversy and debate regarding the optimal time to perform ACL reconstruction in patients with open physes. Similar to nonoperative management, delayed ligament reconstruction can result in progressive development of intra-articular pathology (meniscus tears, chondral damage).[8,9] A study by Lawrence et al.[9] demonstrated that young patients (younger than 14 years) who underwent surgical reconstruction greater than 12 weeks after the initial injury were noted to have an increase in the severity of medial meniscus tears and higher grade lateral and patellofemoral chondral injuries at the time of surgery. A recent meta-analysis has revealed multiple trends that currently favor early surgical stabilization over nonoperative or delayed surgical reconstruction. The authors demonstrated that conservative management resulted in greater pathologic laxity/instability, low rate of return to athletic activity, and an increased prevalence of symptomatic medial meniscus tears.[10] Ultimately, these observations have resulted in a dramatic evolution of modern surgical techniques in order to facilitate early surgical intervention and avoid iatrogenic physeal damage.

Modern operative techniques for pediatric ACL reconstruction can be divided into two primary categories: (1) anatomic and (2) nonanatomic ACL reconstruction. Specifically, anatomic techniques use bone tunnels that are placed within the region of the anatomic footprint of the ACL on both the femoral and tibial sides. Anatomic techniques can use all epiphyseal (physeal sparing), partial transphyseal, or complete transphyseal drilling to create appropriately placed bone tunnels. Conversely, nonanatomic techniques such as the modified McIntosh procedure place the graft in a nonanatomic location with fixation secured to the intermuscular septum along the lateral femur and the periosteum of the anterior tibia.[11] Ultimately, the specific technique used is dictated by individual patient factors, namely, skeletal age and growth remaining. In this chapter, we review the surgical indications and technical considerations for partial transphyseal (hybrid) ACL reconstruction. We also briefly review clinical outcomes and rehabilitation guidelines to facilitate postoperative care.

TREATMENT

Indications/Contraindications

Surgical decision making is based on several patient related factors, including (1) clinical stability of the knee, (2) associated intra-articular pathology, (3) patient activity level and goals, and (4) skeletal age. As previously discussed, current literature suggests both nonoperative and delayed surgical treatment are associated with progressive meniscal and chondral injury.[6–11] Thus, it is important to have a detailed conversation with both the child and parent to determine optimal treatment. A trial of nonoperative management consisting of activity modification, functional bracing, and an accelerated rehabilitation protocol is a reasonable treatment alternative. This approach may be best in a compliant, low-demand child who does not plan on participating in athletic activity. Additionally, some pediatric patients with partial ACL tears may benefit from a trial of nonoperative treatment.[5] Overall, any pediatric patient who demonstrates recurrent instability after a focused rehabilitation program should strongly consider operative intervention. Patients with concomitant meniscus tears or chondral injury should also consider early surgical treatment to prevent progressive injury.

In our experience, partial transphyseal (hybrid) ACL reconstruction is indicated in young adolescents with less than 2 to 3 years of skeletal growth remaining. In general, this typically includes Tanner stage 3 or 4 patients, with boys typically ranging from 13 to 16 years and girls ranging from 12 to 14 years in bone age. The Tanner staging system can be used to classify a patient's physiologic maturity. Assessment of secondary sex characteristics and specific information related to menarche can help determine physiologic age. Skeletal growth (bone age) is routinely determined using a posteroanterior (PA) radiograph of the left hand and wrist for comparison with the Greulich and Pyle atlas. This method relies on a predictable pattern of ossification to estimate skeletal age. Recently, we have transitioned to using the Hospital for Special Surgery Shorthand Bone Age Measurement Scale (see Table 5.2). This method facilitates prediction of bone age without the use of an atlas for comparison, as it relies on the recognition of a few standard radiographic findings to reliably predict bone age with accuracy that has been shown to be equivalent to use of the Greulich and Pyle atlas.[12] We routinely obtain a 51-in anteroposterior (AP) hip-to-ankle radiograph for accurate preoperative assessment of subtle limb length discrepancy and angular deformity. Preoperatively, a growth chart can be used to predict any limb length discrepancy at skeletal maturity with the use of the aforementioned radiographs.

Operative Technique and Outcomes

The partial transphyseal (hybrid) ACL reconstruction technique is a combination of physeal-sparing techniques typically used on the femur and traditional transtibial drilling performed through the physis. In general, smaller bone tunnels are created at a more vertical angle on the tibia to limit the overall cross-sectional area of the physis that is drilled. Studies have demonstrated that the prevalence of growth plate arrest increases when physeal disruption measures greater than 7% of the total physeal volume.[13] Given this unique anatomic consideration, it is possible that graft radius may be a significant contributing factor to the overall volume of physeal injury and subsequent potential for growth arrest. Additionally, some studies have found that increasing the tunnel drill angle to facilitate production of a more vertical tunnel can result in less physeal damage. Specifically, the authors noted a mean 0.2% decrease in physeal volume disrupted for every 5-degree increase in tunnel angle.[14] Given these observations, we tend to use a smaller diameter graft (approximately 7 to 8 mm) that is placed through a slightly vertical tibial tunnel.

In general, clinical outcomes following pediatric ACL reconstruction have demonstrated favorable results with high rates of return to athletic activity. Although the available literature is limited to small case series, studies investigating partial transphyseal (hybrid) techniques have shown excellent outcomes with low rates of postoperative growth arrest secondary to physeal drilling. In the largest series to date, Lipscomb and Anderson[15] reported on 24 skeletally immature children (mean age 13 years) who underwent partial transphyseal ACL reconstruction (transphyseal tibial drilling) using hamstring autograft. At a mean follow-up of 35 months, 83% of patients returned to preoperative activity levels and only one patient (4%) developed a limb length discrepancy (2 cm).[15] Andrews et al.[16] reported on eight patients (mean age 13.5 years) who were treated with hybrid fixation as the authors employed transphyseal tibial drilling and secured the fascia lata or Achilles allograft in the over-the-top position on the femur. At a mean follow-up of 58 months, the authors observed 87.5% good to excellent results with no evidence of limb length discrepancy at final follow-up.[16] A final study by Lo et al.[17] investigated five skeletally immature patients (mean age 12.9 years) who underwent hybrid reconstruction using transtibial drilling (6 mm or smaller drill tunnel) and over-the-top placement of the soft tissue autograft on the femoral side. Overall, there were 80% excellent outcomes and no evidence of limb length discrepancy at a mean follow-up of 7.4 years.

AUTHOR'S PREFERRED TREATMENT

Preoperative Setup

At our institution, we routinely use regional anesthesia prior to initiation of the case. Both fluoroscopic imaging as well as standard knee arthroscopy equipment should be available. In order to avoid inadvertent contamination and crowding of equipment, both the fluoroscopy machine and arthroscopic equipment should be placed at the opposite side of the room (opposite the operative leg). The patient is placed in the supine position on the operating room (OR) table with a sandbag placed at the foot of the bed to facilitate leg positioning throughout the case. This will allow the leg to be positioned at approximately 90 degrees of flexion during femoral and tibial tunnel drilling and precludes the need for the leg to be moved off the side of the bed or the foot of the bed to be lowered throughout the case. A side post is placed at the level of the proximal thigh and a nonsterile tourniquet is routinely applied to the leg. Prior to sterile preparation and draping, a full examination under anesthesia is performed, including anterior/posterior drawer, Lachman, and pivot shift testing as well as varus and valgus stability testing at both 0 and 30 degrees of knee flexion.

Graft Choice and Preparation

In the skeletally immature population, our favored graft source is quadrupled hamstring autograft, consisting of both gracilis and semitendinosus tendons. An allograft source is not typically used, as recent research demonstrates increased rates of graft rupture with allograft tissue in younger, active patients.[18] Following inflation of the nonsterile tourniquet, a 2-cm longitudinal incision is made along the proximal aspect of the medial tibia (2 cm medial to the tibial tubercle) to facilitate hamstring harvest. Each tendon is isolated separately and carefully harvested using a tendon stripper. The graft is subsequently prepared using the GraftLink technique (Arthrex, Naples, FL) on the back table with two suspensory devices attached at each end. We routinely use the ACL TightRope RT (Arthrex) on the femoral side and a TightRope Attachable Button System (ABS) (Arthrex) for tibial fixation. This graft construct provides cortical suspensory fixation on both the tibia and femur and is our favored technique due to the fact that it does not rely on softer epiphyseal bone for secure fixation. The overall graft length should be approximately 65 to 70 mm with a diameter of at least 8 mm. The graft is tensioned at 20 lb for 5 minutes and secured in a sterile plastic bag with a moist gauze on the back table.

Anterior Cruciate Ligament Reconstruction

Diagnostic knee arthroscopy is performed using standard anteromedial and anterolateral portals. Any concomitant pathology, including meniscus tears or chondral lesions, is addressed prior to ligament reconstruction. The torn ACL is identified and débrided to facilitate adequate visualization of the femoral and tibial footprints. We begin by preparing the femoral socket with the use of an outside-in femoral ACL guide (Arthrex) set at approximately 95 degrees within the center of the femoral footprint. This guide is placed through the anterolateral portal and the 30-degree arthroscope is placed through the anteromedial portal to provide adequate visualization during drilling (Fig. 9.1). An appropriately sized FlipCutter based on the size of the graft is then inserted distal to the physis within the epiphyseal region of the lateral condyle (Fig. 9.2). The position of the FlipCutter is confirmed with intraoperative fluoroscopy to ensure that retrograde drilling with the FlipCutter will not encroach on the distal femoral physis (Fig. 9.3). If the position is adequate, the drill sleeve is malleted through the lateral femoral cortex to ensure a minimum bone bridge of 7 mm

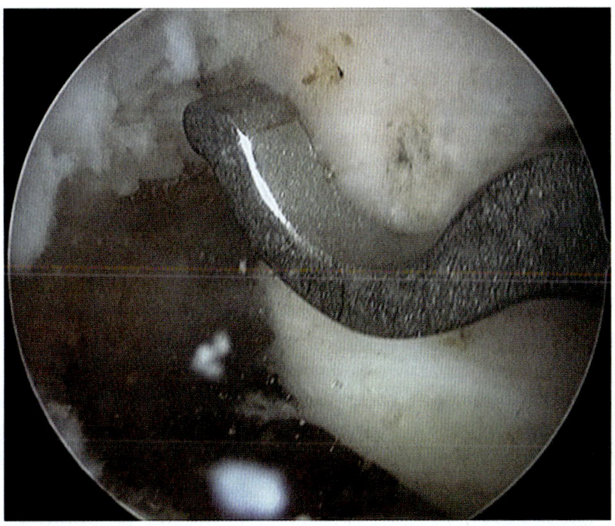

Figure 9.1. The inside-out ACL drilling guide is inserted through the anterolateral portal, and a 30-degree arthroscope is placed in the anteromedial portal to adequately visualize the back wall during drilling. We attempt to preserve a 1.5- to 2-mm back wall during femoral socket drilling.

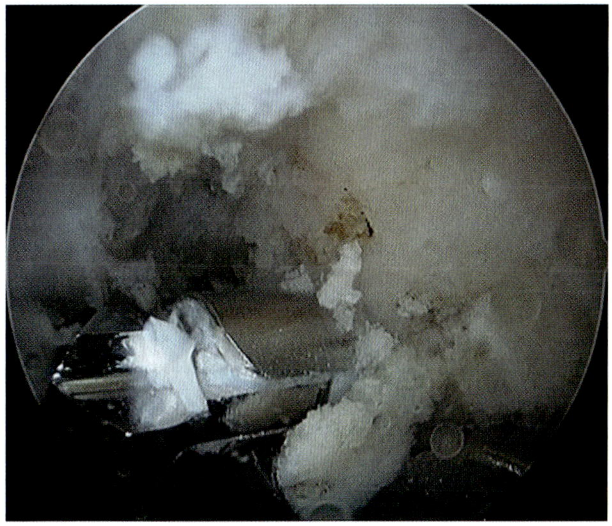

Figure 9.2. The FlipCutter is inserted under arthroscopic visualization.

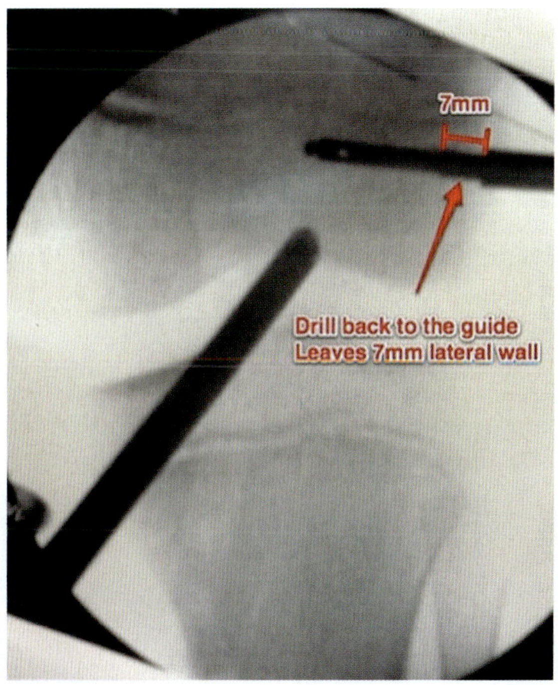

Figure 9.3. Appropriate placement of the FlipCutter is confirmed with fluoroscopic imaging.

is preserved for secure button fixation. The FlipCutter is deployed, and the socket is drilled to a depth of 20 to 25 mm. A FiberStick is inserted through the drill guide and the suture is retrieved through the anteromedial portal and secured for eventual graft passage.

On the tibial side, transtibial drilling can be performed in a retrograde or anterograde fashion using an appropriately sized reamer. We prefer to use a FlipCutter on the tibial side. The tibial ACL guide is set at approximately 55 degrees and inserted through the anteromedial portal. The guide is placed at the center of the tibial footprint, and the aiming arm is placed flush against the proximal tibia to measure the eventual length of the tibial tunnel. We prefer to place this tunnel as vertical as possible to minimize volumetric disruption of the proximal tibial physis. The FlipCutter is inserted under arthroscopic visualization, and the drill sleeve is malleted through the proximal cortical bone prior to drilling (Fig. 9.4). The FlipCutter is advanced as far as possible to provide a long socket (approximately 30 mm) with adequate preservation of the 7-mm bone bridge. It is important to note that the estimated length from the end of the femoral socket to the end of the tibial socket should be at least 10 mm longer than the graft to ensure the graft can be appropriately tensioned (i.e., avoid "bottoming out") (Fig. 9.5). A TigerStick is inserted and retrieved through the anteromedial portal. One important step to note is that the tibial and femoral passing sutures (i.e., FiberStick/TigerSticks) should be retrieved together to avoid creation of a soft tissue bridge that may hinder graft passage.

The graft is initially passed in a retrograde fashion through the anteromedial portal using the femoral passing suture. A 70-degree arthroscope is inserted through the anterolateral portal to visualize the cortical button pass through the femoral socket and deploy along the lateral femoral cortex. Once the button is secured to the cortex, initial graft tensioning to a depth of 10 to 15 mm is performed. We typically place 10- and 20-mm markings on the graft to help determine the amount of graft that is docked within the socket. It is important to note that we do not fully seat the graft within the femoral socket until tibial side graft passage is complete. The TightRope ABS is then secured with a cinch suture to avoid inadvertent tightening of the TightRope as the graft is passed. The tails from the graft are loaded with the cinch suture into the TightRope ABS and the graft is docked within the tibial socket to a depth of approximately 20 mm. The ABS button is secured to the TightRope ABS for secure tibial fixation. We then turn our attention back to the femoral socket, as the TightRope RT is now fully tensioned to completely seat the femoral side of the graft within the socket with the knee in extension. The knee is cycled through full flexion and extension and the tightrope ABS on the tibial side is tightended and secured to the ABS button with standard knot tying techniques. Using an arthroscopic knot pusher, the free ends of the tightrope RT can be sequentially tied down to the femur. The graft is probed to ensure excellent tension, and the knee is placed in full extension to check for graft impingement (Fig. 9.6).

Postoperative imaging is obtained at the first follow-up visit, including AP and lateral radiographs of the knee (Fig. 9.7). Subsequent hip-to-ankle radiographs are obtained at 1 year to evaluate limb length and alignment. A magnetic resonance imaging (MRI) can also be obtained to evaluate the status of the femoral and tibial physes at 1 year (Fig. 9.8).

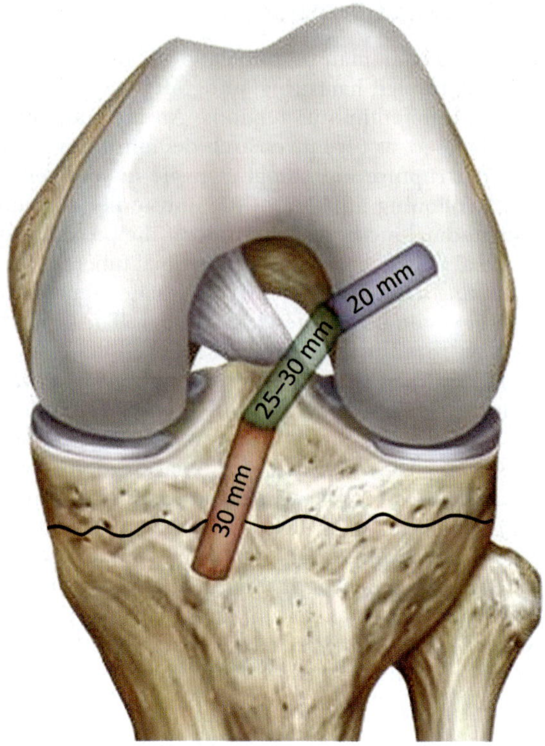

Figure 9.5. It is important to measure the estimated length of the tibial tunnel prior to tibial socket drilling. The overall length of the graft should be at least 10 mm less than the estimated combined length of intra-articular graft (30 mm) and the tibial (30 mm)/femoral (20 mm) sockets.

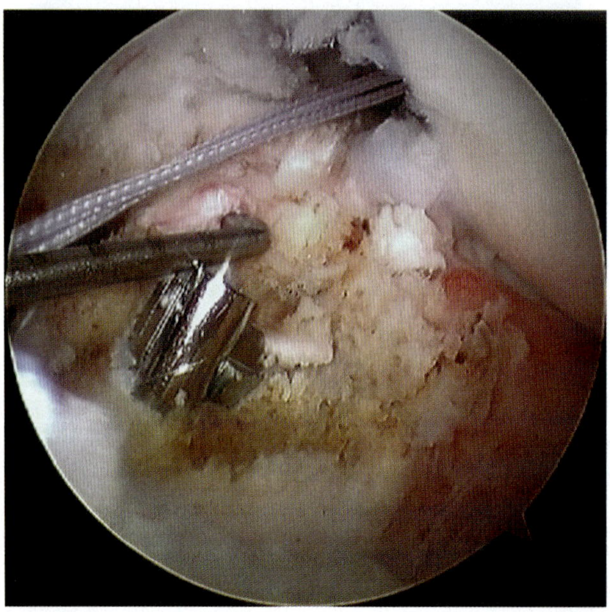

Figure 9.4. The FlipCutter is inserted into the center of the tibial footprint and deployed for drilling.

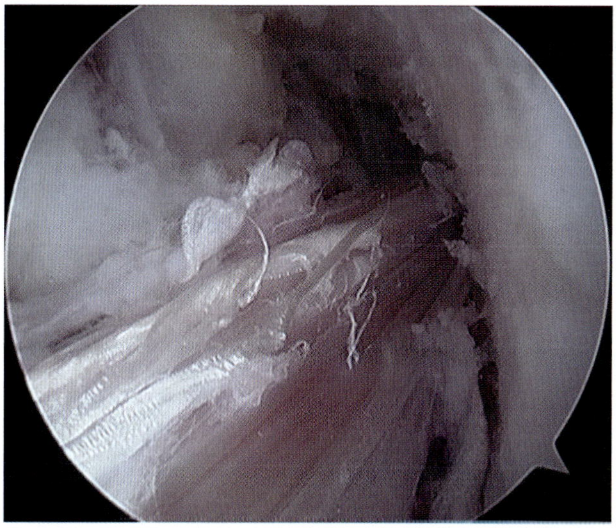

Figure 9.6. The leg is placed into full extension to check for any evidence of notch or wall impingement.

List of Equipment

- Hamstring tendon stripper
- Graft Prep Station
- Arthrex ACL TightRope RT (AR-1588RT)
- TightRope ABS (AR-1588TN)
- TightRope ABS Button (AR-1588TB)
- FiberStick no. 2 (AR-7209)
- TigerStick no. 2 (AR-7209-T)
- Retroconstruction drill guide set for FlipCutter technique (AR-1510S)
- Assorted sizes of FlipCutters (AR-1204AF)

Rehabilitation

In this young patient population, early focused physical therapy is important to ensure successful clinical outcomes. It is important to consider the patient's age and maturity level to guide appropriate management, as compliance with restrictions can be difficult in the pediatric population. A complete description of the postoperative rehabilitation program will be presented in Chapter 12.

REFERENCES

1. DeLee JC, Curtis R. Anterior cruciate ligament insufficiency in children. *Clin Orthop Relat Res.* 1983;172:112–118.
2. Arbes S, Resinger C, Vecsei V, et al. The functional outcome of total tears of the anterior cruciate ligament (ACL) in the skeletally immature patient. *Int Orthop.* 2007;31(4):471–475.
3. Dodwell ER, LaMont LE, Green DW, et al. 20 years of pediatric anterior cruciate ligament reconstruction in New York State. *Am J Sports Med.* 2014;42(3):675–680.
4. McCarroll JR, Rettig AC, Shelbourne KD. Anterior cruciate ligament injuries in the young athlete with open physes. *Am J Sports Med.* 1988;16(1):44–47.
5. Kocher MS, Micheli LJ, Zurakowski D, et al. Partial tears of the anterior cruciate ligament in children and adolescents. *Am J Sports Med.* 2002;30(5):697–703.

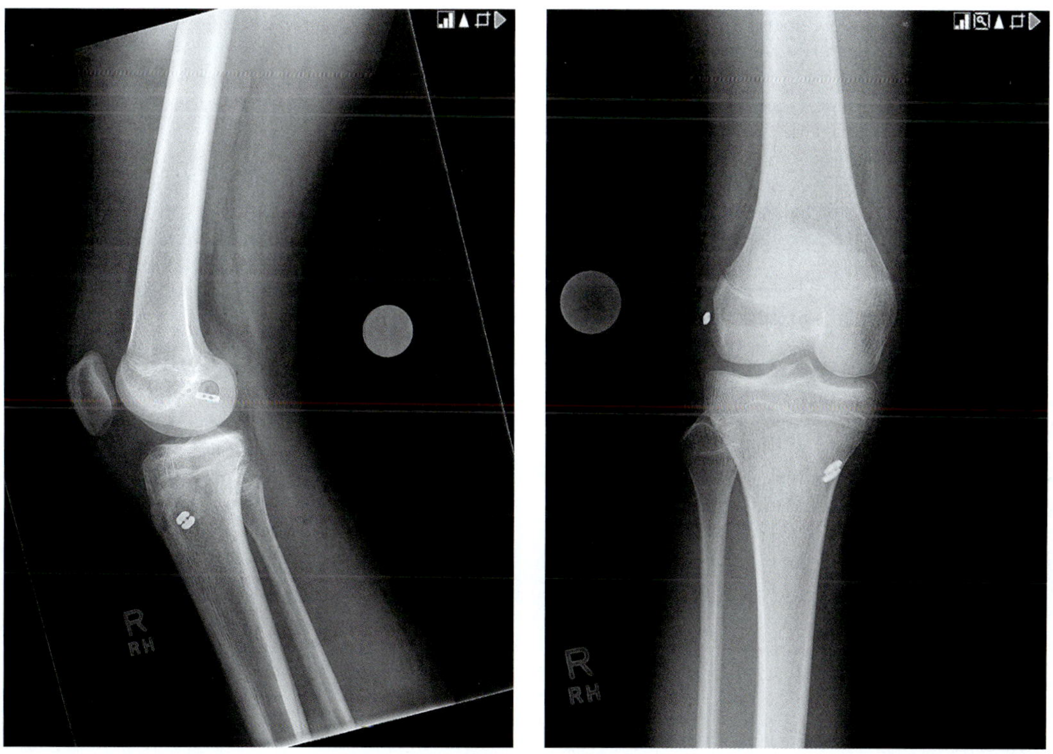

Figure 9.7. AP and lateral radiographs demonstrating appropriately placed femoral fixation within the epiphysis along with a cortical ABS button along the proximal tibia.

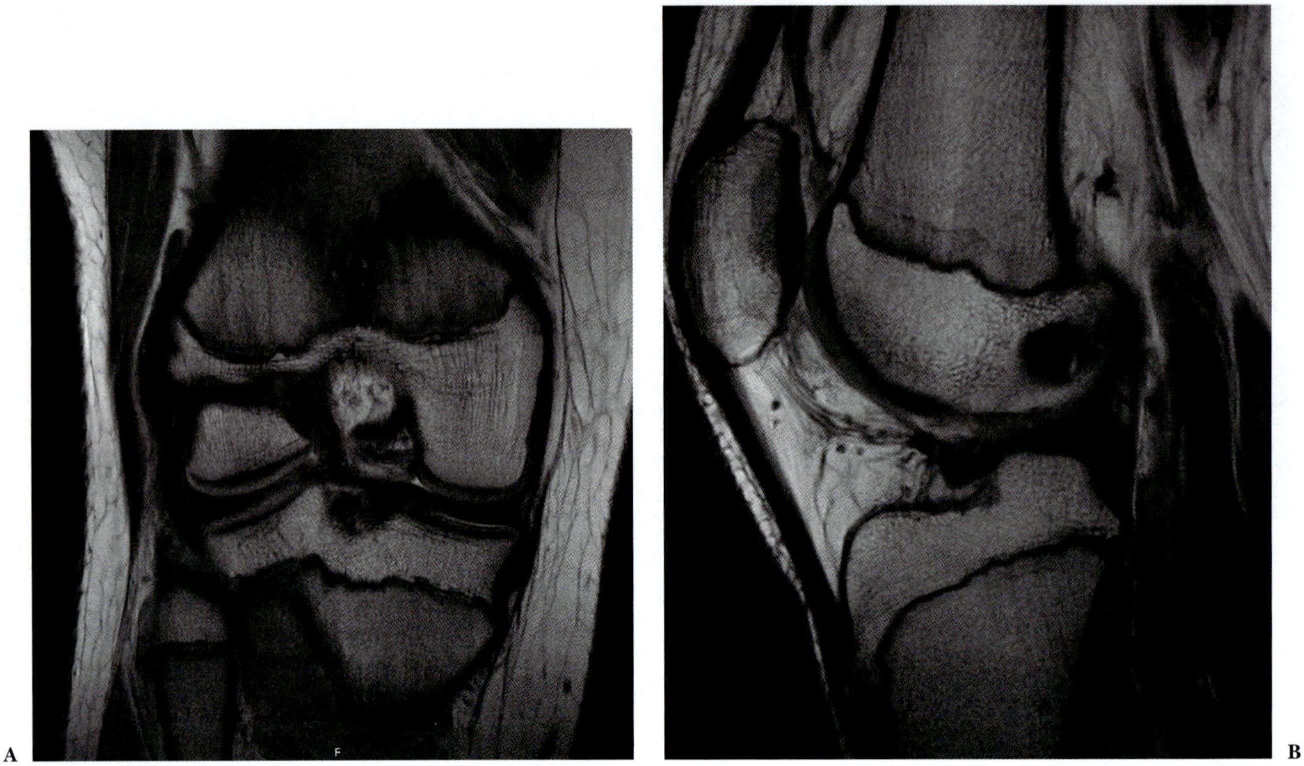

Figure 9.8. **A,B.** MRI (coronal and sagittal views) of the knee obtained at 1 year demonstrates the graft is intact with no evidence of physeal damage/arrest.

6. Graf BK, Lange RH, Fujisaki CK, et al. Anterior cruciate ligament tears in skeletally immature patients: meniscal pathology at presentation and after attempted conservative treatment. *Arthroscopy.* 1992;8(2):229–233.
7. Aichroth PM, Patel DV, Zorrilla P. The natural history and treatment of rupture of the anterior cruciate ligament in children and adolescents. A prospective review. *J Bone Joint Surg Br.* 2002;84(1):38–41.
8. Millett PJ, Willis AA, Warren RF. Associated injuries in pediatric and adolescent anterior cruciate ligament tears: does a delay in treatment increase the risk of meniscal tear? *Arthroscopy.* 2002; 18(9):955–959.
9. Lawrence JT, Argawal N, Ganley TJ. Degeneration of the knee joint in skeletally immature patients with a diagnosis of an anterior cruciate ligament tear: is there harm in delay of treatment? *Am J Sports Med.* 2011;39(12):2582–2587.
10. Ramski DE, Kanj WW, Franklin CC, et al. Anterior cruciate ligament tears in children and adolescents: a meta-analysis of nonoperative versus operative treatment. *Am J Sports Med.* 2014;42(11):2769–2776.
11. Kocher MS, Garg S, Micheli LJ. Physeal sparing reconstruction of the anterior cruciate ligament in skeletally immature prepubescent children and adolescents. *J Bone Joint Surg Am.* 2005; 87(11):2371–2379.
12. Heyworth BE, Osei DA, Fabricant PD, et al. The shorthand bone age assessment: a simpler alternative to current methods. *J Pediatr Orthop.* 2013;33(5):569–574.
13. Guzzanti V, Falciglia F, Gigante A, et al. The effects of intra-articular ACL reconstruction on the growth plates of rabbits. *J Bone Joint Surg Br.* 1994;76(6):960–963.
14. Shea KG, Grimm NL, Belzer JS. Volumetric injury of the distal femoral physis during double-bundle ACL reconstruction in children: a three-dimensional study with use of magnetic resonance imaging. *J Bone Joint Surg Am.* 2011;93(11):1033–1038.
15. Lipscomb AB, Anderson AF. Tears of the anterior cruciate ligament in adolescents. *J Bone Joint Surg Am.* 1986;68(1):19–28.
16. Andrews M, Noyes FR, Barber-Westin SD. Anterior cruciate ligament allograft reconstruction in the skeletally immature athlete. *Am J Sports Med.* 1994;22(1):48–54.
17. Lo IK, Kirkley A, Fowler PJ, et al. The outcome of operatively treated anterior cruciate ligament disruptions in the skeletally immature child. *Arthroscopy.* 1997;13(5):627–634.
18. Kaeding CC, Aros B, Pedroza A, et al. Allograft versus autograft anterior cruciate ligament reconstruction: predictors of failure from a MOON prospective longitudinal cohort. *Sports Health.* 2011;3(1):73–81.

Nathan A. Mall
George A. Paletta, Jr.

CHAPTER

10

Technique: Complete Transphyseal Hamstring Autograft

INTRODUCTION

The number of anterior cruciate ligament (ACL) reconstructions performed in the United States has been increasing, with the most significant rises seen in patients younger than the age of 20 years.[1] Long-term data demonstrates a clear advantage with ACL reconstruction over conservative treatment in terms of risk of surgery for meniscal or cartilage damage, Tegner activity scores, and rotational instability in the knee (positive pivot shift).[2] This data has caused a paradigm shift in which most orthopedic surgeons would recommend surgical intervention for ACL tears even in skeletally immature patients. Previously, the risk of damage to the growth plate was thought to override any risk resulting from an unstable knee and patients were typically given an ACL brace and restricted from sports. Currently, the risk of the irreversible meniscal or cartilage damage is thought to outweigh the small risk of growth plate injury and possible resultant malalignment or limb length discrepancy.[3]

Several techniques have been described for ACL reconstruction in the still skeletally immature athlete. Some authors have proposed algorithms based on skeletal age and projected growth remaining to assist surgeons in determining the proper reconstruction procedure for each individual patient.[4] Each proposed technique has its unique associated technical challenges and potential complications. Transphyseal reconstruction can provide an anatomic type reconstruction and avoid some of the potential complications related to other techniques with minimal risk to the growth plate. This chapter outlines the technical pearls and data supporting transphyseal hamstring autograft reconstruction in the skeletally immature ACL-injured patient.

GRAFT SELECTION

Bone Plug versus Soft Tissue

Bone-patellar tendon-bone (BTB) autografts have been considered as the gold standard ACL graft by many surgeons. However, the characteristics and biomechanical profile of the BTB autograft is not necessarily the closest to that of the native ACL.[5] Some authors have raised concern over placing a bone plug, screw, or both across the physis, believing that this may increase the risk of physeal closure.[6] Two studies, one using periosteum and the other using bone plugs, performed BTB autografts in children with open physes. Neither study reported significant growth disturbance with this technique, although the bone plug or periosteum was placed proximal to growth plate with suspensory cortical fixation. In using these techniques effectively, a soft tissue graft was used across the physis. Although no large studies have evaluated the effect of placing a bone plug across a growing physis, it is generally accepted that this should be avoided, as the risk of formation of a physeal bar would be high. Additionally, harvest of a BTB graft in the skeletally immature would result in violation of the tibial tubercle apophysis with risk of premature closure of the anterior aspect of the proximal tibial physis and the development of a recurvatum deformity. Thus, hamstring grafts have become the gold standard in the skeletally immature patient.[6–9]

Autograft versus Allograft

The literature documents clear differences in revision rates for primary ACLs done with allograft and autograft in young, athletic patients. In a study evaluating 120 cadets entering the U.S. Military Academy, the authors found a 7.7-fold increase in failure rate following ACL reconstruction using allograft as compared with autograft.[10] Ellis et al.[11] found a 15-fold increase in revisions in patients who were skeletally mature but whose age at time of surgery was younger than 18 years when BTB allograft was used as compared with BTB autograft. Another study evaluated risk factors for revision ACL reconstruction and again demonstrated increased graft failure in the young patient (odds ratio, 0.40 for 10-year increase in age) and with allograft tissue (odds ratio, 3.97) used for the ACL reconstruction.[12] Inacio et al.[13] evaluated graft choice and fellowship status as well as case volume, finding that non–fellowship-trained surgeons and low-volume surgeons were more likely to choose allografts. Considering these factors, the authors strongly prefer autograft tissue for ACL reconstruction in the skeletally immature.

Graft Size

Magnussen et al.[14] found that a graft of 8-mm diameter or less produced an odds ratio of 2.20 for failure and subsequent revision. Interestingly, however, the odds ratio for revision of patients younger than the age of 20 years was 18.97. When closely evaluating this study, 16 of the 18 patients requiring revision were both younger than age 20 years and grafts are smaller than 8 mm, making it impossible to differentiate if graft size, age, or both are the true factors in the higher risk of revision. Similarly, a study by the Multicenter Orthopaedic Outcomes Network (MOON) group noted that the only revisions occurred in patients with grafts less than 8 mm; however, 13 of the 14 revisions occurred in patients aged 18 years or younger. Both these studies suggest there may be a higher failure and revision rate in younger patients. The relationship between graft size and failure may not be fully elucidated, as patient age seems to be a confounding factor. However, in the MOON group study, of the 85 patients aged 18 years and younger, only 14 had grafts measuring 8 mm or larger and none of those required a revision.[15]

In fact, grafts too large may also be a problem, leading to graft impingement against the intercondylar notch, lateral wall, or posterior cruciate ligament (PCL).[16–18] Ichiba et al.[18] found that the ACL insertion on the tibia correlated with height and weight of the patient. Both the height and area of the lateral wall of the intercondylar notch have been shown to correlate with the native ACL footprint size on both the femur and the tibia. Another study evaluated the size of various grafts compared with the native footprint, demonstrating that the semitendinosus and gracilis combined hamstring graft may be too big compared to the native ACL. However, this study did not evaluate patient size or bony dimensions in relation to native ACL size or graft size. Thus, perhaps, size of the graft should be based on normative values related to the size of patient. Once these values are noted, augmentation of grafts with cadaveric or suture material may be used for patients with abnormally small hamstring or patellar tendons.

TRANSPHYSEAL DATA

Studies of Effects of Physeal Involvement

Magnetic resonance imaging (MRI) studies of transphyseal techniques demonstrated a mean destruction of the femoral physis of 5.4% using a 9-mm drill. The maximum amount of destruction was 8.8% of the femoral physis, which depended on the obliquity of the tunnel.[19] At the tibial insertion, the mean was 3.8% of the total volume of the physis, with a maximum of 6.6%, again with 9-mm tunnels. In an MRI study of patients undergoing transphyseal reconstruction, the authors found a bone tunnel-to-growth plate ratio of less than 3% in both the femur and the tibia.[20] These numbers are important in light of data from a study performed by Guzzanti et al.[8] in rabbits, which demonstrated injury involving 3% of the cross-sectional area of the femur and 4% of the tibial cross-sectional area as yielding low risk for subsequent deformity. No femoral deformities occurred, and 3 of 21 developed tibial deformities but no epiphysiodesis occurred.[8]

All-epiphyseal techniques require intraoperative fluoroscopy, as the tunnels must be assured to be below the femoral physis. If errant tunnel placement occurs, this could destroy up to 50% of the physis, as the tunnel lies parallel to the physis. An anatomic study of pediatric and fetal femurs demonstrated that the femoral physis was on average about 3 mm from the femoral ACL insertion. The data from this study suggest that transverse tunnels attempting to stay distal to the femoral physis (all-epiphyseal technique) would require at maximum a 5-mm-diameter reamer or less and provide for no margin of error before physeal destruction would occur.[21]

Animal Model Studies

Animal studies can help us better understand the growing physis; however, the typical models use rabbits and dogs whose physes grow faster than in children. Such differences in growth rates can confound some findings and possibly exaggerate any deformity noted. The previously mentioned study by Guzzanti et al.[8] used a rabbit model and found minimal damage to the physis, yet 3 of 21 developed tibial deformity despite no physeal bridge forming. Another study using a canine model cautioned against overtensioning of the graft. In this beagle model, significant valgus deformity of the distal femur and varus deformity of the proximal tibia occurred despite no physeal bar formation when the ACL graft was overtensioned.[22] A study using a canine model demonstrated a protective effect of placing a soft tissue graft across the growing physis. Using fascia lata, the knees with a soft tissue graft had no evidence of bony physeal bridge, whereas the control group where tunnels were drilled and no graft was placed developed a physeal bony bridge.[6] Similar results were demonstrated in a rabbit study where empty tunnels produced a bone bridge, whereas tunnels filled with a soft tissue graft reduced the development of bony bridges and incidence of angular deformity. The addition of mesenchymal stem cells, however, was protective against the development of bone bridges or angular deformities.[23]

Clinical Studies

Clinical studies have demonstrated little risk of growth disturbance with high success rates and high levels of return to sports participation following ACL reconstruction in the skeletally immature.[3,24–32] Several recent studies have evaluated transphyseal reconstructions, following patients until skeletal maturity, and have found little risk of growth disturbance and excellent stability. Many studies have demonstrated that transphyseal reconstruction is safe and effective.[25,29,32–34] In a study of very young patients (Tanner stage 1 or 2), there was only 1 out of 32 patients who developed a very minor valgus deformity not requiring treatment.[35] Gebhard et al.,[33] in a multicenter study, found no difference between hamstring grafts, BTB, quadriceps tendon, and fascia lata grafts in terms of outcomes, failure, or growth disturbance. In the same study, 66 of 68 patients returned to the same level of preoperative sport participation.

CRITICAL PRINCIPLES

There are several critical principles that must be adhered to when performing ACL reconstruction in the skeletally immature individual. Minimizing injury to the physis is the primary principle. Drilling is performed using high-torque, low-speed reamers to minimize potential thermal damage to the physis. Drills should only be passed one time. Multiple drill passes must be avoided. The smallest possible tunnels are used to minimize the cross-sectional area or volume violation of the physes. Ideally, drill bits that vary in size by 0.5 mm are used. Additionally, tunnel obliquity is minimized. The second critical principle is the use of soft tissue grafts placed so that they traverse the physes within the tunnels. This minimizes the risk of premature physeal closure or bar formation. The final key principle is fixation placed away from the physes. Fixation devices traversing the physes must be avoided.

AUTHORS' PREFERRED SURGICAL TECHNIQUE

Our preferred technique is transphyseal hamstring autograft reconstruction using suspensory femoral fixation proximal to the femoral physis and tibial fixation distal to the tibial physis. Once the patient is asleep, we routinely perform an examination under anesthesia. In this setting, the pivot shift examination is more reliable and can be used to confirm rotational instability in the knee, which is important in this population, as partial ACL injuries are quite common. A full examination should be undertaken, including varus and valgus stress testing at 0 and 30 degrees, dial testing, and posterior drawer to rule out associated instability patterns.

Graft Harvest

After confirmation of ACL insufficiency and demonstration of a positive pivot shift, the hamstring tendons are harvested. Hamstring harvest is performed using the standard technique of a longitudinal incision over the insertion of the hamstring tendons on the anteromedial tibia. In thin or small patients, the semitendinosus and gracilis tendons can be palpated. When not easily palpable, a skin incision is created 2 cm medial and 2 cm distal to the tibial tubercle. This location results in an incision that will typically be centered over the tibial insertion of the semitendinosus and gracilis tendons.[36] The oblique incision is used in an attempt to minimize risk of injury to the infrapatellar branches of the saphenous nerve. The semitendinosus and gracilis tendons are located in the second layer of the medial knee, underlying the sartorial fascia. The sartorial fascia is incised along its normal anatomic course in line with the surgical incision. The semitendinosus and gracilis tendons are identified and isolated using a Penrose drain. The tendons are left attached to the tibia until complete harvest has been performed to maximize length of the tendon graft. Care is taken to release all bands to the gastrocnemius muscle to avoid premature transection of the tendon when using the tendon stripper for harvest. Both the semitendinosus and gracilis are then cut sharply from the tibia. The grafts are prepared on the back table. The muscle is removed using the back of a knife handle. The tendon ends are whipstitched. The quadruple strand graft is sized to the nearest 0.5-mm diameter to allow the snuggest fit possible within the tibial and femoral tunnels. The prepared graft is kept in a moist sponge until ready for use.

Arthroscopy and Tunnel Drilling

Standard diagnostic arthroscopy is performed, and any meniscal or cartilage pathology is addressed. A transtibial technique is used to create a slightly less oblique femoral tunnel with the goal of preserving more of the physis. For postmenarche females and Tanner stage 4 or 5 males, we use the same techniques as we would in adults. In the transtibial approach, the tibial tunnel is drilled first. Transtibial techniques have been described that still allow the surgeon to get low on the femoral wall into an anatomic location.[37,38] The tibial drill guide is placed in the appropriate position, using the anterior horn of the lateral meniscus, PCL, and intermeniscal ligament as landmarks. The anterior aspect of the native ACL lies just behind the intermeniscal ligament, and a common mistake is to place this tunnel too far posterior. When performing a transtibial drilling technique, the tibial tunnel is angled slightly from medial to lateral to allow for more lateral position of the femoral tunnel (Fig. 10.1). Most importantly, the tunnel starting point on the proximal medial tibial metaphysis is placed more medially than in the adult to ensure the tibial tubercle is avoided. In addition, the longest tibial tunnel possible is created. Drilling is done using the appropriate drill size to the nearest 0.5 mm. High-torque, low-speed drilling is performed to minimize risk of thermal damage to the physis. The drill is passed one time. Repeated drill passage is avoided.

The femoral tunnel is drilled using a transtibial technique (Fig. 10.2). An over-the-top guide is placed with guide pin centered on the ACL footprint. Some fibers of the ACL are left at the femoral footprint to allow for optimal identification of tunnel placement. A guide pin is placed, and an acorn-type drill bit is used to create the femoral tunnel. The

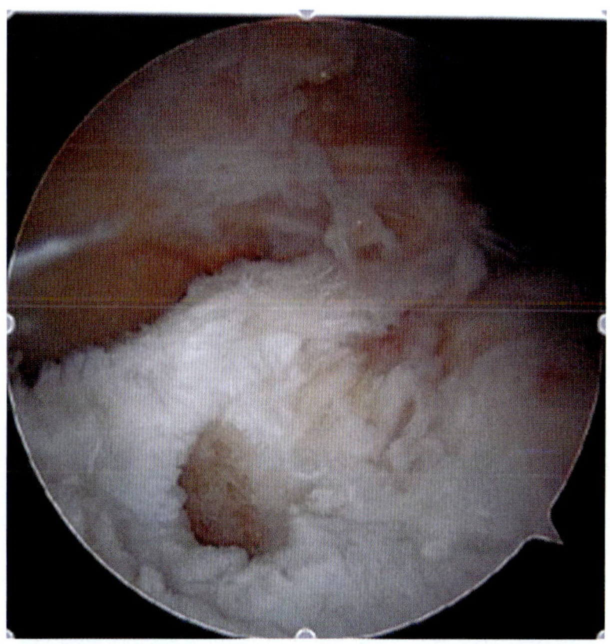

Figure 10.1. Tibial tunnel position for a skeletally immature patient. This will be a transtibial technique, yet the tunnel is quite round.

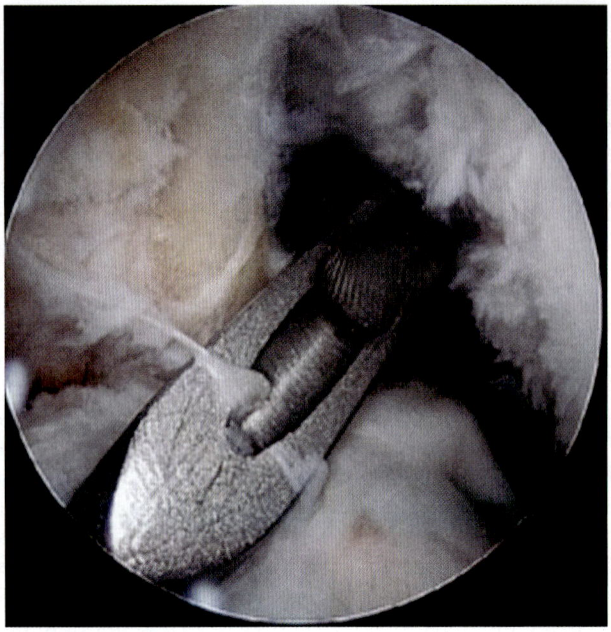

Figure 10.2. Femoral-aiming device through the tibial tunnel for a skeletally immature patient. Note the near-anatomic position; however, the angle is more vertical to minimize the damage to the physis.

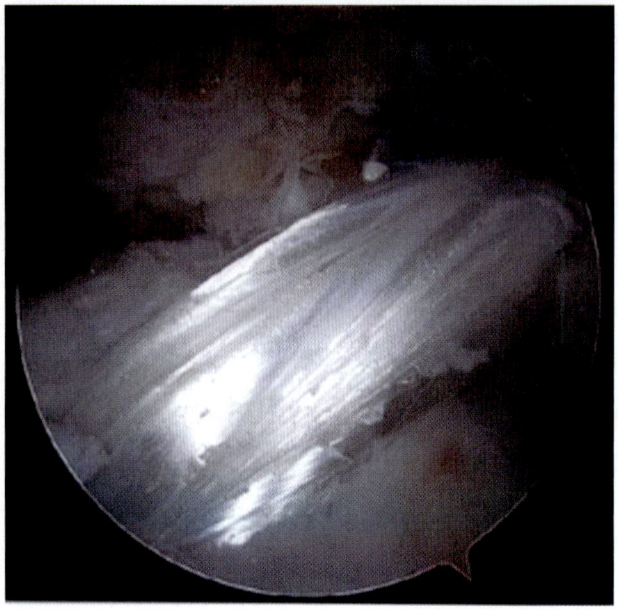

Figure 10.3. Final construct of a skeletally immature ACL reconstruction with a hamstring autograft. The graft maintains good obliquity through the knee joint.

drill is passed by hand through the tibial tunnel. The same principle of high-torque, low-speed drilling is employed. The femoral tunnel is drilled to the lateral femoral cortex without violation of the cortex. This creates a long femoral tunnel that will ensure the hamstring graft will traverse the distal femoral physis.

Graft Passage and Fixation

Once the tunnels have been created, the graft is passed retrograde, under direct arthroscopic visualization, through the tibial tunnel and into the femoral tunnel. Our preferred femoral fixation is the ACL TightRope (Arthrex, Inc., Naples, FL). The arthroscope can be used to make sure the cortical button exits the socket and flips on the femoral cortex. We routinely use intraoperative fluoroscopy to confirm deployment and engagement of the fixation button. The graft is then advanced into the tunnel in a minimum of 25 mm to ensure there is soft tissue traversing the physis. The knee is put through 10 full cycles of flexion and extension while maximally tensioning the graft limbs. This is done to eliminate any graft laxity. The knee is placed in 10 degrees of flexion and a posterior drawer force is placed on the tibia. The graft is manually tensioned. The sutures from the graft can be tied over a post, such as a screw and washer construct, or can be dunked into the bone using a lateral row rotator cuff anchor, such as the SwiveLock (Arthrex, Inc.) anchor. This can be used as either the primary mode of fixation or more commonly used as backup fixation. Our preferred method of tibial fixation is via a post and washer or, if the tibial tunnel is long enough, with interference screw fixation kept below the physis. After final graft fixation, a Lachman and pivot shift tests are performed to assure good knee stability. The arthroscope is reinserted and the graft is palpated (Fig. 10.3). If there is any residual laxity in the graft, it can be further tensioned by advancing the femoral side of the graft using the ACL TightRope. Incisions are then closed with an absorbable suture both in the subcutaneous layer and subcuticular layer. The brace is then applied.

POSTOPERATIVE REHABILITATION AND MONITORING

Rehabilitation Protocol

A postoperative brace is used routinely in this patient population. We have found that children may be less compliant with postoperative instructions and the brace may restrict them from excess activity. The brace is worn locked in full extension at all times except for physical therapy (PT) for weeks 0 to 2. During weeks 3 to 4, it is locked for ambulation, unlocked for sitting set at 0 to 90 degrees, and removed for sleeping. The brace is removed at postoperative week 6 or when good quad control is regained. In this specific patient population, compliance with home exercise programs can be challenging. Formal PT is used, beginning 3 to 5 days postoperatively. The initial phase is directed at swelling reduction and regaining full range of motion. Active, active-assisted, and passive range of motion from 0 to 125 degrees is allowed, without forced passive flexion. Prone hangs are taught and performed as well as patellar mobilization exercises. Strengthening exercises emphasize primarily isometrics or limited closed chain progressive resistive exercises. Quad

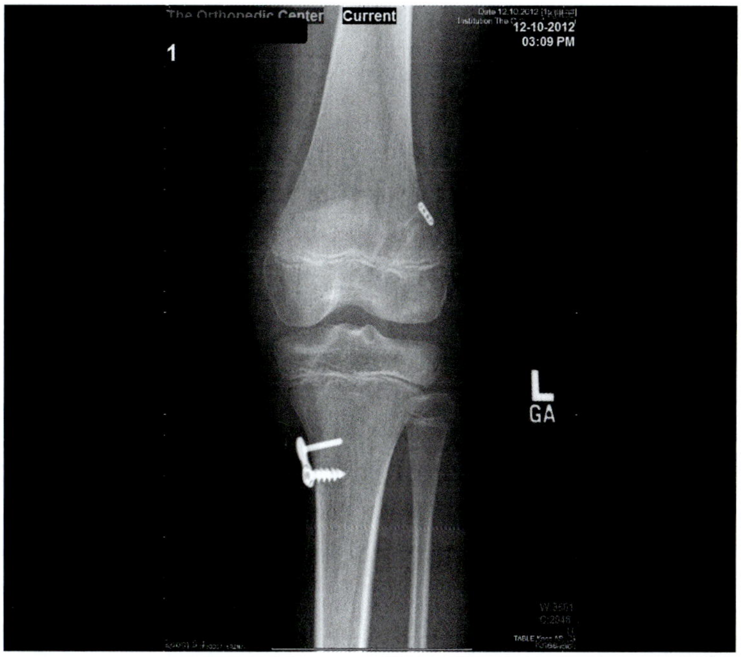

A

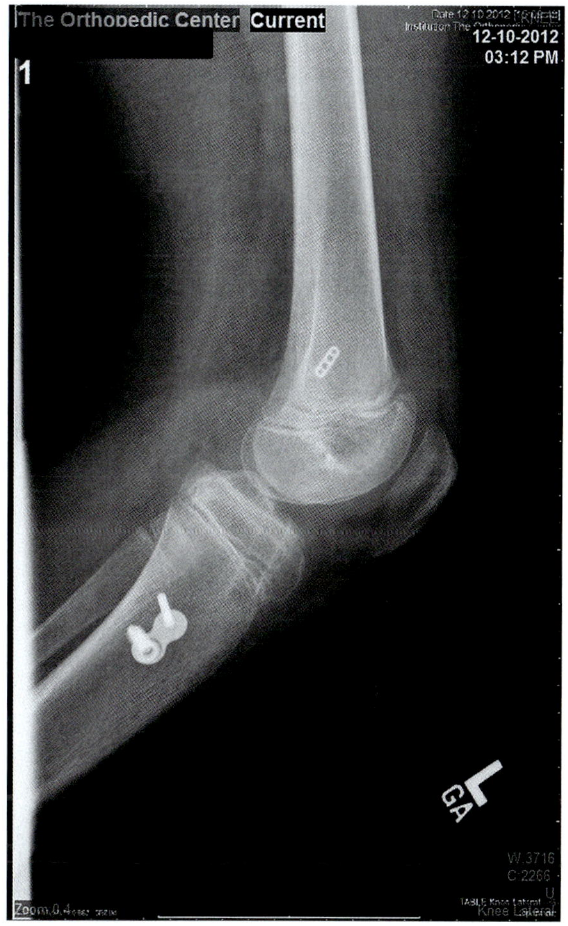

B

Figure 10.4. AP **(A)** and lateral **(B)** radiographs at the first postoperative visit after transphyseal ACL reconstruction in a skeletally immature patient.

sets and leg lifts are initiated during this first phase as well as leg press from 90 to 40 degrees in an eccentric fashion. Active-resisted hamstring exercises at 90 degrees of flexion are initially avoided due to hamstring graft harvest. Short crank bicycle ergometry is allowed.

Phase II (Weeks 6 to 12)

Goals of this phase are to ensure full range of motion, normalize gait, and continue quadriceps strengthening. A squat/step program, wall slides, and leg press are initiated for additional quadriceps strengthening. Treadmill program can be initiated. Proprioception program is started, including balance board, single leg stance, and other balance maneuvers. Nordic track or elliptical trainer can be used as tolerated. Quadriceps isotonics with a proximal pad are allowed in a 90- to 40-degree arc.

Phase III (Weeks 12 to 24)

Goals of the third rehabilitation phase are to restore full lower extremity strength and proprioception, focusing on proper jumping and landing mechanics. In this phase, we aggressively advance agility and functional exercises. We also begin and progress a running program. Limited return to sports is allowed at 16 to 20 weeks, followed by full activity at 20 to 24 weeks. Baseline isokinetic strength testing and functional testing is performed at 16 weeks.

Skeletal Growth Monitoring

Initial postoperative anteroposterior (AP) and lateral radiographs are obtained at the first postoperative visit (Fig. 10.4A,B). Patients should be followed until skeletal maturity is reached to monitor for growth disturbance. Patients are evaluated annually both by clinical examination and radiographic assessment. A full-length standing AP long cassette radiograph of both lower extremities and a lateral radiograph of the affected knee are obtained (Fig. 10.5). These allow for assessment of limb length and angular deformity as well as changes in tibial slope.

CONCLUSION

In conclusion, transphyseal hamstring autograft reconstruction of the ACL is a cost-effective, reproducible, and evidence-based ACL reconstruction technique with excellent clinical results. There is little risk to the growth plate using this technique, and it produces a stable, functional knee required for years of continued sports and activities.

Figure 10.5. Full-length, standing hip to ankle AP radiographs and lateral views are done to evaluate for coronal plane deformity, leg length inequality, and sagittal plane deformity. These are taken annually to monitor for the development of any malalignment or leg length inequality until the patient reaches skeletal maturity. **A.** Full-length, standing hip to ankle AP radiograph taken 6 weeks after surgery demonstrating physiologic bilateral valgus. **B.** Full-length, standing hip to ankle AP radiograph taken at skeletal maturity demonstrating symmetric alignment and no limb length inequality without any ACL reconstruction induced deformity. **C,D.** Corresponding lateral plane radiographs demonstrating no sagittal plane deformity.

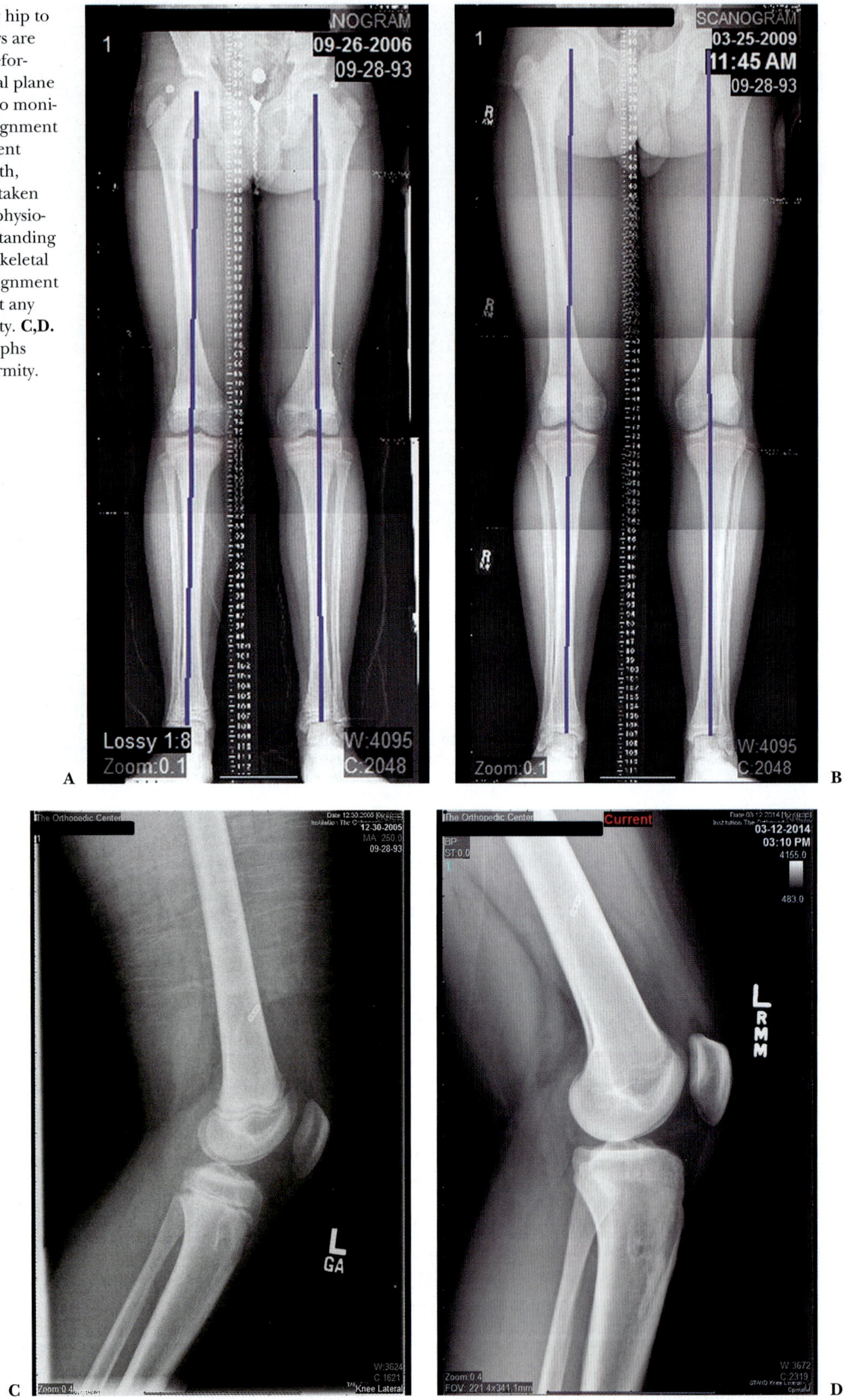

REFERENCES

1. Mall NA, Chalmers PN, Tanaka MJ, et al. Incidence and trends of anterior cruciate ligament reconstruction in the United States. *Am J Sports Med.* 2014;42(10):2363–2370.
2. Chalmers PN, Mall NA, Moric M, et al. Does ACL reconstruction alter natural history?: a systematic literature review of long-term outcomes. *J Bone Joint Surg Am.* 2014;96(4):292–300. doi:10.2106/JBJS.L.01713.
3. Lawrence JT, Argawal N, Ganley TJ. Degeneration of the knee joint in skeletally immature patients with a diagnosis of an anterior cruciate ligament tear: is there harm in delay of treatment? *Am J Sports Med.* 2011;39(12):2582–2587. doi:10.1177/0363546511420818.
4. Milewski MD, Beck NA, Lawrence JT, et al. Anterior cruciate ligament reconstruction in the young athlete: a treatment algorithm for the skeletally immature. *Clin Sports Med.* 2011;30(4):801–810. doi:10.1016/j.csm.2011.08.001.
5. Mall NA, Van Thiel GS, Bedi A, et al. Graft Selection in Anterior Cruciate Ligament Reconstruction. In: ElAttrache NS, Limpivasti O, eds. *Anterior Cruciate Ligament Reconstruction: Evolving Concepts. Monograph Series.* Rosemont, IL: American Academy of Orthopaedic Surgeons; 2013:27–38.
6. Stadelmaier DM, Arnoczky SP, Dodds J, et al. The effect of drilling and soft tissue grafting across open growth plates. A histologic study. *Am J Sports Med.* 1995;23(4):431–435.
7. Aronowitz ER, Ganley TJ, Goode JR, et al. Anterior cruciate ligament reconstruction in adolescents with open physes. *Am J Sports Med.* 2000;28(2):168–175.
8. Guzzanti V, Falciglia F, Gigante A, et al. The effect of intra-articular ACL reconstruction on the growth plates of rabbits. *J Bone Joint Surg Br.* 1994;76(6):960–963.
9. Matava MJ, Siegel MG. Arthroscopic reconstruction of the ACL with semitendinosus-gracilis autograft in skeletally immature adolescent patients. *Am J Knee Surg.* 1997;10(2):60–69.
10. Pallis M, Svoboda SJ, Cameron KL, et al. Survival comparison of allograft and autograft anterior cruciate ligament reconstruction at the United States Military Academy. *Am J Sports Med.* 2012;40(6):1242–1246.
11. Ellis HB, Matheny LM, Briggs KK, et al. Outcomes and revision rate after bone-patellar tendon-bone allograft versus autograft anterior cruciate ligament reconstruction in patients aged 18 years or younger with closed physes. *Arthroscopy.* 2012;28(12):1819–1825.
12. Kaeding CC, Aros B, Pedroza A, et al. Allograft versus autograft anterior cruciate ligament reconstruction: predictors of failure from a MOON perspective longitudinal cohort. *Sports Health.* 2011;3(1):73–81.
13. Inacio MC, Paxton EW, Maletis GB, et al. Patient and surgeon characteristics associated with primary anterior cruciate ligament reconstruction graft selection. *Am J Sports Med.* 2012;40(2):339–345.
14. Magnussen RA, Lawrence JT, West RL, et al. Graft size and patient age are predictors of early revision after anterior cruciate ligament reconstruction with hamstring autograft. *Arthroscopy.* 2012;28(4):526–531.
15. Mariscalco MW, Flanigan DC, Mitchell J, et al. The influence of hamstring autograft size on patient-reported outcomes and risk of revision after anterior cruciate ligament reconstruction: a Multicenter Orthopaedic Outcomes Network (MOON) Cohort Study. *Arthroscopy.* 2013;29(12):1948–1953.
16. Fujimoto E, Sumen Y, Deie M, et al. Anterior cruciate ligament graft impingement against the posterior cruciate ligament: diagnosis using MRI plus three-dimensional reconstruction software. *Magn Reson Imaging.* 2004;22(8):1125–1129.
17. Goss BC, Hull ML, Howell SM. Contact pressure and tension in anterior cruciate ligament grafts subjected to roof impingement during passive extension. *J Orthop Res.* 1997;15(2):263–268.
18. Ichiba A, Kido H, Tokuyama F, et al. Sagittal view of the tibial attachment of the anterior cruciate ligament on magnetic resonance imaging and the relationship between anterior cruciate ligament size and the physical characteristics of patients. *J Orthop Sci.* 2014;19(1):97–103.
19. Shea KG, Belzer J, Apel PJ, et al. Volumetric injury of the physis during single-bundle anterior cruciate ligament reconstruction in children: a 3-dimensional study using magnetic resonance imaging. *Arthroscopy.* 2009;25(12):1415–1422.
20. Yoo WJ, Kocher MS, Micheli LJ. Growth plate disturbance after transphyseal reconstruction of the anterior cruciate ligament in skeletally immature adolescent patients: an MR imaging study. *J Pediatr Orthop.* 2011;31(6):691–696.
21. Behr CT, Potter HG, Paletta GA Jr. The relationship of the femoral origin of the anterior cruciate ligament and the distal femoral physeal plate in the skeletally immature knee. An anatomic study. *Am J Sports Med.* 2001;29(6):781–787.
22. Edwards TB, Greene CC, Baratta RV, et al. The effect of placing a tensioned graft across open growth plates. A gross and histologic analysis. *J Bone Joint Surg Am.* 2001;83-A(5):725–734.
23. Babb JR, Ahn JI, Azar FM, et al. Transphyseal anterior cruciate ligament reconstruction using mesenchymal stem cells. *Am J Sports Med.* 2008;36(6):1164–1170.
24. Anderson AF. Transepiphyseal replacement of the anterior cruciate ligament in skeletally immature patients. A preliminary report. *J Bone Joint Surg Am.* 2003;85-A(7):1255–1263.
25. Courvoisier A, Grimaldi M, Plaweski S. Good surgical outcome of transphyseal ACL reconstruction in skeletally immature patients using four-strand hamstring graft. *Knee Surg Sports Traumatol Arthrosc.* 2011;19(4):588–591.
26. Hui C, Roe J, Ferguson D, et al. Outcome of anatomic transphyseal anterior cruciate ligament reconstruction in Tanner stage 1 and 2 patients with open physes. *Am J Sports Med.* 2012;40(5):1093–1098.
27. Janarv PM, Nyström A, Werner S, et al. Anterior cruciate ligament injuries in skeletally immature patients. *J Pediatr Orthop.* 1996;16(5):673–677.
28. Kim SJ, Shim DW, Park KW. Functional outcome of transphyseal reconstruction of the anterior cruciate ligament in skeletally immature patients. *Knee Surg Relat Res.* 2012;24(3):173–179.
29. Kocher MS, Smith JT, Zoric BJ, et al. Transphyseal anterior cruciate ligament reconstruction in skeletally immature pubescent adolescents. *J Bone Joint Surg Am.* 2007;89(12):2632–2639.
30. Lawrence JT, Bowers AL, Belding J, et al. All-epiphyseal anterior cruciate ligament reconstruction in skeletally immature patients. *Clin Orthop Relat Res.* 2010;468(7):1971–1977.
31. Paletta GA Jr. Complete transphyseal reconstruction of the anterior cruciate ligament in the skeletally immature. *Clin Sports Med.* 2011;30(4):779–788.
32. Redler LH, Brafman RT, Trentacosta N, et al. Anterior cruciate ligament reconstruction in skeletally immature patients with transphyseal tunnels. *Arthroscopy.* 2012;28(11):1710–1717.
33. Gebhard F, Ellermann A, Hoffmann F, et al. Multicenter-study of operative treatment of intraligamentous tears of the anterior cruciate ligament in children and adolescents: comparison of four different techniques. *Knee Surg Sports Traumatol Arthrosc.* 2006;14(9):797–803.
34. Paletta GA. Comparison of trans-physeal vs over-the-top reconstruction: is there a difference? Abstract. ACL Study Group Meeting, Big Sky, MT. 1999.
35. Kumar S, Ahearne D, Hunt DM. Transphyseal anterior cruciate ligament reconstruction in the skeletally immature: follow-up to a minimum of sixteen years of age. *J Bone Joint Surg Am.* 2013;95(1):e1.
36. Solman CG Jr, Pagnani MJ. Hamstring tendon harvesting. Reviewing anatomic relationships and avoiding pitfalls. *Orthop Clin North Am.* 2003;34(1):1–8.
37. Piasecki DP, Bach BR Jr, Espinoza Orias AA, et al. Anterior cruciate ligament reconstruction: can anatomic femoral placement be achieved with a transtibial technique. *Am J Sports Med.* 2011;39(6):1306–1315.
38. Yanke AB, Mall NA, Sherman SL, et al. 5 points on transtibial anterior cruciate ligament reconstruction. *Am J Orthop.* 2013;42(7):305–308.

CHAPTER

11

Frank A. Cordasco
Daniel W. Green

Brief Overview of Surgical Anterior Cruciate Ligament Options: Algorithm Based on Skeletal Age

THE AUTHORS' SURGICAL TREATMENT ALGORITHM

Our surgical treatment algorithm is outlined in the following text. When an anterior cruciate ligament (ACL) tear is confirmed clinically in the pediatric or adolescent athlete, magnetic resonance imaging (MRI) is used to determine the presence of associated pathology and to evaluate the distal femoral and proximal tibial physes. The skeletally immature athlete is then treated immediately with the initiation of activity modification, bracing, and rehabilitation.

Steps 1 and 2

- The patient's physiologic age is determined with use of the methods described in Chapter 38. These methods include a posteroanterior (PA) radiograph of the left hand, an MRI as mentioned earlier, and standing hip/knee/ankle radiographs to assess for limb length discrepancy and alignment.
- The Hospital for Special Surgery (HSS) Shorthand Bone Age Measurement Scale (Fig. 11.1A) is used to determine skeletal age, and the projected remaining growth can be assessed using Anderson-Green growth charts (Fig. 11.1B) as well as other methods (see Chapter 38 for further details).
- The natural history of nonoperative treatment in the ACL-injured skeletally immature athlete has been reviewed completely in Chapters 2 and 5. The indication for ACL reconstruction is predicated on clinical instability, associated intra-articular pathology, the patient's activity level and goals, and skeletal age and growth remaining.

Step 3

- In patients who are prepubescent with more than 6 years of growth remaining, we prefer a physeal-sparing, all-epiphyseal, all-inside reconstruction in young athletes who weigh more than 70 lb or a physeal-sparing modified McIntosh reconstruction for those children weighing less than 70 lb. In the young athlete with 3 to 6 years of growth remaining, we perform an all-inside, all-epiphyseal ACL reconstruction using a hamstring autograft.
- In the young adolescent athlete with 1 to 3 years of remaining growth in whom the proximal tibial physis is approaching closure or beginning to close, we recommend an all-inside partial transphyseal reconstruction with an all-epiphyseal femoral socket and a transphyseal tibial socket.
- For adolescents who are near skeletal maturity (<1 year of remaining growth), we perform a complete transphyseal bone-patellar tendon-bone autograft or an all-inside, complete transphyseal hamstring autograft reconstruction depending on several graft selection factors, which include sport, position, body habitus, and gender (Fig. 11.2).
- When using hamstring autograft, if the diameter of the graft will be less than 8.5 mm, we will either supplement with allograft hamstring or harvest hamstring autograft from the contralateral knee. This is discussed preoperatively with the athlete and family in each case.

Step 1: Determine skeletal age from validated HSS Shorthand Bone Age Measurement Scale.

↓

Step 2: Determine projected remaining growth (Fig. 11.1).

↓

Step 3: Select the indicated surgical reconstruction based on the data above (Fig. 11.2).

Boys (age)	HSS Shorthand Bone Age Measurement Scale	Girls (age)
	AP hand radiograph	
12.5	Appearance of hook of hamate	10
13	Appearance of MP thumb sesamoid bone	11
13.5	Proximal aspect of radial side of radial epiphysis has extended to meet the maximum width of the distal metaphysis, but capping has not occured	
14	Capping of distal radius epiphysis	12
15	Closure[a] of thumb distal phalanx physis	13
15.5	Closure[a] of index finger distal phalanx physis	13.5
16	Closure[a] of index finger proximal phalanx physis	14
	[a]Closure = bridging of ≥50% bone across the physis	

A

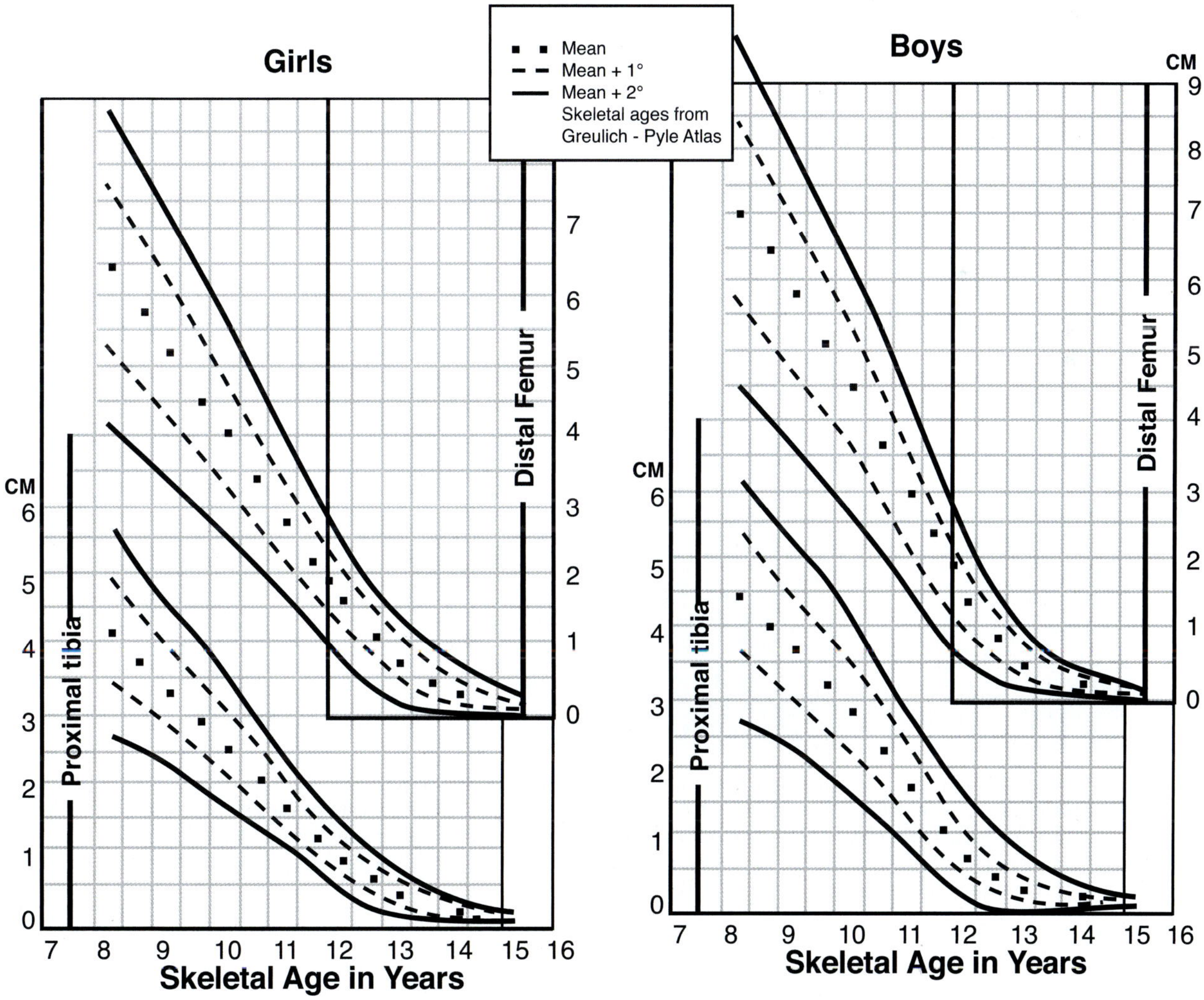

B

Figure 11.1. Predicated on bone age (*not* chronologic age) and projected remaining growth. **A.** Heyworth BE, Osei DA, Fabricant PD, et al. The shorthand bone age assessment: a simpler alternative to current methods. *J Pediatr Orthop.* 2013;33(5):569–574. **B.** Anderson M, Green WT, Messner MB. The classic. Growth and predictions of growth in the lower extremities by Margaret Anderson, M.S., William T. Green, M.D. and Marie Blail Messner, A.B. from the Journal of Bone and Joint Surgery, 45A:1, 1963. *Clin Orthop Relat Res.* 1978;(136):7–21.

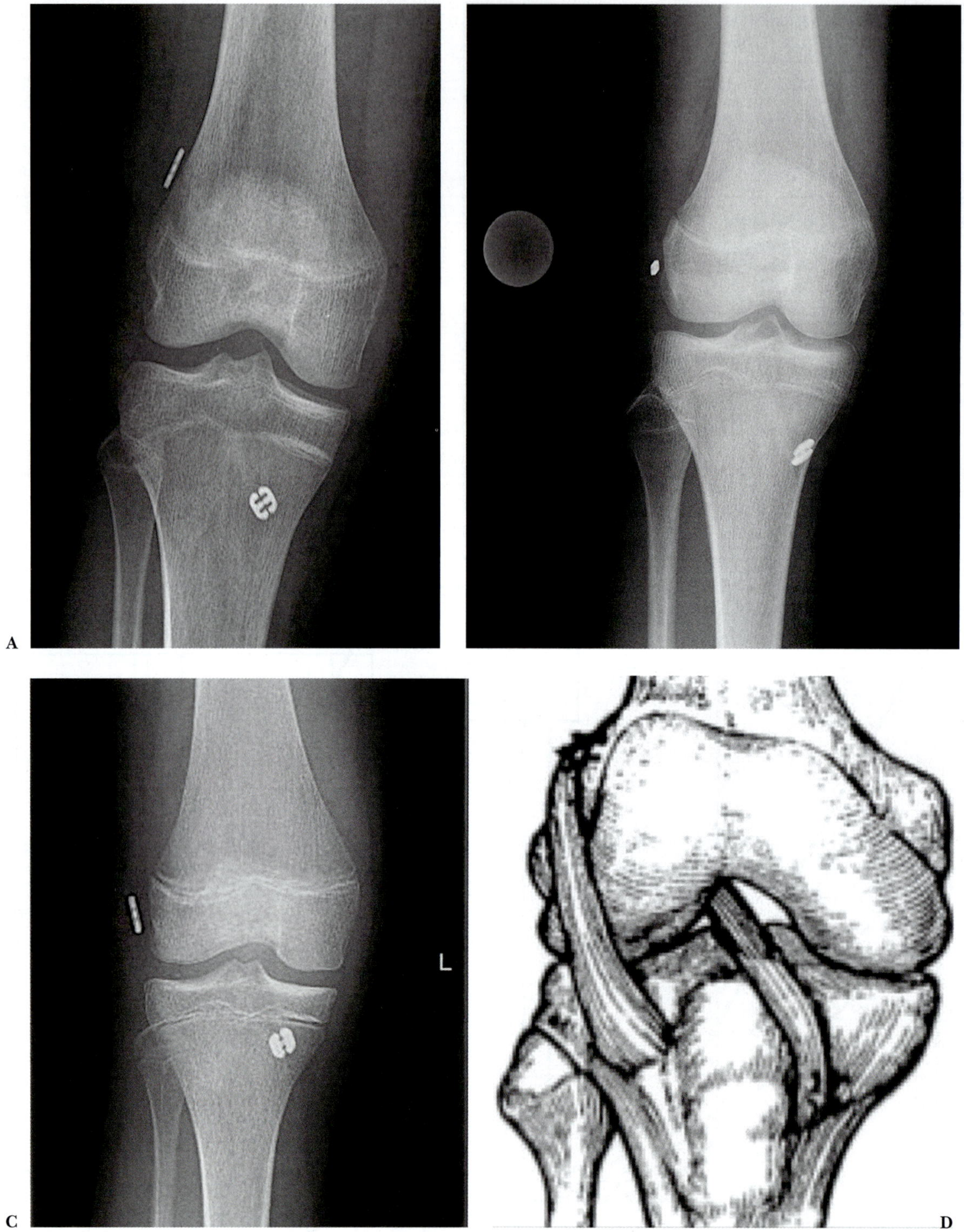

Figure 11.2. Surgical treatment guideline. **A.** One year of remaining skeletal growth. Complete transphyseal (CT) (hamstring vs. bone-patellar tendon-bone). **B.** Two to 3 years of remaining skeletal growth. All-inside partial transphyseal (hamstring). **C.** Three to 6 years of remaining skeletal growth. All-inside all-epiphyseal (hamstring). **D.** More than 6 years of remaining skeletal growth. All-epiphyseal versus physeal-sparing reconstruction (iliotibial band [ITB]) (<65 lb?).

SUGGESTED READING

Cordasco FA. CORR insights: meniscal injury after adolescent anterior cruciate ligament injury—how long are patients at risk? *Clin Orthop Relat Res.* 2014;472:998–1000.

Dodwell ER, Lamont LE, Green DW, et al. 20 years of pediatric anterior cruciate ligament reconstruction in New York State. *Am J Sports Med.* 2014;42(3):675–680.

Fabricant PD, Jones KJ, Delos D, et al. Reconstruction of the anterior cruciate ligament in the skeletally immature athlete: a review of current concepts: AAOS exhibit selection. *J Bone Joint Surg.* 2013;95:e28.

Fabricant PD, McCarthy MM, Cordasco FA, et al. All-inside, all-epiphyseal autograft reconstruction of the anterior cruciate ligament in the skeletally immature athlete. *JBJS Essent Surg Tech.* 2013;3(2):e9.

Graziano J, Green DW, Cordasco FA. Anterior cruciate ligament injury prevention in the young athlete: evidence-based application. *Strength Cond J.* 2013;35:89–97.

Heyworth BE, Osei DA, Fabricant PD, et al. The shorthand bone age assessment: a simpler alternative to current methods. *J Pediatr Orthop.* 2013;33(5):569–574.

McCarthy MM, Graziano J, Green DW, et al. All-epiphyseal, all-inside anterior cruciate ligament reconstruction technique for skeletally immature patients. *Arthrosc Tech.* 2012;1(2):e231–e239.

McCarthy MM, Tucker S, Nguyen J, et al. Contact stress and kinematic analysis of all-epiphyseal and over-the-top pediatric reconstruction techniques for the anterior cruciate ligament. *Am J Sports Med.* 2013;41:1330–1339.

CHAPTER

12

Jessica Graziano

Postoperative Rehabilitation for Pediatric and Adolescent Anterior Cruciate Ligament Reconstruction

With sports participation and specialization on the rise, intrasubstance tears of the anterior cruciate ligament (ACL) in children are now being seen with greater frequency.[1,2] The literature has recently reported on the steady increase in ACL injury in the skeletally immature athlete and has extensively reported on the high incidence in the adolescent female athlete.[3–5] Early specialization, maturation, high-risk movement patterns, and an inadequate strength base all contribute to increased injury rates as well as impact postoperative recovery and decision making.[2,4,6–9]

Postoperative rehabilitation involves progressing athletes through phases of strength and functional mobility as well as addressing growth-related changes that impact postural alignment. In addition, young athletes are returning to higher levels of play with demands for peak performance at earlier ages, causing subsequent higher rates of revision anterior cruciate ligament reconstructions (ACLR).[2,10] Movement patterns play a critical role in ACL injury because they may influence anterior tibial shear force, which strains the ACL.[3,4,8] Therefore, emphasis should be placed on refining movement skills in the final phase of rehabilitation to reduce reinjury risk.

THE EFFECT OF GRAFT SELECTION ON REHABILITATION

In order to reduce reinjury rates, postoperative progression should consider not only the individual's strength but also differences in graft selection and fixation strength. If an athlete is advanced to activities involving excessive loading of the knee, such as plyometrics and running, prior to adequate healing time or without an appropriate strength base to meet the demands of the activity, delayed healing and elongation of the graft may lead to chronic instability.[11]

The most commonly used graft tissues in young athletes are autogenous patellar bone-tendon-bone[12,13] and autogenous hamstring tendons.[14–16] Bone-to-bone healing in the osseous tunnel for patellar tendon grafts occur in approximately 8 weeks. Healing of tendon to bone for hamstring autografts takes approximately 12 weeks.[17,18] Therefore, our rehabilitation progression for hamstring or semitendinosus grafts tends to be less aggressive, and return to running, plyometrics, and sports is slightly slower.[19] In addition, it is important to note that the graft's strength may reach its weakest point at approximately 6 to 8 weeks postoperatively secondary to graft remodeling.[19–22] Although controlled loading in the early phases is important to enhance ligament and tendon healing, excessive loading can damage the healing graft and lead to graft elongation.[21–25] Unfortunately, there is limited data in humans that makes determining timing and optimal loading on healing ACL reconstructions difficult to determine.[23–25]

Multiple techniques for surgical stabilization of the ACL-deficient knee in young athletes have been described. The guidelines to be discussed are a criterion-based progression and take into account general graft healing and incorporate strategies to address physiologic changes incurred by growth and maturation. Surgeon preference for range of motion (ROM) and weight bearing should be respected in the initial acute phase.

REHABILITATION CONSIDERATIONS FOR THE PEDIATRIC AND ADOLESCENT ATHLETE

Advances in graft reconstruction techniques and fixation methods have significantly improved surgical success with ACLR for young athletes.[25–28] Therefore, the potential for an athlete to return to play without reinjury has shifted to be more determined by differences in rehabilitation than by surgical procedure.[11,27–29]

Successful functional outcomes critically depend on a scientifically based rehabilitation program that considers graft healing with respect to joint loading to prevent graft elongation. In addition, outcomes depend on the effects of growth spurts and maturation that have been associated with deficits in core strength, coordination, and neuromuscular control secondary to increased bony lever arms and changes in center of body mass.[3,6,9] A patient may demonstrate proper alignment and neuromuscular control with movement in the early phases of rehabilitation but may need to revisit a movement later on secondary to a growth spurt that affected their center of mass as well as body awareness and alignment.[3,6]

The guidelines to be discussed are the Hospital for Special Surgery's (HSS) ACLR guidelines for the all-epiphyseal technique with hamstring autograft. Special considerations regarding the autogenous patellar tendon graft will be presented for the adolescent population. This is a criterion-based progression, which respects general graft healing and incorporates strategies to address physiologic changes incurred by this special population to improve quality of movement. The decision to return to play is made as a collaborative team effort with the physician, physical therapist, trainer, and coach and is based on both qualitative and quantitative data regarding sports readiness. Surgeon preference for ROM and weight bearing should be respected in the initial acute phase as well as concomitant injury.

POSTOPERATIVE PHASE 1 (WEEKS 0 TO 4): PROTECTION PHASE

Rehabilitation begins immediately after surgery. Patients typically remain in the hospital overnight for observation to allow for control of activity level, pain, and swelling and ensure appropriate start of rehabilitation. If apprehensive with ROM exercises, a continuous passive motion machine is initiated from 0 to 45 degrees while the patient is at the hospital. The initial postoperative visit is vital in establishing a rapport and trust with the patient and their caregivers. Children may be anxious and guarded secondary to pain; therefore, trust needs to be established to create an optimal therapeutic environment.

Rehabilitation in the first month places significant emphasis on protection of the surgical repair, prevention of muscle inhibition caused by effusion, and prevention of postsurgical complications such as arthrofibrosis. The goals are regaining knee extension to 0 degrees, progressive weight bearing, controlling postoperative effusion, gradually restoring flexion ROM, and progressing quadriceps reeducation (Table 12.1).

TABLE 12.1 Phase 1: Protection Phase (Weeks 0–4)

Goals

- Knee extension to 0 degrees
- Flexion ROM ~90 degrees
- Control postoperative effusion/pain
- Straight-leg raise without quadriceps lag
- WBAT with crutches

Criteria to Progress into Phase 2

- Zero degrees of knee extension
- Improved quadriceps strength with ability to perform a straight-leg raise without a quadriceps lag
- At least 90 degrees of flexion ROM
- Able to demonstrate unilateral (involved limb) weight bearing pain-free

Treatment Recommendations

Modalities for Postoperative Pain and Effusion

Controlling postoperative pain and effusion is crucial secondary to their role in muscle inhibition.[30–32] Treatment options for swelling include cryotherapy and joint compression through the use of compression wrap. Cryotherapy, electrical stimulation, and passive range of motion (PROM) may reduce pain.[19,32] In contrast, ultrasound should not be used on the skeletally immature athlete's joint secondary to contraindications on growth plates.[32]

The speed of weight-bearing progression and joint loading may affect pain and swelling. In general, we recommend our patients stay out of school for 3 to 5 days to minimize pain and effusion as well as use bilateral upper extremity crutches for at least 4 weeks to control loading of the knee joint.

Bracing and Ambulation

Advanced fixation techniques allow for immediate weight bearing. Postoperatively, partial weight bearing is instructed with a hinged brace locked in extension to emphasize full knee extension and assist while the quadriceps is inhibited.[17,33,34] Studies have demonstrated improved functional knee scores and proprioception with brace use after surgery.[33,34]

The athletes are advancing to weight bearing as tolerated (WBAT) with an assistive device over the next 2 weeks. Mechanical loading of the knee is progressed with the use of an assistive device over the first 4 to 6 weeks to allow the knee joint to acclimate to increased loads with minimal pain and effusion.

Brace education is reviewed on the initial visit with both the patient and caregiver secondary to its importance for graft protection and maintenance of knee extension ROM. The clinician should encourage frequent brace checks throughout the day as the brace may loosen and slide distally, facilitating a flexed knee gait, which may cause loss of knee extension.

Range of Motion

ROM may begin immediately secondary to graft placement in the native footprint of the ACL[27] and is strongly encouraged to minimize the effects of immobilization such as excessive collagen formation.[35–37] Full passive knee extension is emphasized while flexion is gradually restored. Extension is critical for normalized gait.[38] Flexion contractures cause excessive loading on the patellofemoral joint, leading to pain and quadriceps weakness.[38,39]

Specific exercises targeted toward achieving knee extension are supine hamstring stretches, gastrocnemius stretches with a towel, and towel roll extension. For towel roll extensions, a towel roll is placed under the patient's heel/ankle while lying supine with a low-load, long-duration stretch.

Flexion ROM is gradually progressed and depends on the individual's response to surgery as well as apprehension and age. Constant reassurance should be provided to the child that no damage will occur with ROM exercises. If persistent effusion exists, ROM may advance at a slower pace. ROM should progress gradually in phase 1 rather than aggressively at the expense of increased pain, effusion, and apprehension delaying recovery.

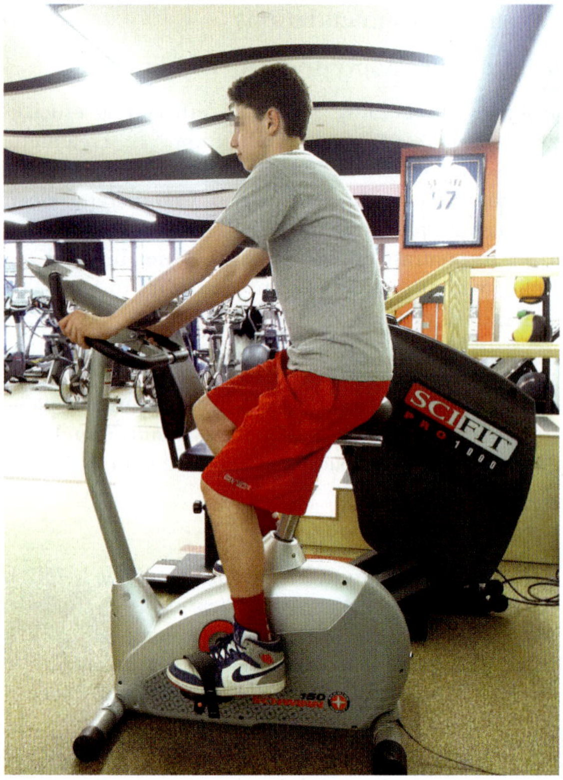

Figure 12.1. Short crank bike being used for ROM, strength, and endurance in phase 1.

Patient and caregiver are instructed on performing seated active-assisted knee flexion/passive extension exercises three to five times per day. When approximately 80 degrees of flexion ROM is achieved, a short crank bike (140 to 180 mm) may be used to develop endurance, strength, and ROM (Fig. 12.1). The shorter crank allows patients to cycle full circles prior to achieving appropriate ROM necessary to start on a standard bike (170 mm).

Patella Mobilizations

Patella mobilizations are performed to minimize decreased ROM and quadriceps inhibition.[39] Loss of mobility may result secondary to excessive scar tissue adhesions along the medial and lateral, fat pad retinacula, and harvesting the patellar tendon for the graft.[39,40] If patellar mobility is lost, infrapatellar contractures may result in ROM complications and difficulty with quadriceps activation.[39–41] Mobilizations are performed in both the medial/lateral and superior/inferior directions, especially for those with a patellar tendon autograft. Superior mobility of the patella is required for complete knee extension and inferior glides for flexion.[39–41]

Strengthening

Reestablishing voluntary quadriceps control is crucial. Quadriceps setting with a towel roll under the knee is used for reeducation and, when combined with neuromuscular electrical stimulation, has been found to be more efficient than exercise alone to improve strength.[42] Once patients demonstrate good quad contraction, they are progressed to straight-leg raises with the brace locked until sufficient quadriceps control is demonstrated. When no quadriceps lag is demonstrated, they may perform straight-leg raises without the brace. When achieved with appropriate endurance, the brace may be unlocked for ambulation.

We recommend incorporating closed kinetic chain (CKC) leg press when ROM is greater than 90 degrees of flexion and quadriceps control improves. Leg press is performed bilaterally inside a pain-free arc (70 to 75 degrees) and advanced to a unilateral exercise using greater ROM in later phases. Closed kinetic exercises are used for strengthening in the early phases, as they have been shown to minimize stress to the ACL.[19,20]

Proximal hip strength is crucial for stability as well as reducing loads at the knee.[2,8,11] Progressive resistance exercise can be performed with cuff weights and isotonic exercises. In later phases, core and proximal hip strength will be crucial for ensuring minimal valgus loading with dynamic activities.

Neuromuscular Training

Neuromuscular training is emphasized because balance deficits have been identified following ACL reconstruction as well as extensive reports in the literature regarding neuromuscular deficits being a risk factor for injury.[3,8,43,44] A rocker board can be used as soon as the patient is 50% weight bearing. Training starts with basic weight shifting in both the medial/lateral direction. A Biodex Balance System (Biodex Medical Systems, Shirley, NY) tends to be fun for young patients and may be used to demonstrate weight shifting and weight bearing (Fig. 12.2).

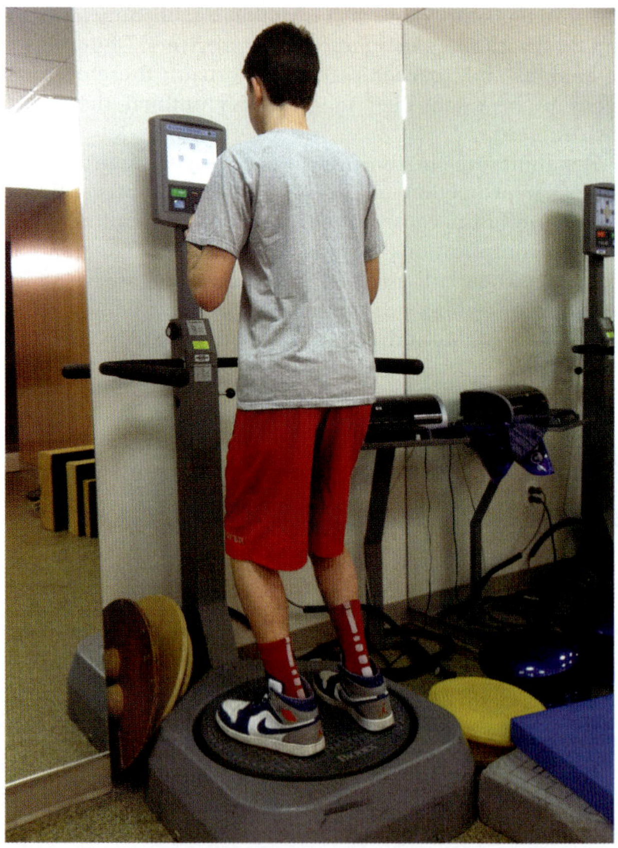

Figure 12.2. Weight shifting and balance training being performed by an adolescent on the Biodex Balance System.

In addition, wall squats may be performed for joint repositioning and weight bearing as well. In later phases, squats may be progressed to unstable surfaces such as a tilt board once the patient exhibits good postural control and lower extremity alignment on solid surfaces.

POSTOPERATIVE PHASE 2 (WEEKS 4 TO 8): INTERMEDIATE PROTECTION PHASE

In phase 2, the graft is not optimal. The literature has reported that the graft undergoes a period of necrosis, revascularization, and remodeling. Graft strength decreases during this period of necrosis and gradually increases as it remodels.[12,14,16,45] Constant reinforcement with activity modification is required to ensure the individual does not push past his or her physiologic capabilities injuring the graft.

The goals are continued emphasis on protection of the surgical repair, controlled effusion, flexion ROM, good patellar mobility, normalized gait, and the ability to ascend a 6- to 8-in step (height dependent) pain-free with good control (Table 12.2).

Treatment Recommendations

Modalities

Cryotherapy continues to be emphasized secondary to gradually increased loads to the joint with activity as well as to minimize quadriceps inhibition. Electrical stimulation for quadriceps reeducation should be discharged at this time secondary to improved quadriceps contraction.

Bracing and Ambulation

As quadriceps strength improves and the patient demonstrates the ability to perform a straight-leg raise without a quadriceps lag, he or she may change to a postoperative brace as per the surgeon's preference. The brace serves as a reminder to the individual and his or her friends to avoid activities that may risk reinjury. Mechanical loading of the knee is progressed during this phase, and the athlete is advanced off of crutches by 6 to 8 weeks, pending normalized gait and extension ROM. We have found that if progressed off of crutches too quickly and without sufficient quad control, patients are at risk of losing knee extension secondary to ambulating on a flexed knee.

Range of Motion

Flexion is gradually progressed to full flexion by 8 to10 weeks postoperatively. This can be achieved by progressing the athlete from seated active-assisted range of motion (AAROM) knee flexion to wall slides (Fig. 12.3A) and a stair stretch (Fig. 12.3B). The clinician should monitor these exercises to ensure compliance with repetitions and sets as well as quality of performance. As ROM progresses from 110 to 115 degrees, cycling is advanced to a standard 170-mm ergometer. Low-peak strain values have been demonstrated on the ACL with stationary cycling.[45,46]

Strengthening

As ROM and strength continues to improve, additional CKC exercises are added such as squats, leg press, advanced

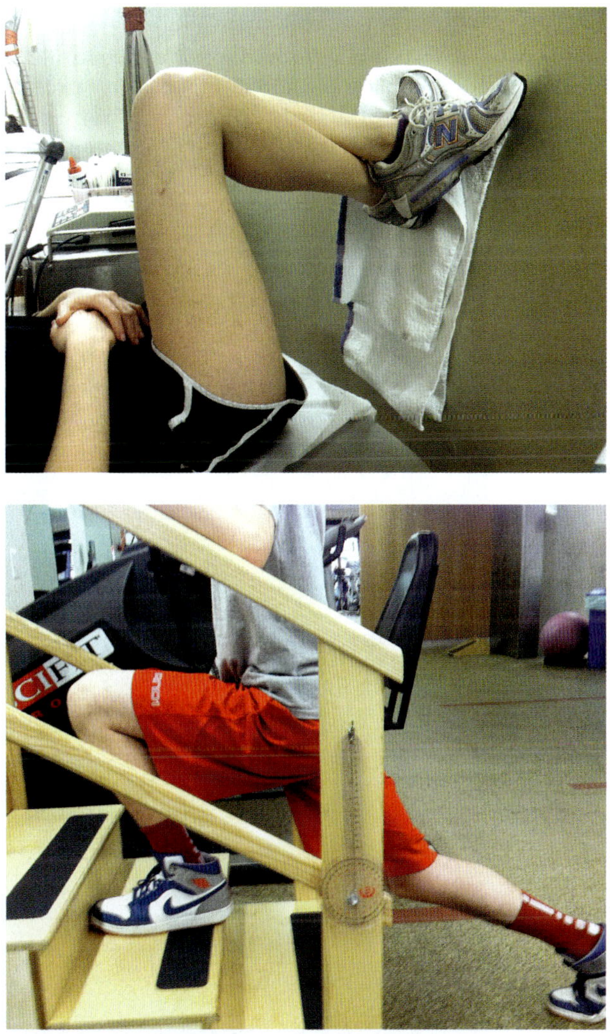

A

B

Figure 12.3. Flexion ROM progression. **A.** Wall slides used for obtaining flexion ROM. The stretch is held by the uninvolved leg for approximately 5 seconds. Then the uninvolved limb is used to slide the leg back up the wall. **B.** Stair stretch being performed by an adolescent with 5- to 8-second holds for flexion ROM.

TABLE 12.2	Phase 2: Moderate Protection Phase (Weeks 4–8)
Goals • Gradually improve knee flexion ROM • Restore patellar mobility • Minimize postoperative pain and effusion • Normalize gait pattern without assistive device • Able to ascend a 6–8-in step with good control	
Criteria to Progress into Phase 3 • ROM (0–130 degrees) • Ability to ascend a 6–8-in step (height dependent) with good control • Minimal to no joint effusion • Normalized gait	

neuromuscular activities, and unilateral CKC exercises. Weight on the leg press is progressed and determined by the athlete's physiologic capabilities as well as quality of movement. Despite popular belief that weight training affects growth plates in children, studies have demonstrated no adverse effects.[47] In contrast, strength training has demonstrated a reduction in the number and severity of knee injuries in adolescent athletes.[48–52] It is recommended that a clinician supervise children at all times while on equipment to ensure safety as well as appropriate weight, repetitions, and quality of movement.[47] Children should be educated to perform movements slowly and controlled with equal weight acceptance to translate over to functional activities.

Squats are progressed from wall slides to free squats. Wall squats and barbell squats have been shown to be effective and safe regarding tensile loads on the ACL. Weight-bearing squats have been reported to have an ACL tensile load of 50 N versus non–weight-bearing knee extensions demonstrating 150 N.[20,53,54] Quality of movement is key to avoid adverse loading of the ACL as well as develop compensatory movement patterns. Anterior knee translation beyond the toes may increase ACL loading during squatting exercises.[20,54] Studies have demonstrated improved lower extremity alignment with verbal feedback and direct supervision in young athletes.[2,55,56] The use of a chair gives the child a cue to sit back and use a hip strategy to prevent anterior knee translation (Fig. 12.4). A mirror may be used for visual feedback if the individual presents with an asymmetrical weight shift. For children who present with weak gluteal musculature and resultant valgus, TheraBands may be used above the knee to activate hip abductors. In addition, it should be understood that the child has potentially never learned proper squatting technique and the clinician may be the first to teach him or her.

Unilateral CKC exercises are added such as contralateral hip abduction and extension with a TheraBand to activate gluteus medius early on as well as address single-leg weight bearing. Forward step-ups are gradually progressed with various step heights for strengthening based on proper alignment and technique. Retrograde treadmill ambulation is used with progressive inclines to facilitate quadriceps strengthening pending patient age and coordination.[57] Proximal hip strengthening exercises are continued and advanced as ROM allows, such as clamshells, bilateral lower extremity bridging, and lateral band walking.

Neuromuscular Training

As proprioception improves, dynamic stabilization drills are progressed to include unilateral weight bearing and multiplanar activities using a rocker board or foam pad. Single-limb activities on flat ground are progressed to unstable surfaces

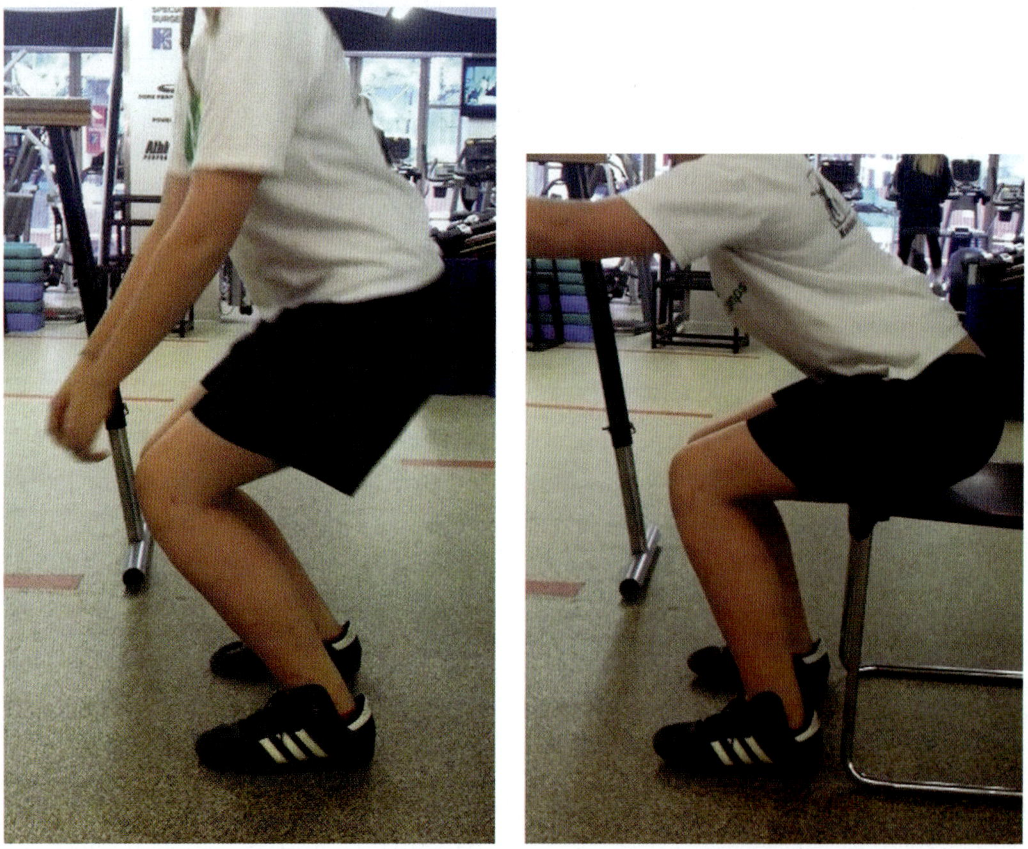

A B

Figure 12.4. Demonstration of impact of cueing on hip strategy **A.** A patient performing a squat with a knee strategy and anterior knee translation beyond the toes. **B.** Same child using a hip strategy after successfully correcting her squat by sitting back into a chair as a cue.

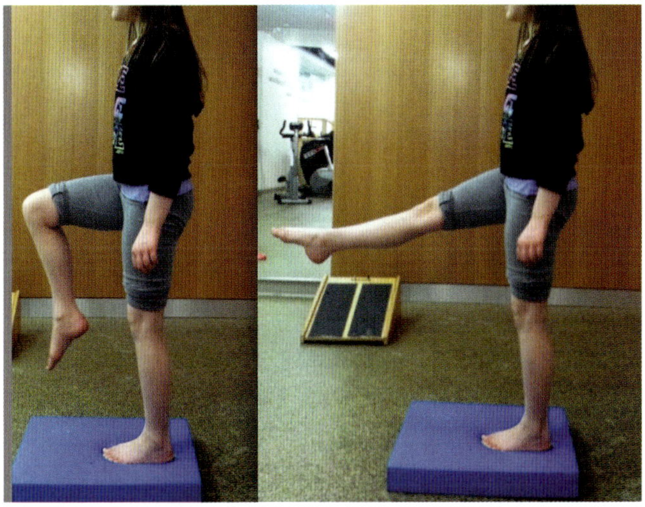

Figure 12.5. Single leg stance being performed with involved limb balancing on foam pad. Balance drill advanced to contralateral knee extension/flexion to promote recruitment of core and lower extremity musculature for dynamic stabilization.

with the knee slightly flexed to encourage agonist/antagonist cocontraction to enhance knee stability. Single-limb stance with uninvolved lower extremity movements is performed as well in the latter part of this phase (Fig. 12.5). These balance drills with extremity movements promote dynamic stabilization and recruit various muscle groups.[19] Improving neuromuscular reaction time to imposed loads will enhance dynamic stabilization around the knee and assist with protecting the graft from reinjury.[19,58] Perturbation training has been proven effective in rehabilitation programs[58–60] and can be performed while the patient is performing double- or single limb balance exercises on an unstable surface.

Flexibility

Quadriceps stretching in the supine and prone position is used to assist with flexion ROM by week 6. Hamstring and calf flexibility should not be neglected secondary to the impact they have on functional mobility. Quadriceps and hamstring flexibility is critical to allow for sufficient knee and hip flexion during sports to reduce ACL strain.[3,61]

PHASE 3: FUNCTIONAL STRENGTHENING AND CORRECTIVE MOVEMENT (8 TO 16 WEEKS)

This phase is dedicated to building a sound strength base to serve as the foundation for advanced movement skills in the next phase. Neuromuscular control, proximal hip strength, core stability, and eccentric quadriceps strength are advanced. Continued focus on proper alignment and control with all movements continues to be emphasized, as athletes will not advance to dynamic sports-specific movement skills unless demonstrated. Running and jumping is not performed until an adequate strength base is achieved to avoid adverse loads to the graft (Table 12.3).

TABLE 12.3	Phase 3: Functional Strengthening and Corrective Movement (Weeks 8–16)
Goals • Restore full ROM • Demonstrates hip strategy and no valgus with squats. Able to self correct symmetry with squat technique. • Demonstrate the ability to descend a 6–8-in step (height dependent) • Improve neuromuscular control • Improve overall lower extremity foundational strength	
Criteria to Progress into Phase 4 • ROM within normal limits (WNL) • Ability to descend a 6–8-in step (height dependent) • Ability to perform single leg stance with knee flexed with good dynamic stability	

Treatment Recommendations

Addressing Range of Motion and Flexibility Deficits

The clinician will typically need to address deficits incurred by growth spurts. Quadriceps, hamstring, and gastrocsoleus flexibility is critical to allow for sufficient knee and hip flexion during maneuvers such as cutting to reduce ACL strain.[2,36,61] Flexibility deficits can result in compensatory movement patterns as well as cause valgus loading of the knee. The inability to dorsiflex at the ankle without the heels lifting up off the ground during a squat (Fig. 12.6A) as well as movements such as foot eversion are indicative of calf tightness (Fig. 12.6B).

Strengthening

Leg press is progressed from bilateral to unilateral as well as eccentric work. For eccentric quadriceps strengthening, the individual is to extend with bilateral lower extremities and slowly lower with one leg. A forward step-down program is introduced with progressive heights (4 to 6 to 8 in). Quality of movement is continually assessed for risk factors that may predispose the athlete to injury as well as guide the clinician to areas that need to be addressed.

Addressing Neuromuscular Imbalances: Reducing Risk Factors

Basic foundational movement patterns are to be perfected prior to advanced agility and plyometrics to avoid adversely loading the ACL. Young athletes demonstrate several measurable neuromuscular imbalances associated with increased injury risk such as quadriceps dominance, leg dominance, and trunk dominance.[3,48,62–64] Children who demonstrate *ligament dominance* tend to stress the ligament before muscular activation to absorb ground reaction forces (GRFs). This may occur secondary to lack of dynamic muscular control, leading to increased valgus moment and potential for high torque at the knee and ACL (Fig. 12.7A,B). *Quadriceps dominance* results from preferential activation of the knee extensors versus the knee flexors during movements leading to hyperextension of the knee and predisposition to ACL injury. *Leg dominance* is a result of imbalances

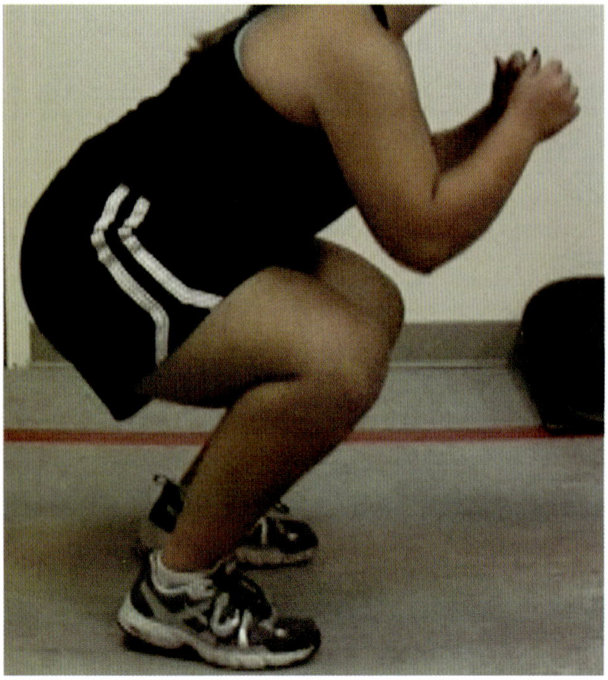

A

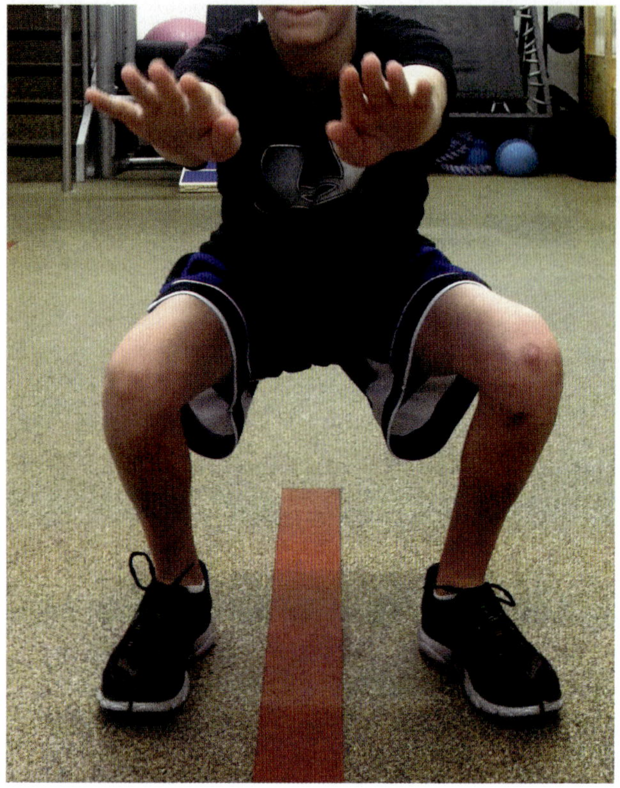

B

Figure 12.6. **A.** Calf tightness demonstrated with the inability to dorsiflex at the ankle with a squat. **B.** Calf tightness demonstrated with left foot eversion with a squat.

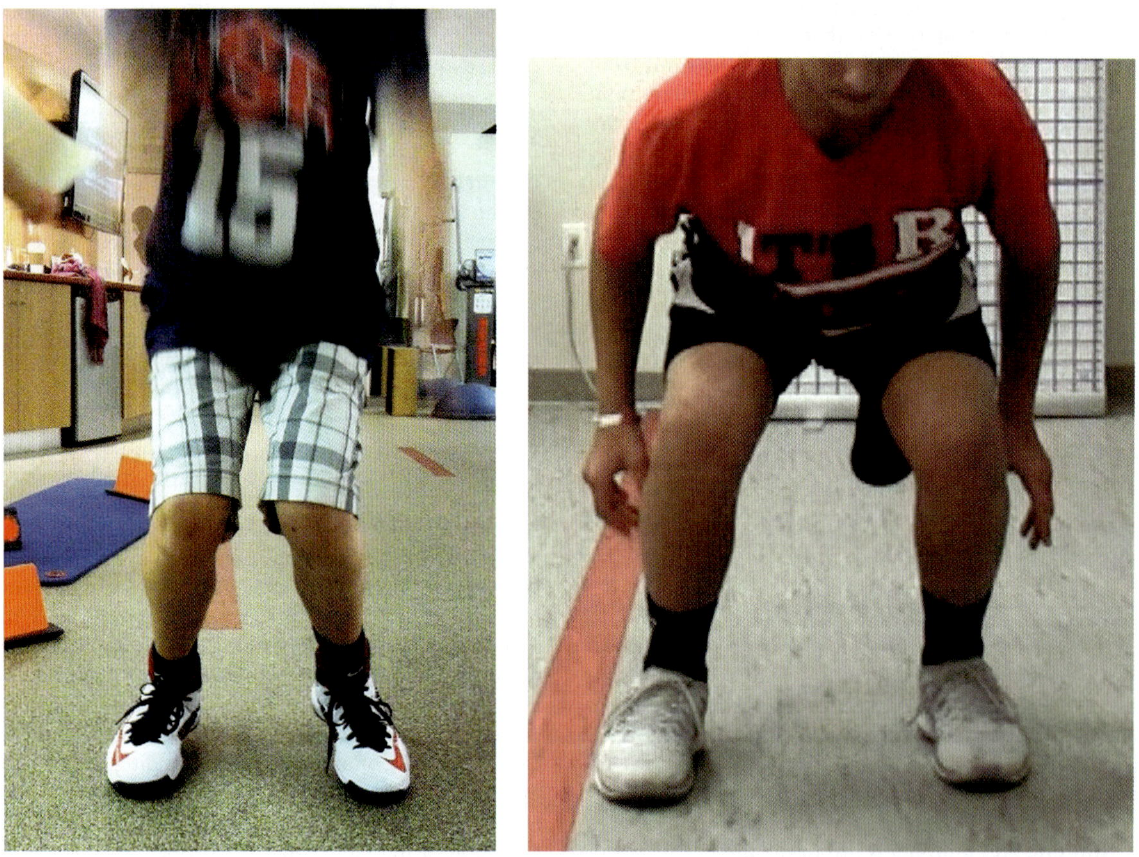

A B

Figure 12.7. Ligament dominance: differences in valgus knee motion during a jump landing. **A.** Increased knee valgus on landing. **B.** Proper knee alignment in a trained individual with no valgus noted.

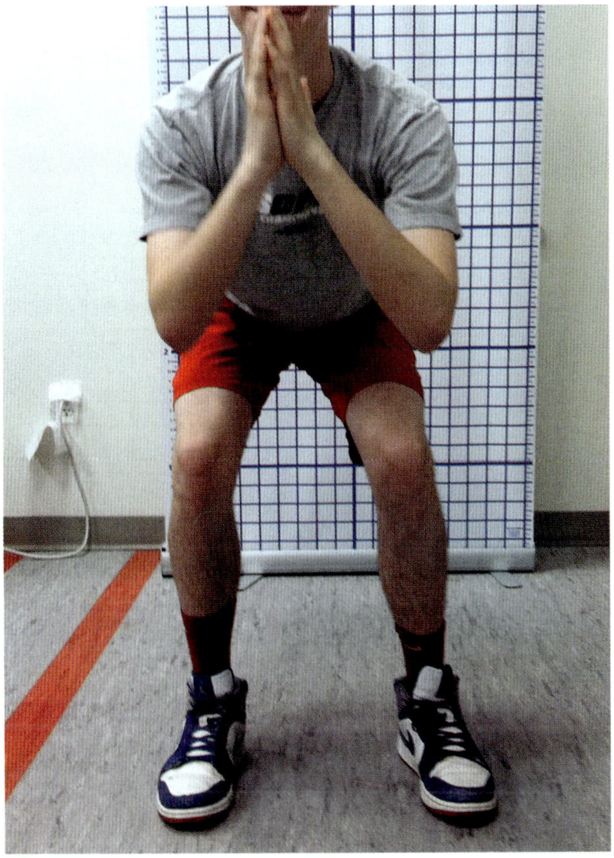

A

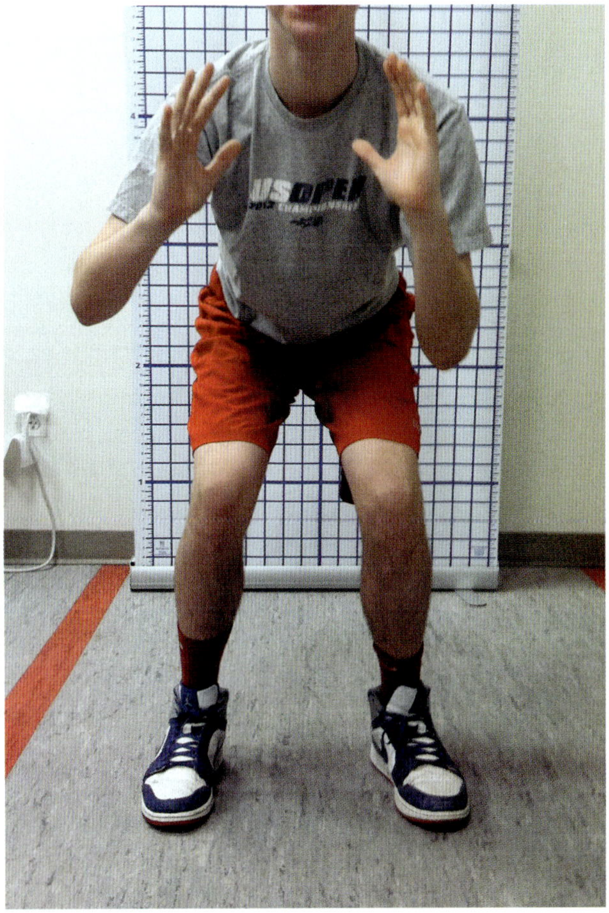

B

Figure 12.8. Leg dominance. **A.** Weight shifted to right limb demonstrating increased loading and dependence. **B.** Weight is equally distributed between both limbs. Modified via visual cueing.

in muscular strength and coordination, which may place either leg at risk. The weaker limb is compromised secondary to the inability to dissipate forces and the stronger limb is subjected to higher forces secondary to increased dependence and loading (Fig. 12.8A,B). *Trunk dominance* pertains to excessive trunk motion in the frontal plane, leading to high GRFs and knee joint abduction loads leaving the knee vulnerable to injury. Trunk dominance may be caused by increased motion of the body's center of mass during single-leg landing, pivoting, or deceleration as well as weak core strength (Fig. 12.9A,B).[3,48,62–64]

Strengthening for Correction of Dynamic Valgus

Strengthening specific areas have been shown to minimize at-risk movement patterns.[47–49,64] Gluteus maximus and medius play a role in preventing dynamic valgus collapse by controlling hip adduction and femoral rotation. Weakness results in inability to maintain the hip in an abducted position during squatting as well as single-leg activities such as landing and cutting. Studies have demonstrated improved control of dynamic valgus collapse with gluteus maximus and medius strengthening.[65,66] Side planks and lateral band walking have been shown to produce sufficient maximal voluntary activation for strengthening of the gluteus medius. Single-limb activities are performed to activate the gluteus medius to maintain a level pelvis.[67] Single-limb squats and deadlifts (Fig. 12.10) have been shown to maximally elicit gluteus maximus. These exercises are progressed from double-limb to single-limb stance when appropriate strength and technique is demonstrated.[2,67] Hamstring weakness and activation deficits have been shown to control dynamic valgus postures by resisting anterior and lateral tibial translation and rotations.[68] Deficits in hamstring strength result in quadriceps dominance secondary to increased knee extensor moments over knee flexor moments, therefore increasing risk of injury.[69–71] Wilk et al.[60] demonstrated improved hamstring and quadriceps activation when a knee-flexed position to 30 degrees was held during an exercise such as balancing.

Strengthening for Correction of Trunk Dominance

Core weakness has been associated with lateral trunk displacement and altered dynamic knee stability in the frontal plane.[8,72–76] We recommend using core stabilization exercises and core proprioceptive neuromuscular training to address body sway, which predisposes the knee to valgus. Plank and side plank progressions are used and appropriate feedback is provided for proper alignment and core stabilization for neutral spine (Fig. 12.11A–D). In addition, we have found proprioceptive exercises such as holding a squat position on a rocker board with unexpected perturbations to be effective in

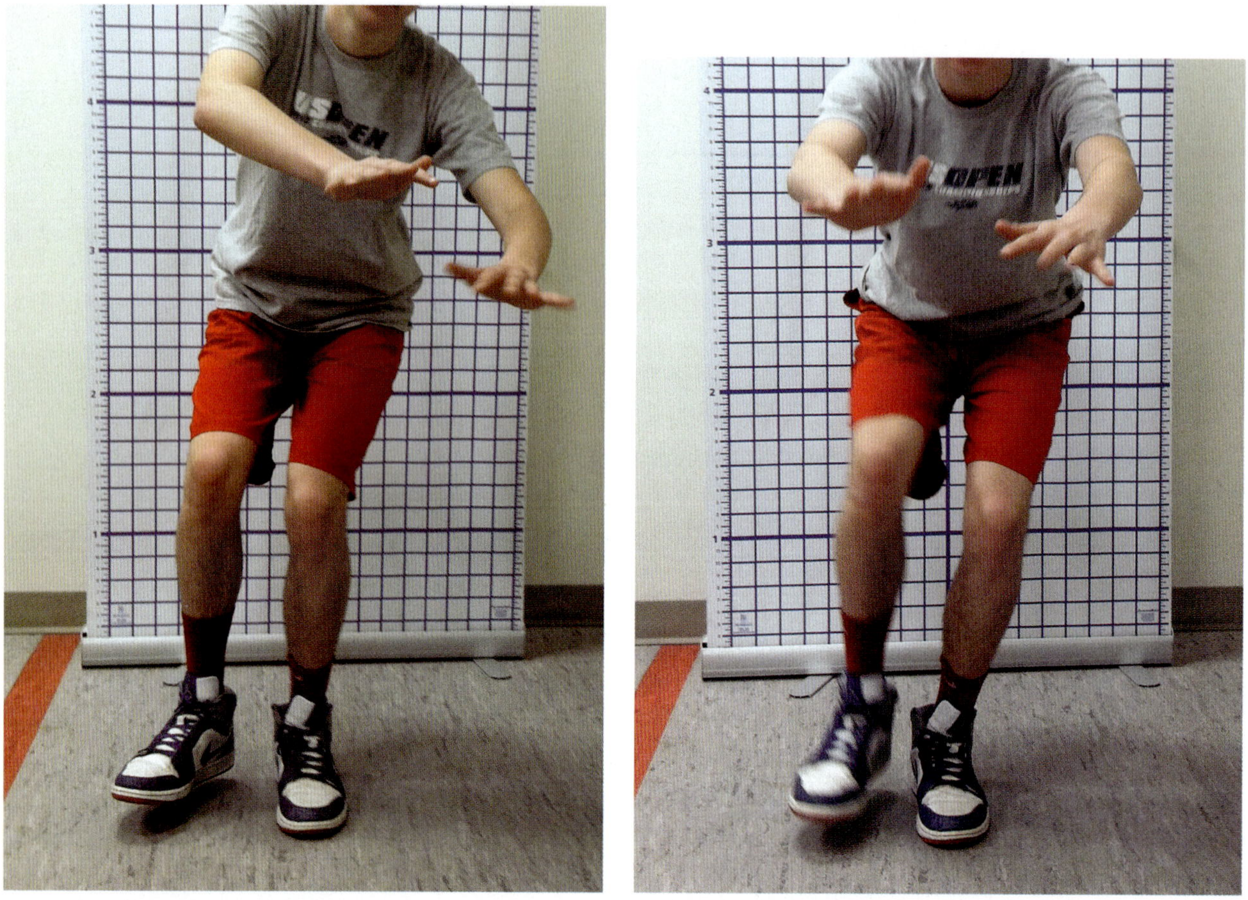

Figure 12.9. Trunk dominance. **A.** Increased lateral displacement of the body's center of mass causing valgus loading of the knee. **B.** Balanced body's center of mass with neutral trunk, hip, knee, and foot/ankle alignment.

reducing postural sway with functional activities. Perturbation may be performed by tapping the hips and trunk to provide postural disturbances[19] with advanced activities that include balancing on less stable surfaces (half foams, DynaDiscs, etc.) to further challenge the neuromuscular system. A ball toss against a trampoline alters the position of the center of mass by incorporating random unexpected movement of the upper extremities while standing on one limb. We recommend addressing both the involved and uninvolved limb moving forward secondary to the increased risk of contralateral injury.[7]

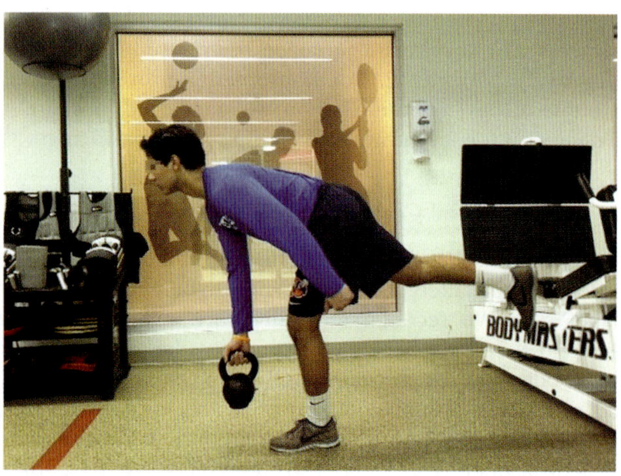

Figure 12.10. Single-leg deadlift with kettlebell weight. Adolescent is standing on the involved limb.

Technique Monitoring and Feedback for Correction of Leg Dominance and Alignment

Leg dominance may result from weakness, flexibility deficits, and/or pain avoidance.[2,3,72] If dominance is noted, the clinician should focus on each leg in isolation. In addition, children should be monitored to ensure safe and proper technique.[48] Studies have demonstrated that young athletes were able to make positive changes in landing mechanics and performance after brief verbal instruction and feedback as well as while under direct supervision.[55–77]

Addressing Deficits with a Squat: Athletic Stance

The ability to perform a squat with proper symmetry, depth, alignment, and strategy is the key fundamental position for dynamic movements such as jumping and as well as the athletic ready position for basically every sport. Patients are expected to demonstrate a symmetrical squat with no leg or ligament dominance (Fig. 12.12A) to a depth of 90 degrees with a hip

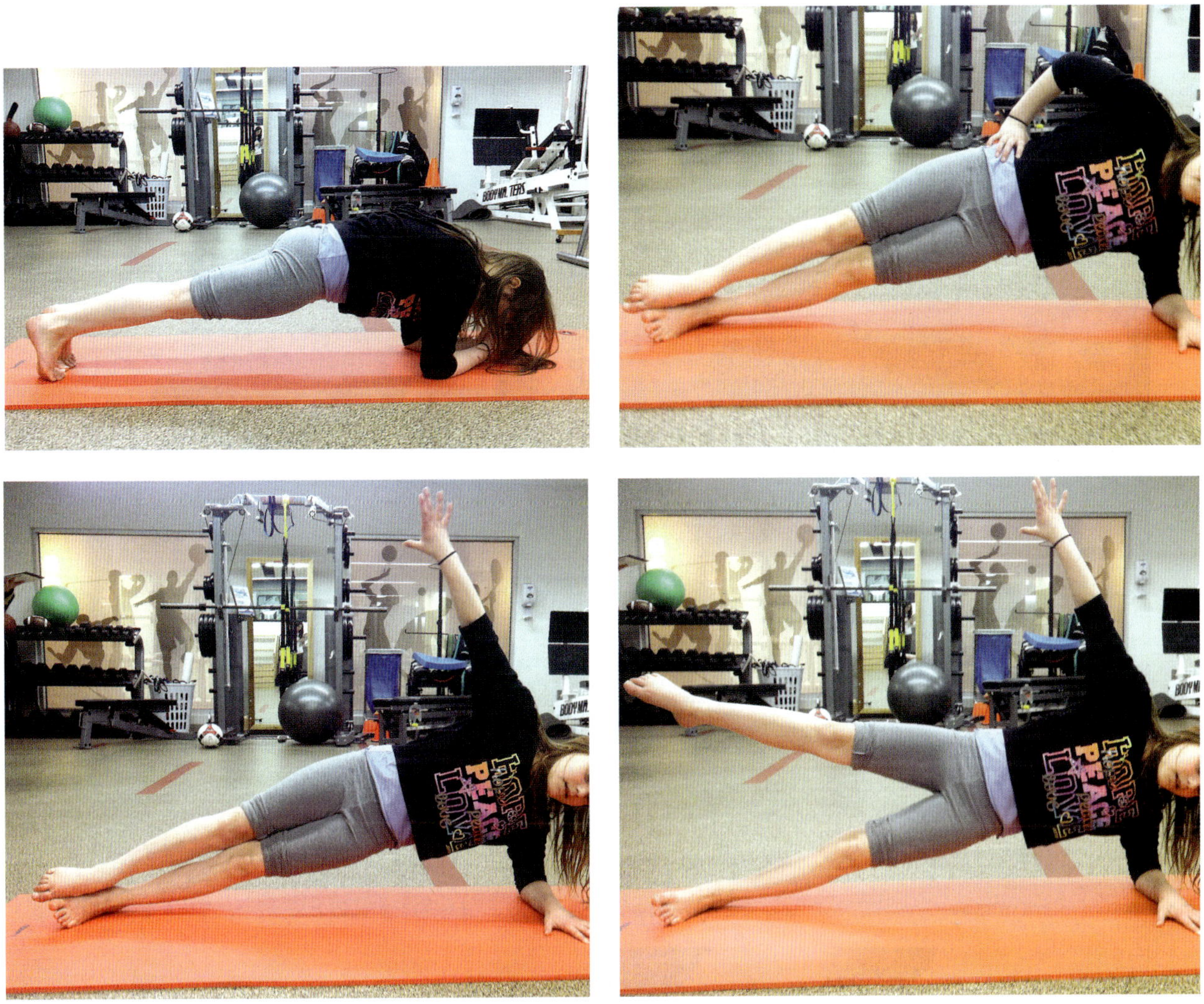
A B C D

Figure 12.11. Plank progression. **A.** Standard plank with proper alignment and core stabilization for neutral spine. **B.** Side plank with proper alignment of spine, hips, and lower extremity **C.** Side plank progressed with upper extremity movement shoulder abduction **D.** Side plank progressed to start with upper extremity and lower extremity abduction, challenging the core for maximal stability.

strategy (Fig. 12.12B) to ensure appropriate strength for dynamic movement progression with jumps and changes in direction. Individuals who demonstrate any of the mentioned compensatory movements will not advance into the next phase of plyometrics (Fig. 12.12C) secondary to risk of injury. Squats may be progressed to unstable surfaces once the patient exhibits good postural control and lower extremity alignment on solid surfaces. Squats held on a tilt board positioned to move in either the medial/lateral or anterior/posterior direction (Fig. 12.13) have been demonstrated to address cocontraction of quadriceps and hamstrings.[19]

PHASE 4: ADVANCED ACTIVITY PHASE (WEEKS 16 TO 24)

This phase is dedicated to advancing dynamic movement patterns with a continued focus on proper alignment, improved neuromuscular control, and maximizing strength and flexibility. Pending an appropriate strength base, those who received autogenous patellar tendon grafts may progress to basic plyometrics and running between months 4 and 5, whereas those who received autogenous hamstring grafts via all-epiphyseal technique may progress at approximately month 5.

Prior to initiation of sports-specific training, the athlete must demonstrate sufficient strength to undertake high joint-loading activities to avoid stretching the graft.[78] In addition, care should be taken to ensure that sports-specific movement patterns and training loads do not exceed the child's physiologic capabilities.[2] The clinician should take into consideration that an athlete may master a skill prior to a growth spurt but may need to revisit that skill to refine alignment secondary to changes body mass[2] (Table 12.4).

Treatment Recommendations

Strengthening

Lower extremity and core strengthening should continue to be progressed. Isotonic knee extension may be performed to full arc as long as the athlete is pain-free and crepitus-free.

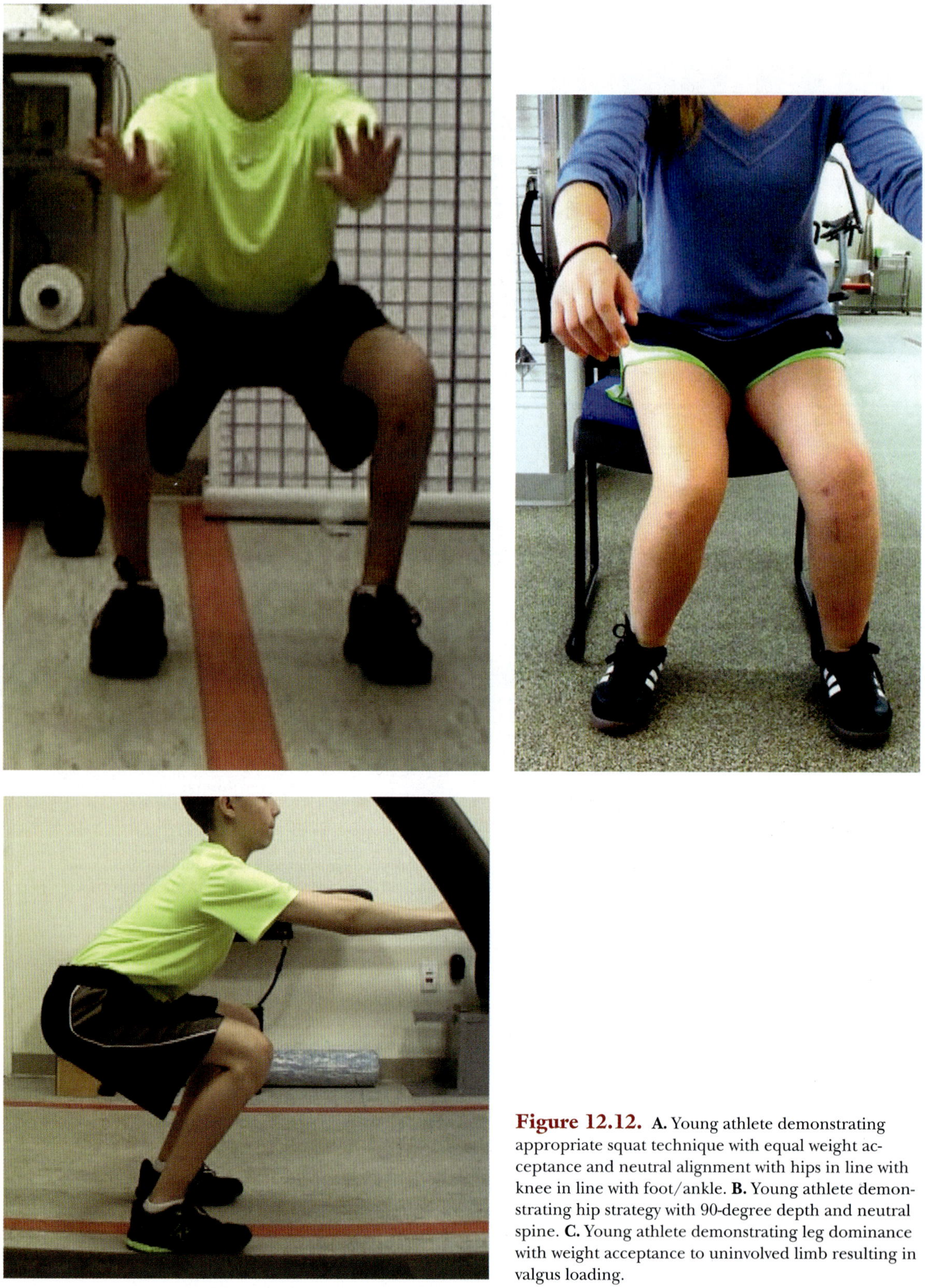

A

C

B

Figure 12.12. **A.** Young athlete demonstrating appropriate squat technique with equal weight acceptance and neutral alignment with hips in line with knee in line with foot/ankle. **B.** Young athlete demonstrating hip strategy with 90-degree depth and neutral spine. **C.** Young athlete demonstrating leg dominance with weight acceptance to uninvolved limb resulting in valgus loading.

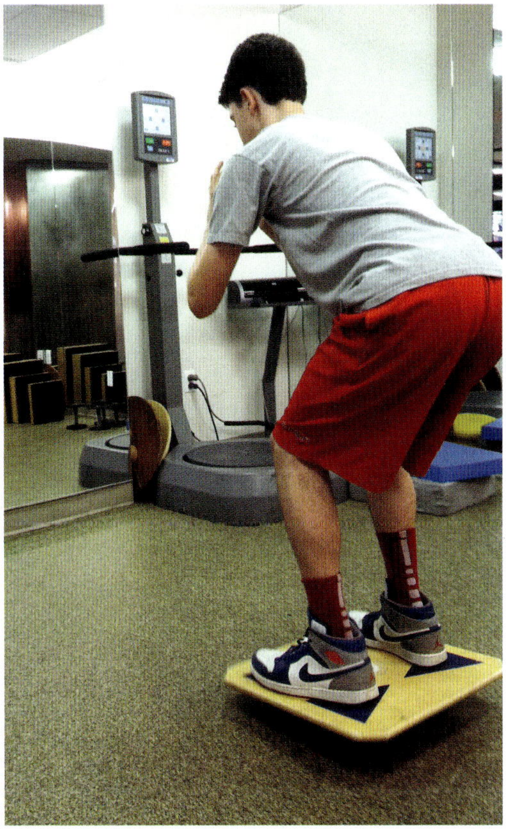

Figure 12.13. Adolescent challenging the neuromuscular system by holding a mini-squat on a rocker board as well as receiving visual feedback on alignment from a mirror in front of him. Neutral spine with a level pelvis, hips, knees, and ankles in alignment.

Single-limb weight-bearing strength and power are improved at increasingly greater knee flexion angles with exercises such as lunges and single leg squatting with quality of movement constantly emphasized and addressed (Fig. 12.14A–C). A mirror to allow for visual feedback is a great tool.

TABLE 12.4	Phase 4: Advanced Activity Phase (Weeks 16–24)
Goals • Maximize strength and flexibility to meet demands of activities of daily living/running • Maximize core strength • Improve neuromuscular control • Movement correction: proper alignment with squats for jump training • Pain-free running progression	
Criteria to Progress into Phase 5 • Functional progression pending functional assessment, alignment, and control • Solid lower extremity and core strength base • Demonstrates athletic ready position with proper alignment and control without cueing for all plyometric and agility movement • Asymptomatic with running progression	

Motor Learning Strategy

Motor learning strategy is essential when teaching a movement skill to allow appropriate integration without frustration. Children have different learning styles. Therefore, a clinician should provide three forms of communication: visual, auditory, and kinesthetic. When teaching a jump in place, one can provide a visual demonstration, an auditory instruction (sound of landing on the balls of their feet), and a kinesthetic element (land lightly). Timing of the feedback is critical and should be presented instantly and frequently when learning a new task. As the child progresses, feedback is less frequent, allowing the individual to become less dependent on the clinician and able to process his or her own feedback. Eventually, feedback is withdrawn without affecting performance. Once the child develops the motor skill, repetitions and speed are advanced as long as alignment is maintained.[79]

Plyometric Progression

Plyometric training has been shown to be effective in decreasing peak GRFs, reducing abduction/adduction moments at the knee during landing, and increasing hamstring–quadriceps ratio in adolescent athletes.[19,73] Much focus is spent on takeoff and landing technique to work on control, prevention of valgus loading, and force dissipation to avoid injury (Fig. 12.15A–D). Instructions to land softly on the toes and keep the knees slightly flexed to avoid knee hyperextension are provided.[72,80–82] One must first work on technique, then developing strength, power, and agility. In the technique phase, low repetitions are performed with feedback.[80]

The individual must demonstrate the ability to perform a symmetrical squat with appropriate depth, alignment, and hip strategy prior to advancing to two-legged jumps to prevent overloading the contralateral limb. In this phase, a jump progression includes vertical jumps progressed to horizontal jumps pending ability. All exercises should be performed equally on each leg with proper alignment. Our vertical jump progression involves squat to jump which involves starting and finishing in a squat position (Fig. 12.16). Athletes are then progressed to jumping up onto a platform (with progressive heights) and stepping down (Fig. 12.17). They then advance to jumps in place and jumps down. The ability to absorb the downward acceleration is crucial for reducing GRFs and risk of lower extremity injury. To effectively slow down the body's center of mass, the athlete is instructed to use a toe-to-heel and triple flexion technique during landing.[81] This allows the foot/ankle, knee, and hips to effectively slow down the body's center of mass over a longer period of time. The initial contact at the foot/ankle complex is made by the ball of the foot and followed immediately by dorsiflexion at the ankle.[80,81] The hips and knees must coordinate and flex simultaneously during forefoot contact in order to allow the knees to stay behind the toes, avoiding knee strategy to reduce anterior shear forces at the knee.[72,80–82] Feedback is constantly provided to ensure no valgus on takeoff or landing as well as symmetrical movements.

Agility Training

Agilities should begin with simple movements and progress to more advanced skills, pending symptoms, strength, and physiologic capabilities. An agility ladder is a great way to develop basic movement skills and footwork. A simple progression is one

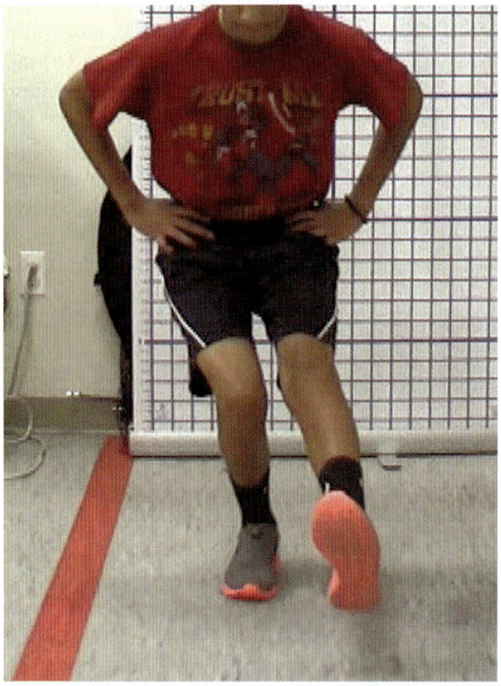

A

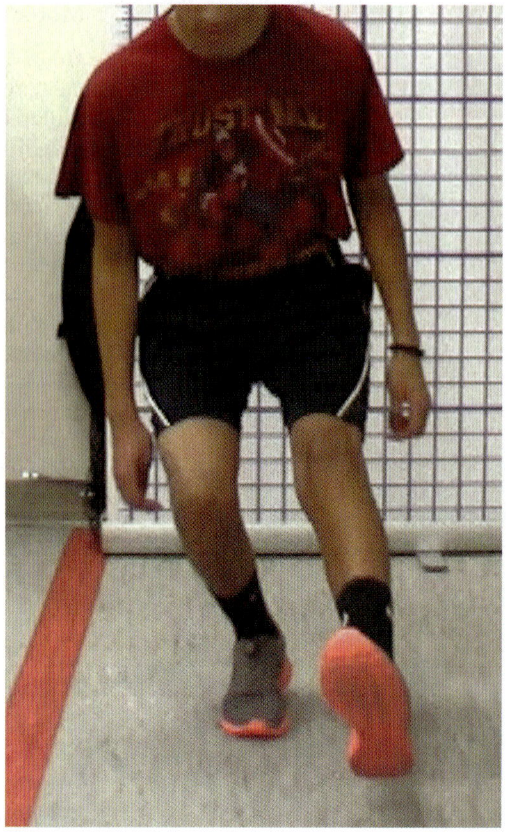

B

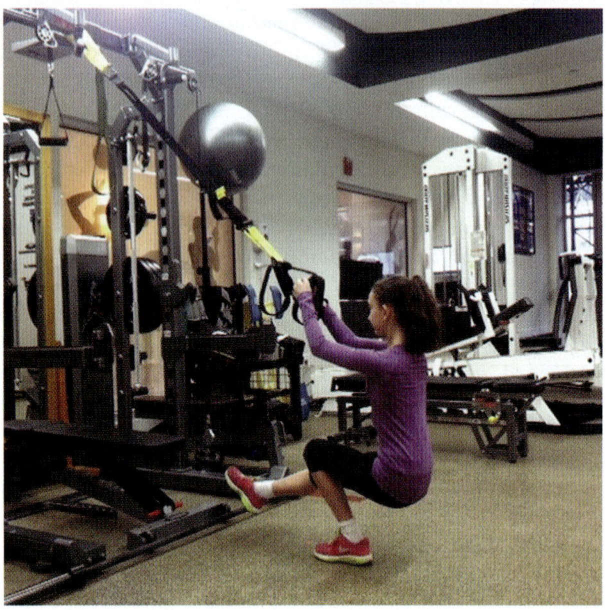

C

Figure 12.14. Single-leg squat progression. **A.** Single-leg squat: poor alignment with valgus loading of the knee. Movement should be corrected with strengthening and cueing prior to performance. **B.** Single-leg squat: proper alignment with trunk, hip, knee, and foot ankle in alignment with same athlete with verbal and visual cueing. **C.** TRX band may be used to provide assist with single-leg squat early on with use of a mirror to provide feedback.

in the hole, two in the hole, lateral two in the hole (Fig. 12.18A), forward jumps two in and two out (Fig. 12.18B), and Ickey Shuffle (Fig. 12.18C). The clinician should ensure the athlete leads with both feet and does not depend on one versus the other.

The proper athletic position should be maintained with all movements and includes face forward, neutral spine, hips and knees slightly bent, and weight on the balls of their feet.[83] Asymmetries early on may cause some children to struggle with footwork going to their involved side or starting with a particular foot. If asymmetry is noted, feedback is provided and the pace is slowed down until the movement is improved.[79,83] Side shuffling, running forward and backward, high steps, and butt kicks may be performed in this phase as well.

Neuromuscular Training

The clinician should continue with a well-structured neuromuscular training program to eliminate uncoordinated movement

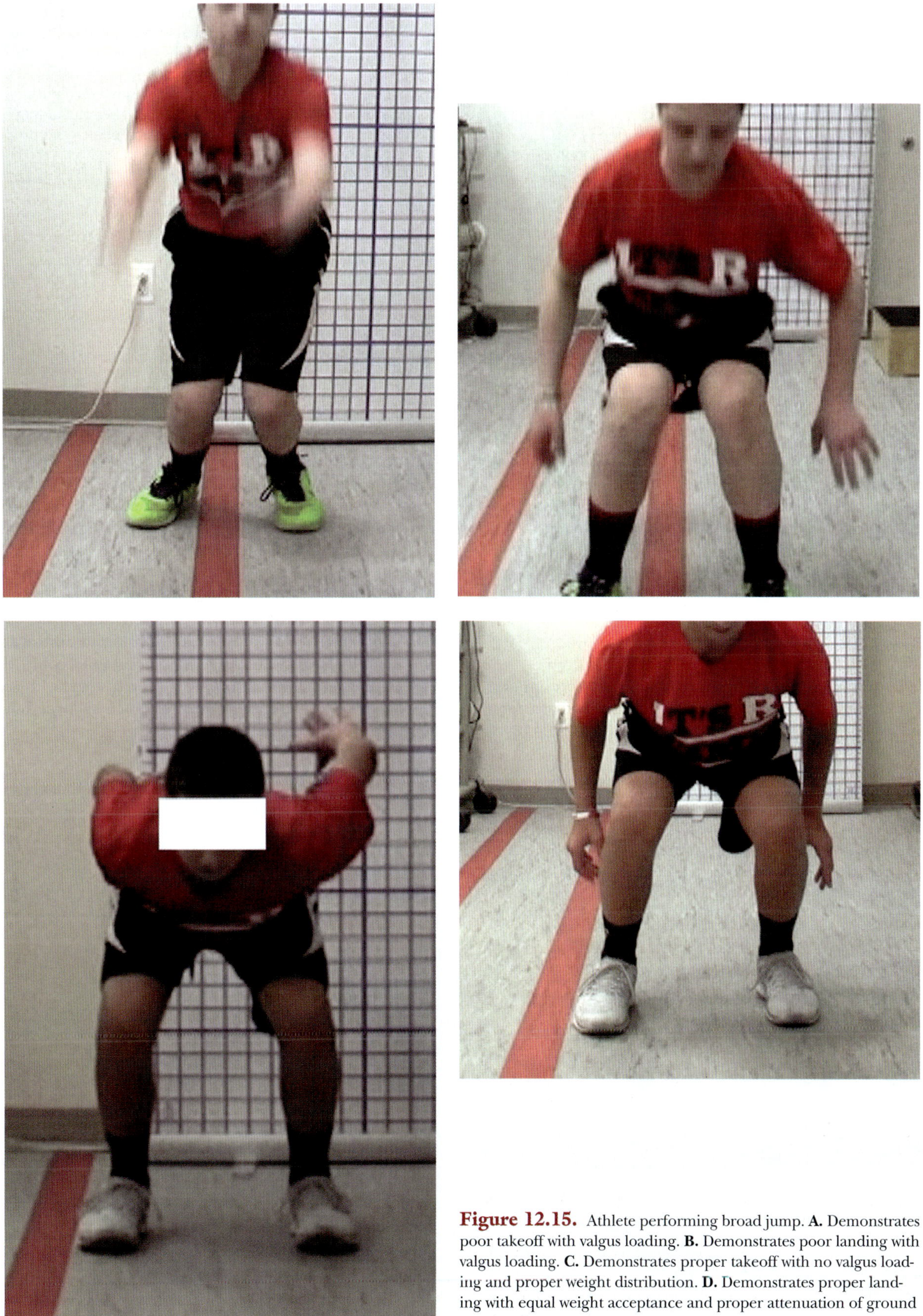

A B C D

Figure 12.15. Athlete performing broad jump. **A.** Demonstrates poor takeoff with valgus loading. **B.** Demonstrates poor landing with valgus loading. **C.** Demonstrates proper takeoff with no valgus loading and proper weight distribution. **D.** Demonstrates proper landing with equal weight acceptance and proper attenuation of ground reaction forces.

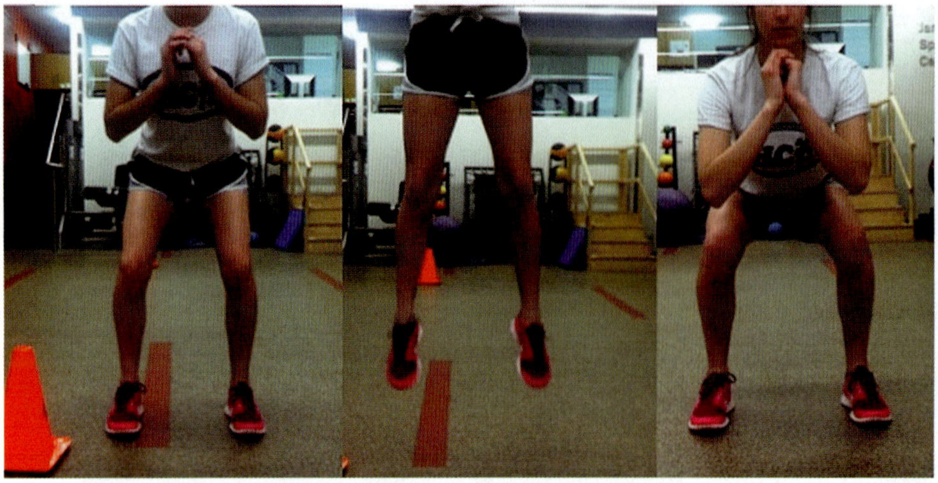

Figure 12.16. Squat to jump demonstrated by an adolescent female. **A.** Assumes start squat position **B.** Takes off with focus on proper alignment, weight distribution, equal push-off, and no valgus. **C.** Focuses on landing with equal weight acceptance and proper alignment.

which are predictive of another injury.[3,80] Proprioceptive and neuromuscular control has been shown to diminish once muscular fatigue has occurred.[19,84–86] Therefore, one can perform these exercises at the start of the session when the dynamic stabilizers are fresh or choose to challenge the neuromuscular control of the knee at the end of the session when the dynamic stabilizers are fatigued as long as one ensures appropriate alignment is maintained.

Running Progression

An athlete may progress to running when the appropriate strength and control is demonstrated as well as their doctors clear them. We assess their strength and control with the performance of an 8-in step-down assessment. Athletes are to stand on an 8-in step with hands on hips. They are asked to slowly lower themselves and step completely off the box. Quality of movement is assessed in terms of alignment for valgus loading as well as an eccentric drop which would indicate weak eccentric quadriceps strength.[45,87] If an athlete demonstrates any of the described deficits, running is withheld to avoid adverse loading of the knee and the graft.[45] If satisfactory results, then retro-running is started prior to forward running secondary to decreased patellofemoral joint compression forces.[88] A forward running program is progressed with an emphasis on speed over shorter distances (such as three bouts of

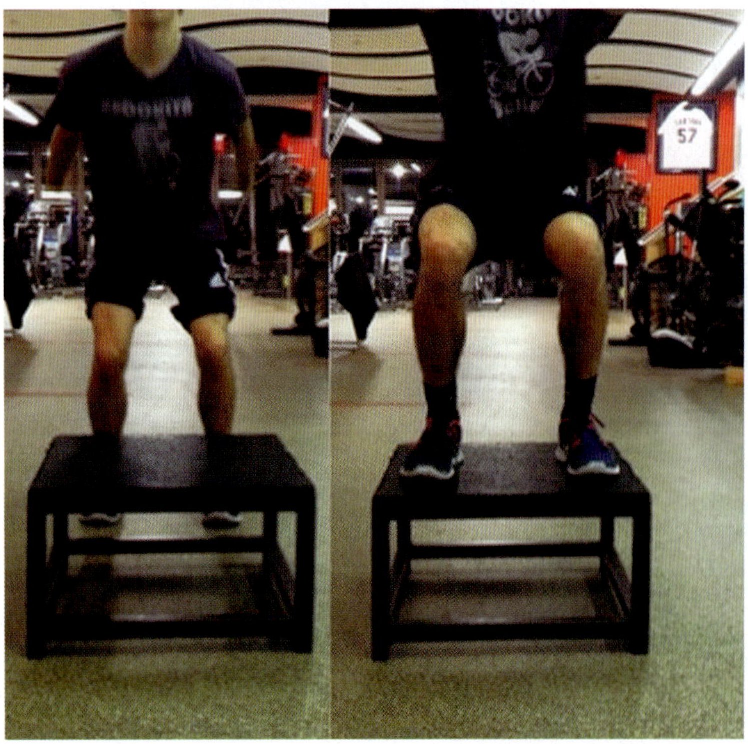

Figure 12.17. Adolescent male jumping onto box with soft landing and proper alignment.

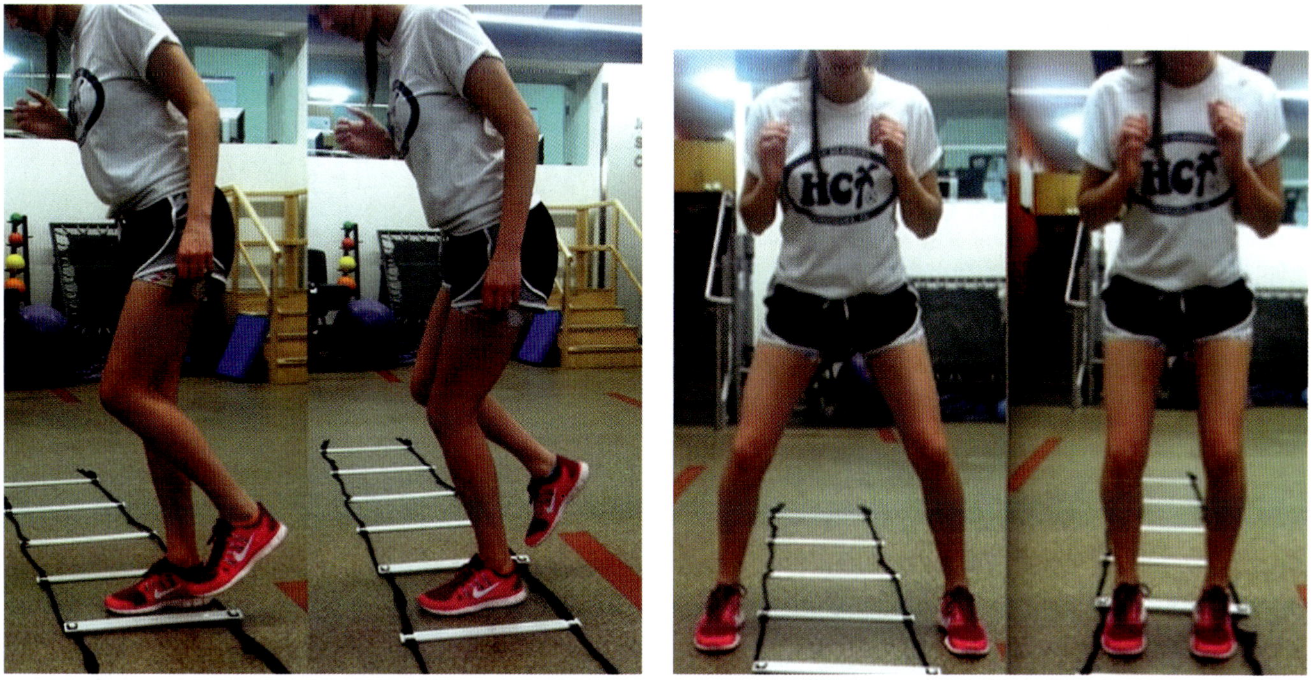

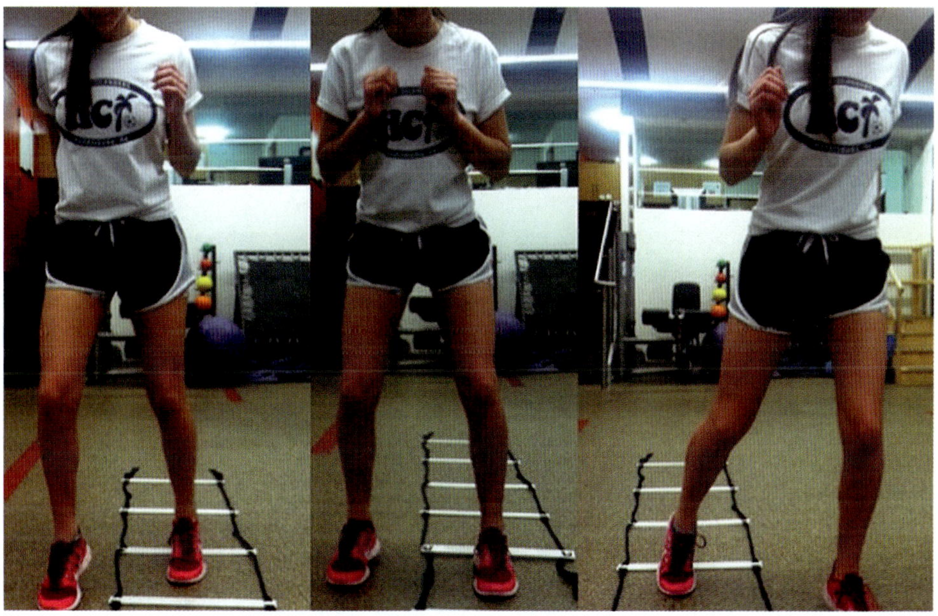

Figure 12.18. Adolescent female performing agility ladder progression with reciprocal arm swing, soft feet, and flexed knees **A.** Lateral two in the hole. **B.** Ickey Shuffle. **C.** Jumps with two feet in and two feet out.

30 seconds at 5.5 to 6.0 mph) versus slower distance running. Treadmill running depends on age and coordination. If pain-free and no effusion the same or next day, the program may progress with increased time.

PHASE 5: RETURN TO PLAY PREPARATION (6 TO 8 MONTHS)

The emphasis of this phase is on assessing and refining quality of movement prior to advanced sports-specific skills; maximizing flexibility, strength, and endurance; advanced neuromuscular control drills; and progressing basic sports-specific training drills. Before entering this phase, individuals must achieve the predetermined criteria to progress to advanced sports-specific drills (Table 12.5). Those who received the all-epiphyseal–sparing technique typically enter this phase at month 6, whereas the adolescents who received patellar tendon grafts typically enter at month 5.

There is a paucity of evidence in the literature regarding guidelines for return to play. Our team believes in preparing individuals to have the ability to meet the sports-specific demands imposed on them when returned to play in an effort to reduce reinjury rates. Successful return is based not

TABLE 12.5	Phase 5: Return to Play Preparation 1 (Months 6–8)

Goals
- Demonstrate pain-free running
- Demonstrate control and alignment with jump takeoff and landings with increased repetitions
- Maximize strength and flexibility to meet demands of sport
- Return to Play assessment demonstrating satisfactory results to progress without risk

Criteria to Progress into Phase 6
- Symptom-free running
- Good control and alignment with two-legged jump takeoffs and landing
- Able to perform single-leg squat with proper alignment and control
- KT-1000 (within 2 mm side-to-side difference)
- Pain-free with all activities

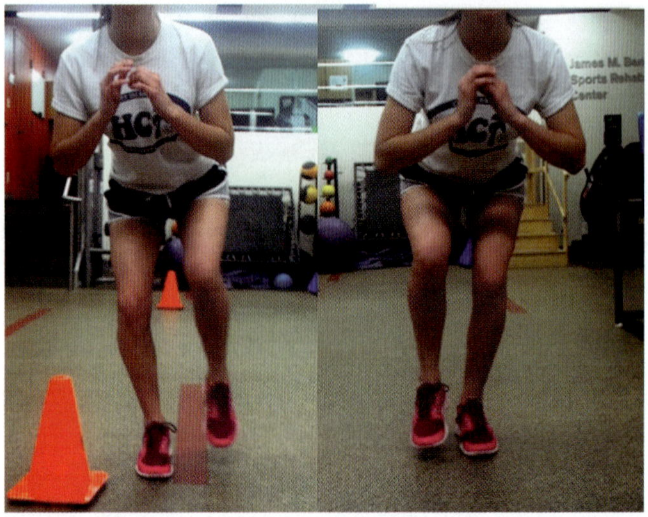

Figure 12.19. Lateral jumps: Start position with knee flexed and jumps laterally, landing softly with knee flexed.

on speed of recovery but return to sport without reinjury. Considering our work with young athletes, the goal is not always to return them to prior activity level, as oftentimes, this level included a poor strength base which was unable to meet the demands of the sport. Our goals is to maximize strength, endurance, and sports-specific skills to allow them to meet the demands of whatever activity they choose to do safely.

Dynamic Movement Assessment

The athletes participate in the Dynamic Movement Assessment program at HSS Sports Rehabilitation and Performance Center, which uses Dartfish software to analyze quality of movement with specific tasks. The analysis is reviewed by the team as well as the physician who is caring for the patient. An isokinetic assessment, performed at 180 degrees per second and 300 degrees per second, and a knee arthrometer to assess knee stability are performed on the same day. The qualitative assessment serves as a guide to performing specific strengthening exercises selected to correct deficits and advance plyometrics and neuromuscular drills, single-leg strength and power, and sports-specific training drills based on the findings. The knee arthrometer score should be comparable with the uninvolved knee (within 2 mm).

Muscular Coactivation for Dynamic Stabilizers

Because quadriceps dominance has been noted as a risk factor in the literature, rehabilitation's goals is to train the athlete to use the coactivation pattern of the quadriceps and hamstrings to stabilize the knee.[2,3,89,90] ACL injury typically occurs during a deceleration, cutting/pivoting maneuver, or landing with the knee in a hyperextended position.[2,3,72] Therefore, hamstring coactivation is crucial to train the athlete to land, cut, and change directions with a flexed knee, and repetitive training with landing on a flexed knee has been shown to improve coactivation.[90–93] Lateral lunges with a resistance cord applied have been shown to assist with coactivation. The athlete progresses to lateral jumps landing with the knees flexed to approximately 25 to 30 degrees and feedback is provided as needed (Fig.12.19) to reduce risk factors and loading of the ACL as demonstrated with the valgus loading in Figure 12.20.

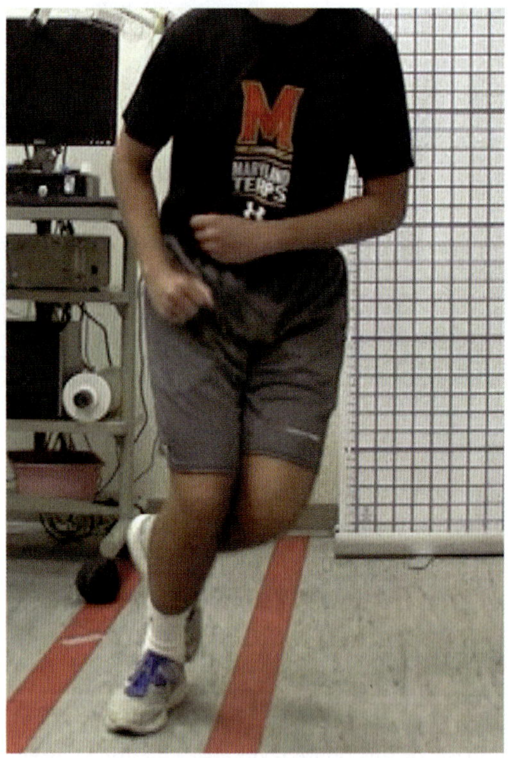

Figure 12.20. Adolescent male performing lateral jumps with valgus knee moment.

Training for Reaction Time

Once athletes have demonstrated proper alignment with movements, they are trained at faster speeds. Reaction time is important for stabilizing muscles of the knee joint.[94] It is important to keep in mind that the literature reports females generate muscular force more slowly than males, which may leave them predisposed to injury.[92] Some examples of drills used are rapid line drills progressing from two feet forward and back, to two feet side to side, to one-foot forward and back, to one foot laterally (Fig. 12.21).

Advanced Agility and Plyometric Training

Drills are progressed with agility ladder to focus on limb isolation. Plyometric exercises are progressed in terms of speed of performance and endurance. Complexity of the task is advanced with single-limb jumps both forward and back as well as laterally. Agility focuses on speed as well as maintaining alignment. Athletes are progressed to switch between movement patterns, for example, side shuffle to a cone, sprint forward at the subsequent cone, and side shuffle to the next cone. Athletes are then advanced in the latter part of this phase to changes in direction and deceleration with unanticipated visual, verbal, and auditory cueing to prepare for gamelike situations.

Changes in direction, cutting, and decelerating are taught and progressed by performing the movements at 25% and progressing to 100% speed by the end of the phase. The emphasis is on trunk, hip, and knee flexed position with hip, knee, and foot/ankle in alignment. Cones are used as visual cues to get the individual to flex forward for changes in direction (Fig. 12.22) or with cutting.

During this phase, athletes typically are cleared to begin some activities with their team, however, in noncontact situations. They are allowed to participate in an active warm-up and may participate in ball skills such as dribbling, passing, shooting, and throwing. If returning to a sport, it is important that the individual progress back into the basic sports skills during this phase such as dribbling, passing, or throwing.

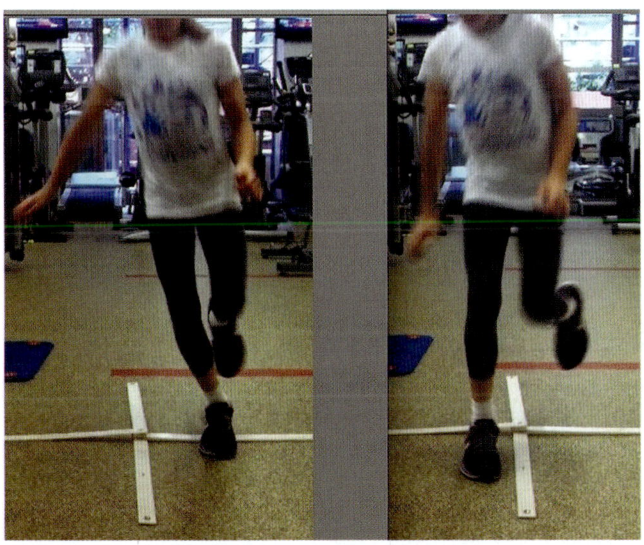

Figure 12.21. Female performing single hops for speed. She jumps laterally, back, laterally, forward, etc. Maintains soft knee bend.

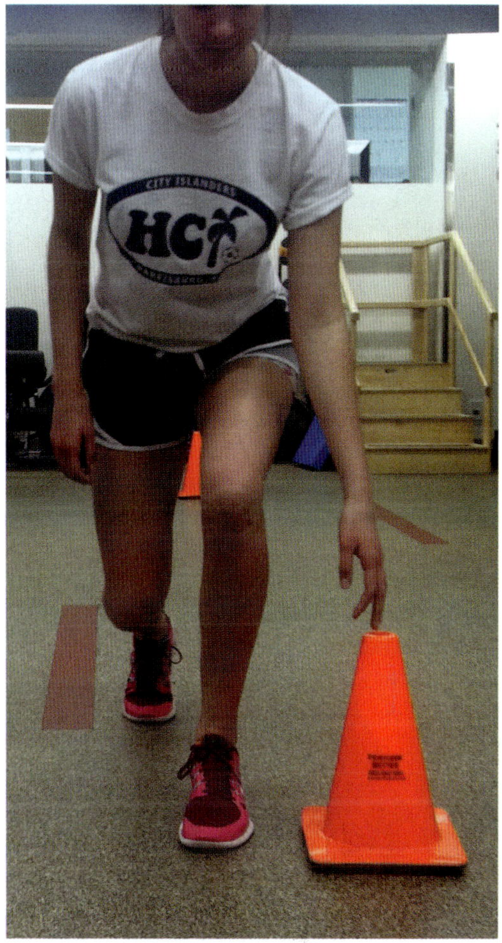

Figure 12.22. Athlete runs to cone; touches cone to enforce flexed trunk, hip, and knee; then backpedals.

PHASE 6: RETURN TO PLAY CLEARANCE

Once athletes have improved quality of movement with an athletic stance; double-limb and single-limb jumping (takeoff and landing); changes in direction, acceleration, and deceleration; and cutting maneuvers, they are to be assessed for their final movement assessment. If there are deficits that need to be worked on, they are relayed to the treating therapist/trainer. If they demonstrate satisfactory results as well as greater than 90% limb symmetry with a single-leg hop test, they are then cleared to progress toward more advanced drills with their team. In the previous phase, they were participating in noncontact drills, and now they are to progress with scrimmage and gamelike play after clearance by the physician.

This phase is geared toward maximizing endurance, neuromuscular control, and strength of the knee stabilizers with advanced sports-specific exercises (Fig. 12.23). Sports-specific agility training with variations in running, turning, cutting maneuvers, acceleration, and deceleration are progressed (Fig. 12.24A,B).

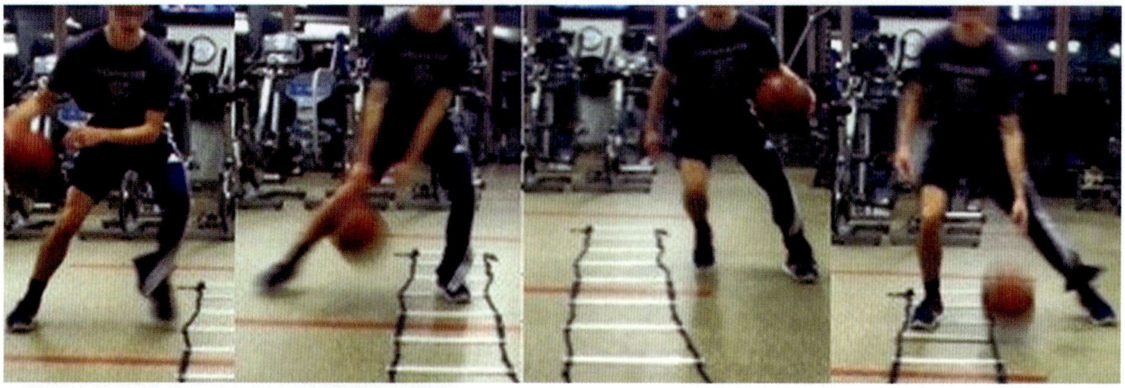

Figure 12.23. Sports-specific drill incorporated as part of the agility ladder. Patient performs drill for speed, while dribbling, as well as maintaining proper alignment of flexed knee, stable and upright trunk, and no valgus.

A

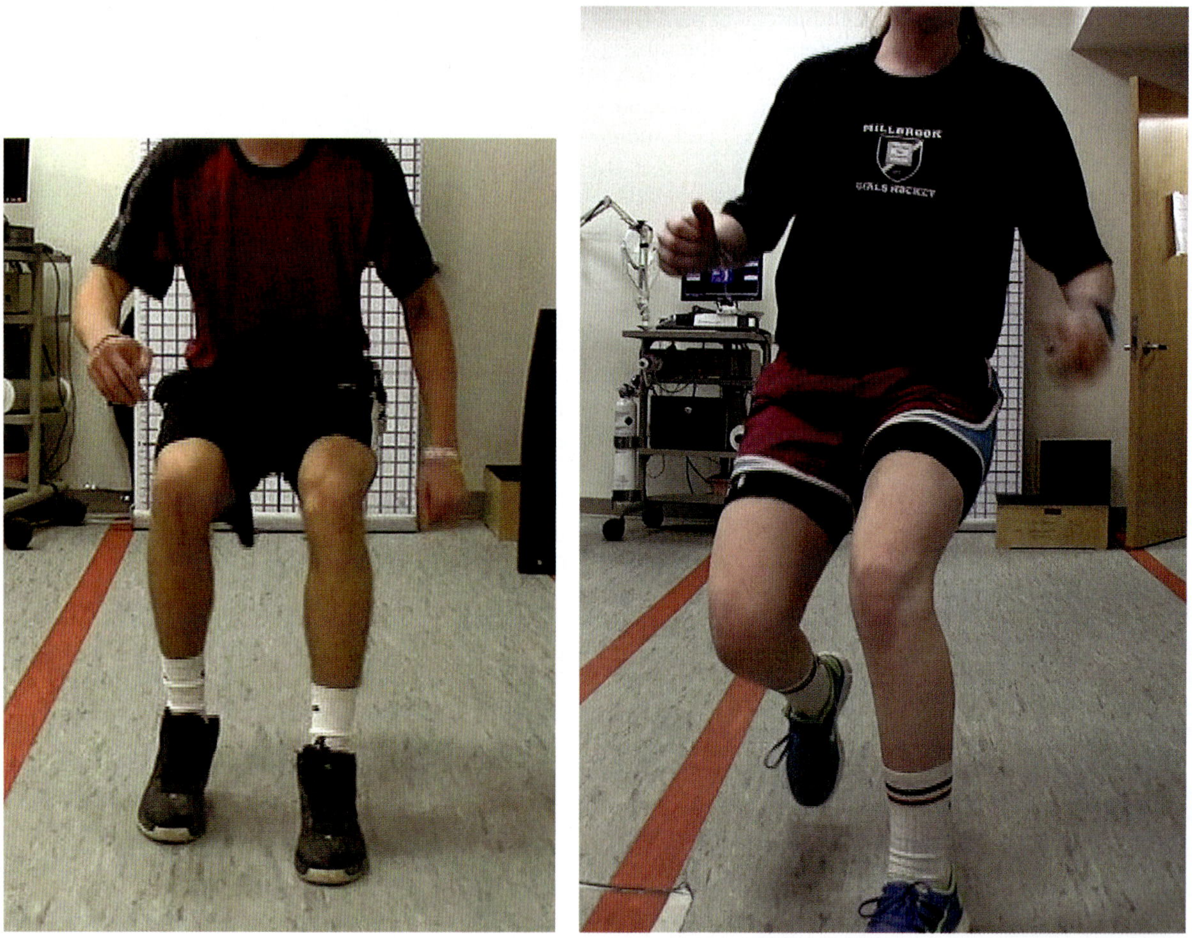

B

Figure 12.24. Unanticipated deceleration. Patients are to sprint forward and decelerate on command, and then backpedal. **A.** Individual with correct form with flexed knees, no valgus, flexed hip/trunk, feet pointing forward, no loss of balance. **B.** Individual with poor form: valgus on deceleration as well as difficulty stopping and trunk shifts over her left leg.

TABLE 12.6	Phase 6: Return to Play (Months 8–12)
Goals • Lack of apprehension and risk factors with sports-specific movements • Demonstrate control, alignment, and power with single-leg jumps • Satisfactory results on second HSS Return to Play assessment • Maximize strength and endurance • Single-leg hop test >90% limb symmetry	
Criteria to Progress to Return to Play/Contact • Symptom-free running • Good control and alignment with one- and two-legged jump takeoffs and landing • Demonstrates ability to performing cutting maneuvers and decelerate with unanticipated cueing with proper alignment and technique • Single-leg hop test >90% limb symmetry • Pain-free with all activities	

Endurance training is vital secondary to increased risk of injury toward the later half of games secondary to fatigue and therefore resultant decrease in quality of movement[95] (Table 12.6)

Advanced drills include sports-specific movements to include higher impact drills as appropriate. The desired adaptation to these drills is that quality and speed of movement are improved.[26,94,95]

Dynamic Cutting

During dynamic cutting tasks, individuals post-ACLR have been shown to use a cutting strategy with decreased knee flexion angles.[26,93–95] Exercises and feedback to incorporate appropriate biomechanical techniques with deeper knee flexion angles (Fig. 12.25A) and core and hip stability for prevention of trunk dominance and valgus (Fig. 12.25B) assist in avoiding reinjury with return to sport.

The goal of this rehabilitation program is to enhance outcomes as well as incorporate a preventive program to reduce incidence of reinjury rates. We have used this particular program with early clinical success in terms of reduced reinjury rates with successful return to play. We strongly encourage the use of both qualitative and quantitative assessments focused on both limbs and a focus on sports symmetry training in the latter phases of rehabilitation to optimize safe return and gradual return to activity.

ACKNOWLEDGMENTS

The author would like to acknowledge the expert care of physicians, physical therapists, and the performance team at Hospital for Special Surgery in their continued efforts to provide the pediatric and adolescent population with the most up-to-date care to allow for successful return to activity and everyday living.

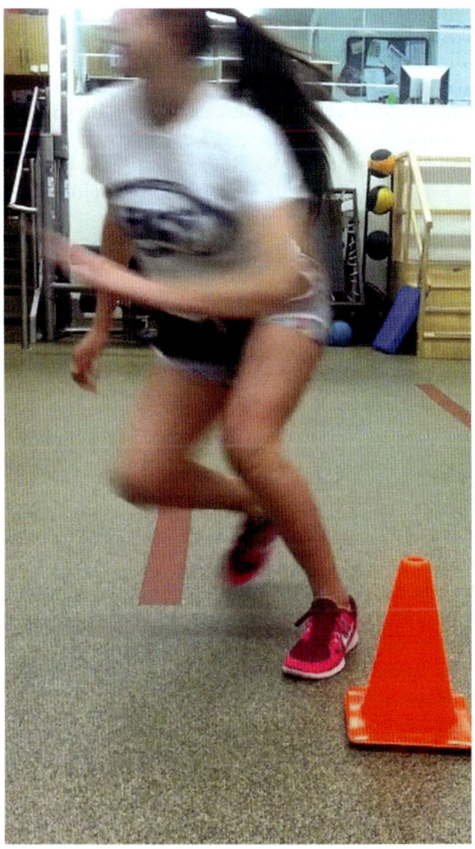

A

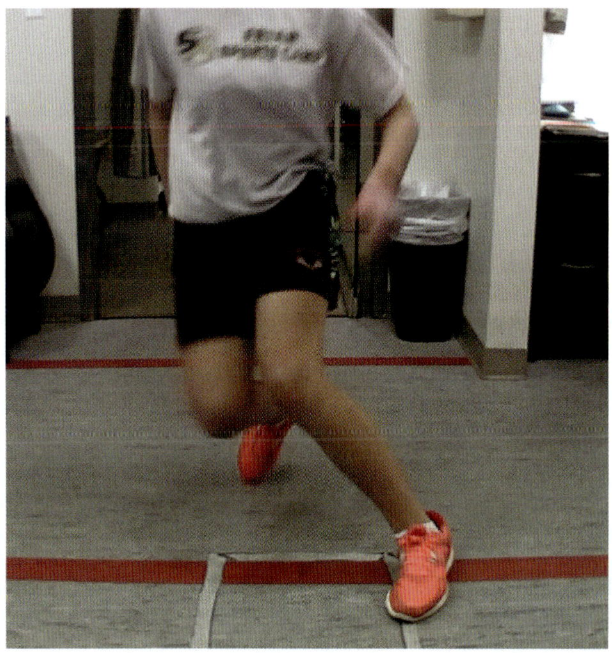

B

Figure 12.25. Cutting technique. **A.** Individual with correct form: No valgus, good trunk control and stability, flexed hip and knee. **B.** Individual with poor technique demonstrating trunk shift and valgus.

REFERENCES

1. Kocher MS, Mandiga R, Klingele K, et al. Anterior cruciate ligament injury versus tibial spine fracture in the skeletally immature knee: a comparison of skeletal maturation and notch width index. *J Pediatr Orthop.* 2004;24:185–188.
2. Graziano J, Green DW, Cordasco FA. Anterior cruciate ligament injury prevention in the young athlete: evidence-based application. *Strength Cond J.* 2013;35(3):89–97.
3. Hewett TE, Myer GD, Ford KR, et al. The 2012 ABJS Nicolas Andry Award: the sequence of prevention: a systematic approach to prevent anterior cruciate ligament injury. *Clin Orthop Relat Res.* 2012;470:2930–2940.
4. DiStefano LJ, Blackburn TJ, Marshall SW, et al. Effects of an age-specific anterior cruciate ligament injury prevention program on lower extremity biomechanics in children. *Am J Sports Med.* 2011;39(5):949–957.
5. Ladenhauf HN, Graziano J, Marx RG. Anterior cruciate ligament prevention strategies: are they effective in treating young athletes? Current concepts and review of the literature. *Curr Opin Pediatr.* 2012;25(1):65–71.
6. Hass CJ, Schick Ea, Tillman MD, et al. Knee biomechanics during landings: comparison of pre- and postpubescent females. *Med Sci Sports Exerc.* 2005;37(1):100–107.
7. Henja W, Rosenberg A, Buturusis D, et al. The prevention of sports injuries in high school students through strength training. *J Strength Cond Res.* 1982;4:28–31.
8. Hewett TE, Stroupe AL, Nance TA, et al. Plyometric training in female athletes. Decreased impact forces and increased hamstring torques. *Am J Sports Med.* 1986;24:765–773.
9. Gianotti SM, Marshall SW, Hume PA, et al. Incidence of anterior cruciate ligament injury and other knee ligament injuries: a national population-based study. *J Sci Med Sport.* 2009;12(6):622–627.
10. Paterno MV, Rauh MJ, Schmitt LC, et al. Incidence of contralateral and ipsilateral anterior ACL reconstruction and return to sport. *Clin J Sport Med.* 2012;22(2):116–121.
11. Myer GD, Paterno MV, Ford KR, et al. Rehabilitation after anterior cruciate ligament reconstruction: criteria-based progression through the return-to-sport phase. *J Orthop Sports Phys Ther.* 2006; 36(6):385–402.
12. Clancy WB Jr, Nelson DA, Reider B, et al. Anterior cruciate ligament reconstruction using one-third of the patellar ligament, augmented by extra-articular tendon transfers. *J Bone Joint Surg Am.* 1982;64:352–359.
13. Shelbourne KD, Gray T. Anterior cruciate ligament reconstruction with autogenous patellar tendon graft followed by accelerated rehabilitation. A two- to nine-year followup. *Am J Sports Med.* 1997;25:786–795.
14. Aglietti P, Buzzi R, Menchetti PM, et al. Arthroscopically assisted semitendinosus and gracilis tendon graft in reconstruction for acute anterior cruciate ligament injuries in athletes. *Am J Sports Med.* 1996;24:726–731.
15. MacDonald PB, Hedden D, Pacin O, et al. Effects of an accelerated rehabilitation program after anterior cruciate ligament reconstruction with combined semitendinosus-gracilis autograft and a ligament augmentation device. *Am J Sports Med.* 1995;23:588–592.
16. Yasuda K, Tsujino J, Ohkoshi Y, et al. Graft site morbidity with autogenous semitendinosus and gracilis tendons. *Am J Sports Med.* 1995;23:706–714.
17. Rodeo SA, Kawamura S, Kim HJ, et al. Tendon healing in a bone tunnel differs at the tunnel entrance versus the tunnel exit: an effect of graft-tunnel motion? *Am J Sports Med.* 2006;34:1790–1800.
18. Suzuki T, Shino K, Nakagawa S, et al. Early integration of a bone plug in the femoral tunnel in rectangular tunnel ACL reconstruction with a bone-patellar tendon-bone graft: a prospective computed tomography analysis. *Knee Surg Sports Traumatol Arthosc.* 2001;19(suppl 1):29–35.
19. Wilk KE, Macrina LC, Cain EL, et al. Recent advances in the rehabilitation of anterior cruciate ligament injuries. *J Orthop Sports Phys Ther.* 2012;42(3):153–171.
20. Wilk KE, Escamilla RF, Fleisig GS, et al. A comparison of tibiofemoral joint forces and electromyographic activity during open and closed kinetic chain exercises. *Am J Sports Med.* 1996;24:518–527.
21. Butler DL, Grood ES, Noyes FR, et al. Mechanical properties of primate vascularized vs. nonvascularized patellar tendon grafts; changes over time. *J Orthop Res.* 1989;7:68–79.
22. Arem AJ, Madden JW. Effects of stress on healing wounds: I. Intermittent noncyclical tension. *J Surg Res.* 1976;20:93–102.
23. Bair GR. The effect of early mobilization versus casting on anterior cruciate ligament reconstruction. *Trans Orthop Res Soc.* 1980;5:108.
24. Beynnon BD, Johnson RJ, Toyama H, et al. The relationship between anterior-posterior knee laxity and the structural properties of the patellar tendon graft. A study in canines. *Am J Sports Med.* 1994;22:812–820.
25. Ballock RT, Woo SL, Lyon RM, et al. Use of patellar tendon autograft for anterior cruciate ligament reconstruction in the rabbit: a long-term histologic and biomechanical study. *J Orthop Res.* 1989;7: 474–485.
26. Cascio BM, Culp L, Cosgarea AJ. Return to play after anterior cruciate ligament reconstruction. *Clin Sports Med.* 2004;23:395–408, ix.
27. Delay BS, Smolinksi RJ, Wind WM, et al. Current practices and opinions in ACL reconstruction and rehabilitation: results of a survey of the American Orthopaedic Society for Sports Medicine. *Am J Knee Surg.* 2001;14:85–91.
28. Nawabi DH, Jones KJ, Lurie B, et al. Physeal-specific MRI analysis of growth plate disturbance following all-inside anterior cruciate ligament reconstruction in skeletally immature patients: does a physeal-sparing technique offer any advantage? *Orthop J Sports Med.* 2013;1(4).
29. Kvist J. Rehabilitation following anterior cruciate ligament injury: current recommendations for sports participation. *Sports Med.* 2004;34:269–280.
30. Young A, Stokes M, Shakespeare DT, et al. The effect of intra-articular bupivacaine on quadriceps inhibition after meniscectomy. *Med Sci Sports Exerc.* 1983;15:154.
31. Spencer JD, Hayes KC, Alexander IJ. Knee joint effusion and quadriceps reflex inhibition in man. *Arch Phys Med Rehabil.* 1984;65:171–177.
32. DeLisa JA, Gans BM, Walsh NE. *Physical Medicine and Rehabilitation: Principles and Practice.* 4th ed. Vol 1. Philadelphia, PA: Lippincott Williams & Wilkins; 2005:258–259.
33. Birmingham TB, Kramer JF, Kirkley A, et al. Knee bracing after ACL reconstruction: effects on postural control and proprioception. *Med Sci Sports Exerc.* 2001;33:1253–1258.
34. Risberg MA, Holm I, Steen H. The effect of knee bracing after anterior cruciate ligament reconstruction. A prospective, randomized study with two years' follow-up. *Am J Sports Med.* 1999;27:76–83.
35. Akeson WH, Woo SLY, Amiel D. The connective tissue response to immobilization: biomechanical changes in periarticular connective tissue of the immobilized rabbit knee. *Clin Orthop Relat Res.* 1973;93:356–362.
36. Noyes FR, Mangine RE, Barber S. Early knee motion after open and arthroscopic ACL reconstruction. *Am J Sports Med.* 1987;15(2): 149–160.
37. Salter RH, Simmonds DF, Malcolm BW, et al. The biological effect of continuous passive motion on healing of full-thickness defects in articular cartilage. *J Bone Joint Surg.* 1980;62(8):1232–1251.
38. Perry J, Antonelli D, Ford W. Analysis of knee-joint forces during flexed-knee stance. *J Bone Joint Surg.* 1975;57(7):961–967.
39. Ahmad CS, Kwak SD, Ateshian GA, et al. Effects of patella tendon adhesion to the anterior tibia on knee mechanics. *Am J Sports Med.* 1998;26:715–724.
40. Atkinson TS, Atkinson PJ, Mendenhall HV, et al. Patellar tendon and infrapatellar fat pad healing after harvest of an ACL graft. *J Surg Res.* 1998;79:25–30.

41. Benum P. Operative mobilization of stiff knees after surgical treatment of knee injuries and posttraumatic conditions. *Acta Orthop Scand.* 1982;53:625–631.
42. Kim KM, Croy T, Hertel J, et al. Effects of neuromuscular electrical stimulation after anterior cruciate ligament reconstruction on quadriceps strength, function, and patient-oriented outcomes: a systematic review. *J Orthop Sports Phys Ther.* 2010;40:383–391.
43. Jerosch J, Schäffer C, Prymka M. Proprioceptive abilities of surgically and conservatively treated knee joints with injuries of the cruciate ligament [in German]. *Unfallchirurg.* 1998;101(1):26–31.
44. Paterno MV, Gelb ID, Hewett TE, et al. The return of neuromuscular coordination after anterior cruciate ligament reconstruction. *J Orthop Sports Phys Ther.* 1998:27(1):96.
45. Cavanaugh J. Anterior cruciate ligament reconstruction. In: Cioppa-Mosca J, Cahill JB, Cavanaugh JT, et al, eds. *Postsurgical Rehabilitation Guidelines for the Orthopedic Clinician.* St. Louis, MO: Mosby Elsevier; 2006: 425–438.
46. Fleming BC, Beynnon BD, Renstrom PA, et al. The strain behavior of the anterior cruciate ligament during bicycling. An in vivo study. *Am J Sports Med.* 1998;26(1):109–118.
47. Faigenbaum AD. Strength training for children and adolescents. *Clin Sports Med.* 2000;19(4):593–619.
48. Hewett TE, Johnson DL. ACL prevention programs: fact or fiction? *Orthopedics.* 2010;33:36–39.
49. Cahill B, Griffith E. Effect of preseason conditioning on the incidence and severity of high school football knee injuries. *Am J Sports Med.* 1978;6:180–184.
50. Mizner RL, Kawaguchi JK, Chmielewski TL. Muscle strength in the lower extremity does not predict postinstruction improvements in the landing patterns of female athletes. *J Orthop Sports Phys Ther.* 2008;38:353–361.
51. Mizuta H, Kubota K, Shiraishi M, et al. The conservative treatment of complete tears of the anterior cruciate ligament in skeletally immature patients. *J Bone Joint Surg Br.* 1995;77:890–894.
52. Swartz EE, Decoster LC, Russell PJ, et al. Effects of developmental stage and sex on lower extremity kinematics and vertical ground reaction forces during landing. *J Athl Train.* 2005;40(1): 9–14.
53. Escamilla RF, Fleisig GS, Zheng N, et al. Biomechanics of the knee during closed kinetic chain and open kinetic chain exercises. *Med Sci Sports Exerc.* 1998;30:556–569.
54. Escamilla RF, Fleisig GS, Zheng N, et al. Effects of technique variations on knee biomechanics during the squat and leg press. *Med Sci Sports Exerc.* 2001;33:1552–1566.
55. Padua DA, Distefano LJ. Sagittal plane knee biomechanics and vertical ground reaction forces are modified following ACL injury prevention programs: a systematic review. *Sports Health.* 2009;1(2): 165–173.
56. Prapavessis H, McNair PJ. Effects of instruction in jumping technique and experience jumping on ground reaction forces. *J Orthop Sports Phys Ther.* 1999;29(6):352–356.
57. Cipriani DJ, Armstrong CW, Gaul S. Backward walking at three levels of treadmill inclination: an electromyographic and kinematic analysis. *J Orthop Sports Phys Ther.* 1995;22(3):95–102.
58. Ardern CL, Webster KE, Taylor NF, et al. Return to sport following anterior cruciate ligament reconstruction surgery: a systematic review and meta-analysis of the state of play. *Br J Sports Med.* 2011;45:596–606.
59. Markolf KL, Graff-Radford A, Amstutz HC. In vivo knee stability. A quantitative assessment using an instrumental clinical testing apparatus. *J Bone Joint Surg Am.* 1978;60:664–674.
60. Wilk KE, Arrigo C, Andrews JR, et al. Rehabilitation after anterior cruciate ligament reconstruction in the female athlete. *J Athl Train.* 1999;34:177–193.
61. Renström P, Arms SW, Stanwyck TS, et al. Strain within the anterior cruciate ligament during hamstring and quadriceps activity. *Am J Sports Med.* 1986;14(1):83–87.
62. Ebben WP, Fauth ML, Petushek EJ, et al. Gender-based analysis of hamstring and quadriceps muscle activation during jump landings and cutting. *J Strength Cond Res.* 2010;24:408–415.
63. Ford KR, Shapiro R, Myer GD, et al. Longitudinal sex differences during landing in knee abduction in young athletes. *Med Sci Sports Exerc.* 2010;42:1923–1931.
64. Hewett TE, Stroupe AL, Nance TA, et al. Plyometric training in female athletes. Decreased impact forces and increased hamstring torques. *Am J Sports Med.* 1996;24:765–773.
65. Mascal CL, Landel R, Powers C. Management of patellofemoral pain targeting hip, pelvis, and trunk muscle function: 2 case reports. *J Orthop Sports Phys Ther.* 1978;33:647–674.
66. Myer GD, Ford KR, Hewett TE. Rationale and clinical techniques for anterior cruciate ligament injury prevention among female athletes. *J Athl Train.* 2004;39:352–364.
67. Krause DA, Jacobs RS, Pilger KE, et al. Electromyographic analysis of the gluteus medius in five weight bearing exercises. *J Strength Cond Res.* 2009;23:2689–2694.
68. Alentorn-Geli E, Myer GD, Silvers HJ, et al. Prevention of non-contact anterior cruciate ligament injuries in soccer players. Part 1: mechanisms of injury and underlying risk factors. *Knee Surg Sports Traumatol Arthrosc.* 2009;17:705–729.
69. Myer GD, Ford KR, Divine JG, et al. Longitudinal assessment of noncontact anterior cruciate ligament injury risk factors during maturation in a female athlete: a case report. *J Athl Train.* 2009;44: 101–109.
70. Kaminski TW, Wabbersen CV, Murphy RM. Concentric versus enhanced eccentric hamstring strength training: clinical implications. *J Athl Train.* 1998;33:216–221.
71. Mjølsnes R, Arnason A, Østhagen T, et al. 10 week randomized trial comparing eccentric vs. concentric hamstring strength training in well-trained soccer players. *Scand J Med Sci Sports.* 2004;14: 311–317.
72. Bien DP. Rationale and implementation of anterior cruciate ligament injury prevention warm-up programs in female athletes. *J Strength Cond Res.* 2011;25:271–285.
73. Boden BP, Dean GS, Feagin JA Jr, et al. Mechanisms of anterior cruciate ligament injury. *Orthopedics.* 2000;23:573–578.
74. Zazulak BT, Hewett TE, Reeves NP, et al. The effects of core proprioception on knee injury: a prospective biomechanical-epidemiologic study. *Am J Sports Med.* 2007;35:368–373.
75. Zazulak BT, Ponce PL, Straub SJ, et al. Gender comparison of hip muscle activity during single-leg landing. *J Orthop Sports Phys Ther.* 2005;35:292–299.
76. Zebis MK, Bencke J, Anderson LL, et al. The effects of neuromuscular training on knee joint motor control during sidecutting in female elite soccer and handball players. *Clin J Sport Med.* 2005;18:329–337.
77. Mizner RL, Kawaguchi JK, Chmielewski TL. Muscle strength in the lower extremity does not predict post-instruction improvements in the landing patterns of female athletes. *J Orthop Sports Phys Ther.* 2008;38:353–361.
78. Lewek M, Rudolph K, Axe M, et al. The effect of insufficient quadriceps strength on gait after anterior cruciate ligament reconstruction. *Clin Biomech (Bristol Avon).* 2002;17:56–63.
79. Jeffreys I. Motor learning-applications for agility, part 2. *Strength Cond J.* 2006;28(6):10–14.
80. Hewett TE, Lindenfeld TN, Riccobene JV, et al. The effect of neuromuscular training on the incidence of knee injury in female athletes: a prospective study. *Am J Sports Med.* 1999;27(6):699–706.
81. Iida Y, Kanehisa H, Inaba Y, et al. Short-term landing training attenuates landing impact and jump height in landing-to-jump movement. *J Strength Cond Res.* 2013;27:1560–1567.
82. Yu B, Lin CH, Garrett WE. Lower extremity biomechanics during the landing of a stop-jump. *Clin Biomech.* 2006;21:297–305.
83. Young W, Farrow D. A review of agility: practical applications for strength and conditioning. *Strength Cond J.* 2006;28(5):24–29.

84. Lattanzio PJ, Petrella RJ. Knee proprioception: a review of mechanisms, measurements, and implications of muscular fatigue. *Orthopedics.* 1998;21:463–470.
85. Lattanzio PJ, Petrella RJ, Sproule JR, et al. Effects of fatigue on knee proprioception. *Clin J Sport Med.* 1997;7:22–27.
86. Skinner HB, Wyatt MP, Hodgdon JA, et al. Effect of fatigue on joint position sense of the knee. *J Orthop Res.* 1986;4:112–118.
87. Cavanaugh JT, Stump TJ. Forward step down test. *J Orthop Sports Phys Ther.* 2000;30(1):A–46.
88. Flynn TW, Soutas-Little RW. Patellofemoral joint compressive forces in forward and backward running. *J Orthop Sports Phys Ther.* 1995;21(5):277–282.
89. Ageberg E, Zatterstrom R, Moritz U, et al. Influence of supervised and nonsupervised training on postural control after an acute anterior cruciate ligament rupture: a three-year longitudinal prospective study. *J Orthop Sports Phys Ther.* 2001;31:632–644.
90. Barratta R, Solomonow M, Zhou BH, et al. Muscular coactivation: the role of the antagonist musculature in maintaining knee stability. *Am J Sports Med.* 1988;16:113–122.
91. Perry J, Anontelli D, Ford W. Analysis of knee joint forces during flexed-knee stance. *J Bone Joint Surg Am.* 1975;57:961–967.
92. Wilk KE, Arrigo C, Andrews JR, et al. Rehabilitation after anterior cruciate ligament reconstruction in the female athlete. *J Athl Train.* 1999;34(2):177–193.
93. McCarty L, Bach B. Rehabilitation after patellar tendon autograft anterior cruciate ligament reconstruction. *Tech Orthop.* 2005;20:439–451.
94. Risberg M, Mork M, Jenssen H, et al. Design and implementation of a neuromuscular training program following anterior cruciate ligament reconstruction. *J Orthop Sports Phys Ther.* 2001;31:620–631.
95. Silvers H, Mandelbaum B. Prevention of anterior cruciate ligament injury in the female athlete. *Br J Sports Med.* 2007;41(1):52–59.

Polly de Mille
Theresa A. Chiaia

CHAPTER 13

Controversies in Return to Play

INTRODUCTION

Scope of Problem

Roughly 2 million anterior cruciate ligament (ACL) injuries occur worldwide each year, 200,000 in the United States. ACL reconstruction (ACLR) is the sixth most common procedure in orthopedics in the United States and the standard of care for athletes who wish to return to their previous level of play.

The rate of primary ACL injury has increased at an alarming rate over the past two decades and shows no signs of diminishing. Lyman et al.[1] showed that ACLRs increased in New York (NY) State by 21.5% and up to 67.8% nationwide over a 9-year period. In a study of NY State hospital admissions, Dodwell et al.[2] reported a steady increase in the rate of ACLR over the past 20 years in the 3- to 20-year-old age group. ACLR increased from 17.6 per 100,000 in 1990 to 50.9 in 2009, with the greatest rate and greatest increase of ACLR occurring in the 15- to 18-year-old age group.

The rate of ACLR differs between genders particularly in the second decade of life. Young female athletes are at 2.6 times greater overall risk in this age group. A meta-analysis of basketball players indicates that this discrepancy diminishes as maturity and level of play increases. The female-to-male ratio of noncontact ACL injuries decreases at the college level and approaches 1:1 at the professional level.[3]

More than 38 million children and adolescents participate in sports each year in the United States, and nearly three-quarters of US households with school-age children have at least one child who plays organized sports.[4] More than 7.8 million high school students, 42% females, participate in organized sports.[5] Compare that to the roughly 8% of high school athletes who go on to play at the college level.[6]

For a long time, injury to the ACL in the skeletally immature athlete was not a concern. With increased intensity of participation in organized sports, recreational activities and exercise, along with increased recognition, the number of injuries to the ACL in this younger population are increasing. Early on, the focus of the discussion centered on whether this injury should be treated operatively or nonoperatively as adequate protection of the graft in this perpetually active population seemed impossible. The results of nonoperative treatment yielded poor outcomes. Concerns for the immediate trauma to the individual and injury to the knee's menisci and articular cartilage with recurrent episodes of instability, as well as the long-term health of the knee with the looming consequence of osteoarthritis (OA), have made surgical reconstruction of the ACL the treatment of choice in the individual with a torn ACL. The advent of more skeletal age–appropriate surgical techniques has made reconstruction of the ACL in this population a more attractive option.

The combination of greater numbers of athletes with less refined skills, greater accessibility to play, and physiologic changes associated with growth and development contribute to a unique constellation of risk factors for the pediatric and adolescent athlete who has sustained an ACL injury and wishes to return to play.

Injury to the ACL impacts the life of a child and adolescent in ways different than it impacts an adult. The cost of an ACL injury in the young athlete is not only measured in dollars but also in quality of life issues: social skill acquisition, dependence/independence, identity development, self-esteem, academic performance, and emotional well-being, in addition to the potential loss of scholarship dollars. The injured pediatric individual presents unique concerns related to development, both physical and psychological.

The conundrum of when to return the pediatric athlete to play will be presented. Returning an athlete to sport is the fundamental core of sports medicine.

Consider this: A 12-year-old boy tears his ACL while playing basketball in January. He is an avid lacrosse player in the spring and soccer player in the fall. Following 1 month of prehabilitation, he undergoes an ACLR in February. Immediately, he begins his lengthy postoperative rehabilitation. During this time, this young boy does not go to "gym" class, does not play outside with his friends (free play), does not run around during recess, and does not play in organized sport teams or athletic activities. He is only absent from school for a week, by conservative estimates; however, his grades suffer. During his rehabilitation, he grows 4 in and gains 20 lb. He now must learn to control a new body. The application of the current statistics suggests that this boy may have an arthritic knee by the age of 22 years.[14]

RISK OF REINJURY

The pediatric and adolescent athlete who returns to sport following ACLR faces a substantial risk of retear. The estimated rate of rerupture or failure in patients younger than 20 years of age who return to play following ACLR is 18% to 23%.[7] In a study of 90 patients 15 years postisolated ACL tear, Hui et al.[8] reported that patients younger than 18 years of age had a seven times greater odds of contralateral ACL rupture than those older than 18 years of age. The Multicenter ACL Revision Study (MARS) group also found the ACL revision rate highest in young athletes reporting a 22% risk in the 12- to 18-year-old age group.[9] The significantly elevated risk of injury to the ipsilateral or contralateral knee in young athletes is well-documented and presents a challenge to those involved in return to play decisions for young athletes.[8,10–12] Although there does not seem to be a gender difference in the rate of rerupture,[12] the risk of a contralateral tear appears to be greater in females. Paterno et al.[13] reported that 88% of documented ACL injuries to the contralateral limb occurred in female athletes.

TABLE 13.1 Return to Play Statistics for Professional Athletes

	Time to RTP (Months)	*Athletes who RTP (%)*
NFL	10.8	63
NBA	11.6	86
WNBA	11.8	78
UEFA	12	89

RTP, return to play; NFL, National Football League; NBA, National Basketball Association; WNBA, Women's National Basketball Association; UEFA, Union of European Football Associations.

RATE OF RETURN

The ACL is the main stabilizing ligament of the knee. The goal of ACLR is to restore function of the knee, thereby reducing symptoms (pain, instability), improving quality of life (active lifestyle), and minimizing complications (short term [meniscus, articular cartilage] and long-term [degenerative OA] health of the knee) so the individual can return to sport. This is never truer than in the pediatric population, whose existence centers around free play and organized sports and who has many decades of an active lifestyle ahead. For one reason or another, however, these goals have not consistently been met. Even with surgical reconstruction, the risk of developing degenerative knee OA is still a concern.[14]

There is considerable data suggesting limited success in returning athletes to their preinjury level of play. A systematic review demonstrated that although 82% of athletes returned to sports, only 63% returned to preinjury level.[15]

In a study of 503 competitive athletes, Arden et al.[16] reported that two-thirds had not returned to play at 12 months and less than half were planning on returning despite good functional outcome on International Knee Documentation Committee. The mean age in this cohort was 27.2 years, so it may not be representative of the pediatric and adolescent athlete. Shah et al.[17] reported 63% (31 of 49) National Football League (NFL) athletes with a mean age of 26.2 years returned to NFL game play at an average of 10.8 months following primary ACLR. Sixty-four National Basketball Association (NBA) players (mean age of 25.7 years) with 69 ACL tears were identified with return to sport and performance data between 1975 and 2012.[18] Harris et al.[18] reported that 86% (55 knees) of these players returned to play in the NBA at an average of 11.6 months. Guards had the most difficulty returning to play. Seventy-eight percent of Women's NBA athletes who tore their ACL returned to play with only a slight decrease in performance.[19] Elite professional soccer players in the Union of European Football Associations (UEFA) following ACLR need 7 months to return to first training, 10 months to return to regular training, and 12 months to return to match play[20] (Table 13.1).

In a follow-up study of 314 athletes (mean age 32.7 years), less than half (45%) of these athletes had returned to sport at greater than 3 years after ACLR. However, younger athletes were found to return to preinjury levels of play at a greater rate. Of the 43 athletes younger than 18 years of age, 72% had attempted playing their preinjury sport which was the highest percentage of any of the groups (18 to 25 years, 26 to 32 years, >32 years) but only 49% reported playing at their preinjury level at follow-up.[21]

The Multicenter Orthopaedic Outcomes Network (MOON) group reported 85% of 100 soccer athletes (mean age ♂ 27.7 ♀ 19.8 years) returned to preinjury level of play.[22] Shelbourne et al.[23] provided further evidence that age is inversely related to the likelihood of return to competition. In a study of 413 high school basketball and soccer athletes with mean age of 15.5 years, Shelbourne et al.[23] reported that 87% of the basketball athletes (both boys and girls) returned to high school competition and 93% of the females and 80% of the male soccer athletes returned to competition.

PSYCHOLOGICAL FACTORS

"Other interests" and fear were cited as the primary reasons for failure to return to play rather than physical symptoms in high school and college football players following ACLR.[24]

Psychological factors may play a significant role in a greater likelihood of return to preinjury level of activity in adolescent athletes following ACLR. In a study comparing adolescent and adult psychological readiness for ACL surgery, Udry et al.[25] found that adolescents reported not only higher preoperative mood disturbance levels than adults but also higher levels of "psychological readiness" for surgery. Adolescents reported more pros associated with surgery and used a greater number of cognitive and behavioral processes of change than adults. The greater mood disturbances prior to surgery and the greater "readiness" for surgery may be the result of the central role that physical activity may play in their life at this stage. Adolescents may be more disturbed by the disruption in their usual activities and separation from their peers and more invested in returning to their previous level of activity.

Both organized sports and social play and games play an important developmental role in the child and adolescent athlete. Acceptance by peer groups takes on critical importance at this stage as the child develops his or her sense of identity independent of his or her family. Sports provide a way to learn to interact socially, work toward a collective goal, follow rules, and understand the concept of fair play.[26] When children and adolescents are sidelined by injury, they are not only deprived of the pleasure of playing a sport they enjoy but also deprived of the opportunities for personal growth and development that is provided by the social aspect of organized sports and free play.

In a study of the influence of patient outcomes following ACLR, younger patients had significantly higher self-efficacy scores which are related to greater perceived knee function, postoperative sports activity levels, and knee-related quality of life.[27] The patient's preinjury level of activity was also found to be predictive of the probability of returning to preinjury levels of activity.

The greater availability of sports for middle and high school athletes, the social role that sports may play in this age group in which teammates form a key social support system, and psychological factors may all play a role in the greater return to play rates in pediatric and adolescent athletes following ACLR.

An ACL injury at a young age is a life-changing event. In addition to surgery and many months of rehabilitation, the time lost from school and play can have significant effects on the athlete's mental health and academic performance.[28] Elective knee ligament reconstruction performed on a school day results in more difficulties than surgery performed during a school holiday or summer break; therefore, a child's daily school life should be accounted for in the surgical decision-making process.[29] The consequences are far more reaching than being sidelined from their sport; they are often sidelined from their life, or perceive it that way.

FACTORS ASSOCIATED WITH RISK OF SECOND INJURY

The psychological makeup of a pediatric patient combined with the physical challenges they must overcome following ACLR is a recipe for increased risk of a second injury.

Given that pediatric and adolescent ACL patients are more likely to return to sport and face a high risk of a second injury, what specific factors have been identified as risk factors?

Not surprisingly, risk is related to activity levels. For each increase of 4 points on the Marx Activity Scale, the risk of retear increases threefold.[30] Age is also a key factor; risk of reinjury is estimated to drop by 50% for each decade of life, placing the pediatric and adolescent athlete squarely in the highest risk group.[31] In discussing RTP, it must be remembered that top-level athletes may well have exceptional neuromuscular skills and therefore be reasonably well prepared to meet the demands of safe return to sport. It is, however, the clumsy or unskilled player who returns to a low level of sport who may be at greater risk of reinjury.[32]

Biomechanical factors that have been identified as risk factors for primary ACL tear are, not surprisingly, found to be associated with risk of secondary ACL tear.[11,13,33–37] Paterno et al.[11] performed 3-day analysis of drop vertical jump (DVJ), postural stability analysis by Biodex, and a KT-1000 on 56 athletes aged 13 to 20 years returning to level 1 sports; 13 athletes went on to suffer a second ACL tear in the first year following return to play. Athletes who demonstrated deficits in postural stability on the involved limb were two times more likely to retear. Findings from the 3-day analysis of DVJ were even more predictive of second injury. Side-to-side differences in sagittal knee moment at initial contact and greater frontal plane knee motion during landing were correlated with a three-fold or greater increase in likelihood to tear, whereas those demonstrating hip rotation at the initial 10% of landing were more than eight times more likely to suffer a second ACL injury.

In a follow-up study of the incidence of second ACL injury 2 years after primary ACL injury and return to sport, Paterno et al.[38] reported 15 times greater risk of ACL tear during the first year compared to a 6 times greater risk than controls in the second year following return to sport.

The influence of biomechanical factors and neuromuscular control on risk of sustaining a second ACL injury, either ipsilateral or contralateral, indicates the need for evaluation of these factors in the return to play decision-making process in this high-risk population.

CURRENT MODELS OF RETURN TO PLAY DECISION MAKING

Quantitative measures have historically played the principal role in determining when an athlete is cleared for play following ACLR. A systematic review from 2001 to 2011 was conducted to identify factors used to determine unrestricted return to play after ACLR.[39] Of 264 articles, 40% failed to provide any criteria, 32% used amount of time postoperatively as the only criterion, and only 13% noted objective criteria required for return to athletics. These included muscle strength (9%), single-leg hop test (4%), general knee examination (6%), knee stability (1%), and validated questionnaire (1%). Only 2 studies out of 264 surveyed reported using three to four criteria to determine readiness to return to unrestricted activity. The criteria included strength, single-leg hop tests, absence of effusion, full range of motion (ROM), and 90% limb symmetry index (LSI). There is a discrepancy between functional and physical measures and the rate of return. Ardern et al.[15] reported that despite 90% of patients achieving normal or near-normal outcomes on impairment-based measures of knee function, only 44% returned to competitive sports. This suggests that factors other than knee function could be contributing to return to sport. It also may suggest that LSI, in this population, may not be a good indicator of readiness. The contralateral limb is not the standard to which the index limb should be held. The commonly used functional tests may not be sensitive enough or demanding enough to identify deficits. Perhaps, the element of fatigue is not addressed sufficiently. Again, the role of psychological readiness cannot be overstated.

In a 2013 survey of 274 experienced arthroscopic surgeons, the most common measures used to determine clearance for play included Lachman test, pivot shift, anterior drawer, and ROM.[40] Over 85% reported using no clinical measures whatsoever.

Barber-Westin and Noyes[39] recommended a multifaceted approach to determining readiness to return to play: less than 10% LSI with isokinetic testing, less than 15% LSI with single-leg hop testing, less than 3 mm increased anteroposterior tibial displacement on Lachman or arthrometer testing, greater than 60% knee separation distance with DVJ, no effusion, full knee ROM, normal patellar mobility, no or minimal patellar crepitus, and no pain or swelling with all activities. In addition, single-leg squat, multistage fitness test, and 60-second sit-up test are considered.

A multifaceted approach has been proposed by several clinicians; however, it seems their criteria are still heavily weighted toward quantitative data. Myer et al.[41] at the Cincinnati Children's Hospital propose an algorithm for a safe return to sport. In order to enter the return to sport phase, the athlete must have no postsurgical history of giving-way, an International Knee Documentation Committee score of 70, and minimum baseline strength of knee extension peak torque to body mass: 30% females, 40% males at 300 degrees per second; 50% females, 60% males at 180 degrees per second. They propose a four-stage criteria-based return to sport progression, which incorporates measures of side-to-side symmetry in strength and landing force as well as measures of dynamic stability and mechanics of jumping and landing.

Wilk et al.[42] proposed a return to sport progression over 20 to 30 weeks of rehabilitation based on fulfillment of specific criteria including results of KT-1000, isokinetic testing, proprioception, hop test, and practical specific tests.

Criteria used at the University of Delaware include quadriceps strength index (QSI), LSI on four hop tests, Knee Injury and Osteoarthritis Outcome Score (KOOS), and Global Rating Scale before entering the return to sport phase.[43]

Given the high rate of reinjury, the ideal criteria to determine readiness to return to play has yet to be identified. Quantitative measures combined with the eagerness of the child and family to return to activity may result in clearing an athlete who demonstrates all of the qualitative risk factors for retear (postural instability, hip internal rotation, etc.) despite "passing" the quantitative thresholds. Often, these young individuals have not trained formally prior to their injury. The adolescent has only focused on skill development—playing soccer, etc. The optimum performance pyramid as described by Cook[44] has a broad base of functional movement, with a slightly smaller level in the middle of functional performance and an even smaller level on top of sport-specific skill. Movement patterns, movement efficiency, and sport skill are balanced and adequate in the optimum performance pyramid (Fig. 13.1). In our experience, the adolescent and the injured athlete's pyramids are often out of balance. As mentioned, the adolescent athlete focuses on the very top of the pyramid, where the focus for the rehabilitating athlete is too often the middle part of the pyramid. There may also be instances when the athlete does not feel ready to return to play despite meeting all clinical criteria. Patient reported outcome measures (PROM) specific to this population should be administered.

A GENERAL MODEL OF RETURN TO PLAY

Creighton et al.[45] proposed a three-step decision-based model for return to play after injury, not specifically ACL rupture. Evaluation of health status is step 1 and includes such measures as medical history, symptoms, physical exam, lab tests, functional tests, psychological state, potential seriousness, and patient demographics. Step 2, evaluation of participation risk, involves examining the type of sport (contact vs. noncontact),

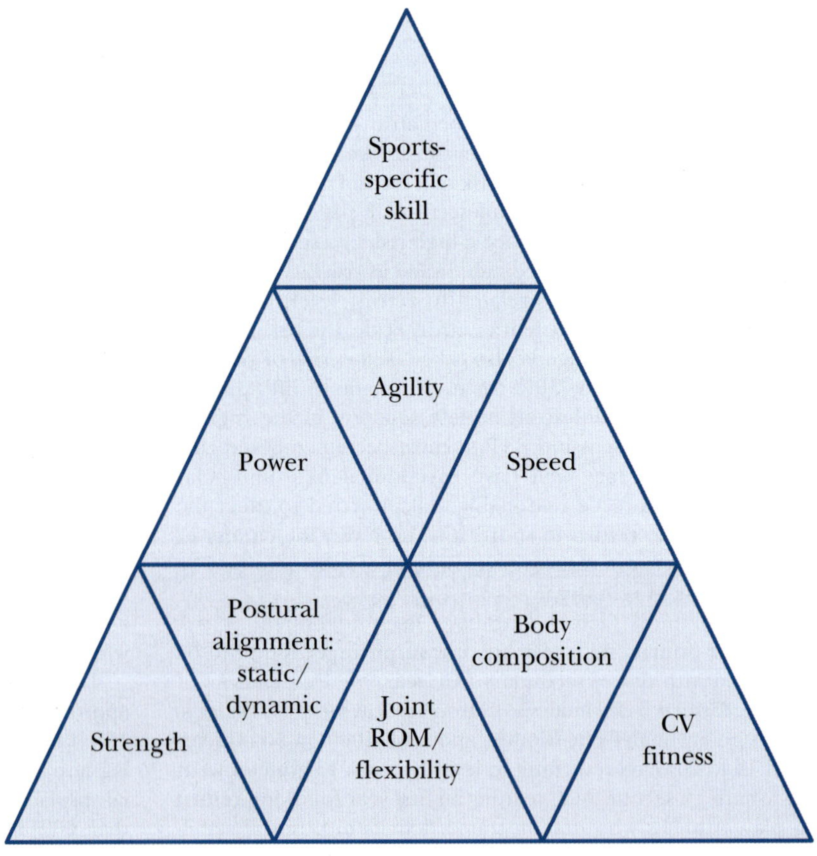

Figure 13.1. The performance pyramid adapted for return to play (RTP) demonstrating specific pyramids at each level. *ROM*, range of motion; *CV*, cardiovascular.

position played, limb dominance, competitive level, and ability to protect the injured limb. The final step, step 3, is evaluating the "decision modifiers," which include timing and season, pressure from the athlete, external pressure, conflict of interest, fear of litigation, and masking the injury. This model takes into account the wide range of factors involved in clearing an athlete to return to play.

In applying this model to ACLR in the pediatric population (Fig. 13.2), step 1 in Creighton's model would involve reviewing the mechanism of injury (contact vs. noncontact),

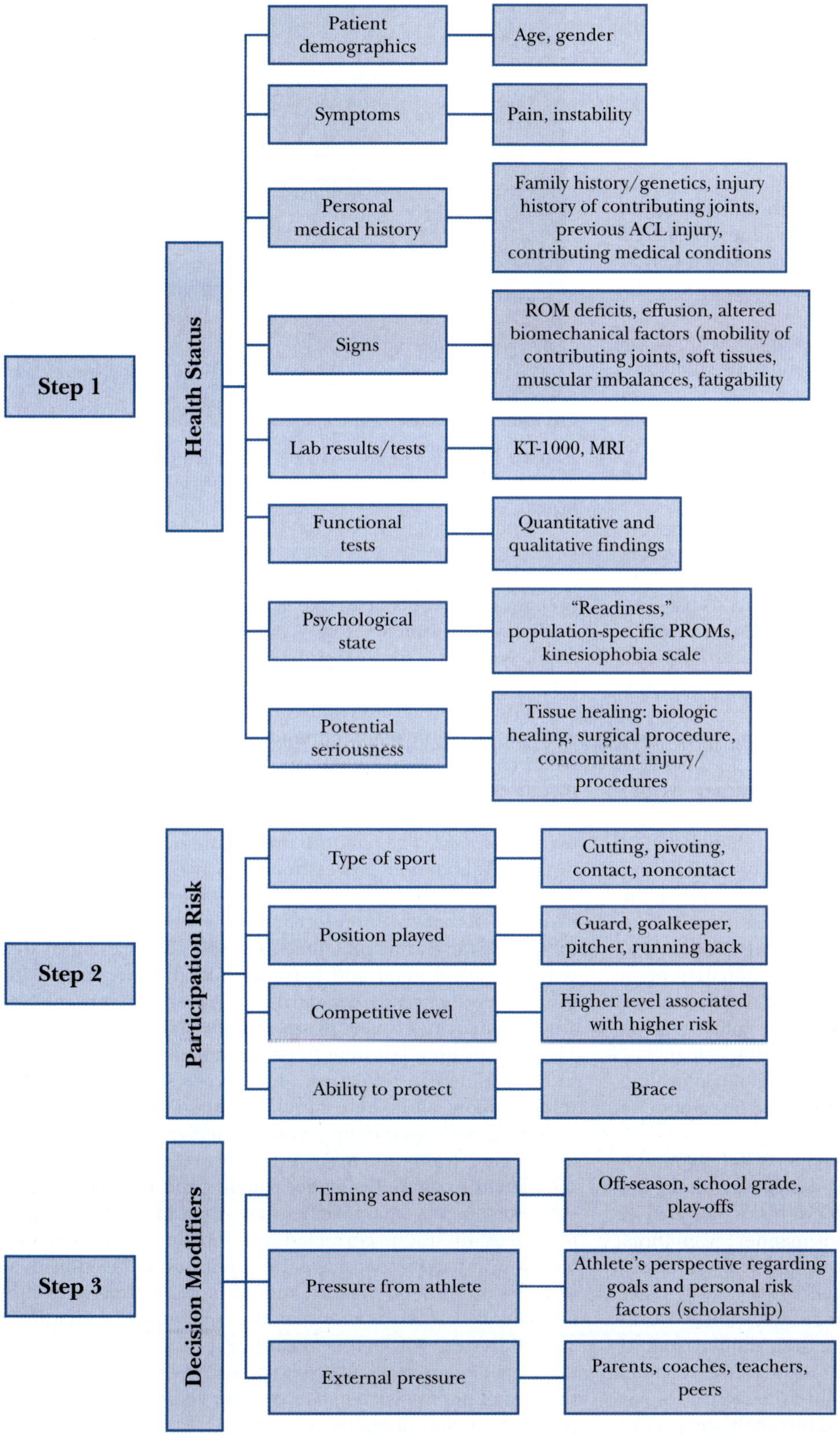

Figure 13.2. The decision-based return to play (RTP) model adapted for RTP following ACLR in the pediatric population. *ACL*, anterior cruciate ligament; *ROM*, range of motion; *MRI*, magnetic resonance imaging; *PROMs*, patient-reported outcomes.

medical history (previous ACL injuries, musculoskeletal injuries, can impact current movement patterns) current symptoms/signs (pain, effusion, ROM deficits, muscular imbalances, fatigability, etc.), tests (KT-1000, isokinetic testing, hop tests), age, and growth since time of injury. The surgical procedure (graft, fixation, concomitant injuries/procedures) must be taken into account. Also included in this step should be qualitative measures (alignment, control, etc.). A more extensive test battery is suggested to measure both qualitative and quantitative aspects of functional performance following ACLR.[46] Monson and Arendt[47] demonstrates in their functional assessment during patella rehabilitation that tests have a qualitative as well as quantitative component.

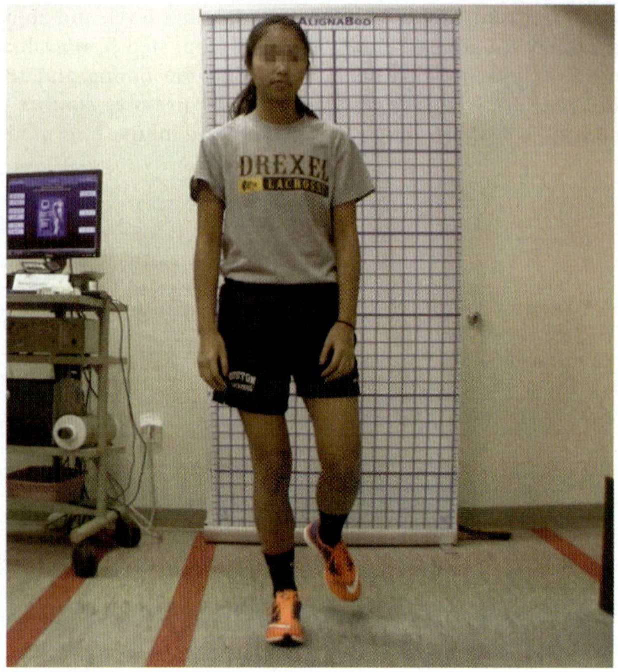

Figure 13.3. Single limb stance = alignment (qualitative) + stability (quantitative). Notice the femoral internal rotation and valgus.

The evaluation of participation risk would allow the clinician to view the findings from step 1 through the lens of the specific demands that would be placed on the athlete if cleared to return: level of sport (cutting, contact), the position played (goalkeeper, running back, cross country runner), and the competitive level.

The final step would involve not only the decision modifiers identified by Creighton but also the potential psychological and social effects of being sidelined from activity at an age when engagement with peer groups is so critical. The benefits and risks of returning an athlete to play versus the benefits and risks of keeping the athlete from participation must be carefully considered. In addition, the concerns of the patient, parents, coach, therapist, and trainer are also important to consider when evaluating what is in the best interest of the young patient after ACLR. It is our observation that the parents are torn between risk of reinjury if their child returns to play versus the risk of psychological/emotional decline if their child is held from activity. This model allows the clinician to weigh all the factors—pros and cons—to guide the final decision regarding clearance.

Obtaining both quantitative and qualitative measures by a multidisciplinary team beginning at 6 months postoperative is our current model at Hospital for Special Surgery (HSS) (Figs. 13.3 and 13.4). In fact, a continuum of care is initiated preoperatively. The patient, if not being rehabilitated at our institution, returns for follow-up at monthly checkpoints. This model allows for informed guidance in minimizing the risk associated with returning to play. Readiness to return to play includes many factors: full ROM, the absence of pain and swelling; flexibility; joint mobility; strength/functional strength; appropriate movement strategies; symmetrical movement patterns; alignment; balance; stability; endurance; agility; control; and the ability to jump, land, and decelerate. Physiologic factors that are not visible to the patient such as biologic healing (graft, articular cartilage), joint homeostasis, and integration of neural input must not be ignored.

The Return to Play Program at HSS Sports Rehabilitation and Performance Center, currently, is designed to help the athlete at any level of competition achieve his or her goal of returning to play in a safe and efficient manner. A multidisciplinary team that includes the surgeon, physical therapists, certified strength and conditioning specialists, and a registered clinical exercise physiologist/registered nurse works together with the patient's physical therapist, trainer, and, of course, the patient to guide the patient through the rehabilitation process, evaluate his or her readiness to return to play through movement analysis (video), and then help the patient prepare to meet his or her goals. Movement analysis includes qualitative assessment of movement strategy, depth of movement, symmetry, control, and alignment in various planes of motion (frontal, transverse, sagittal). Low rate of failure (5%) was observed in 38 skeletally immature athletes who underwent an all-epiphyseal technique and were returned to play based on movement quality, as well as standard quantitative measures, at short-term follow-up.[48] These outcomes support the use of qualitative measures in the return to play decision-making process. The 6-month mark is an important milestone in the rehabilitation process for many reasons: It is the time that is referenced regularly by patients as to when they expect to return to sports; therefore, it is the time table by which these individuals measure their progress. The patient at this point is feeling good and is feeling like they are done with this process; benefits from third-party payers are running out and it demarcates a new phase of the rehabilitation process. This demarcation is a time to pause with all the stakeholders, so the athlete can reflect on where he or she is, in terms of rehabilitation, and where he or she wants to go (goals). By gathering both quantitative and qualitative information, the health care team can make informed recommendations to the patient to guide his or her training and rehabilitation in the return to play phase. Deficits may exist in quality of movement that will not be corrected with repetition only. The biomechanical factors that may have predisposed this individual to injury may still be present, and/or movement patterns that may have developed as a result of this injury must be identified and addressed. All factors regarding health status (physical and physiologic), participation risk, and decision modifiers, to the best of our knowledge, are considered a multifactorial approach by a multidisciplinary team.

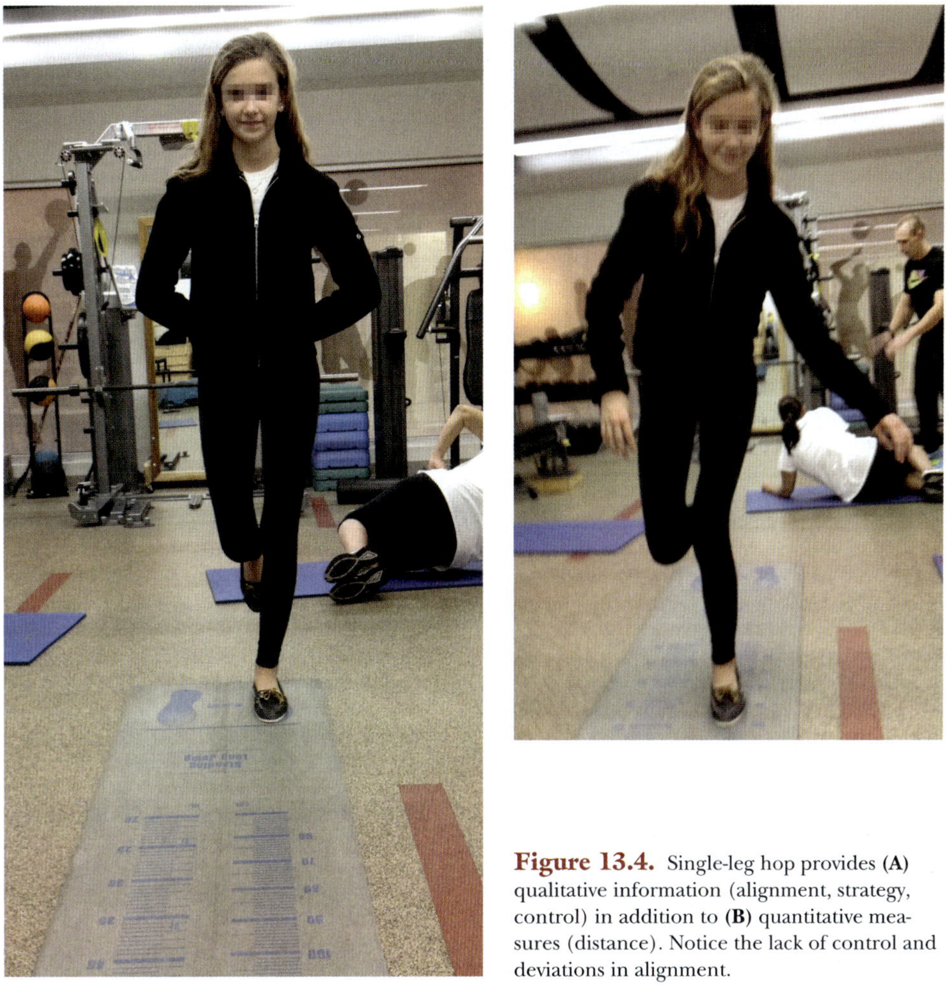

A B

Figure 13.4. Single-leg hop provides **(A)** qualitative information (alignment, strategy, control) in addition to **(B)** quantitative measures (distance). Notice the lack of control and deviations in alignment.

CONCLUSION

The psychological makeup of pediatric patients combined with the physical challenges they must overcome following ACLR places this population at an increased risk of a second injury. The decision to return an athlete to play must take a multidisciplinary and multifactorial approach. Expectations regarding time to return to play and criteria—quantitative and qualitative, physical, physiologic, and psychological—that influences the decision must be communicated from the outset to minimize frustration. As the incidence of this injury and surgery continue to rise, postoperative rehabilitation must address the predisposing factors and not just the deficits resulting from injury and surgery to ensure a safe return to previous level of activity. More importantly, injury prevention strategies that include education against early specialization, incorporation of training principles which includes rest, training for participation, and preparing this population for this increased level and intensity of participation are paramount.

REFERENCES

1. Lyman S, Koulouvaris P, Sherman S, et al. Epidemiology of anterior cruciate ligament reconstruction: trends, readmissions, and subsequent knee surgery. *J Bone Joint Surg Am.* 2009;9(10):2321–2328.
2. Dodwell ER, Lamont LE, Green DW, et al. 20 years of pediatric anterior cruciate ligament reconstruction in New York State. *Am J Sports Med.* 2014;42(3):675–680.
3. Prodromos CC, Han Y, Rogowski J, et al. A meta-analysis of the incidence of anterior cruciate ligament tears as a function of gender, sport, and a knee injury-reduction regimen. *Arthroscopy.* 2007;23(12):1320–1325.e6.
4. Adirim TA, Cheng TL. Overview of injuries in the young athlete. *Sports Med.* 2003;33(1):75–81.
5. National Federation of State High School Associations. *Book 2013–2014 High School Athletics Participation Survey Results.* Indianapolis, IN: National Federation of State High School Associations; 2012.
6. O'Rourke P. ScholarshipStats.com. 2014. Retrieved from http://www.scholarshipstats.com/about.html
7. Kocher MS, Saxon HS, Hovis WD, et al. Management and complications of anterior cruciate ligament injuries in skeletally immature patients: survey of the Herodicus Society and the ACL Study Group. *J Pediatr Orthop.* 2002;22(4):452–457.
8. Hui C, Salmon LJ, Kok A, et al. Fifteen-year outcome of endoscopic anterior cruciate ligament reconstruction with patellar tendon autograft for "isolated" anterior cruciate ligament tear. *Am J Sports Med.* 2011;39(1):89–98.
9. Wright RW, Huston LJ, Spindler KP, et al. The MARS Group. Descriptive epidemiology of the Multicenter ACL Revision Study (MARS) cohort. *Am J Sports Med.* 2010;38(10):1979–1986.
10. Salmon L, Russell V, Musgrove T, et al. Incidence and risk factors for graft rupture and contralateral rupture after anterior cruciate ligament reconstruction. *Arthroscopy.* 2005;21(8):948–957.

11. Paterno MV, Schmitt LC, Ford KR, et al. Biomechanical measures during landing and postural stability predict second anterior cruciate ligament injury after anterior cruciate ligament reconstruction and return to sport. *Am J Sports Med.* 2010;38(10):1968–1978.
12. Shelbourne KD, Gray T, Haro M. Incidence of subsequent injury to either knee within 5 years after anterior cruciate ligament reconstruction with patellar tendon autograft. *Am J Sports Med.* 2009;37(2):246–251.
13. Paterno MV, Rauh MJ, Schmitt LC, et al. Incidence of contralateral and ipsilateral anterior cruciate ligament (ACL) injury after primary ACL reconstruction and return to sport. *Clin J Sport Med.* 2007;22(2):116–121.
14. Lohmander LS, Englund PM, Dahl LL, et al. The long-term consequence of anterior cruciate ligament and meniscus injuries: osteoarthritis. *Am J Sports Med.* 2010;35(10):1756–1769.
15. Ardern CL, Webster KE, Taylor NF, et al. Return to sport following anterior cruciate ligament reconstruction surgery: a systematic review and meta-analysis of the state of play. *Br J Sports Med.* 2011;45(7):596–606.
16. Arden CL, Webster KE, Taylor NF, et al. Return to the preinjury level of competitive sport after anterior cruciate ligament reconstruction surgery: two-thirds of patients have not returned by 12 months after surgery. *Am J Sports Med.* 2011;39(3):538–543.
17. Shah VM, Andrews JR, Fleisig GS, et al. Return to play after anterior cruciate ligament reconstruction in National Football League athletes. *Am J Sports Med.* 2010;38(11):2233–2239.
18. Harris JD, Erickson BJ, Bach BR Jr, et al. Return-to-sport and performance after anterior cruciate ligament reconstruction in National Basketball Association players. *Sports Health.* 2013;5(6): 562–568.
19. Namdari S, Scott KB, Milby A, et al. Athletic performance after ACL reconstruction in the Women's National Basketball Association. *Phys Sports Med.* 2011;39(1):36–41.
20. Walden M, Hagglund M, Magnusson H. ACL injury is rather uncommon in elite football. *Knee Surg Sports Traumatol Arthrosc.* 2011;19:11–19.
21. Ardern CL, Taylor NF, Feller JA, et al. Return-to-sport outcomes at 2 to 7 years after anterior cruciate ligament reconstruction surgery. *Am J Sports Med.* 2012;40(1):41–48.
22. Brophy RH, Schmitz L, Wright RW, et al. Return to play and future ACL injury risk after ACL reconstruction in soccer athletes from the Multicenter Orthopaedic Outcomes Network (MOON) group. *Am J Sports Med.* 2012;40(11):2517–2522.
23. Shelbourne KD, Sullivan AN, Bohard K, et al. Return to basketball and soccer after anterior cruciate ligament reconstruction in competitive school-aged athletes. *Sports Health.* 2009;1(3):236–241.
24. McCullough KA, Phelps KP, Spindler KP, et al. Return to high school- and college-level football after anterior cruciate ligament reconstruction: a Multicenter Orthopaedic Outcomes Network (MOON) cohort study. *Am J Sports Med.* 2012;40(11):2523–2529.
25. Udry E, Shelbourne K, Gray T. Psychological readiness for anterior cruciate ligament surgery: describing and comparing the adolescent and adult experiences. *J Athl Train.* 2003;38(2):167–171.
26. Tremayne P, Tremayne R. Children and sport psychology. In: Morris T, Summers J, eds. *Sport Psychology: Theory, Applications and Issues.* 2nd ed. Brisbane, Australia: John Wiley & Sons; 2004.
27. Brand E, Nyland J. Patient outcomes following anterior cruciate ligament reconstruction: the influence of psychological factors. *Orthopedics.* 2009;32(5):335.
28. LaBella CR, Hennrikus W, Hewett TE; Council on Sports Medicine and Fitness, and Section on Orthopaedics. Anterior cruciate ligament injuries: diagnosis, treatment, and prevention. *Pediatrics.* 2014;133(5):e1437–e1450.
29. Trentacosta NE, Vitale MA, Ahmad CS. The effects of timing of pediatric knee ligament surgery on short-term academic performance in school-aged athletes. *Am J Sports Med.* 2009;37(9):1684–1691.
30. Kaeding CC, Aros B, Pedroza A, et al. Allograft versus autograft anterior cruciate ligament reconstruction: predictors of failure from a MOON prospective longitudinal cohort. *Sports Health.* 2011;3(1):73–81.
31. Shelbourne KD, Sullivan AN, Bohard K, et al. Return to basketball and soccer after anterior cruciate ligament reconstruction in competitive school-aged athletes. *Sports Health.* 2009;1(3):236–241.
32. Renström PA. Eight clinical conundrums relating to anterior cruciate ligament (ACL) injury in sport: recent evidence and a personal reflection. *Br J Sports Med.* 2013;47(6):367–372.
33. Hewett TE, Myer GD, Ford KR, et al. Biomechanical measures of neuromuscular control and valgus loading of the knee predict anterior cruciate ligament injury risk in female athletes: a prospective study. *Am J Sports Med.* 2005;33(4):492–501.
34. Myer GD, Ford KR, Hewett TE. Tuck jump assessment for reducing anterior cruciate ligament injury risk. *Athl Ther Today.* 2008;13(5):39–44.
35. Zazulak BT, Hewett TE, Reeves NP, et al. The effects of core proprioception on knee injury: a prospective biomechanical-epidemiological study. *Am J Sports Med.* 2007;35(3):368–373.
36. Leys T, Salmon L, Waller A, et al. Clinical results and risk factors for reinjury 15 years after anterior cruciate ligament reconstruction: a prospective study of hamstring and patellar tendon grafts. *Am J Sports Med.* 2012;40(3):595–605.
37. Rudolph KS, Axe MJ, Buchanan TS, et al. Dynamic stability in the anterior cruciate ligament deficient knee. *Knee Surg Sports Traumatol Arthrosc.* 2001;9(2):62–71.
38. Paterno MV, Rauh MJ, Schmitt LC, et al. Incidence of second ACL injuries 2 years after primary ACL reconstruction and return to sport. *Am J Sports Med.* 2014;42(7):1567–1573.
39. Barber-Westin SD, Noyes FR. Factors used to determine return to unrestricted sports activities after anterior cruciate ligament reconstruction. *Arthroscopy.* 2011;27(12):1697–1705.
40. Petersen W, Zantop T. Return to play following ACL reconstruction: survey among experienced arthroscopic surgeons (AGA instructors). *Arch Orthop Trauma Surg.* 2013;133(7):969–977.
41. Myer GD, Paterno MV, Ford KR, et al. Rehabilitation after anterior cruciate ligament reconstruction: criteria-based progression through the return-to-sport phase. *J Orthop Sports Phys Ther.* 2006; 36(6):385–402.
42. Wilk KE, Macrina LC, Cain EL, et al. Recent advances in the rehabilitation of anterior cruciate ligament injuries. *J Orthop Sports Phys Ther.* 2012;42(3):153–171.
43. Adams D, Logerstedt DS, Hunter-Giordano A, et al. Current concepts for anterior ligament reconstruction: a criterion-based rehabilitation progression. *J Orthop Sports Phys Ther.* 2012;42(7):601–614.
44. Cook G. *Athletic Body in Balance: Optimum Movement Skills and Conditioning for Performance.* Champaign, IL: Human Kinetics; 2003.
45. Creighton DW, Shrier I, Shultz R, et al. Return-to-play in sport: a decision-based model. *Clin J Sport Med.* 2010;20(5):379–385.
46. Engelen-van Melick N, van Cingel RE, Tijssen MP, et al. Assessment of functional performance after anterior ligament reconstruction: a systematic review of measurement procedures. *Knee Surg Sports Traumatol Arthrosc.* 2013;21(4):869–879.
47. Monson J, Arendt EA. Rehabilitative protocols for select patellofemoral procedures and nonoperative management schemes. *Sports Med Arthrosc.* 2012;20(3):136–144.
48. Nawabi DH, McCarthy M, Graziano J, et al. Return to play and clinical outcomes after all-inside, anterior cruciate ligament reconstruction in skeletally immature athletes. Paper presented at: 2014 Annual Meeting of the American Orthopaedic Society for Sports Medicine; July 10–13, 2014; Seattle, WA.

Jessica Graziano
Aisling M. Toolan

CHAPTER 14

Anterior Cruciate Ligament Injury Prevention Programs

INTRODUCTION

Anterior cruciate ligament (ACL) injury in young athletes continues to be one of the most debilitating injuries despite extensive research on injury prevention. Sports participation is on the rise, and we live in an era of specialization where children are training year-round and at earlier ages. ACL injuries in children were once rare; however, they are now being seen with increased incidence paralleling the trend in specialization at younger ages.[2–5] ACL injury has a significant physical and psychosocial impact resulting in time lost from play, interaction with teammates, loss of college scholarships, and decreased performance in the academic arena.[1,2]

The literature has extensively reported on the high incidence of ACL injury in high school female athletes.[3–5] With the rise in intrasubstance tears of the ACL in the prepubescent athlete, much attention is being paid to the injuries' effects on general health.[5–9] Sports injuries in children may threaten general health maintenance efforts, lead to arthritis, as well as contribute to obesity.[10] In addition, the reinjury rate is highest amongt young athletes and has been reported to be 15 times more likely within the first year and 6 times more likely within the first 24 months after return to sports activity.[11]

Given the serious impact this injury may have on young individuals, considerable effort has been directed toward prevention programs and is a rising area of interest to physicians, trainers, coaches, physical therapists, and caregivers. Approximately 70% of ACL tears occur from noncontact mechanisms such as during a jump landing or sharp deceleration.[12,13] Because risk factors such as poor movement patterns and alignment with jump landings and changes in direction have been demonstrated to be modifiable, these mechanisms of injury are theoretically preventable.[12,13] This chapter reviews the prevention programs centered on modifiable noncontact ACL mechanisms of injury. In order to have a better understanding of these programs, evidence-based mechanisms of injury and risk factors will be reviewed.

MECHANISM OF INJURY

Athletes may injure their knee via a contact or noncontact mechanism. A contact injury occurs when physical contact is made with another athlete. A noncontact injury is one that occurs without physical contact with another athlete.[13] A noncontact ACL injury may occur as a result of combined motions at the knee joint, for example knee valgus and femoral internal rotation.[14] Typically, these forces occur in sports during a sudden deceleration, jump landing (Fig. 14.1), and/or cutting maneuver (Fig. 14.2).

Female athletes have demonstrated the highest risk of ACL injury compared to their male counterparts, with incidence being two to eight times higher than males in soccer, basketball, and volleyball.[2,15,18] Increased attention is being paid to prepubescent young athletes secondary to at-risk movement patterns being seen in children as young as 10 years of age as well as increased incidence of injury.[11,16–18] Stanitski et al.[19] found that ACL injury was associated in 47% of children 7 to 12 years of age who had acute knee effusions.[19] Movement patterns play a critical role in ACL injury by creating the potential for anterior tibial shear force, which directly strains the ACL.[11,20,21]

Both modifiable and nonmodifiable risk factors have been described in the literature. Modifiable risk factors are the premise for ACL prevention programs secondary to the potential to induce change on specific variables. Therefore, this chapter focuses on modifiable risk factors and their role in injury prevention programs.

RISK FACTORS SPECIFIC TO YOUNG ATHLETES

Early Specialization

Preadolescent and adolescent athletes are a special population secondary to the growth and development that occurs as they are trying to meet the demands of sports. Early specialization, maturation, undeveloped physical skills, high-risk movement patterns, and an inadequate strength base are all contributing factors to increased injury rates.[11,22] However, children do not master complex motor skills until late childhood (age 10 to 12 years) and demonstrate increased risk of injury when age-appropriate skill set does not meet the demands imposed on them by coaches and sport.[11,23] If emphasis is placed on strengthening and the development of fundamental motor skills, as opposed to sports-specific training, then injuries sustained may be reduced.[11]

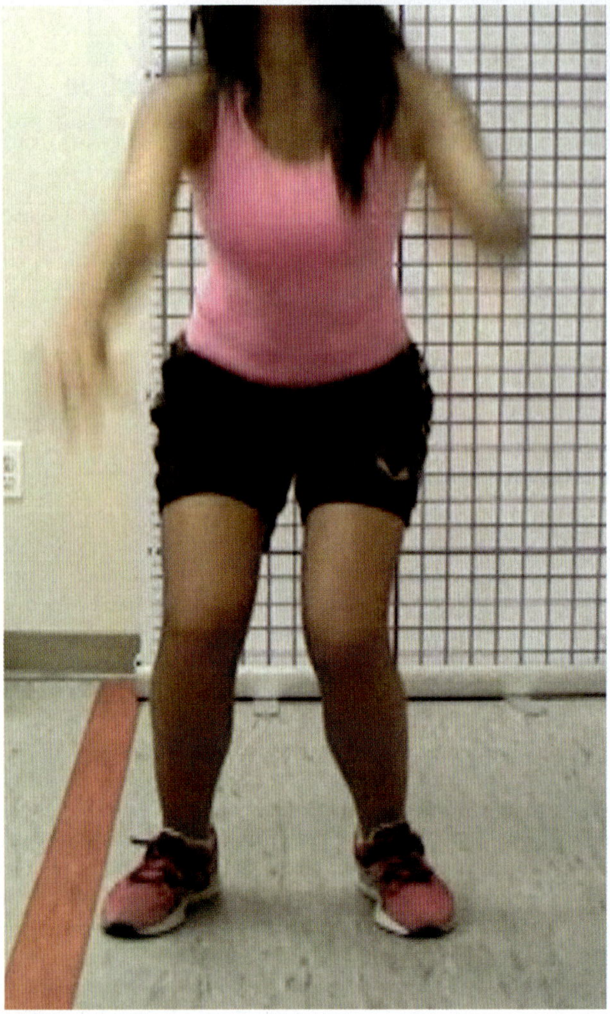

Figure 14.1. An adolescent female athlete landing from a jump, demonstrating valgus (inward collapse) moments to bilateral knees, predisposing the athlete to risk of noncontact injury.

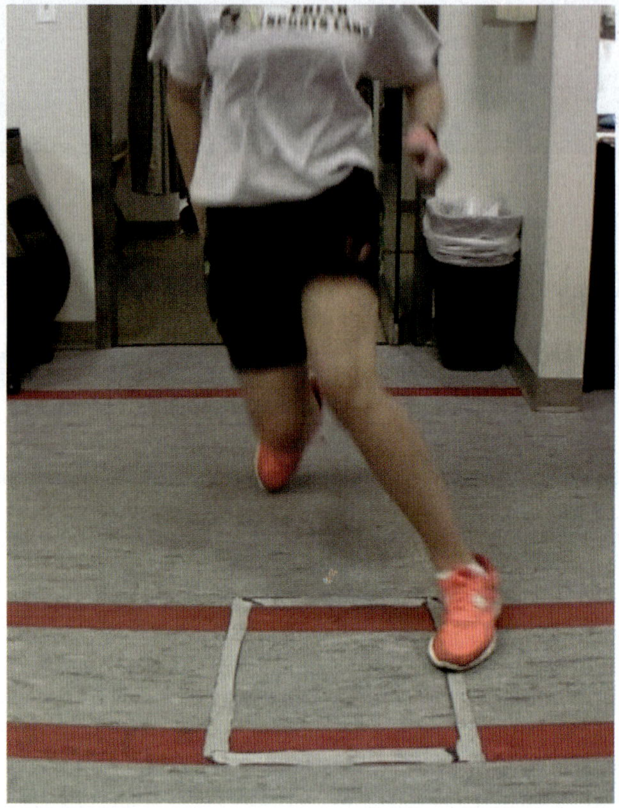

Figure 14.2. Female athlete performing a cutting maneuver and demonstrating risk of injury secondary to a trunk lean with knee valgus and rotation.

Growth Spurts and Maturation

Growth-related factors such as growth spurts, maturity-associated variation, and immature or underdeveloped coordination predispose young athletes to injury.[24–26] These factors may exert their influence with more frequent and intensive training and competition seen today.[11,21] There have been no differences in incidence in ACL tears reported between preadolescent males and females; however, differences become marked following maturation, with adolescent females demonstrating the most risk.[11,28,29] Puberty has been associated with deficits and delays in core stability and neuromuscular regression, and many sex-related differences emerge that have been associated with ACL injury.[18–21,27–30]

Adolescent female athletes demonstrate measurable neuromuscular imbalances following the onset of maturation. Hewett et al.[31] reported that female athletes landed with significantly more medial knee motion and greater maximum lower extremity valgus than male athletes following the onset of maturation. Males appear to have a neuromuscular spurt in strength, power, and coordination during puberty, which allows them to adapt to increased bony lever arms and a greater mass where females show little change (Fig. 14.3A,B).[31–33] Core stability declines during growth spurts and may predispose athletes to at-risk movements secondary to mechanical breakdown throughout the kinetic chain.[11,22] During growth spurts, there is an increase in bony lever arms and the body's center of mass changes which impacts postural alignment and neuromuscular control.[22] Therefore, core strength, neuromuscular ability, coordination, and proprioception become imbalanced and contribute to risk of injury.[21,22,30]

Increased demand for peak performance is expected at younger ages during a time of major physiologic change.[10,21] Care should be taken to ensure demands such as expected sports-specific movement patterns or training loads placed on the athlete's body does not exceed their physiologic capabilities. In addition, a child may master a skill prior to their growth spurt but may need to revisit that skill later on in order to refine the movement patterns secondary to the changes they incur. To successfully reduce the incidence of ACL injuries in young athletes, one must demonstrate an understanding of modifiable risk factors specific to injury prevention programs.

MODIFIABLE RISK FACTORS: COMPONENTS OF ANTERIOR CRUCIATE LIGAMENT PREVENTION PROGRAMS

Many risk factors have been described in the literature. The most effective prevention programs combine a multifaceted approach to address various components. These components

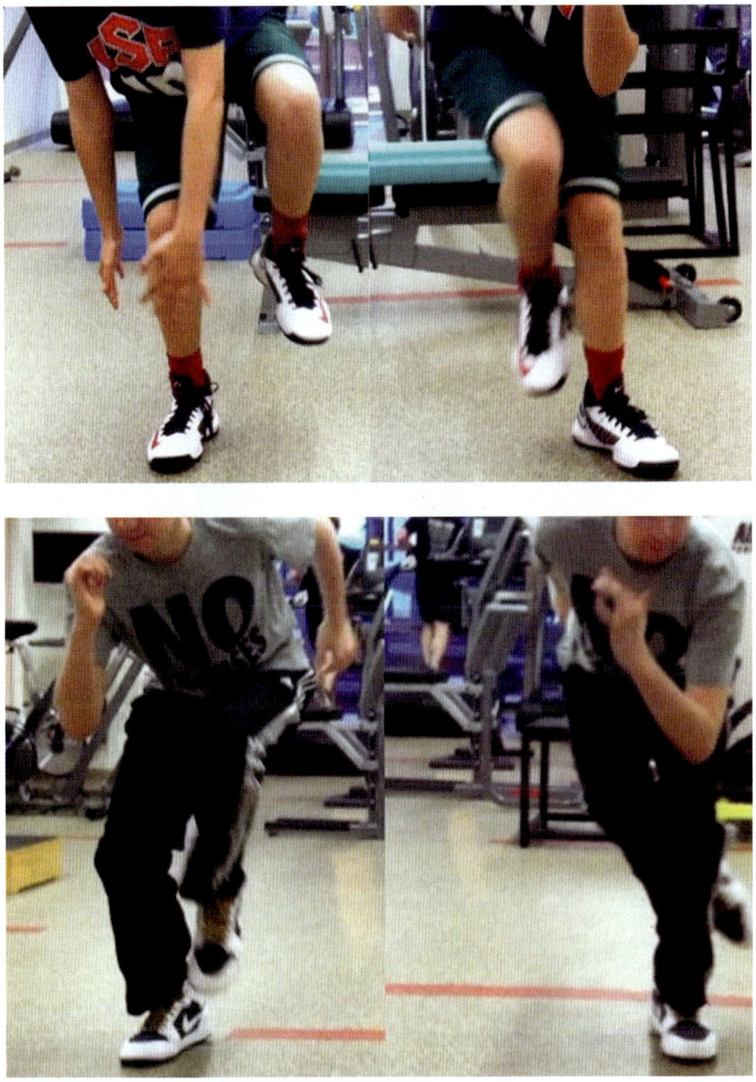

A

B

Figure 14.3. **A.** Prepubescent male performing lateral jumps with trunk shift over his right lower extremity and overall decreased control. **B.** Same male after puberty performing lateral jumps with good control, proper alignment, and more power.

include neuromuscular training, plyometric training, resistance training, flexibility, proprioception training, and technique monitoring and feedback. Neuromuscular training has received a lot of attention in the literature secondary to demonstrating the most promise in terms of altering movement patterns and decreasing ACL injuries.[14,15] Athletes may display movement patterns, which put them at risk because of one or more imbalances that can be easily addressed with interventions. Hewett et al.[29] describe several modifiable risk factors, which have been demonstrated to reduce risk of ACL injury when addressed: ligament dominance, quadriceps dominance, leg dominance, and trunk dominance. Identification of these risk factors allows individuals potentially at risk to be identified and prevention strategies to be provided.

NEUROMUSCULAR CONTROL

Ligament Dominance

Ligament dominance is defined as the tendency for valgus collapse secondary to neuromuscular imbalances and lack of muscular support about the knee affecting the ability to absorb ground reaction forces[29] (Fig. 14.4A,B). Therefore, the static restraints about the knee including bone, cartilage, and ligaments take the increased force.[14] An athlete is at high risk when displaying substantial medial knee motion in the coronal plane combined with a low knee flexion angle.[34–37] Gluteals, hamstrings, and gastrocnemius-soleus strength are critical components in prevention of ACL injury, and improper recruitment during landing tasks result in high abduction moments with increased strain on the ACL.[34–37] In addition, several studies have demonstrated that high school female athletes demonstrate greater maximum knee valgus angle and greater ground reaction forces with a drop vertical jump than males and uninjured athletes, which may explain the higher prevalence of ACL injury in that population.[35,36]

Female athletes have been shown to exhibit greater hip adduction and internal rotation with decreased knee flexion during tasks such as walking, running, anticipated and unanticipated cutting, and landing.[38–40] Increased hip adduction and internal rotation predispose the athlete to valgus collapse at the knee. Gluteus maximus and medius play a role in prevention of dynamic valgus collapse by controlling hip adduction and femoral rotation. Weakness has been associated as a predictor

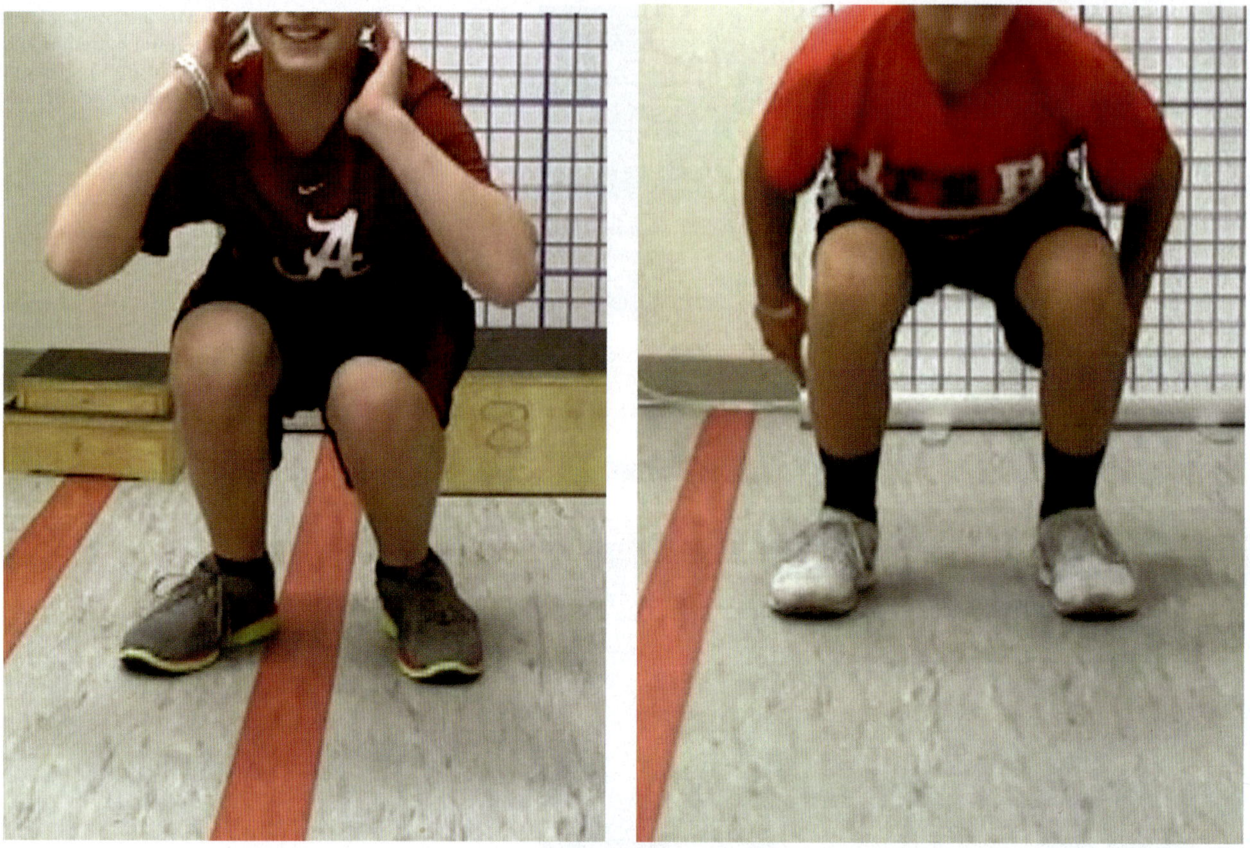

A B

Figure 14.4. Ligament dominance. **A.** Young athlete performing jumps in place and demonstrating valgus loading bilaterally. **B.** Same young athlete demonstrating proper alignment with jump landings 2 months after receiving intervention and feedback.

of injury secondary to inability of the weak musculature to keep the hip abducted during high-level single-leg activities such as landing and cutting.[38–40] Studies have demonstrated improved control of dynamic valgus collapse of the knee with gluteus maximus and medius strengthening.[11,13,38] Several electromyographic studies have reported that side-lying hip abduction, side planks, and lateral band walks elicit sufficient maximal voluntary activation for strengthening of gluteus medius (Fig. 14.5A).[41] Side-lying hip abduction may be performed during a side plank if appropriate control and stability can be maintained (Fig. 14.5B). Single-leg squats and single-leg deadlifts have also been demonstrated to maximally elicit gluteus maximus.[41]

Quadriceps Dominance

Quadriceps dominance occurs during sports maneuvers such as cutting or jumping when preferential activation of knee extensors over flexors occurs.[29] The quadriceps acts as an antagonist, exerting maximum strain to the ACL in the last 30 degrees of knee extension.[39] In addition, it has been demonstrated that preferential activation of the quadriceps while landing in an erect position exerts anterior shear stress to the knee (Fig. 14.6A–C).[28,29,34,37] Hamstring activation has been shown to play a role in controlling dynamic valgus by resisting anterior and lateral tibial translation and rotation.[11,27,34,37,39] In addition, hamstring activation with a jump landing or during a cutting maneuver results in a flexed knee posture (Fig. 14.7A–C) and is more protective to the ACL.[37,39]

Studies have demonstrated the effectiveness of neuromuscular training with improved dynamic valgus control and decreased strain on the anteromedial bundle of the ACL with prelanding and landing activation.[27,32,34,36,40] It has been reported extensively in the literature that females demonstrate a lower hamstring-to-quadriceps ratio, resulting in greater risk of injury.[27,29,34,36,37] Ebben et al.[37] reported females' hamstring-to-quadriceps ratio was lower and they sustained quadriceps activation longer during cutting. Other studies have reported that females have the tendency to preferentially activate their quadriceps more than males with jump landings resulting in stiff-legged landings, which do not allow absorption of ground reaction forces.[35] Hewett et al.[32] demonstrated the effectiveness of a plyometric training program designed to increase hamstring-to-quadriceps torque and a 22% decreased impact force. The studies mentioned highlight the importance of neuromuscular and plyometric training to address hamstring strength and neuromuscular deficits in prevention programs.

Leg Dominance

Leg dominance relates to side-to-side symmetry, balance, and muscular strength, which may place both limbs at risk.[29] The weaker limb is compromised in its ability to dissipate forces, whereas the stronger limb is subjected to higher forces

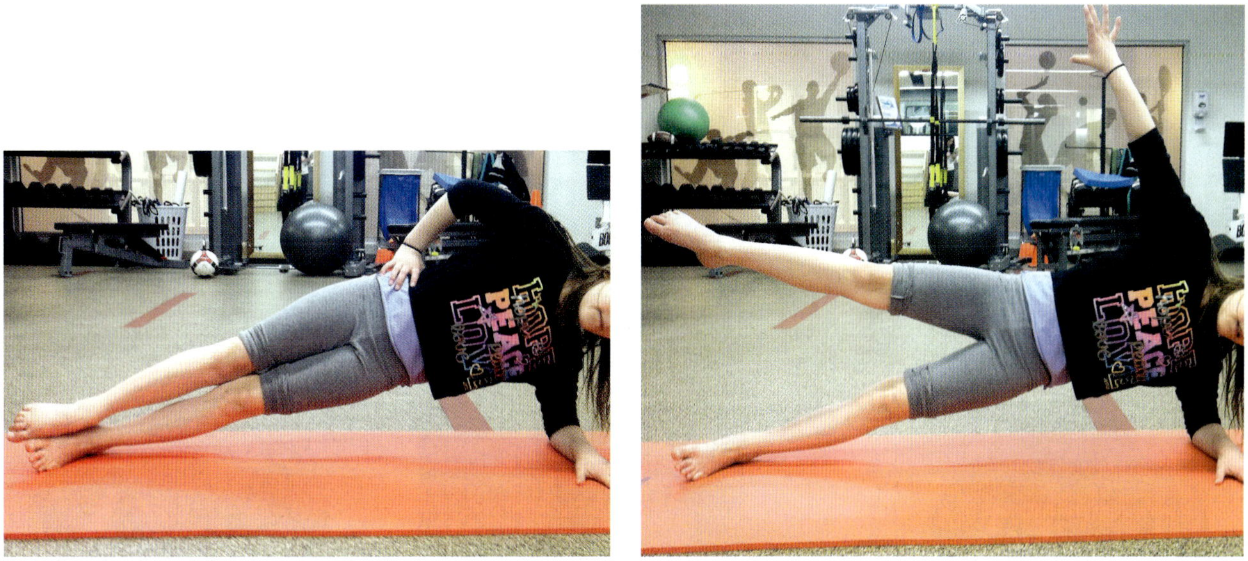

A B

Figure 14.5. Gluteus medius strengthening for correction of dynamic valgus. **A.** Side plank. **B.** Side plank performed with hip abduction of the top leg while maintaining proper core stabilization.

secondary to increased dependence and excessive loading (Fig. 14.8A–F).[29] Hewett et al.[28] reported that females tended to favor one leg more than the other when compared to their male counterparts. Ford et al.[35] found that high school female basketball players landed from a vertical jump with significantly greater maximum valgus knee angle on their nondominant side in comparison to their dominant side. In addition, leg dominance may be secondary to asymmetrical muscle weakness and/or pain avoidance. In order to address leg dominance, training should progress from emphasis on quality of double leg movements to single leg movements. For example, if an individual has an asymmetrical squat, they will carry the asymmetry over to their broad jumps. If they do not produce equal force output through each leg, they will then have a difficult

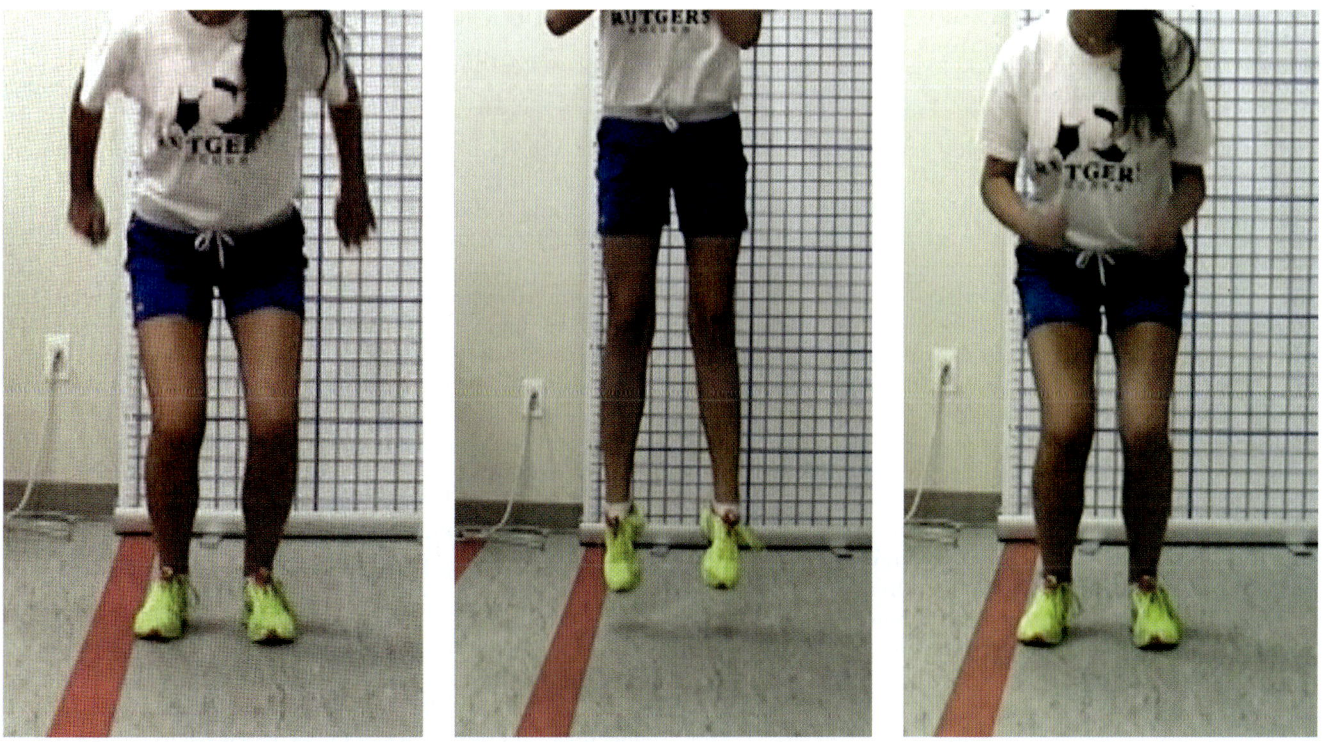

A, B C

Figure 14.6. Quadriceps dominance. **A.** Female adolescent athlete in takeoff position for jump in place. **B.** Athlete pushes off into the air. **C.** Athlete landing with minimal knee flexion, preferential activation of quadriceps bilaterally, and valgus loading of the knees bilaterally.

A, B

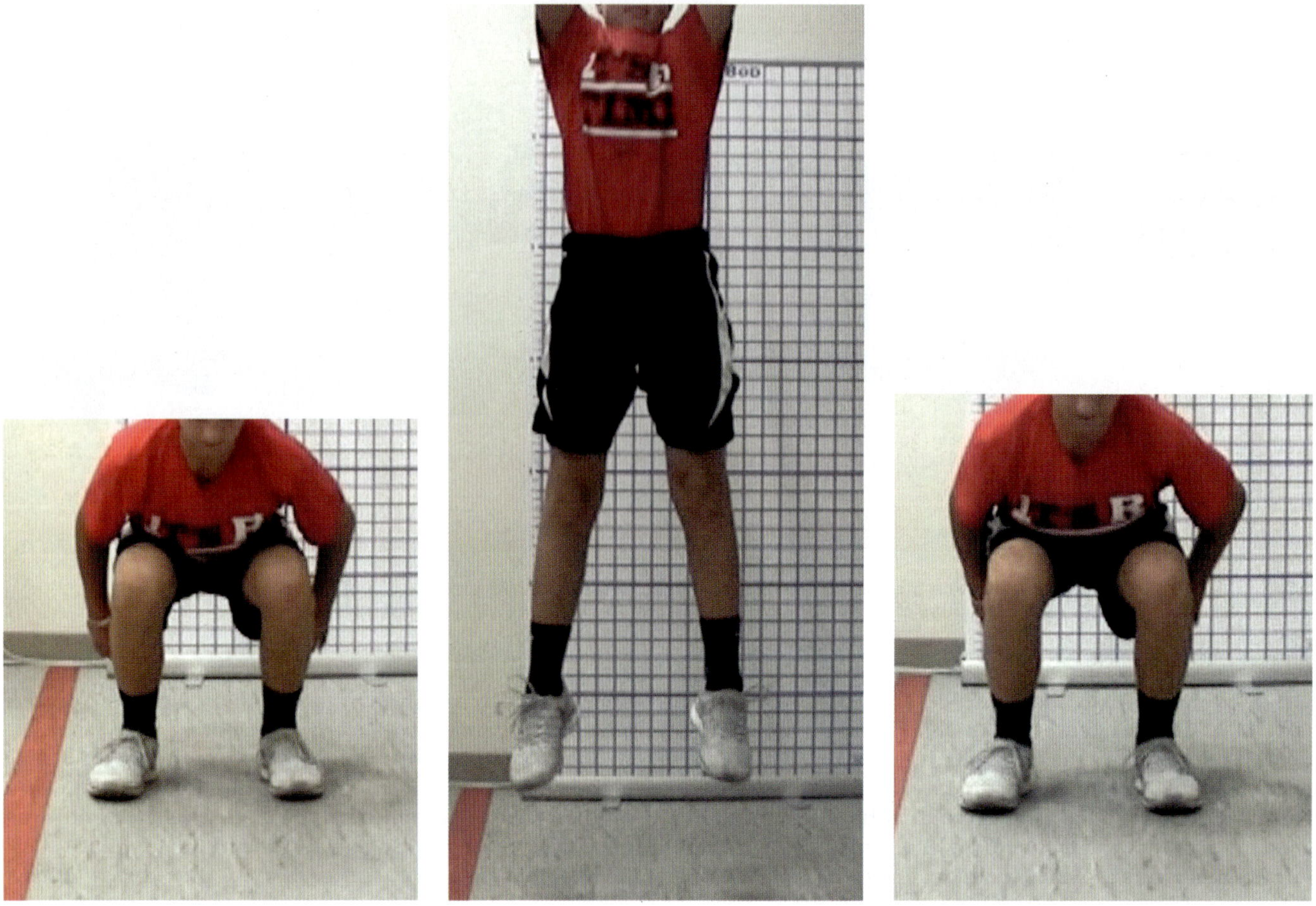

C

Figure 14.7. **A.** Jump takeoff position by adolescent male athlete with proper lower extremity alignment and flexed knee posture **B.** Athlete jumps into air with equal push-off. **C.** Athlete lands with hamstring activation and knee flexed posture.

time maintaining proper positioning and posture during the jump takeoff and landing. This will reduce performance outcomes as well as increase risk of injury. The weaker leg will have to work harder to maintain an equal position during jumping. Moreover, quality is always more important than quantity. Myers et al.[42] discusses the importance of ensuring an athlete does not drop one leg posterior to the other leg during a jump because this facilitates imbalances by overloading the stronger (posterior) leg and unloading the weaker leg. Interventions should focus on ensuring each limb works independently. Some examples of effective exercises are single leg squats, single leg hops, bounding, and single leg balance on unstable surfaces (Fig. 14.9A,B). More complex movement patterns require greater coordination in side-to-side performance and lead to greater balance in side-to-side muscle recruitment as well as ensuring bilateral coordination and power. In order to efficiently correct for leg dominance, the athlete must coordinate multijoint actions and multiplanar movements into power movements that are to be used in competition.[42]

Trunk Dominance

Trunk dominance is caused by increased motion of the body's center of mass during single-leg landing, pivoting, or deceleration due to decreased core strength and neuromuscular control (Fig. 14.10A,B).[11,28,37,40] Athletes without sufficient core strength and trunk control lack the dynamic stability to control excessive trunk motion in the frontal plane. Core deficits and proprioception have been associated with lateral trunk displacement, altered dynamic knee stability, and predicted injury risk.[11,13,28,32,40] Young athletes experience growth spurts, which cause changes in bony levers and center of body mass, making muscular control of the trunk more difficult. Therefore, young athletes are more susceptible to injury during growth spurts secondary to imbalanced core strength, neuromuscular control, and coordination deficits that occur during this time.[43] Maintaining core strength during growth spurts is vital for young athletes.

Fatigue

Dynamic stability may decrease secondary to fatigue of the major stabilizing muscle groups, placing increased risk of strain on the ACL. Chappell et al.[44] found significant increases in peak proximal tibial anterior shear forces, increased valgus moments, and decreased knee flexion angles in athletes who performed three stop-jump tasks after completing a fatigue exercise as compared with when they performed the tasks in a non-fatigued

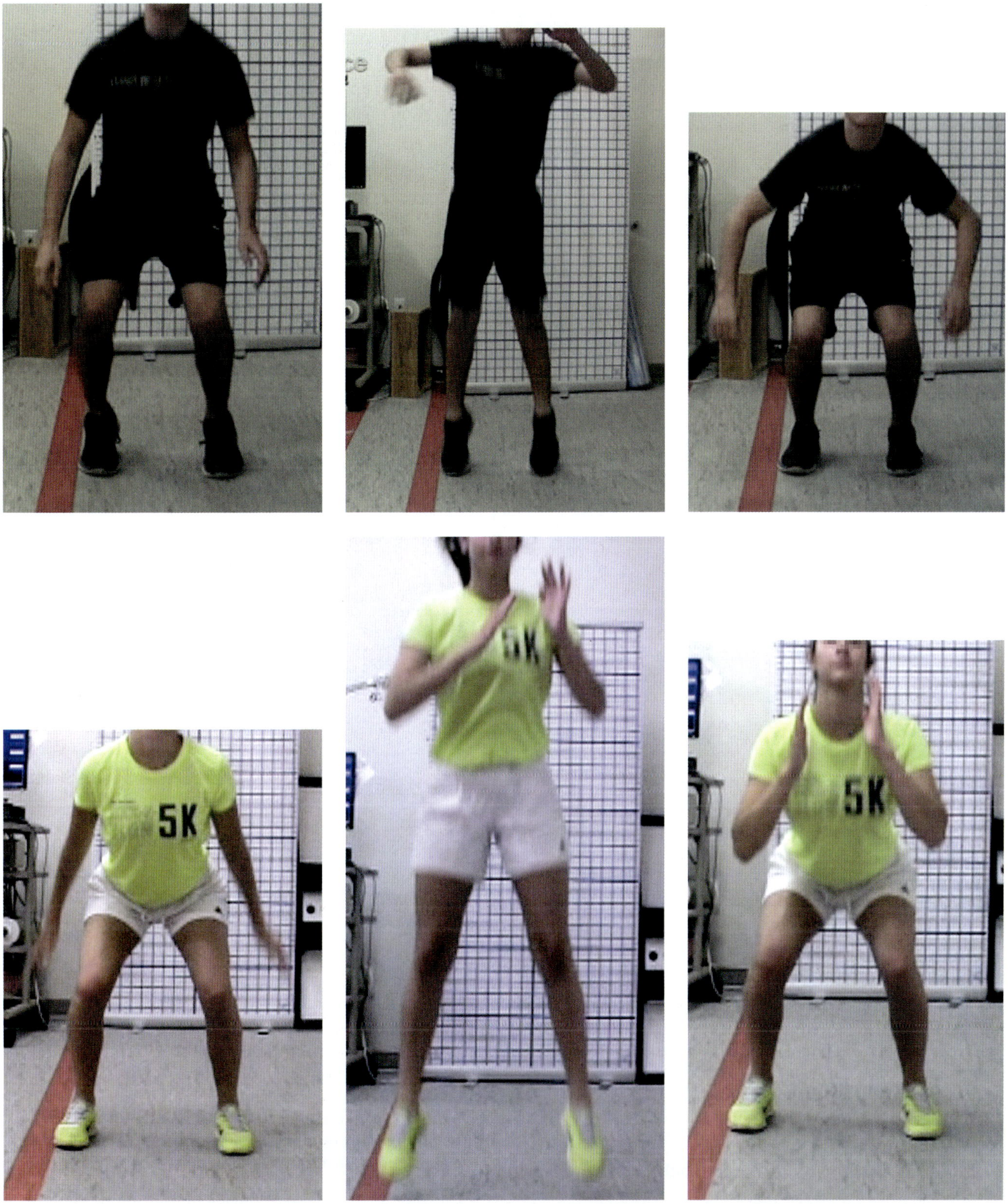

A, B C

D, E F

Figure 14.8. Leg dominance. **A.** Young athlete shifts to right leg during takeoff phase of a squat jump demonstrating excessive loading of one leg over the other. **B.** Athlete pushes off for jump with right leg dominance. **C.** Athlete lands with increased loading of right lower extremity over left. **D.** Athlete demonstrating equal weight bearing for takeoff. **E.** Athlete demonstrating symmetrical push-off. **F.** Athlete demonstrating symmetrical landing of bilateral lower extremities.

Figure 14.9. Exercises to improve single leg strength and recruitment to prevent leg dominance. **A.** Single-leg X-hop: The athlete starts on one leg in a quadrant and hops to each quadrant with appropriate knee flexed position, trunk position, and control. **B.** Athlete performs hopping onto opposite leg and maintains appropriate knee flexion, trunk, and lower extremity control on landing.

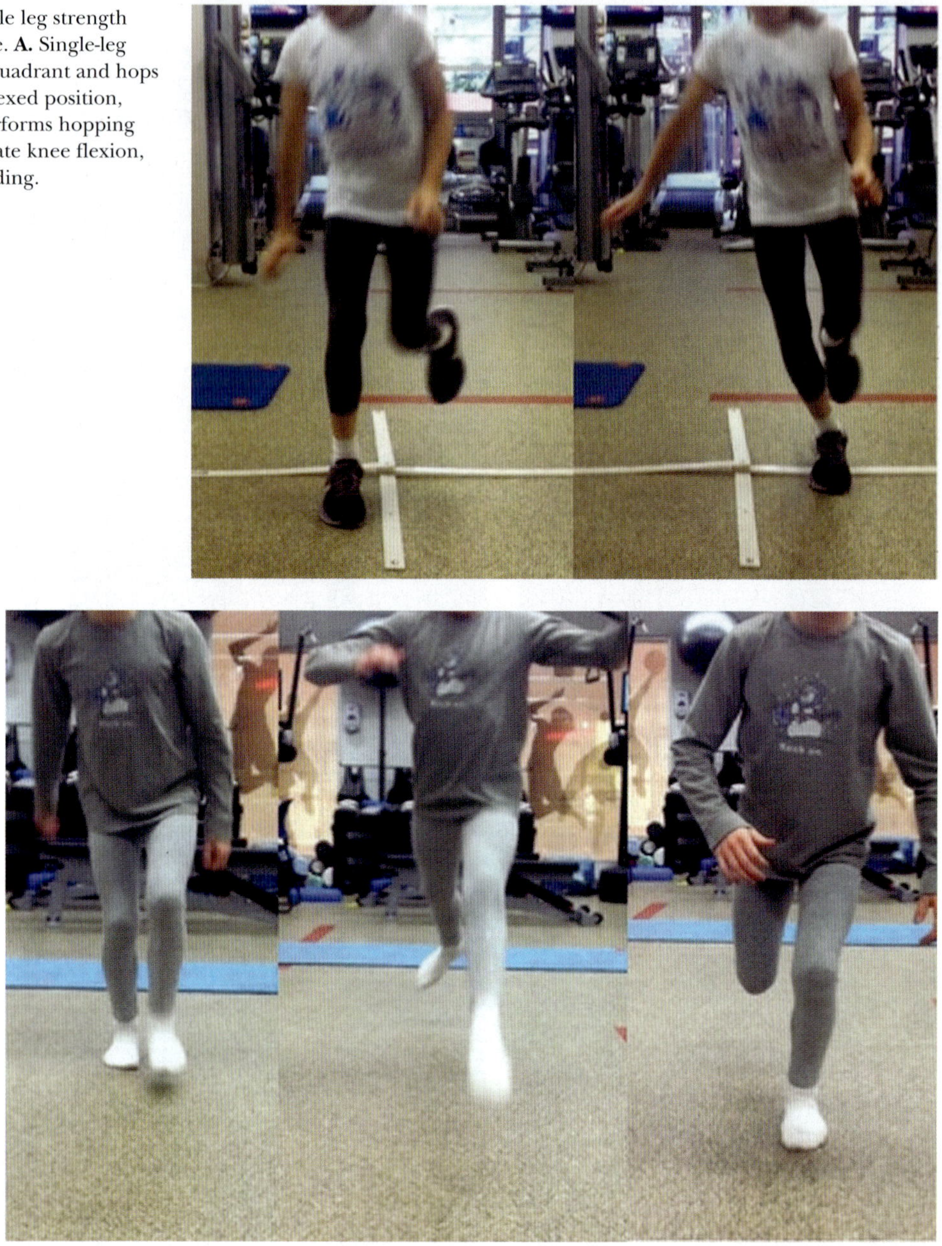

A

B

state. The literature has repeatedly reported increased risk of injury during the later portion of games in a variety of sports. Moreover, during running and rapid stop tasks, the late onset of quadriceps and hamstring muscle activation occurred with fatigue.[44] Fatigue may be supported as a risk factor; however, there is a paucity of research to validate this theory.

Technique Monitoring and Feedback

Children have decreased attention spans in comparison to adults and therefore should be actively monitored to ensure proper and safe technique. Studies have demonstrated that young athletes were able to make significant changes in landing mechanics in repeat trials after being given brief verbal cueing and feedback such as a decrease in peak ACL forces and increased hip and knee flexion.[45] Padua et al.[46] demonstrated that vertical ground reaction forces (GRFs) associated with ACL injury were decreased when athletes were provided verbal instruction and feedback for proper landing technique, and auditory cues for minimizing landing forces under direct supervision and on a regular basis. Studies that did not note change were those that did not incorporate regular verbal or auditory feedback nor provide direct supervision on a regular basis.[46] Even more impressive is a study presented by Prapavessis and McNair[48] where they demonstrated a decrease in GRF with jumping via altered technique after only one feedback session.

ANTERIOR CRUCIATE LIGAMENT INJURY PREVENTION PROGRAMS

ACL injuries are prevalent in young athletes and prevention is vital for reduction of long-term sequelae. Neuromuscular

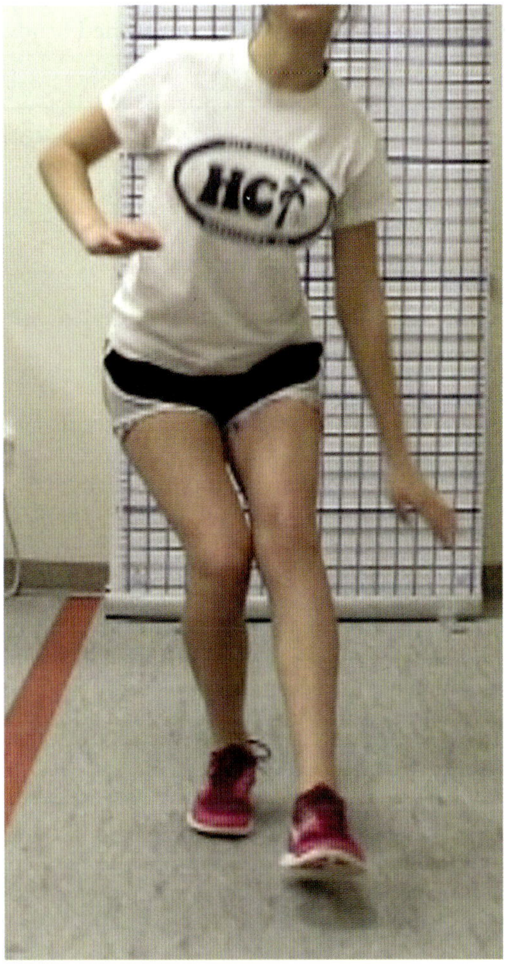

A

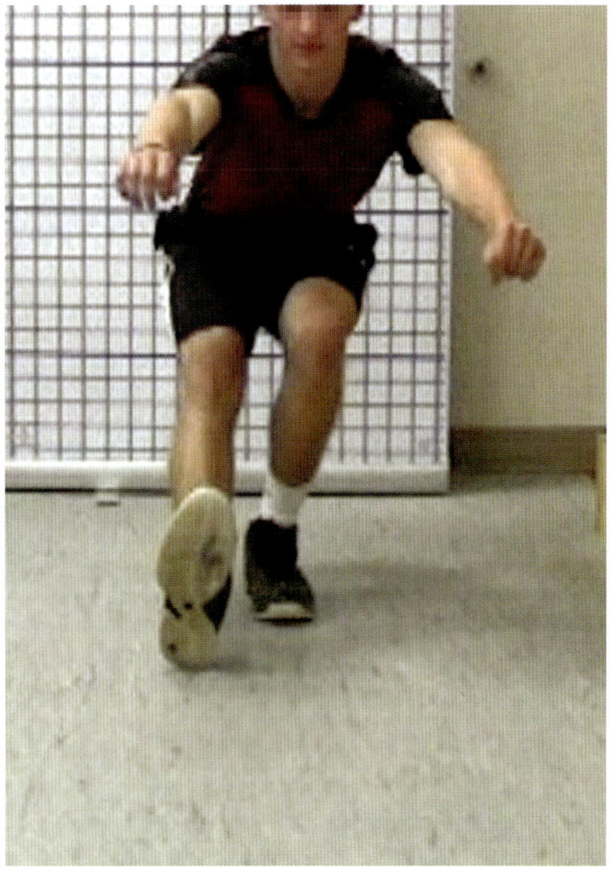

B

Figure 14.10. Trunk dominance. **A.** Trunk shifts over the athlete's center of mass during a single-leg hop resulting in valgus collapse at the knee. **B.** Proper alignment of the trunk, hip, knee, and ankle during a single-leg hop

and biomechanical characteristics that contribute to risk factors have received attention in the literature secondary to their potential to modify lower extremity alignment through prevention programs.[35,36,42,43,47,49] As noted previously in this chapter, athletes who land with knee valgus, have greater quadriceps to hamstring activation during sports-specific maneuvers, and demonstrate trunk dominance are at risk for ACL injury. Numerous injury prevention programs have been developed to modify neuromuscular and biomechanical characteristics in order to reduce incidence of ACL injury. Programs that take on a multifaceted approach and include components such as proprioception training, neuromuscular training, plyometric training, and strengthening have demonstrated biomechanical changes and therefore a reduction of ACL injury.[29,40]

Proprioception is the awareness of a body segment's orientation and positioning. Proprioception training works to improve the athlete's coordination, positioning, and balance in multiple planes of motion with or without perturbations.[50] One of the first studies to demonstrate the importance of proprioception training on ACL injury prevention was conducted in Italy. Caraffa et al.[50] performed a prospective controlled study of 600 soccer players in semiprofessional or amateur teams. They studied the preventive effect of gradually increasing proprioceptive training on four different types of wobble boards over three soccer seasons. The training was performed in the preseason, and each phase consisted of 2 to 6 days of training. In phase 1, balance training was performing without a board.[50] In phase 2, training was performing on each leg using a rectangular balance board. Phase 3 consisted of training on a round board. In phase 4, the athletes were trained on a combined round and rectangular board, and in phase 5, they were progressed to a BAPS board (Camp. Jackson, MI).[50] Each phase consisted of two subphases: anterior up-step and posterior up-step exercises. Three hundred athletes were trained 20 minutes per day with five different phases of increasing difficulty (Table 14.1), whereas a control group trained for their regular season without special balance training.[50] ACL injuries were documented. The training group demonstrated a reduction in incidence of ACL injuries in comparison to the control group.[50] Other effective ways to train proprioception in young athletes include balance exercises on a balance board, on varying unstable surfaces, as well as progression from double- to single-limb stance (Fig. 14.11).

TABLE 14.1 Proprioception Training Described in Caraffa et al.'s Prospective Controlled Study

Phases of Difficulty	*Balance Training Progression on Four Types of Wobble Boards*
1	Training without a balance board; instructed to stand alternately on one leg for 2.5 min four times per day
2	Training on a rectangular balance board; same time period as phase 1
3	Training on a round board; same time period as phase 1
4	Training on a combined round and rectangular board; same time period as phase 1
5	Training on a BAPS board; same time period as phase 1

Plyometric training exercises are explosive and are designed to build power, strength, and speed. They involve jumping, landing, and cutting maneuvers in various planes of motion at varying intensity levels.[51] The most important component to consider with plyometric training is alignment of the body (trunk and lower extremities) with the landing. The literature has demonstrated several risk factors for ACL injury, such as knee valgus moments, trunk dominance, and ligament dominance.[47] Plyometric training for ACL injury prevention focuses on strength, power, and speed while ensuring appropriate alignment throughout the progression. If an athlete performs plyometrics for quantity as opposed to quality, they may be performing the movement with poor alignment, develop poor habits, and put themselves at risk during sports-specific situations (Fig. 14.12A,B).

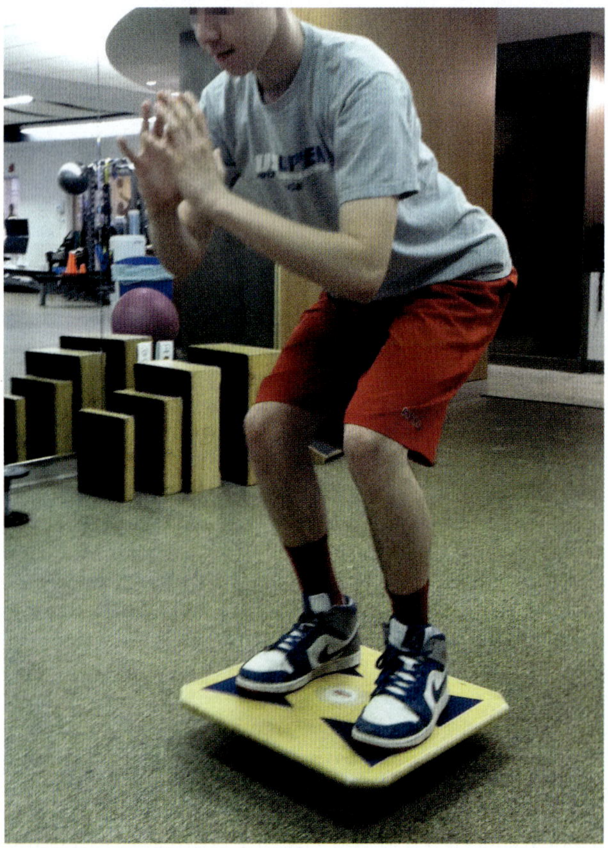

Figure 14.11. Adolescent athlete training proprioceptive awareness on a balance board.

Neuromuscular training programs are designed to enhance joint stability and improve joint position sense to prevent injury.[51] They have demonstrated a significant effect on the reduction of ACL injury risk in adolescent female athletes in both landing and cutting sports secondary to addressing neuromuscular deficits, which predisposes them to injury (ligament dominance, leg dominance, quadriceps dominance, and trunk dominance). Neuromuscular control may be the greatest contributor to dynamic knee stability and therefore offer the greatest potential for injury prevention. Dynamic neuromuscular training programs have demonstrated reduced sex-related differences in force absorption, active joint stabilization, muscle imbalances, and functional biomechanics while increasing strength of structural tissues such as bone, ligaments, and tendons.[26–32] Other components of prevention programs include technique-movement awareness and flexibility training.[36,51]

The practicality and effectiveness of ACL prevention programs has been questioned secondary to time constraints and needed equipment. As a result, some programs have implemented neuromuscular training in a warm-up format.[49,51] A drawback of warm-up formats is the lack of ability to measure athletic performance enhancement which affects compliance.[13,40] Alentorn-Geli et al.[49] reported improved compliance when the training targeted improved performance measures.

Prevention programs vary in terms of exercise combinations, compliance, and timing (preseason/postseason), which affect the outcomes of these programs.[51] Studies have demonstrated the importance of multifaceted training programs that incorporate sports-specific plyometrics, neuromuscular training, agility training, strengthening, and an emphasis on technique as part of a warm-up. Although the programs to be discussed differ in how they combine and implement the latter components, there are several common themes in how each program addresses modifiable risk factors for noncontact ACL injury (Table 14.2). Several well-known programs are discussed as well as their various components and current research.

Sportsmetrics Anterior Cruciate Ligament Injury Prevention Program

Hewett at al.[27] published the first prospective, nonrandomized clinical study which examined the protective effects of a neuromuscular training program in 1999. They followed

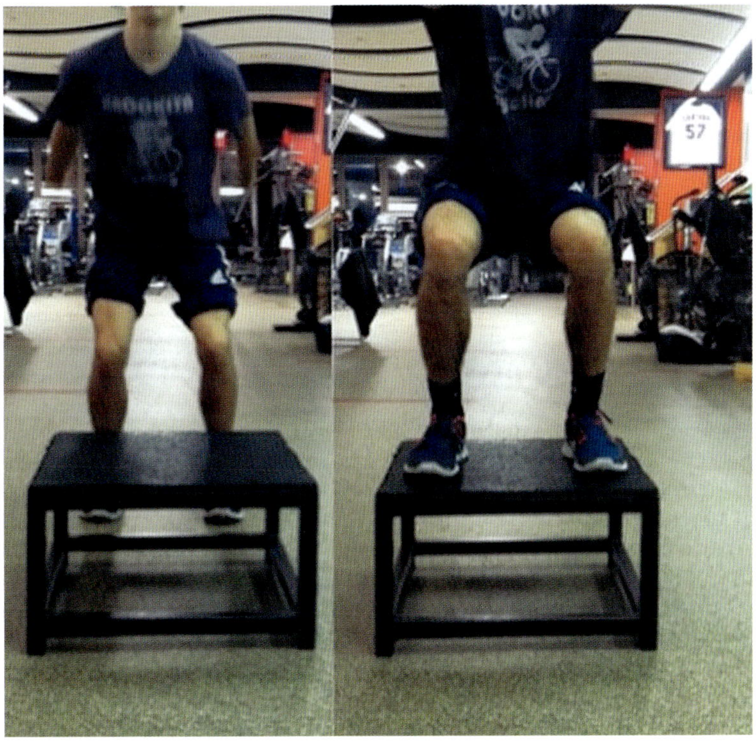

A

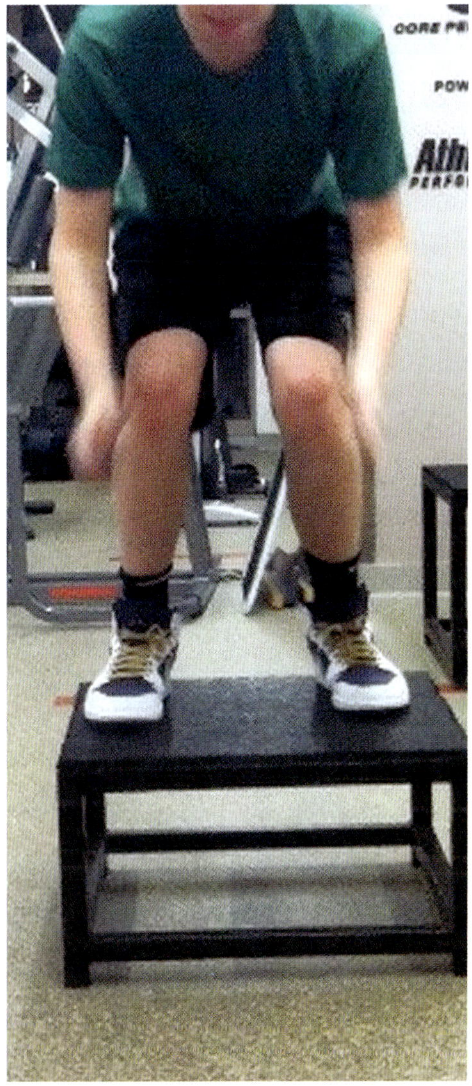

B

Figure 14.12. Ensuring proper alignment with plyometrics. **A.** Young athlete performs a box jump with proper alignment; hips level and hip/knee/ankles in proper alignment with landing. **B.** Young athlete performs box jump with valgus landing to bilateral lower extremities.

1,263 soccer, volleyball, and basketball high school athletes for 1 year.[27] They divided the athletes into a trained and untrained female group and an untrained male group. The trained group underwent a preseason neuromuscular training program, now known as the *Sportsmetrics ACL Injury Prevention Program* (Dr. Frank Noyes, Cincinnati Sports Medicine, Cincinnati, OH). The training group focused on flexibility, plyometrics, and weight training and emphasized proper technique.[27] The untrained female group demonstrated a significantly increased incidence of injuries when compared with the trained female group (3.6 times), and there was no significant difference between the untrained male and trained female groups.[27] The program consists of a dynamic warm-up, plyometrics and jump training, strength training, and flexibility (Table 14.3) and is extensively used today.[27] The jump training phase consists of subphases. Phase 1 being

TABLE 14.2 **Injury Prevention Program Components**

	Warm-up	*Flexibility*	*Hip/Leg Strength*	*Core Strength*	*Plyometrics*	*Agility*	*Balance*
Sportsmetrics	✓	✓	✓	✓	✓	✓	
PEP	✓	✓	✓		✓	✓	✓
Myklebust ACL Program							✓
FIFA 11+	✓	✓	✓	✓	✓	✓	✓

TABLE 14.3 Sportsmetrics Program

Components	*Purpose*
Dynamic warm-up	The warm-up improves flexibility and coordination as well as prepares the individual for sports-specific activities.
Plyometrics/jump training	Emphasis is placed on technique and improving strength and control.
Strengthening	Emphasis is on alignment and form for all exercise prescriptions. Focus is on core strength and muscular efficiency.
Flexibility	Muscle lengthening of all muscle groups to allow for proper alignment with movements and for power

the technique phase where proper jump technique is demonstrated and practiced. The fundamentals phase focuses on building a base of strength, power, and agility. The performance phase focus on achieving maximum vertical height. The program is recommended for 60 to 90 minutes, three times per week for 6 weeks.[27]

The Sportsmetrics Warm-Up for Injury Prevention and Performance (WIPP) program was created secondary to an understanding of time constraints. It contains the four components of Sportsmetrics for muscle preparation, plyometrics, strength, and flexibility but is shorter in duration for each phase. The added agility drills (2 minutes) at the end of the warm-up work to transition into practice activities. Each exercise session is recommended to last 20 minutes.[52]

Prevent Injury and Enhance Performance Program

The Prevent Injury and Enhance Performance (PEP) program was devised by the Santa Monica Sports Medicine Research Foundation and consists of five phases: a dynamic warm-up, strengthening, plyometrics, agility training including deceleration, and stretching for the lower extremities (Table 14.4).[53] The PEP program was designed to replace the normal warm-up routine and consists of education, stretching, strengthening, plyometrics, and soccer agility drills.[53] The program is designed to address deficits in strength and coordination of the musculature support around the knee. Technique is emphasized during all exercises, specifically a soft landing and deep hip and knee flexion as opposed to landing with a flat foot with knee extension. The program is to be performed three times per week, before practice, and all exercises should be completed in 15 to 20 minutes.[52,53]

Mandelbaum et al.[53] performed a prospective, nonrandomized cohort study to examine the effectiveness of the PEP program in young female soccer players aged 14 to 18 years. Over the course of two seasons, a total of 1,885 soccer players took part in the PEP program. Controls consisted of age and skill-matched athletes in the same league. The intervention group demonstrated an 88% reduction in the first season, and a 74% reduction in the second, in the rate of ACL injury.[53]

Gilchrist et al.[54] examined the effects of the PEP program in collegiate female soccer players. This randomized controlled trial included 583 National Collegiate Athletic Association (NCAA) Division 1 athletes in the PEP group and 852 in the control. Overall, the rate of noncontact ACL injury was significantly less in the PEP group, with the rate of noncontact ACL injury being 3.3 times greater in the control group.[54]

Myklebust's Anterior Cruciate Ligament Injury Prevention Program

Myklebust et al.[55] published a prospective nonrandomized study in 2003, which examined the effectiveness of an ACL injury prevention program in 1,705 Norwegian handball players.[55] The program consisted of three sets of exercises: running and cutting with partner feedback, wobble board exercises (disc diameter, 38 cm; Norpro, Notodden, Norway) of increasing difficulty, and mat balance exercises (40 × 50 cm, 7 cm thick; Alusuisse Airex, Sins, Switzerland) of increasing intensity with partner perturbations. The focus of the exercises was to improve awareness and knee control during standing, cutting, jumping, and landing activities. Over the course of three seasons, there was no statistically significant difference between the control and intervention groups, although there

TABLE 14.4 Prevent Injury and Enhance Performance Program

Phase	*Purpose*
Warm-up	Prepares the athlete for training and sports-specific movements
Strengthening: legs	Quadriceps, hamstrings, calves
Plyometrics	Increases power and strength as well as emphasizes neuromuscular control
Agilities	Increases dynamic stability of ankle-knee-hip as well as encourages avoidance of valgus positioning; increases hip flexion strength for power and speed
Flexibility	Lengthening of calves, quadriceps, adductors, hamstrings, hip flexors

was a trend toward a reduction in the overall incidence of ACL injury in the intervention group (P = .06).[55] The program is recommended to take approximately 15 minutes and be performed three times per week for 5 to 7 weeks preseason and 1 time per week while in season.[55]

Federation Internationale de Football Association 11+

The Federation Internationale de Football Association (FIFA) 11+ program is an injury prevention program designed by the FIFA medical committee to reduce the incidence of injuries in soccer, including ACL injury.[56] "The 11" program consisted of exercises focusing on core stability, balance, dynamic stabilization, and eccentric hamstring strength.[57] Steffan et al.[57] had examined the effect of "The 11" over a season among 2,000 female players aged 13 to 17 years in a randomized controlled trial. They found no difference in injury risk between the intervention group and control group secondary to low compliance.[57] They followed up this study by developing an exercise program to improve the preventive effects of the program by improving compliance of the coaches and players.[58] An expert group convened by FIFA, with representatives from Oslo Sports Trauma Research Center, the Santa Monica Orthopaedic and Sports Research Foundation, and the FIFA Medical Assessment and Research Centre revised the program and added an additional running component best suited as a comprehensive warm-up. The revised program, FIFA 11+, consists of three parts with a total of 15 exercises, which should be performed in a specified sequence at the beginning of each training session.[56,58] Proper technique is emphasized throughout the program. The first component includes multidirectional running exercises combined with dynamic stretching and controlled partner contacts. Part two consists of six sets of exercises focusing on core, hip, general lower extremity strength, balance, and plyometric exercises, with increasing levels of difficulty depending on the abilities of each player. Part 3 includes running exercises at a moderate to high speed combined with change of direction and cutting movements.[58]

It should be noted that the FIFA 11+ program was designed to reduce the incidence not only of ACL injury but also of other common soccer-related injuries. In a recently published abstract, Silvers et al.[56] found that the FIFA 11+ program significantly reduced injury rates and time lost in the male collegiate soccer players. More research must be conducted to examine the effect of the FIFA 11+ on ACL injury rates specifically as well as their effect on young athletes.

A number of ACL injury prevention programs are currently being used by young athletes today and each are composed of various elements and applications. There are, however, several common themes as to which elements of program design may be most effective. In a 2010 meta-analysis performed by Yoo et al.,[59] the authors concluded that the most effective program for ACL injury prevention was a preseason and in-season neuromuscular training program with an emphasis on plyometrics and strength training exercises. These programs are most effective when implemented in female athletes younger than 18 years of age.[59] It would appear from this and other meta-analyses performed by Hewett et al.[60] and Sadoghi et al.[61] that the most effective ACL injury prevention programs should combine preseason and in-season training and include strength and plyometric exercises rather than balance training alone.

CONCLUSION

Most ACL injury prevention programs take a multifaceted approach and target dynamic neuromuscular and proprioceptive deficits. The focus lies on noncontact mechanisms of injury, jump, and landing techniques and improving movement patterns during pivoting, cutting, and change in direction secondary to the high incidence. It has been demonstrated in the literature that adolescent female athletes are predisposed to injury secondary to neuromuscular deficits. In addition, it has been demonstrated that these neuromuscular deficits can be corrected and effectively reduced with implementation of neuromuscular training programs. However, the effectiveness of these programs in skeletally immature athletes has not been studied, and therefore its' potential effectiveness remains to be proven. It is encouraged that young athletes partake in preseason training programs focused on strengthening, flexibility, neuromuscular, and proprioceptive training under appropriate supervision of qualified personnel to reduce the risk of ACL injury. Training programs should emphasize proper technique and be performed year-round for maintenance. Coaches, parents, trainers, and physical therapists should emphasize proper technique and alignment throughout all movement patterns, appropriate foundational strength and flexibility for the young athlete to meet the demands of their sport, as well as appropriate conditioning to allow the athlete to perform while maintaining quality of movement. It is encouraged that prevention programs be incorporated at earlier ages (potentially ages 9 to 12 years) to allow for appropriate training prior to changes in neuromuscular control secondary to maturation.

ACKNOWLEDGMENTS

The authors would like to acknowledge those who have been pioneers in the field of ACL prevention and research such as Greg Meyers, Timothy Hewett, as well as Dr. Frank Noyes. The diligent research produced in this field will continue to assist in the prevention of ACL injuries to young athletes to come. We would also like to acknowledge the passion of Dr. Frank Cordasco and Dr. Daniel Green and the work they do on a daily basis for the well-being of their pediatric and adolescent athletes.

REFERENCES

1. Freedman KB, Glasgow MT, Glasgow SG, et al. Anterior cruciate ligament injury and reconstruction among university students. *Clin Orthop Relat Res.* 1998;(356):208–212.
2. Daniel DM, Stone ML, Dobson BE, et al. Fate of the ACL-injured patient. A prospective outcome study. *Am J Sports Med.* 1994;22: 632–644.
3. Agel J, Arendt EA, Bershadsky B. Anterior cruciate ligament injury in national collegiate athletic association basketball and soccer: a 13-year review. *Am J Sports Med.* 2005;33(4):524–530.
4. Arendt E, Dick R. Knee injury patterns among men and women in collegiate basketball and soccer. NCAA data and review of literature. *Am J Sports Med.* 1995;23(6):692–701.

5. Mihata LC, Beutler Al, Boden BP. Comparing the incidence of anterior cruciate ligament injury in collegiate lacrosse, soccer, and basketball players: implications for anterior cruciate ligament mechanism and prevention. *Am J Sports Med.* 2006;34(6): 899–904.
6. Kocher MS, Foreman ES, Micheli LJ. Laxity and functional outcome after arthroscopic reduction and internal fixation of displaced tibial spine fractures in children. *Arthroscopy.* 2003;19:1085–1090.
7. Rang M, ed. *Children's Fractures.* 2nd ed. Philadelphia: Lippincott; 1983.
8. Kocher MS, Mandiga R, Klingele K, et al. Anterior cruciate ligament injury versus tibial spine fracture in the skeletally immature knee: a comparison of skeletal maturation and notch width index. *J Pediatr Orthop.* 2004;24:185–188.
9. Eiskjaer S, Larsen ST, Schmidt MB. The significance of hemarthrosis of the knee in children. *Arch Orthop Trauma Surg.* 1988;107: 96–98.
10. Graziano J, Green DW, Cordasco FA. Anterior cruciate ligament injury prevention in the young athlete: evidence-based application. *Strength Cond J.* 2013;35(3):89–97.
11. Paterno MV, Rauh MJ, Schmitt LC, et al. Incidence of second ACL injury after primary ACL reconstruction and return to sport. *Am J Sports Med.* 2014;42(7):1567–1573.
12. McNair PJ, Marshall RN, Matheson JA. Important features associated with acute anterior cruciate ligament injury. *N Z Med J.* 1990;103(901):537–539.
13. Bien BP. Rationale and implementation of anterior cruciate ligament injury prevention warm-up programs in female athletes. *J Strength Cond Res.* 2001;25:271–285.
14. Shimokochi Y, Shultz SJ. Mechanisms of noncontact anterior cruciate ligament injury. *J Athl Train.* 2008;43:396–408.
15. Mandelbaum BR, Silvers HJ, Watanabe DS, et al. Effectiveness of a neuromuscular and proprioceptive training program in preventing anterior cruciate ligament injuries in female athletes: 2-year follow-up. *Am J Sports Med.* 2005;33:1003–1010.
16. Ford KR, Myer GD, Hewett TE. Valgus knee motion during landing in high school female and male basketball players. *Med Sci Sports Exerc.* 2003;35:1745–1750.
17. Ford KR, Myer GD, Smith RL, et al. A comparison of dynamic coronal plane excursion between matched male and female athletes when performing single leg landings. *Clin Biomech (Bristol, Avon).* 2006;21:33–40.
18. Ford KR, Myer GD, Toms HE, et al. Gender differences in the kinematics of unanticipated cutting in young athletes. *Med Sci Sports Exerc.* 2005;37:124–129.
19. Stanitski CL, Harvell JC, Fu F. Observations on acute knee hemarthrosis in children and adolescents. *J Pediatr Orthop.* 1993;13: 506–510.
20. Kidd PS, McCoy C, Steenbergen L. Repetitive strain injuries in youth. *J Am Acad Nurse Pract.* 2000;12:413–426.
21. DiStefano LJ, Padua DA, DiStefano MJ, et al. Influence of age, sex, technique, and exercise program on movement patterns after an anterior cruciate ligament injury prevention program in youth soccer players. *Am J Sports Med.* 2009;37(32):495–504.
22. Carter CW, Micheli LJ. Training the child athlete: physical fitness, health and injury. *Br J Sports Med.* 2011;45:880–885.
23. Jurimae T, Jurimae J. *Growth, Physical Activity, and Motor Development in Prepubertal Children.* Boca Raton, FL: CRC Press LLC; 2000.
24. Giugliano DN, Solomon JL. ACL tears in female athletes. *Phys Med Rehabil Clin N Am.* 2007;18(3):417–438.
25. Gianotti SM, Marshall SW, Hume PA, et al. Incidence of anterior cruciate ligament injury and other knee ligament injuries: a national population-based study. *J Sci Med Sport.* 2009;12(6):622–627.
26. Gomez E, DeLee JC, Farney WC. Incidence of injury in Texas girls' high school basketball. *Am J Sports Med.* 1996;24:684–687.
27. Hewett, TE, Lindenfeld TN, Riccobene JV, et al. The effect of neuromuscular training on the incidence of knee injury in female athletes. A prospective study. *Am J Sports Med.* 1999;27:699–706.
28. Hewett TE, Ford KR, Hoogenbaum BJ, et al. Understanding and preventing ACL injuries: current biomechanical and epidemiologic considerations. *Am J Sports Med.* 2007;35(2):235–241.
29. Hewett TE, Myer GD, Ford KR, et al. The 2012 ABJS Nicolas Andry Award: the sequence of prevention: a systematic approach to prevent anterior cruciate ligament injury. *Clin Orthop Relat Res.* 2012;470:2930–2940.
30. Hewett TE, Paterno MV, Myer GD. Strategies for enhancing proprioception and neuromuscular control of the knee. *Clin Orthop Relat Res.* 2002;402:76–94.
31. Hewett TE, Myer GD, Ford KR. Decrease in neuromuscular control about the knee with maturation in female athletes. *J Bone Joint Surg Am.* 2004;86(8):1601–1608.
32. Hewett TE, Stroupe AL, Nance TA, et al. Plyometric training in female athletes. Decreased impact forces and increased hamstring torques. *Am J Sports Med.* 1996;24:765–773.
33. Jurimae T, Jurimae J. *Growth, Physical Activity, and Motor Development in Prepubertal Children.* Boca Raton, FL: CRC Press LLC; 2000.
34. Chappell JD, Creighton RA, Giuliani C, et al. Kinematics and electromyography of landing preparation in vertical stop-jump: risks for noncontact anterior cruciate ligament injury. *Am J Sports Med.* 2007;35(2):235–241.
35. Ford KR, Myer GD, Hewett TE. Valgus knee motion during landing in high school female and male basketball players. *Med Sci Sports Exerc.* 2003;35(10):1745–1750.
36. Hewett TE, Myer GD, Ford KR, et al. Biomechanical measures of neuromuscular control and valgus loading of the knee predict anterior cruciate ligament injury risk in female athletes: a prospective study. *Am J Sports Med.* 2005;33(4):492–501.
37. Ebben WP, Fauth ML, Petushek, et al. Gender-based analysis of hamstring and quadriceps muscle activation during jump landings and cutting. *J Strength Cond Res.* 2010;24:408–415.
38. Mascal CL, Landel R, Powers C. Management of patellofemoral pain targeting hip, pelvis, and trunk muscle function: 2 case reports. *J Orthop Sports Phys Ther.* 1978;33:647–674.
39. Quatman CE, Hewett TE. The anterior cruciate ligament injury controversy: is "valgus collapse" a sex-specific mechanism? *Br J Sports Med.* 2009;43:328–335.
40. Ladenhauf HN, Graziano J, Marx RG. Anterior cruciate ligament prevention strategies: are they effective in young athletes—current concepts and review of literature. *Curr Opin Pediatr.* 2013;25:64–71.
41. Krause DA, Jacobs RS, Pliger KE, et al. Electromyographic analysis of the gluteus medius in five weight bearing exercises. *J Strength Cond Res.* 2009;23:2689–2694.
42. Myer GD, Ford KR, Hewett TE. Rationale and clinical techniques for anterior cruciate ligament injury prevention among female athletes. *J Athl Train.* 2004;39(4):353–364.
43. Myer GD, Chu DA, Brent JE, et al. Trunk and hip control neuromuscular training for the prevention of knee joint injury. *Clin Sports Med.* 2008;27(3):425–428, ix.
44. Chappell JD, Herman DC, Knight BS, et al. Effect of fatigue on knee kinetics and kinematics in stop-jump tasks. *Am J Sports Med.* 2005;33(7):1022–1029.
45. Mizner RL, Kawaguchi JK, Chmielewski TL. Muscle strength in the lower extremity does not predict postinstruction improvements in the landing patterns of female athletes. *J Orthop Sports Phys Ther.* 2008;38:353–361.
46. Padua DA, Distefano LJ. Sagittal plane knee biomechanics and vertical ground reaction forces are modified following ACL injury prevention programs: a systematic review. *Sports Health.* 2009;1:165–173.
47. Zebis MK, Benchke J, Anderson LL, et al. The effects of neuromuscular training on knee joint motor control during sidecutting in female elite soccer and handball players. *Clin J Sport Med.* 2008;18:329–337.
48. Prapavessis H, McNair PJ. Effects of instruction in jumping technique and experience jumping on ground reaction forces. *J Orthop Sports Phys Ther.* 2003;33:2004–2207.

49. Alentorn-Geli E, Myer GD, Silvers HJ, et al. Prevention of noncontact anterior cruciate ligament injuries in soccer players. Part 2: a review of prevention programs aimed to modify risk factors and to reduce injury rates. *Knee Surg Sports Traumatol Arthrosc.* 2009;17:859–879.
50. Caraffa A, Cerulli G, Projetti M, et al. Prevention of anterior cruciate ligament injuries in soccer. A prospective controlled study of proprioceptive training. *Knee Surg Sports Traumatol Arthrosc.* 1996;4(1):19–21.
51. Postma WE, West RV. Anterior cruciate ligament injury-prevention programs. *J Bone Joint Surg Am.* 2013;95:661–669.
52. Grandstrand SL, Pfeiffer RP, Sabick MB, et al. The effects of a commercially available warm-up program on landing mechanics in female youth soccer players. *J Strength Cond Res.* 2006;20(2):331–335.
53. Mandelbaum BR, Silvers HJ, Watanabe DS, et al. Effectiveness of a neuromuscular and proprioceptive training program in preventing anterior cruciate ligament injuries in female athletes: 2-year follow up. *Am J Sports Med.* 2005;33(7):1003–1010.
54. Gilchrist J, Mandelbaum BR, Melancon H, et al. A randomized controlled trial to prevent noncontact anterior cruciate ligament injury in female collegiate soccer players. *Am J Sports Med.* 2008;36(8):1476–1483.
55. Myklebust G, Engebretsen L, Braekken IH, et al. Prevention of anterior cruciate ligament injuries in female team handball players: a prospective intervention study over three seasons. *Clin J Sports Med.* 2003;13(2):71–78.
56. Silvers H, Mandelbaum B, Bizzini M, et al. Abstracts from the IOC World Conference on Prevention of Injury & Illness in Sport, Monaco 2014: the efficacy of the FIFA 11+ program in the collegiate male soccer player (USA). *Br J Sports Med.* 2014;48:662.
57. Steffan K, Myklebust G, Olsen OE, et al. Preventing injuries in female youth football—a cluster randomized controlled trial. *Scand J Med Sci Sports.* 2008;18(5):605–614.
58. Soligard T, Myklebust G, Andersen TE. Comprehensive warm-up programme to prevent injuries in young female footballers: cluster randomized controlled trial. *BMJ.* 2008;337:2469.
59. Yoo JH, Lim BO, Ha M, et al. A meta-analysis of the effect of neuromuscular training on the prevention of the anterior cruciate ligament injury in female athletes. *Knee Surg Sports Traumatol Arthrosc.* 2010;18(6):824–830.
60. Hewett TE, Ford KR, Myer GD. Anterior cruciate ligament injuries in female athletes: part 2, a meta-analysis of neuromuscular interventions aimed at injury prevention. *Am J Sports Med.* 2006;34(3):490–498.
61. Sadoghi P, von Keudell A, Vavken P. Effectiveness of anterior cruciate ligament injury prevention programs. *J Bone Joint Surg Am.* 2012;94(9):769–776.

SECTION

2

Patellofemoral Instability

Amy L. McIntosh

CHAPTER 15

Overview, Pathomechanics, Epidemiology, and Assessment of Patellar Dislocation

INTRODUCTION

Patellofemoral instability (PFI) is a relatively common condition in children and adolescents with an incidence estimated to be approximately 43 per 100,000.[1] In a recent study by Abbasi et al.,[2] 31% of 131 adolescent patients presenting with an acute traumatic knee effusion who underwent magnetic resonance imaging (MRI) were diagnosed with a patellofemoral dislocation. Patellofemoral dislocation was more commonly the causative factor for the knee effusion in children aged 10 to 14 years, compared to anterior cruciate ligament (ACL) disruption for those aged 15 to 18 years.[2]

Surgical treatment for PFI with anatomic medial patellofemoral ligament (MPFL) reconstruction has risen dramatically in the last decade.[3] However, the pathomechanics that contribute to PFI are multifactorial. Therefore, a combination of options exists for surgically treating PFI. This chapter helps to provide an understanding of the relevant risk factors for recurrent PFI and reviews the clinical and radiographic tests that are necessary to determine optimal surgical or nonsurgical treatment of patients presenting with PFI.

Consider reviewing the pediatric patellar dislocation classification described by Weeks et al.[3a] in the 2013 review article in *Sports Medicine and Arthroscopy Review (SMAR)*

PATHOMECHANICS

The stability of the patellofemoral joint relies on the integration of static (bony configuration), passive (capsule/ligament), and dynamic (muscle) stabilizers.[4] Pathology in any of the stabilizers can quickly disrupt the balance and lead to PFI.

In full knee extension, the patella is located slightly superior and lateral to the trochlear groove. Between 10 and 30 degrees of knee flexion, the patella starts to make contact with the trochlea and slides into the sulcus.[5] The MPFL is a portion of the medial soft tissue complex of the knee and is the main stabilizer of the patellofemoral joint in extension and lower degrees of knee flexion (0 to 3 degrees). Warren and Marshall[6] described a three-layered structure of the medial soft tissue complex of the knee joint. The MPFL is in the second layer and has a "sail-like" appearance with two functional portions: (1) inferior straight bundle and (2) superior oblique bundle (SOB).[7] The MPFL originates from the medial femoral condyle just proximal to the femoral attachment of the medial collateral ligament and distal to the adductor tubercle. It inserts on the superomedial border of the patella.[8] In children and adolescents with open physes, the femoral insertion is located slightly distal (4 to 5 mm) to the medial femoral physis.[9,10] During 0 to 30 degrees of knee flexion, the MPFL contributes more than 60% of the medial stability of the patella and isolated insufficiency leads to increased lateralization or dislocation.[11]

As the knee continues past 30 degrees of flexion, the depth of the trochlea increases and the bony anatomy becomes the major stabilizer of the patellofemoral joint.[12] Past 90 degrees of knee flexion, the patella is located in the notch. The vastus medialis obliquus (VMO) is the most important dynamic stabilizer. However, it only affects patellofemoral stability in flexion greater than 60 degrees, when the fibers run perpendicularly to the patellar motion, and an intact connection exists between the SOB of the MPFL and the quadriceps tendon.[4]

In extended positions, when the patella is not engaged in the trochlea, the MPFL is the only structure that resists lateralizing forces. Therefore, a functionally deficient MPFL contributes greatly to the pathomechanics of PFI. Recently, two studies have shown MRI evidence of pathologic alteration of the MPFL in the majority (78% to 94%) of children and adolescents who had sustained a recent patellofemoral dislocation.[10,13]

One may question: How does a patella dislocate without an MRI demonstrating evidence of MPFL injury? In a recent article,[4] senior author Schoettle describes a condition that he termed *early and chronic PFI*. I prefer the term *early-onset PFI*.

Early-onset PFI occurs when the MPFL becomes chronically insufficient due to underlying bony malalignment. The bony malalignment is often related to trochlear dysplasia, patella alta, valgus mechanical axis, excessive internal femoral rotation (excessive anteversion), and/or excessive external tibial torsion. The combination of excessive anteversion and external tibial torsion is called *miserable malalignment*.[14] These congenital bony pathologies combine and lead to lateral shift and tilt of the patella. This places persistent traction on the MPFL, which then results in a stretched and nonfunctional passive stabilizer. A "normal" MPFL does not develop due to the persistent traction, and the major restraint to PFI in low knee flexion angles is (functionally) absent.[4]

Early-onset PFI can also occur in patients with hyperlaxity syndromes (Ehlers-Danlos syndrome). The genetic alterations in the tissue that form the MPFL lead to stretching and insufficiency with the forces of daily activity. Even without the underlying bony pathology, these hyperlaxity in patients have a "functionally absent" MPFL leading to PFI at low flexion angles.

EPIDEMIOLOGY AND RISK FACTOR ASSESSMENT

PFI is a common but complex condition. It can occur as an isolated event (acute, first-time dislocation) or it can be chronic condition. The instability can also occur as a traumatic or nontraumatic injury. Most traumatic PFI occurs in sports that involve cutting and pivoting, such as soccer, football, or basketball. The involved limb often is in a position of significant internal rotation and valgus stress.[4] Nontraumatic dislocations occur with minimal force during activities of daily living and often reduce spontaneously. Patients with nontraumatic recurrent instability will often subluxate their patella on multiple occasions between dislocation events.

It is important to take a detailed history to help distinguish between acute traumatic PFI and chronic nontraumatic PFI because the risks for recurrent PFI differ when the two groups are compared.

Two studies have recently been published that investigate pediatric/adolescent (18 years old or younger) patients presenting with an acute, first-time patellofemoral dislocation.[1,13] The rate of recurrent PFI ranges between 30% and 38%. In other words, during the study periods, 62% to 70% of patients successfully completed nonoperative treatment and did not experience a subsequent episode of PFI.

However, a similar and important conclusion arose from both studies. Younger patients between the ages of 11 and 13 years with immature growth plates had a statistically significant higher rate of recurrent PFI.

In the study by Seeley et al.,[13] the overall rate of recurrent PFI was 30.6%, with the highest rate (43%) occurring in patients between the ages of 11 and 13 years. Lewallen et al.[1] concluded that the rate of recurrent PFI was 38% for the group as a whole. However, skeletally immature patients with open growth plates and trochlear dysplasia had a recurrence rate of 69%.[1] Trochlear dysplasia increased the risk of recurrent PFI by a factor of 2.2, and combining trochlear dysplasia with immature physes increased that risk by a factor of 3.3 (Table 15.1).

Fithian et al.[15] investigated acute, first-time PFI. However, his patient population included both pediatric and adult patients. He also found that younger patients, age 10 to 17 years, were more likely to develop recurrent PFI than older adult patients.[15]

Interestingly, Lewallen et al.[16] demonstrated that patients older than the age of 40 years presenting with an acute, first-time patellofemoral dislocation had a PFI recurrence rate of 0%.[16] A positive family history for PFI was a risk factor for recurrent PFI after first-time patellofemoral dislocation in a study by Palmu et al.[17] It was also a risk factor for the development of contralateral knee PFI in studies by Fithian et al.[15] and Palmu et al.[17]

Female sex is not a risk factor for developing recurrent PFI after an acute first-time patellofemoral dislocation.[1,13,15,17]

Fithian et al.[15] demonstrated that patients presenting with a previous history of PFI (chronic nontraumatic PFI) are more likely to be older (median age of 21 years) and female (70%). They are also 6.6 times more likely to have recurrent PFI compared to patients presenting with an acute first-time patellofemoral dislocation.

CLINICAL ASSESSMENT

A detailed clinical evaluation and the supplemental use of radiographic tests are crucial to determine the appropriate diagnosis, risks for recurrent instability episodes, and treatment for patients presenting with PFI. This assessment should also be divided into those patients presenting with an acute, first-time patellofemoral dislocation and those presenting with a previous history of PFI.

FIRST-TIME PATELLOFEMORAL DISLOCATION

This is usually a traumatic and painful injury. Occasionally, the reduction of the patella requires anesthesia or sedation. To avoid damage to the patellar and trochlear cartilage, the

TABLE 15.1 Analysis of Maximum Likelihood Estimates[a]

	Hazard Ratio (95% CI)	*P Value*
Open/closing physes and trochlear dysplasia	3.3 (1.8–6.0)	<.001
Closed physes and trochlear dysplasia	2.2 (0.97–4.9)	.06
Open/closing physes and no trochlear dysplasia	1.2 (0.6–2.5)	.54
Closed physes and no trochlear dysplasia	1.0 (Ref)	

[a]CI, confidence interval; Ref, reference statistic.

From Lewallen LW, McIntosh AL, Dahm DL. Predictors of recurrent instability after acute patellofemoral dislocation in pediatric and adolescent patients. *Am J Sports Med.* 2013;41(3):575–581.

reduction should be performed by extending the knee while holding the patella in the lateral dislocation position. Reduction attempts with the knee in higher degrees of flexion should be avoided.[4]

The physical exam can be difficult in these patients due to pain from the recent trauma. It is important to assess the medial soft tissue complex of the knee. The MPFL and VMO are often torn. Special attention should be paid to any swelling or ecchymosis in this area. A large hemarthrosis can develop if an osteochondral fracture of the patella or trochlea occurred during the dislocation or reduction events. A recent study demonstrated that 38% (46/122) of adolescent patients with an acute patellofemoral dislocation had a displaced osteochondral fracture.[18]

Radiographs of the knee (anteroposterior [AP], lateral, and Merchant views) should be obtained to assess for osteochondral fractures and the status of the physis. The distal femoral and proximal tibial physes should be graded as open, closing, or closed. The radiographs can also be assessed for patellar height and trochlear dysplasia. For both to be assessed accurately, a perfect lateral radiograph (medial and lateral posterior condyles overlapping) of the femur should be obtained with the knee in 30 degrees of flexion.

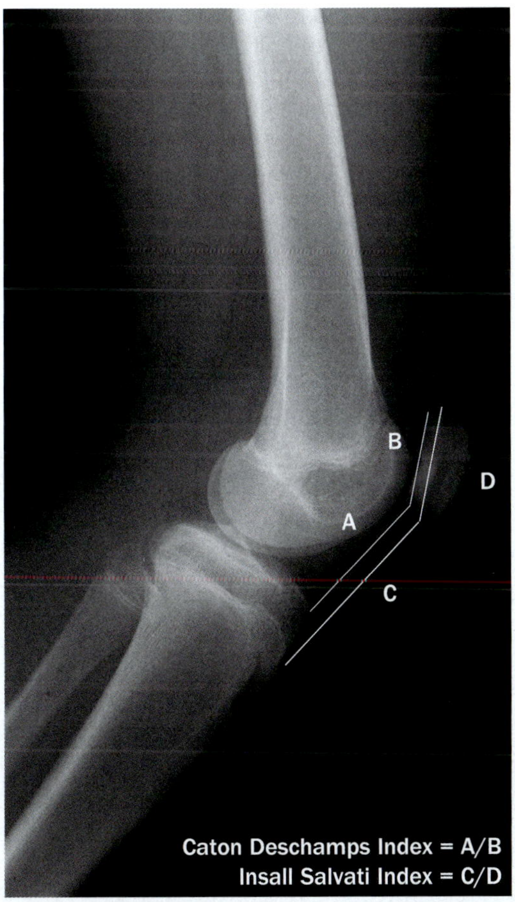

Figure 15.1. Lateral knee x-ray of a skeletally immature patient demonstrating measurement techniques for Caton-Deschamps (*A,B*) and Insall-Salvati (*C,D*) to determine patellar height. A ratio greater than 1.2 is considered patella alta.

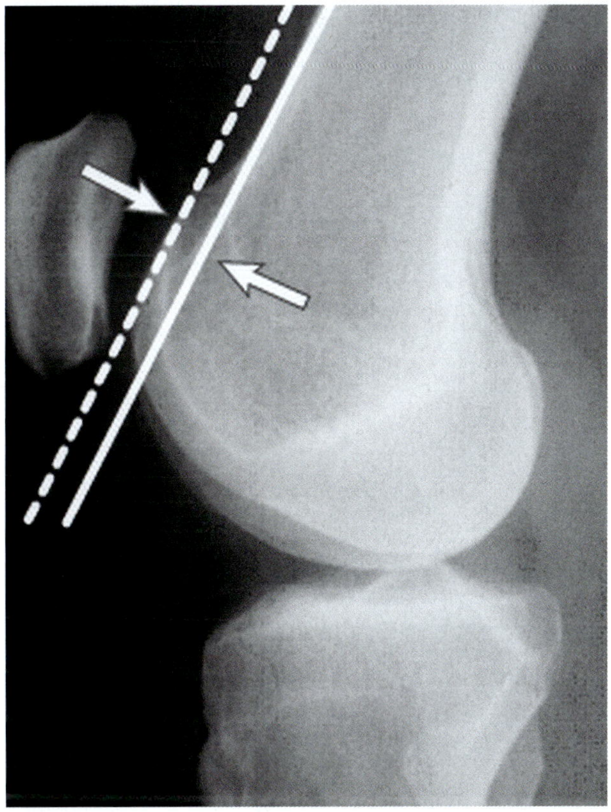

Figure 15.2. The crossing sign occurs when the line representing the trochlear floor crosses the anterior border of the femoral condyles. It indicates a deficient proximal trochlea with decreased relative height of the lateral trochlear wall.

The Caton Deschamps (C-D) index has been validated to assess patellar height in children and adolescents.[19] The mean C-D index in normal children and adolescents was 1.06 ± 0.21. Intraobserver and interobserver reliability studies showed excellent reliabilities with an intraclass correlation coefficient that was between 0.930 and 0.944 (95% confidence interval). A C-D index greater than 1.2 is considered to be diagnostic for patella alta. The Insall-Salvati index can also be used, but it is not validated in children and adolescents (Fig. 15.1).

The Dejour classification is used to determine if a patient has trochlear dysplasia.[20] Type A dysplasia is characterized by a shallow trochlea. On the Merchant (axial) view, the shallow trochlea will have a sulcus angle that measures greater than 145 degrees. The lateral x-ray will demonstrate a **crossing sign**. The **crossing sign** occurs when the line representing the trochlear floor crosses the anterior border of the femoral condyles. It indicates a deficient proximal trochlea with decreased relative height of the lateral trochlear wall[21] (Fig. 15.2).

Type B dysplasia is characterized by a flat trochlea on the axial radiographs and a **supratrochlear spur** on lateral x-rays. The **supratrochlear spur** is an extension of the trochlear groove above the anterior cortex of the femur (Fig. 15.3).

Type C dysplasia is characterized by the presence of a crossing sign and a **double contour** on the lateral x-ray as well as medial hypoplasia and lateral convexity on the axial x-ray.

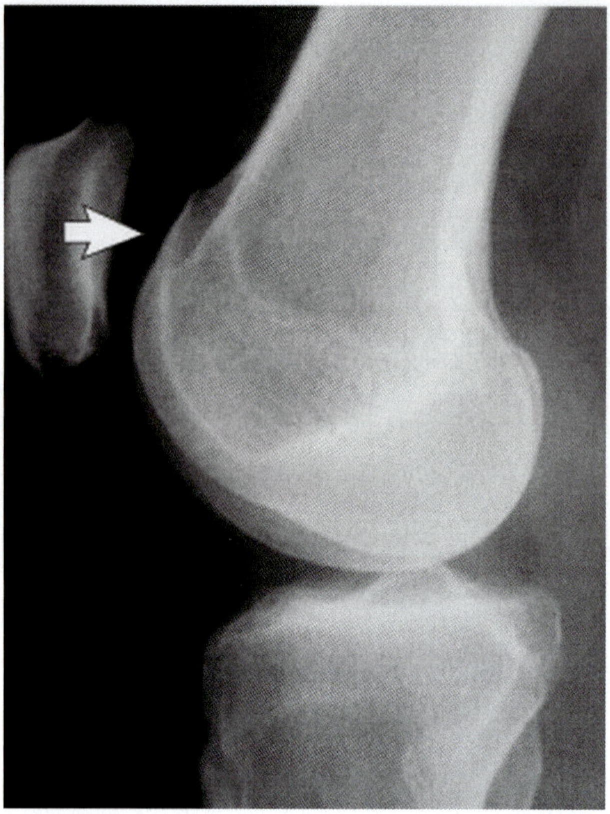

Figure 15.3. A supratrochlear spur is an extension of the trochlear groove above the anterior cortex of the femur.

A **double contour** is seen on the lateral x-rays as a double line at anterior aspect of condyles. This occurs because the medial trochlea is hypoplastic.

Type D dysplasia is a severe form of trochlear dysplasia. There is significant asymmetry between the large lateral trochlea and hypoplastic medial trochlea as well as a cliff between the trochlear facets. This leads to a **double contour** and **supratrochlear spur** on the lateral x-ray. The Dejour classification has not been validated in patients with skeletally immature physes.

Should an MRI be obtained to evaluate a patient with a first-time patellofemoral dislocation? In my practice, I obtain an MRI if the patient has osteochondral fracture on x-rays, a noticeable joint effusion/hemarthrosis, or if the history and physical exam are unclear.

Seeley et al.[18] demonstrated that 44% of the patients with osteochondral fractures had plain radiographs that were negative.[18] The osteochondral fracture was only diagnosed after the MRI was obtained. If the osteochondral fracture is large enough to treat operatively, then the location of the MPFL rupture is important to determine preoperatively. Kepler et al.[10] demonstrated that 61% of pediatric and adolescent patients with PFI had MRI evidence of injury to the patellar attachment of the MPFL. Twelve percent injured the femoral attachment, 12% injured both the patellar and femoral attachments, 9% had midsubstance injuries, and 6% had no identifiable injury to the MPFL.[10]

The MRI can also be used to assess trochlear dysplasia and the tibial tubercle to trochlear groove (TT-TG) distance.

Lippacher et al.[22] recently compared lateral x-rays with MRI for determining trochlear dysplasia in patients with PFI. A two-grade system divided into low-grade (type A) and high-grade (types B to D) trochlear dysplasia was compared to the traditional four-grade system. The four-grade analysis showed fair intraobserver and interobserver agreements (24% to 78%), whereas the two-grade analysis showed good to excellent agreement (56% to 96%). The best overall agreement was found for the two-grade analysis on MRI scans (62% to 96%). The lateral radiographs tended to underestimate the severity of trochlear dysplasia compared with axial MRI.[22]

The TT-TG distance is a useful tool in guiding management for patients with recurrent lateral patellar instability (Fig. 15.4). Current recommendations for tibial tubercle transfer are based on TT-TG distance thresholds derived from adult populations. Recurrent patellar instability, however, frequently affects children, but normal and pathologic TT-TG values have not been established for pediatric patients. Recently published work by Dickens et al.[23] sought to (1) confirm that MRI measurements for TT-TG distance in a pediatric population are reliable and reproducible, (2) determine whether the TT-TG distance changes with age, (3) define normal TT-TG distances in a pediatric population, and (4) confirm that a subgroup of pediatric patients with patellar instability have higher TT-TG distances.[23] There were 618 MRIs retrospectively collected for patients who were 9 months to 16 years old. TT-TG distance changed with chronologic age in the pediatric population. Therefore, a percentile-based growth chart was developed in order to better depict normal TT-TG distances in the

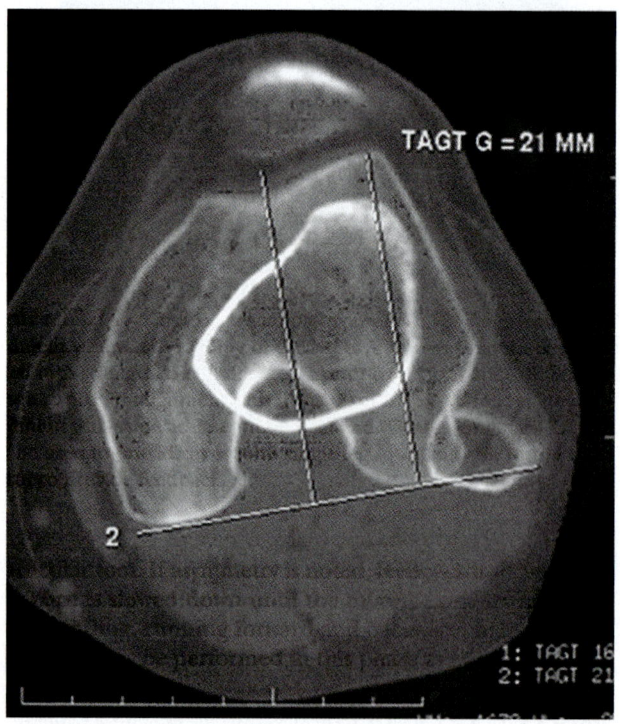

Figure 15.4. Radiographic measurement of the TT-TG distance occurs in the axial plane. It represents the distance that the tibial tubercle is lateralized from the center of the trochlea.

pediatric population. The median TT-TG distance for patients without patellar instability in this pediatric population was 8.5 mm (mean and 95% confidence interval, 8.6 ± 0.3 mm). Patients with patellar instability had higher TT-TG distances (median, 12.1 mm; $P < .001$).[23] This percentile-based growth chart should be used to help direct surgical decision making regarding tibial tubercle transfer in pediatric and adolescent patients.

RECURRENT PATELLOFEMORAL INSTABILITY

In these patients, it is very important to evaluate the extremities clinically and radiographically in the standing position. The foot progression angle should be determined while watching the normal gait cycle. The standing mechanical axis should be assessed, with particular attention paid to valgus mechanical alignment. Pelvic obliquity/leg length discrepancy should be determined by placing both hands on the patient's iliac crests while the patient is standing with his or her feet positioned shoulder-width apart. The patient should then be directed to lie down on the table in the prone position. Femoral internal and external rotation should be documented as well as tibial torsion. Next, the patient should be placed in a sitting position and asked to bring their knee through a normal range of motion. Particular attention should be paid to the development of the "J sign." The flexion angle at which the patella shifts laterally should be documented. The patient should then lie in the supine position. Lateral patellar glide should be assessed by pushing the patella laterally while the knee is fully extended. The distance of lateral glide can be divided into quadrants based on the width of the patella. One quadrant represents when the patella lateralizes one-fourth width of the patella. Two quadrants → one-half of the patella, three quadrants → three-fourths of the patella, and four quadrants → the patella subluxates off the trochlea or dislocates. The patient's face should be evaluated during this maneuver to determine if he or she fears a subluxation/dislocation. If the patient becomes very uncomfortable, then a positive apprehension sign has occurred.

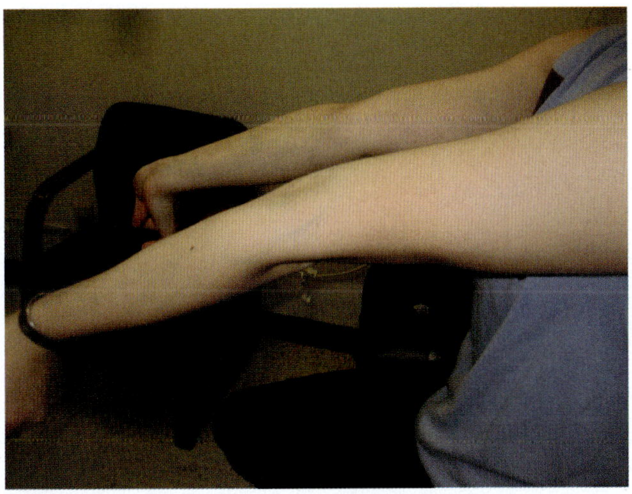

Figure 15.5. Hyperextension of the elbow may indicate an underlying connective tissue disorder

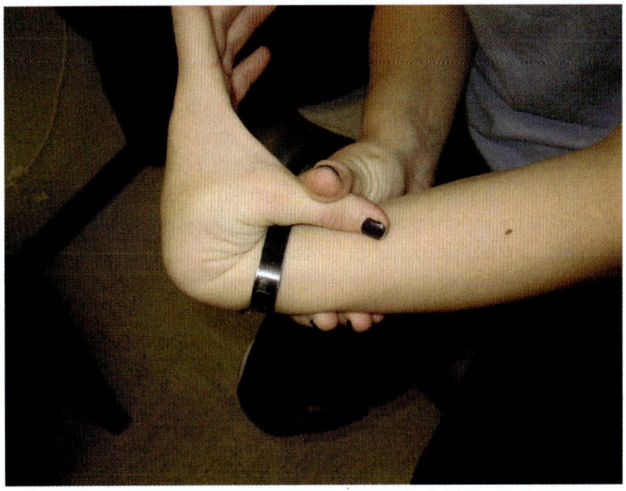

Figure 15.6. The ability to touch your thumb to your forearm may indicate an underlying connective tissue disorder.

The patient should also be assessed for ligamentous laxity by using the Beighton test which was validated in children.[24] The Beighton score is calculated as follows:

1. One point if while standing forward bending, you can place palms on the ground with legs straight.
2. One point for each elbow that bends backward (Fig. 15.5)
3. One point for each knee that bends backward
4. One point for each thumb that touches the forearm when bent backward (Fig. 15.6)
5. One point for each little finger that bends backward beyond 90 degrees (Fig. 15.7)

A score of 5 or more indicates ligamentous laxity and a genetics consultation should be considered.

Standing AP lower extremity radiographs from hip to ankle should be obtained to document mechanical axis as well as standing AP, lateral, and Merchant views of the involved knee. The x-rays should be assessed for maturity of the physis, patellar height, and trochlear dysplasia. If excessive femoral anteversion or external tibial torsion is demonstrated on clinical exam, then computed tomography (CT) or EOS three-dimensional (3-D) modeling can be used to verify the rotational abnormality radiographically. MRI should also be performed to assess TT-TG, trochlear dysplasia, and chronic damage to the patellar and trochlear cartilage.

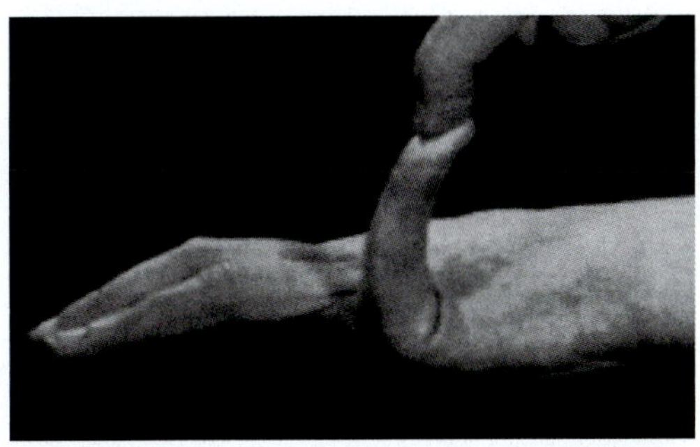

Figure 15.7. The ability to extend your small finger past 90 degrees may indicate an underlying connective tissue disorder.

CONCLUSION

PFI is a common but complex condition. First-time patellofemoral dislocation and chronic recurrent PFI should be considered separately to help to clarify risks factors for recurrent PFI and to optimize management. By participating in comprehensive rehabilitation program, 62% to 70% of pediatric and adolescent patients who experience a first-time patellofemoral dislocation will avoid a recurrent dislocation. However, younger patients between the ages of 11 and 13 years, with immature growth plates and trochlear dysplasia, have a statistically higher rate of recurrent PFI.

Pediatric patients presenting with recurrent PFI need a comprehensive clinical and radiographic evaluation, as they are unlikely to gain patellar stability without operative intervention. Particular attention needs to be paid to ligamentous laxity, valgus mechanical alignment, patella alta, excessive femoral anteversion and/or tibial torsion, trochlear dysplasia, and abnormal TT-TG. Each patient's individual pathoanatomy and risk factors for recurrence will help guide treatment. The treatment recommended should be tailored to each patient's unique presentation.

REFERENCES

1. Lewallen LW, McIntosh AL, Dahm DL. Predictors of recurrent instability after acute patellofemoral dislocation in pediatric and adolescent patients. *Am J Sports Med.* 2013;41(3):575–581.
2. Abbasi D, May MM, Wall EJ, et al. MRI findings in adolescent patients with acute traumatic knee hemarthrosis. *J Pediatr Orthop.* 2012;32(8):760–764.
3. Schöttle PB, Schmeling A, Rosenstiel N, et al. Radiographic landmarks for femoral tunnel placement in medial patellofemoral ligament reconstruction. *Am J Sports Med.* 2007;35(5):801–804.

3a. Weeks KD, Fabricant PD, Ladenhauf HN, et al. Surgical options for patellar stabilization in the skeletally immature patient. *Sports Med Arthrosc.* 2012;20(3):194–202.

4. Hensler D, Sillanpaa PJ, Schoettle PB. Medial patellofemoral ligament: anatomy, injury and treatment in the adolescent knee. *Curr Opin Pediatr.* 2014;26(1):70–78.
5. Tecklenburg K, Dejour D, Hoser C, et al. Bony and cartilaginous anatomy of the patellofemoral joint. *Knee Surg Sports Traumatol Arthrosc.* 2006;14(3):235–240.
6. Warren LF, Marshall JL. The supporting structures and layers on the medial side of the knee: an anatomical analysis. *J Bone Joint Surg Am.* 1979;61(1):56–62.
7. Kang HJ, Wang F, Chen BC, et al. Functional bundles of the medial patellofemoral ligament. *Knee Surg Sports Traumatol Arthrosc.* 2010;18(11):1511–1516.
8. Tuxøe JI, Teir M, Winge S, et al. The medial patellofemoral ligament: a dissection study. *Knee Surg Sports Traumatol Arthrosc.* 2002; 10(3):138–140.
9. Shea KG, Polousky JD, Jacobs JC Jr, et al. The relationship of the femoral physis and the media; patellofemoral ligament in children: a cadaveric study. *J Pediatr Orthop.* 2014;34(8):808–813.
10. Kepler CK, Bogner EA, Hammoud S, et al. Zone of injury of the medial patellofemoral ligament after acute patellar dislocation in children and adolescents. *Am J Sports Med.* 2011;39(7): 1444–1449.
11. Desio SM, Burks RT, Bachus KN. Soft tissue restraints to lateral patellar translation in the human knee. *Am J Sports Med.* 1998; 26(1):59–65.
12. Senavongse W, Amis AA. The effects of articular, retinacular, or muscular deficiencies on patellofemoral joint stability: a biomechanical study in vitro. *J Bone Joint Surg Br.* 2005;87(4):577–582.
13. Seeley M, Bowman KF, Walsh C, et al. Magnetic resonance imaging of acute patellar dislocation in children: patterns of injury and risk factors for recurrence. *J Pediatr Orthop.* 2012;32(2):145–155.
14. Bruce WD, Stevens PM. Surgical correction of miserable malalignment syndrome. *J Pediatr Orthop.* 2004;24(4):392–396.
15. Fithian DC, Paxton EW, Stone ML, et al. Epidemiology and natural history of acute patellar dislocation. *Am J Sports Med.* 2004;32(5): 1114–1121.
16. Lewallen LW, McIntosh AL, Dahm DL. *Risk Factors for Recurrent Instability Following Acute Patellofemoral Dislocation.* Paper presented at: 2013 American Academy of Orthopaedic Surgeons Annual Meeting; March 19–23, 2013; Chicago, IL.
17. Palmu S, Kallio PE, Donell ST, et al. Acute patellar dislocation in children and adolescents: a randomized clinical trial. *J Bone Joint Surg Am.* 2008;90(3):463–470.
18. Seeley MA, Knesek M, Vanderhave KL. Osteochondral injury after patellar dislocation in children and adolescents. *J Pediatr Orthop.* 2013;33(5):511–518.
19. Thévenin-Lemoine C, Ferrand M, Courvoiser A, et al. Is the Caton-Deschamps index a valuable ratio to investigate patellar height in children? *J Bone Joint Surg Am.* 2011;93(8):e35.
20. Dejour D, Le Coultre B. Osteotomies in patello-femoral instabilities. *Sports Med Arthrosc.* 2007;15(1):39–46.
21. Bollier M, Fulkerson JP. The role of trochlear dysplasia in patellofemoral instability. *J Am Acad Orthop Surg.* 2011;19(1):8–16.
22. Lippacher S. Dejour D, Elsharkawi M, et al. Observer agreement on the Dejour trochlear dysplasia classification: a comparison of true lateral radiographs and axial magnetic resonance images. *Am J Sports Med.* 2012;40(4):837–843.
23. Dickens AJ, Morrell NT, Doering A, et al. Tibial tubercle-trochlear groove distance: defining normal in a pediatric population. *J Bone Joint Surg Am.* 2014;96(4):318–324.
24. van der Giessen LJ, Liekens D, Rutgers KJ, et al. Validation of beighton score and prevalence of connective tissue signs in 773 Dutch children. *J Rheumatol.* 2001;28(12):2726–2730.

Gregory Pinkowsky
William Hennrikus

CHAPTER 16

Technique: Quad Tendon Medial Patellofemoral Ligament Reconstruction

INTRODUCTION

Treatment of a first-time acute patellofemoral dislocation in the adolescent athlete is usually nonsurgical unless associated with an articular cartilage fracture. In the setting of recurrent patellar instability, surgical reconstruction is indicated after nonoperative treatment has failed. The medial patellofemoral ligament (MPFL) is the primary restraint to patellofemoral instability at 0 to 30 degrees of flexion and provides more than 50% of the medial restraint to the patella.[3,22] The patella is most prone to dislocate from 0 to 30 degrees of knee flexion.[25] The MPFL helps to guide the patella into the trochlear groove during early knee flexion. Once the patella is in the trochlea groove, the slope of the lateral patella facet provides the primary restraint to lateral translation.[10,13] The origin of the MPFL is near the adductor tubercle on the medial femoral epicondyle at or just distal to the distal femoral physis.[15,17] In children and adolescents, a large drill hole in this area risks physeal injury.[14] The MPFL originates about 1 cm distal to the superior pole of the patella on the upper third of the medial patella. The MPFL is about 55 mm long and 15 mm wide.[31] The MPFL is torn during acute lateral patellar dislocations in the majority of patients.[24,26]

Surgical treatment of patellofemoral instability in the adolescent athlete has evolved from nonanatomic extensor mechanism realignment procedures to anatomic restorative procedures based on reconstitution of the MPFL.

TREATMENT—BRIEF LITERATURE REVIEW

Many surgical procedures have been described for treatment of recurrent patellar instability.[1,20] The surgical approach should be individualized for each patient and should address the pathoanatomy contributing to the repeat dislocations. Often, combinations of procedures are needed to correct all patellofemoral problems.[28] No single procedure has been shown to be indicated in all patients with patellar dislocations. Surgical options for patellofemoral instability in adolescents includes proximal realignment, distal realignment, lateral release, MFPL reconstruction, guided growth with tension band plates, and combinations of the earlier procedures.[14] Osteotomies of the proximal tibia or distal femur are reserved for older teenagers who have demonstrated closure of the growth plates.[18] The goal of MPFL reconstruction is to reestablish the normal checkrein against lateral motion of the patella. When reconstructing the MPFL, it is important to replicate the native anatomy. In most chronic cases, reconstruction is recommended rather than MPFL repair because the chronically injured medial retinacular tissues are usually insufficient to reestablish the normal tether to prevent lateral dislocation. Multiple graft choices have been used for MPFL reconstruction including hamstrings,[16] patellar tendon,[5,15] adductor magnus,[30] allografts, and the quadriceps tendon.[12,20,32]

Isolated MPFL reconstruction may not be sufficient to prevent recurrent dislocation if other risk factors such as patella alta, patella tilt, an increased Q angle, a tibial tuberosity–trochlear groove (TT-TG) distance of more than 20 mm, or trochlear dysplasia are also present.[7,9,34] Treatment of the other risk factors can be combined with an MPFL reconstruction.

INDICATIONS AND CONTRAINDICATIONS

Indications for surgical treatment of patellar instability in the adolescent athlete include repeat patellar dislocations that have failed nonoperative treatment.[14] The essential lesion in chronic lateral is patellofemoral instability insufficiency of the MPFL.[19] The ideal indications for an isolated MPFL reconstruction in a child or adolescent would be a recurrent lateral patellar dislocation without valgus malalignment, patella alta, or trochlear dysplasia.

OPERATIVE: AUTHORS' PREFERRED TREATMENT

For the adolescent athlete with recurrent patellar dislocations, we prefer an anatomic MPFL reconstruction using the medial quadriceps tendon. This technique avoids injury to the

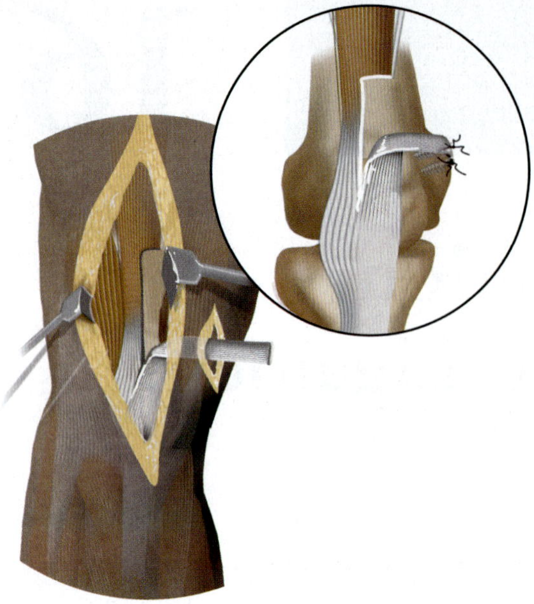

Figure 16.1. Illustration of quadriceps tendon graft passed medially to femoral epicondyle.

growth plates and is particularly applicable to the skeletally immature pediatric and adolescent athlete. This technique is a combination of previously described techniques by Noyes and Albright,[20] Steenson et al.,[32] and Goyal.[12] An 8- × 70-mm full-thickness strip of medial quadriceps tendon is used to reconstruct the MPFL. The quadriceps graft is left attached to the superomedial border of the patella. The free end of the graft is passed between the synovium and the retinaculum and is sutured to the medial intermuscular septum adjacent to the medial femoral epicondyle (Figs. 16.1 and 16.2). Femoral fixation is augmented with a small absorbable suture anchor placed via C-arm direction to ensure accurate placement of the graft. The remaining medial retinaculum is imbricated when the quadriceps tendon harvest site is closed. This technique avoids large patella and femoral drill holes and minimizes the risk of patellar fracture or injury to the distal femoral physis.

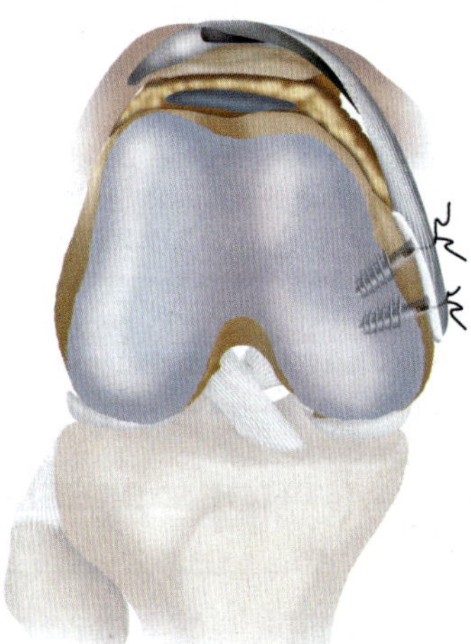

Figure 16.2. Illustration of graft with suture anchor attached to femur.

The graft is tensioned at 30 to 45 degrees of knee flexion. A lateral release is added if tightness of the lateral retinaculum prevents normal medial patellar translation or in cases of abnormal patellar tilting.

The goal of MPFL reconstruction is to replace the torn ligament with a graft that is stronger than the native MPFL and with a tension similar to the native ligament. Normal patellar motion allows about two patella quadrants of lateral translation.[2] Graft tensioning should be performed with the knee in about 30 to 45 degrees of flexion.[11,16] In addition, we use the C-arm to help locate the femoral attachment site. Schöttle et al.[27] and Redfern et al.[23] have described radiographic landmarks to locate the anatomic femoral position of the MPFL. The femoral attachment site is very important for achieving a good outcome.[25] For example, in cadaver studies, Steensen et al.[31] and Stephen et al.[33] demonstrated that the position of the MPFL graft femoral attachment substantially influenced the graft length change pattern. The patellar attachment site, on the other hand, had little effect. The most common error in graft placement is to fix the graft too far anteriorly on the femur which may lead to graft laxity in extension and graft tension in flexion. This graft malposition can lead to overloading of the medial patellofemoral cartilage, anterior knee pain, and loss of flexion.[4,8,35] In addition, Camp et al.[6] reported that a nonanatomic MPFL femoral attachment site can result in a high rate of recurrent patellar dislocation following MPFL reconstruction. An overtightened graft combined with a lateral release can result in iatrogenic medial patellar subluxation in flexion.[4] After graft fixation, knee motion should be equal to the opposite knee and there should be a good end point to lateral patellar translation from 0 to 30 degrees of knee flexion.

OUR SURGICAL TECHNIQUE IS AS FOLLOWS

Preoperative Planning

The operation should be performed with the patient under general anesthesia and in the supine position. A radiolucent operating room (OR) table (Fig. 16.3), such as the OSI flat top (Mizuho OSI, Union City, CA), is used with the C-arm positioned on the opposite side of the injured extremity. A thorough examination under anesthesia is performed to confirm incompetence of the MPFL. Lateral translation of the patella is assessed with the knee at 0 and 30 degrees of knee flexion (Fig. 16.4). Greater than 50% lateral translation of the patella

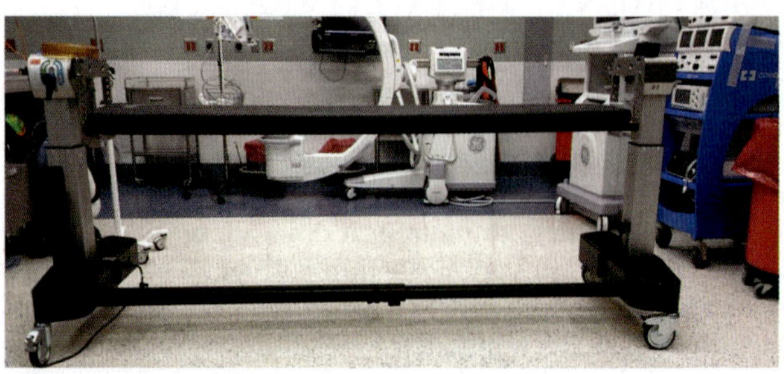

Figure 16.3. OSI flat-top table is used for the procedure.

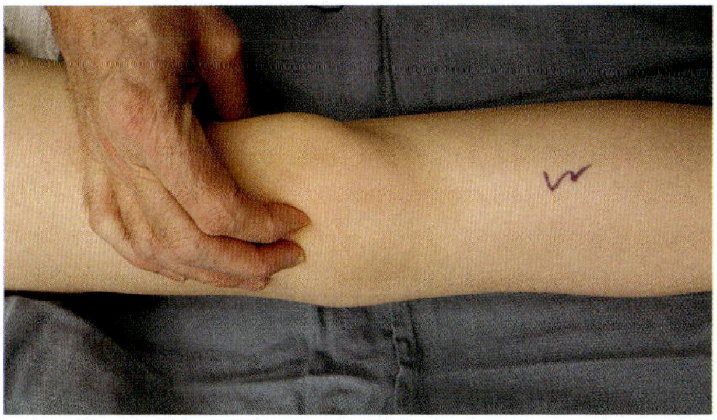

Figure 16.4. Lateral translation on the patella reveals greater than 50% translation.

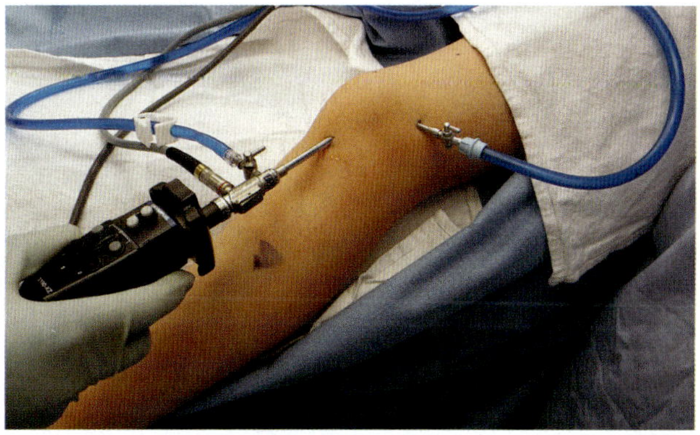

Figure 16.6. Standard diagnostic arthroscopy is performed to determine any concomitant injury and grade any cartilage damage.

is diagnostic of MPFL rupture; in the illustrated case, the patella could be completely dislocated (Fig. 16.5). Assessment of a tight lateral retinaculum is also assessed to determine the need for a lateral release.

Surgical Approach

The patient is prepped and draped in the usual sterile fashion. Perioperative antibiotics are administered. A preoperative time-out is performed. A nonsterile tourniquet is placed on the proximal thigh and inflated during the procedure. Standard diagnostic knee arthroscopy is performed, documenting any associated injuries and concomitant articular cartilage damage is graded (Fig. 16.6). Medial and lateral translation of the patella is again assessed under arthroscopy (Fig. 16.7). If it is determined, a lateral release is needed; this is performed with use of a radiofrequency ablation wand. This is performed from the 10 o'clock position (right knee), or 2 o'clock position (left knee), and extended distally until release deemed adequate. Once the arthroscopic evaluation is complete, the equipment is removed from the knee joint and the open MPFL reconstruction is performed.

Technique

A longitudinal incision is made from the superior pole of the medial patella extending 5 to 6 cm proximally (Fig. 16.8). Full-thickness flaps are developed and dissected down to the quadriceps tendon and its insertion on the patella. An Army-Navy retractor is used to retract the soft tissue, and the insertion of the VMO on the quadriceps tendon is identified (Fig. 16.9). Next, an 8- × 70-mm full-thickness graft is harvested, leaving the patellar insertion intact (Fig. 16.10). The proximal free end of the graft is sutured with a whipstitch using no. 2 Ethibond (Ethicon, Johnson & Johnson, Menlo Park, CA) suture to prepare for passage of the graft.

The knee is then flexed to about 40 degrees over a radiolucent triangle (Fig. 16.11). A 2-cm incision is made over the medial femoral epicondyle based on fluoroscopy and palpation. Fluoroscopic imaging is used to identify the MPFL insertion just distal to the femoral physis and just proximal to the posterior aspect of the femur (Fig. 16.12). Dissection is performed down to bone. A soft tissue tunnel is made using a large hemostat between the medial retinaculum and the synovium. The graft is then rotated 90 degrees medially and passed distally through the medial incision (Fig. 16.13). Next, a 2.5-mm bioabsorbable suture anchor with 3-0 FiberWire suture on a needle (Arthrex, Naples, FL) is placed at the femoral insertion (Fig. 16.14). A pilot stitch is placed to hold the tendon graft in place while the tension and patellar tracking are checked with gentle range

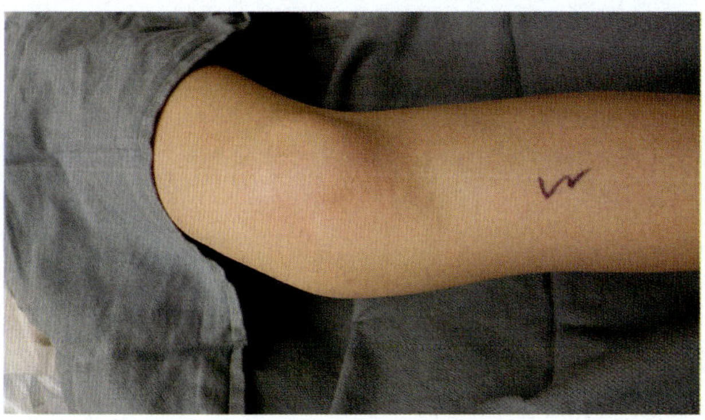

Figure 16.5. Illustrative case demonstrating complete dislocation of patella.

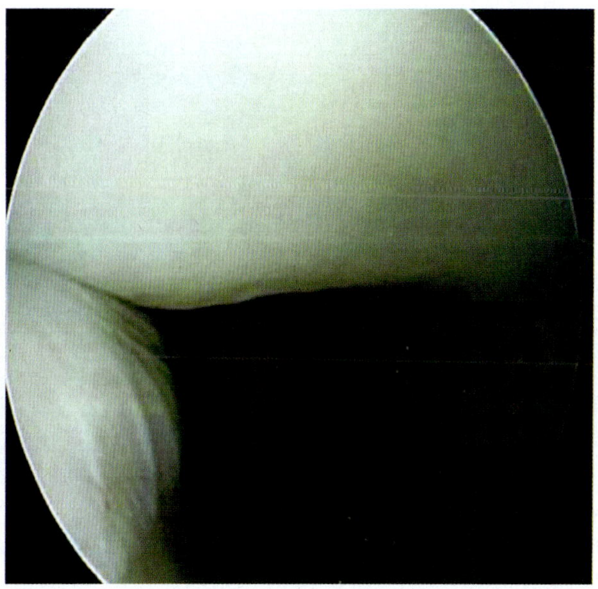

Figure 16.7. Arthroscopic image of laterally translated patella.

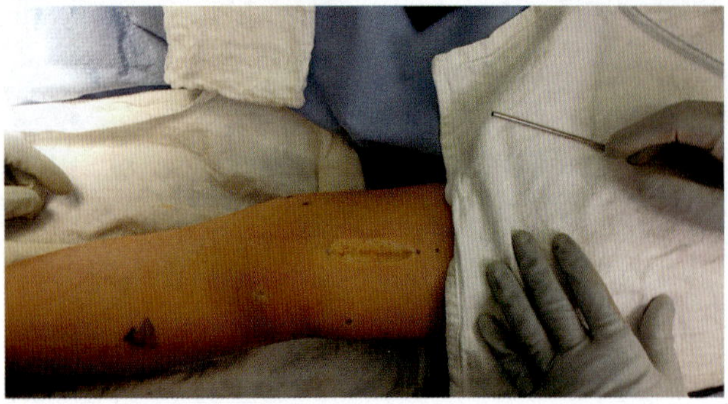

Figure 16.8. A 5- to 6-cm longitudinal incision is made from the superior pole of the medial patella extending proximally.

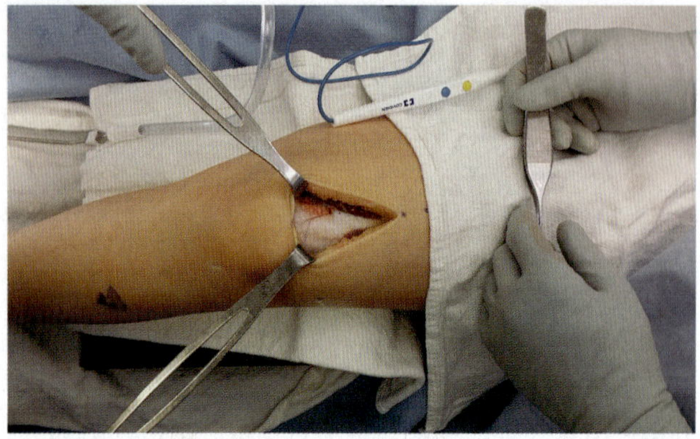

Figure 16.9. VMO insertion on patella is clearly identified prior to graft harvest.

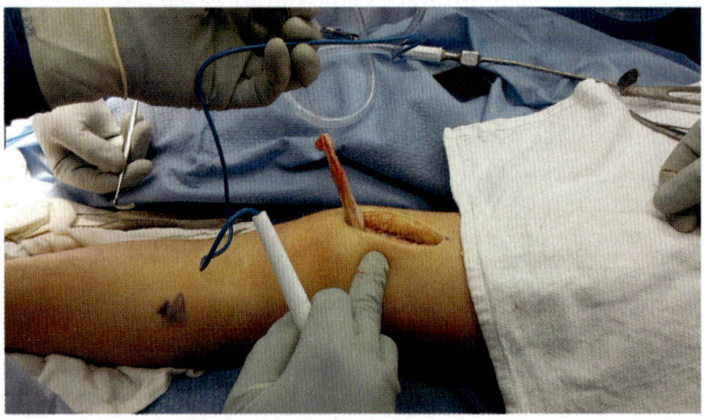

Figure 16.10. Quadriceps tendon harvest.

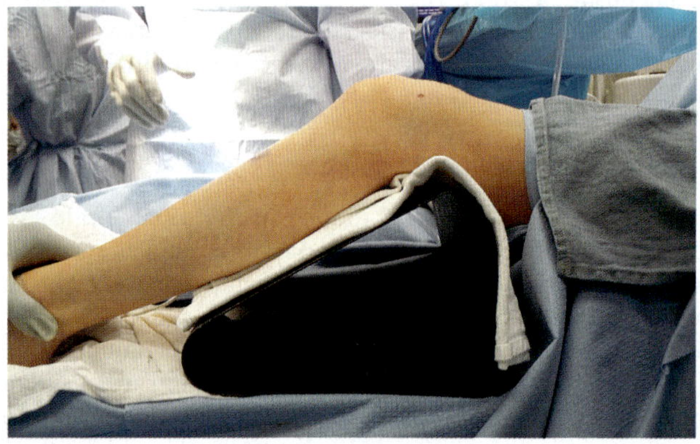

Figure 16.11. Knee held in 40 degrees of flexion with radiolucent triangle.

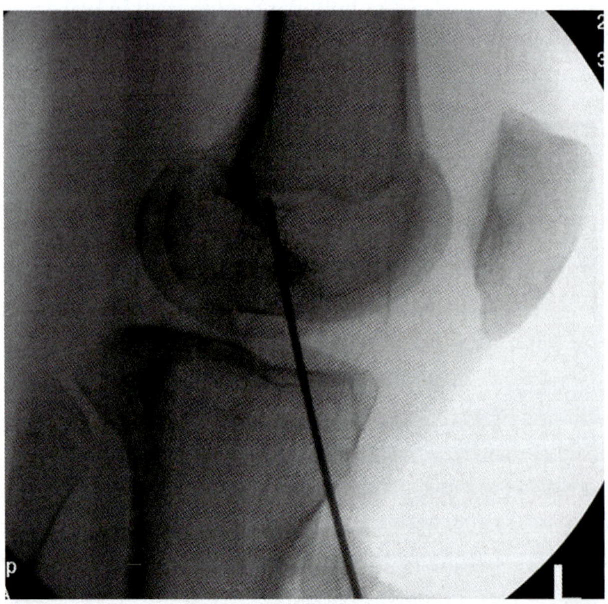

Figure 16.12. Lateral radiograph with proper femoral tunnel placement, just anterior to the posterior femoral cortex and just distal to the physis.

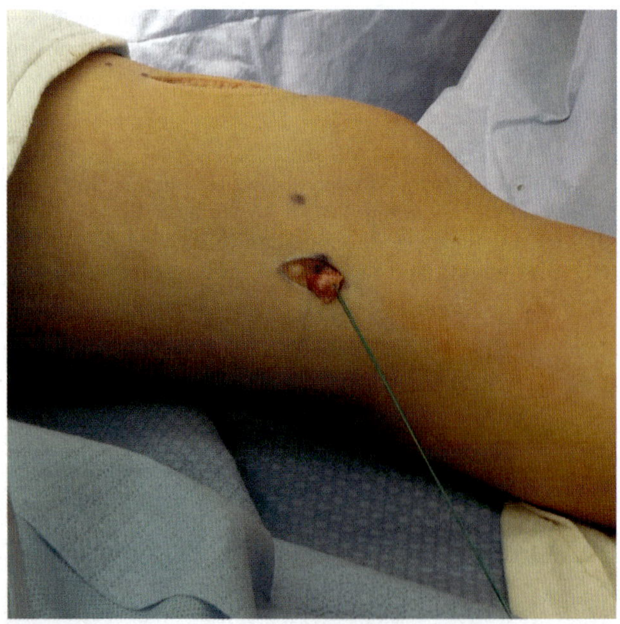

Figure 16.13. Quadriceps tendon graft pulled through the medial incision.

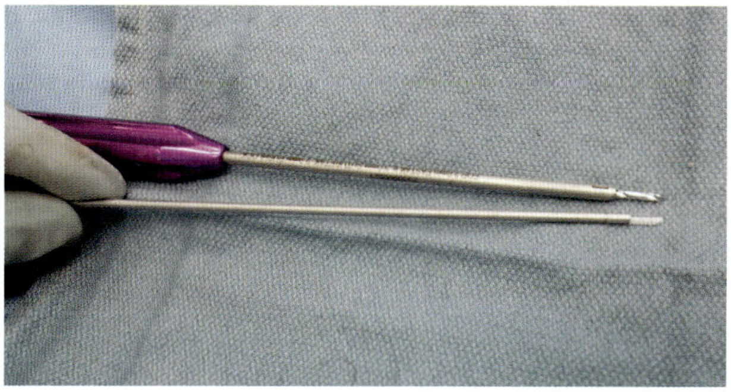

Figure 16.14. Arthrex 2.5-mm suture anchor drill with anchor.

of motion. Be sure that the patella can still be manually moved laterally about 10 mm to prevent overtensioning. The goal is to maintain the patellar tracking centrally in the trochlea without any sign of medial subluxation. The quadriceps tendon graft is then sutured in place to the medial femoral epicondyle using the FiberWire from the suture anchor, below the growth plate (Fig. 16.15). Reinforcement of the fixation is made with no. 2 Ethibond suture to the medial intermuscular septum. In addition, imbricate and attach the quadriceps tendon and medial retinaculum to the patella with no. 2 Ethibond sutures. This is done in conjunction with medial reefing of the patella to the graft with no. 2 Ethibond suture.

The knee is then placed through range of motion and patellar tracking is assessed. The wounds are then irrigated, and the knee joint is injected with 0.25% Marcaine for postoperative pain relief. The quadriceps tendon graft site is closed with interrupted absorbable Vicryl sutures. Subcutaneous tissues are also closed with Vicryl, and the skin is then closed with a Monocryl subcuticular suture (Fig. 16.16).

The patient is placed in a knee immobilizer in extension postoperatively (Fig. 16.17). Partial weight bearing of the extremity is allowed as tolerated in the immobilizer (Table 16.1).

List of Equipment Used

See Table 16.2.

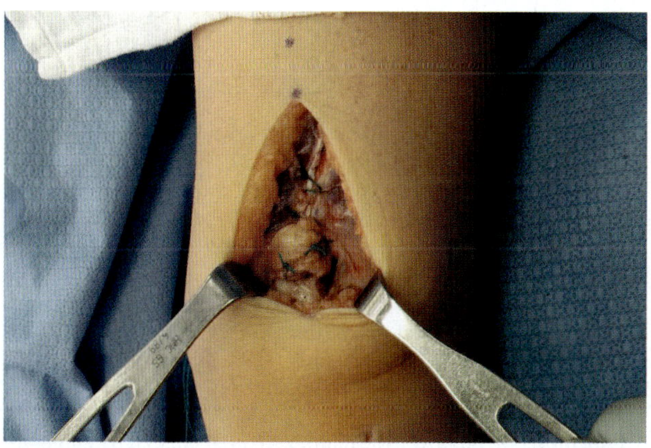

Figure 16.15. Quad tendon graft sutured into place with suture anchor.

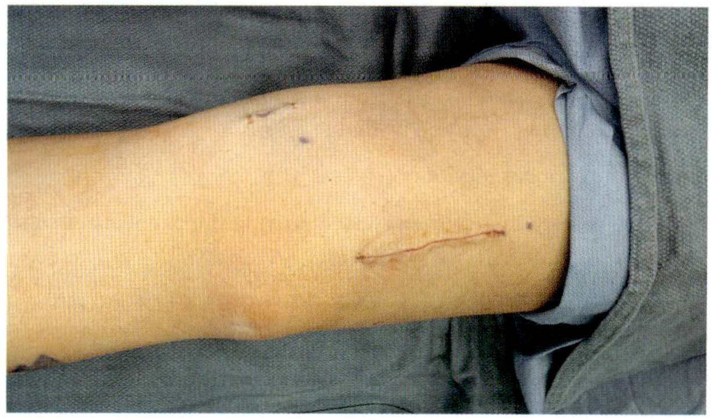

Figure 16.16. Final closure of wounds.

Rehabilitation

The goal of rehabilitation is to protect the MPFL reconstruction while knee motion and strength are regained. A knee immobilizer brace is used for 4 weeks and gradually weaned to allow for gradual increase in motion during this time. Ice packs and ice massage after surgery are helpful. Partial weight bearing is allowed immediately postoperatively and is progressed to full weight bearing over 1 week. Initial quadriceps isometric exercises are supplemented with patella mobility exercises and straight-leg raises. At 1 week, the brace is removed three times per day to work on knee range of motion. At 4 weeks, the brace is discontinued and full knee motion is allowed as tolerated. Closed kinetic exercises such as half squats and stationary biking are then added. Most patients can be expected to jog by 3 to 4 months and return to full sports activity by 5 to 6 months.

Pearls to Avoid Complications

The complication rate for MPFL reconstruction is high at up to 26%.[21,29] Complications following treatment of patellofemoral instability in adolescents include recurrent instability, patellofemoral pain, osteoarthritis, knee stiffness, wound infection, patellar fracture, medial instability, neuroma, and growth plate injury. Proper patient selection and attention to technical details are key to good outcomes.

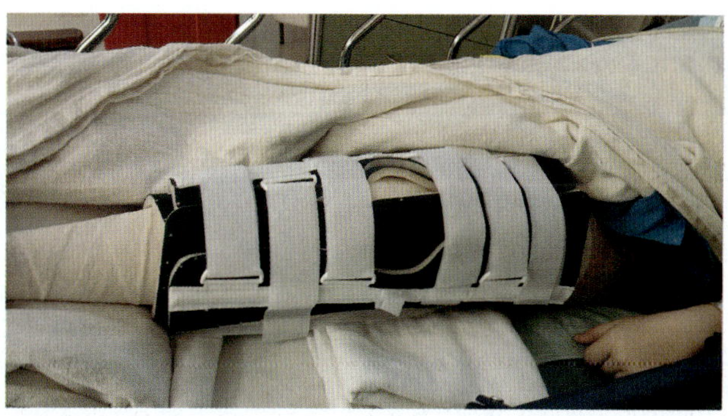

Figure 16.17. Postoperative knee immobilizer with knee in extension.

TABLE 16.1	Surgical Steps
Longitudinal incision is made from the superior pole of the medial patella extending 5–6 cm proximally.	
Identify quadriceps tendon.	
Quadriceps tendon graft is harvested, leaving the patellar insertion intact.	
Medial incision over medial epicondyle, create tunnel, and pass graft.	
Identify MPFL femoral insertion using lateral fluoroscopy.	
Place suture anchor in femoral insertion and suture graft to anchor.	
Perform medial reefing; imbricate and attach the quadriceps tendon and medial retinaculum to the patella.	
Assess patellar tracking through range of motion.	
Closure of wounds and skin	

Pearls

- Careful preoperative clinical evaluation, including Q angle, tibial torsion, femoral torsion, ligamentous laxity, gait, range of knee motion
- Complete radiographic and magnetic resonance imaging (MRI) evaluation of the knee, including evaluation of skeletal maturity
- Avoid malposition of the femoral attachment site—use the C-arm to confirm this location when making the medial skin incision and when placing the suture anchor.
- A 6-cm incision started at the medial border of the patella
- Harvest a medial quadriceps graft of sufficient length of 8 × 70 mm.
- Leave 2 mm of quadriceps tendon with the VMO for later closure.
- Dissect quadriceps graft subperiosteally down the patella, about 1 cm, with care not to amputate the graft.
- After this turndown of the quadriceps graft, reinforce this subperiosteal dissection site with additional no. 2 Ethibond stay sutures. Place a whipstitch using no. 2 Ethibond at the free proximal end of the graft.
- Dissect a wide path between the retinaculum and the synovium down to the medial epicondyle.
- Make a 2-cm incision centered on the medial epicondyle. Puncture the medial retinaculum with a large snap, anterior to the medial intermuscular septum adjacent to the medial epicondyle. Pass the graft using the whipstitch and a snap from the 6-cm anterior incision to the 2-cm medial incision.
- Imbricate and attach the quadriceps tendon and medial retinaculum to the patella with no. 2 Ethibond sutures.
- Avoid inadequate tensioning or overtensioning of the graft. Set the tension of the MPFL reconstruction with the patella reduced and the knee placed at about 30 to 45 degrees of flexion.
- Place a 3-mm absorbable suture anchor using C-arm imaging just distal to the physis and anterior to the posterior femoral cortex.
- Place a pilot stitch to hold the tendon graft, and check tensioning and patellar tracking by gently flexing and extending the knee. Be sure that the patella can still be manually moved laterally about 10 mm to prevent overtensioning. The goal is to maintain the patellar tracking centrally in the trochlea without any sign of medial subluxation.
- Secure the graft to the suture anchor sutures. Add additional no. 2 Ethibond sutures to repair the graft to the intermuscular septum and surrounding retinaculum.
- Selectively perform a judicious lateral release in cases of residual abnormal patellar tilt. Avoid overrelease.
- Selectively combine MPFL reconstruction with additional procedures to address other risk factors such as an abnormal Q angle, increased TT-TG distance, or patella alta.

TABLE 16.2	Preoperative Planning
OR table: OSI flat top	
Position/positioning aids: supine; radiolucent triangle under knee	
Fluoroscopy location: opposite the side of the injured extremity	
Equipment: basic arthroscopy set, basic orthopedic set, K-wires, 2.5-mm bioabsorbable suture anchor with 3-mm FiberWire suture, no. 2 Ethibond sutures	
Tourniquet: nonsterile	
Etc.: knee immobilizer for postoperative care	

Pitfalls

- Overtensioning the graft
- Failure to recognize and address underlying malalignment
- Excessive lateral release

SUMMARY

Acute patellofemoral dislocation is the most common knee disorder in children and adolescents. In the setting of recurrent instability that has failed conservative treatment, surgical reconstruction is recommended. MPFL reconstruction using the quadriceps tendon is a prudent alternative for chronic patellofemoral instability in the skeletally immature athlete. The technique is simple, safe, and avoids drill holes in the patella and femur and therefore minimizes the risk of patellar fracture of physeal injury.

REFERENCES

1. Andrish J. The management of recurrent patellar dislocation. *Orthop Clin North Am.* 2008;39(3):313–327.
2. Arendt EA. Medial side patellofemoral anatomy. Surgical implications in patellofemoral instability. In: Zaffagninn S, Dejour D, Arendt EA, eds. *Patellofemoral Pain, Instability, and Arthritis.* Berlin, Germany: Springer; 2010:149–152.
3. Bicos J, Fulkerson JP, Amis A. Current concepts review: the medial patellofemoral ligament. *Am J Sports Med.* 2007;35(3):484–492.
4. Bollier M, Fulkerson J, Cosgarea A, et al. Technical failure of medial patellofemoral ligament reconstruction. *Arthroscopy.* 2011;27(8): 1153–1159.
5. Camanho GL, Bitar AC, Hernandez AJ, et al. Medial patellofemoral ligament reconstruction: a novel technique using the patellar ligament. *Arthroscopy.* 2007;23(1):e1–e108.

6. Camp CL, Krych AJ, Dahm DL, et al. Medial patellofemoral ligament repair for recurrent patellar dislocation. *Am J Sports Med.* 2010;38(11):2248–2254.
7. Dejour H, Walch G, Nove-Josserand L, et al. Factors of patellar instability: an anatomic radiographic study. *Knee Surg Sports Traumatol Arthrosc.* 1994;2(1):19–26.
8. Elias JJ, Cosgarea AJ. Technical errors during medial patellofemoral ligament reconstruction could overload medial patellofemoral cartilage: a computational analysis. *Am J Sports Med.* 2006;34(9): 1478–1485.
9. Erasmus PJ. The medial patellofemoral ligament: function, injury, and treatment [in German]. *Orthopade.* 2008;37(9):858, 860–863.
10. Farahmand F, Tahmasbi MN, Amis AA. Lateral force displacement behavior of the human patella and its variation with knee flexion—a biomechanical study in vitro. *J Biomech.* 1998;31(12):1147–1152.
11. Farr J, Schepsis AA. Reconstruction of eh medial patellofemoral ligament for recurrent patellar instability. *J Knee Surg.* 2006;19(4): 307–316.
12. Goyal D. Medial patellofemoral ligament reconstruction: the superficial quad technique. *Am J Sports Med.* 2013;41:1022–1029.
13. Heegaard J, Leyvraz PF, Van Kampen A, et al. Influence of soft structures on patellar three-dimensional tracking. *Clin Orthop Relat Res.* 1994;(299):235–243.
14. Hennrikus W, Pylawka T. Patellofemoral instability in skeletally immature athletes. *J Bone Joint Surg.* 2013;95(2):176–183.
15. Kepler CK, Bogner EA, Hammound S, et al. Zone of injury of the medial patellofemoral ligament after acute patellar dislocation in children and adolescents. *Am J Sports Med.* 2011;39(7): 1444–1449.
16. LeGrand AB, Greis PE, Dobbs RE, et al. MPFL reconstruction. *Sports Med Arthrosc.* 2007;15(2):72–77.
17. Nelitz M, Dornacher D, Dreyhaupt J, et al. The relation of the distal femoral physis and the medial patellofemoral ligament. *Knee Surg Sports Traumatol Arthrosc.* 2011;19(12):2067–2071.
18. Nelitz M, Dreyhaupt J, Lippacher S. Combined trochleoplasty and medial patellofemoral ligament reconstruction for recurrent patellar dislocations in severe trochlear dysplasia. *Am J Sports Med.* 2013;41(5):1005–1012.
19. Nomura E. Classification of lesions of the medial patella-femoral ligament in patellar dislocation. *Int Orthop.* 1999;23(5):260–263.
20. Noyes FR, Albright JC. Reconstruction of the medial patellofemoral ligament with autologous quadriceps tendon. *Arthroscopy.* 2006;22:904.e1–e7.
21. Parikh SN, Nathan ST, Wall EJ, et al. Complications of medial patellofemoral ligament reconstruction in young patients. *Am J Sports Med.* 2013;41(5):1030–1038.
22. Philippot R, Chouteau J, Wegrzyn J, et al. Medial patellofemoral ligament anatomy: implications for its surgical reconstruction. *Knee Surg Sports Traumatol Arthrosc.* 2009;(5):495–479.
23. Redfern J, Kamath G, Burks R. Anatomical confirmation of the use of radiographic landmarks in medial patellofemoral ligament reconstruction. *Am J Sports Med.* 2010;38(2):293–297.
24. Sallay PI, Poggi J, Speer KG, et al. Acute dislocation of the patella. A correlative pathoanatomic study. *Am J Sports Med.* 1996; 24:52–60.
25. Sanchis-Alfonso V. Guidelines for medial patellofemoral ligament reconstruction in chronic lateral patellar instability. *J Am Acad Orthop Surg.* 2014;22:175–182.
26. Sanders TG, Morrison WB, Singleton BA, et al. Medial patellofemoral ligament injury following acute transient dislocations of the patella: MR findings with surgical correlation in 14 patients. *J Comput Assist Tomogr.* 2001;25:957–962.
27. Schöttle PB, Schmeling A, Rosenstiel N, et al. Radiographic landmarks for femoral tunnel placement in medial patellofemoral ligament reconstruction. *Am J Sports Med.* 2007;35(5):801–804.
28. Scuderi GR. Surgical treatment for patellar instability. *Orthop Clin North Am.* 1992;23(4):619–630.
29. Shah JN, Howard JS, Flannigan DC, et al. A systematic review of complications and failures associated with medial patellofemoral ligament reconstruction for recurrent patellar dislocations. *Am J Sports Med.* 2012;40(8):1916–1923.
30. Sillanpää PJ, Mäenpää H, Mattila VM, et al. A mini-invasive adductor magnus tendon transfer technique for medial patellofemoral ligament reconstruction: a technical note. *Knee Sports Traumatol Arthrosc.* 2009;17(5):508–512.
31. Steensen RN, Dopirak RM, McDonald WG III. The anatomy and isometry of the medial patellofemoral ligament: implications for reconstruction. *Am J Sports Med.* 2004;32:1509–1513.
32. Steenson RN, Dopirak RM, Maurus PB. A simple technique for reconstruction of the medial patellofemoral ligament using a quadriceps tendon graft. *Arthroscopy.* 2005;21:365–370.
33. Stephen JM, Lumpaopong P, Deehan DJ, et al. The medial patellofemoral ligament: location of femoral attachment and length change patterns resulting from anatomic and non-anatomic attachments. *Am J Sports Med.* 2012;40(8):1871–1879.
34. Tateishi T, Tsuchiya M, Motosugi N, et al. Graft length change and radiographic assessment of femoral drill hole position for medial patellofemoral ligament reconstruction. *Knee Surg Sports Traumatol Arthrosc.* 2011;19(3):400–407.
35. Thaunat M, Erasmus PJ. Management of over tight medial patellofemoral ligament reconstruction. *Knee Surg Sports Traumatol Arthrosc.* 2009;17(5):480–483.

CHAPTER

17

Elizabeth B. Gausden
Daniel W. Green

Medial Patellofemoral Ligament Reconstruction: Hamstring Technique

INTRODUCTION

Patellofemoral instability (PFI) is a complex disorder that most commonly occurs in children and adolescents. Patellar dislocation can result from isolated trauma, but in some cases, anatomic abnormalities, including patella alta, trochlear dysplasia, or laxity of the soft tissue restraints of the knees, predispose certain patients to more frequent patellofemoral dislocation. We typically categorize pediatric patellar dislocation into four types, which include traumatic dislocation, fixed patellar dislocation, obligatory patellar dislocation, and syndromic types such as cases associated with Ehlers-Danlos syndrome and Marfan syndrome. This review focuses on traumatic dislocation.

Incidence of patellar dislocation is reported to be 43 in 100,000 individuals.[19] The peak age of dislocation is 15 years, and females tend to dislocate more than males. The rate of recurrent instability and/or recurrent dislocation has been widely studied, but the reported rates vary widely from 14% to 71%[20–25] (Table 17.1).

Risk factors such as family history and younger age at first dislocation have been associated with recurrent instability. As expected, abnormal anatomy including patellofemoral malalignment as measured by increased Q angle, trochlear dysplasia, and abnormal patellar configuration are also associated with recurrent dislocations or instability.[20,21,24]

The patellofemoral joint is stabilized against lateral instability by both osseous and soft tissue structures. In patients with normal trochlea anatomy, the patella enters the osseous confines of the trochlea at 30 degrees of knee flexion which provides static stability, whereas in extension, the medial patellofemoral ligament (MPFL) is the most important stabilizer of the patellofemoral joint. As opposed to the cruciate ligaments, the MPFL has relatively low tension throughout flexion and extension, between 2 N and 10 N.[1] Furthermore, the MPFL remains isometric throughout flexion from 0 to 110 degrees and then becomes slack past 110 degrees of flexion.[2] This biomechanical data suggests that the MPFL acts as a "checkrein" for the patella in that it is a main stabilizer against lateral patellar dislocation when an outside force is exerted on the knee in extension. When put to the test in this action of forced lateral subluxation, the native MPFL can withstand a tension of approximately 200 N.[3] Studies have shown that when the patella dislocates from trauma, the MPFL is torn in approximately 90% of patients.[4] The zone of injury of the MPFL tear, whether it tears off of the patella or its femoral insertion, has been the topic of a number of radiographic studies.[4–10] The studies isolated to adolescent patients[5–7] have found that the MPFL more commonly is torn near its patellar insertion. In a study of 43 children with acute patellar dislocation, as confirmed by magnetic resonance imaging (MRI), 61% had tears isolated to the patellar insertion.[7]

The MPFL lies in the second layer of the knee as described by Warren and Marshall.[11] The patellar attachment is a fan-like attachment at the junction between the proximal and middle thirds of the superomedial border of the patella.[12] A recent anatomic study investigated the patellar insertion of the MPFL in eight cadavers and found the proximal fibers of the MPFL were mainly attached to the vastus intermedius tendon, whereas its distal fibers were inserted partially on the medial retinaculum.[13] The authors proposed that this anatomic relationship allows the MPFL to pull both the patella and the patellar tendon, albeit indirectly, medially to keep the patella engaged in the trochlea throughout flexion and extension. The femoral attachment of the MPFL is bounded by the adductor tubercle proximally and the femoral attachment of the medial collateral ligament (MCL) distally.[12] In the anterior to posterior dimension, it lies approximately 1.3 mm anterior to a line drawn along the posterior cortex of the femoral diaphysis.[14]

Surgically addressing the MPFL has become a mainstay of treating PFI given both the biomechanical importance of the MPFL as a restraint to lateral dislocation as well as the high frequency of MPFL injury following traumatic patellar dislocation. Similar to the experience with anterior cruciate ligament repair, repairing the remaining ends of a torn MPFL has not been a successful surgical option.[15,16] Dozens of different techniques of MPFL reconstruction have been reported in the literature, and there is still no consensus supporting one technique over another.[17] Although MPFL reconstruction in the skeletally mature patient is well described in the literature, there are fewer studies that focus on patients with open growth plates.[17,18]

INDICATIONS

A recent patellar dislocation can be confirmed with MRI. Transchondral fracture and bone marrow edema pattern,

TABLE 17.1 Major Studies Reporting Natural History following Primary Patellar Dislocation

Study	*N*	*Percent with Recurrent Dislocation*	*Included Adults*	*Risk Factors*
Cofield and Bryan[20] (1977)	48	44%	Yes	Did not assess risk factors; 13 patients later underwent surgical treatment
Hawkins et al.[21] (1986)	27	71%	No	Patellofemoral malalignment, abnormal patellar configuration
Palmu et al.[22] (2008)[a]	28	44%	Yes	Positive family history of redislocation
Sillanpää et al.[25] (2008)[a]	21	48%	Yes	No associated risk factors identified
Lewallen et al.[24] (2013)	198	38.4%	No	Trochlear dysplasia, immature physes

[a]These studies were done as trials, and the data presented in this table is from the nonoperative treatment arm of the study.

increased signal intensity in the lateral femoral condyle on fluid-sensitive imaging, and short T1 inversion recovery (STIR) sequencing are indicative of an acute dislocation.[7] In addition, cartilage-sensitive magnetic resonance (MR) sequencing is useful in identifying an MPFL tear as well as the zone of injury of such a tear. Finally, MRI also can identify an osteochondral lesion or a loose body that needs to be addressed surgically. Guerrero et al.[26] found that 49% of patellar dislocations were associated with an osteochondral lesion and 13% incurred a loose body in the joint.

First-time dislocators are treated with a trial of nonoperative management that includes quadriceps and core strengthening. If this treatment fails and the patient experiences recurrent instability or recurrent episodes of patellar dislocation, then MPFL reconstruction is recommended. Patients with additional risk factors, younger age or family history, as well as those with osteochondral lesions or loose bodies for surgery may be indicated for surgery after their first dislocation event.

Generally, distal realignment procedures are reserved for skeletally mature patients with pathologic patellofemoral anatomy that predisposes to PFI, such as patients with large Q angle (>20 degrees), large J signs, or increase tibial tubercle–trochlear groove distances (TT-TG). A TT-TG distance of over 20 mm is typically used to indicate adults for a tibial tubercle osteotomy (TTO) or other distal realignment procedure. However, recently published literature reported that TT-TG in children increases with age, and an increase in TT-TG should be expected as a child matures.[27]

If a patient has underlying anatomic pathology, it is important to address this surgically in addition to MPFL reconstruction to achieve a good outcome. For instance, in cases of fixed or obligatory dislocation, part of the etiology is a tight quadriceps mechanism. This must be addressed surgically with a quadriceps release in order to prevent recurrence.

TECHNIQUES DESCRIBED IN LITERATURE

Although over 100 different techniques for reconstructing the MPFL have been described, this section focuses on the six common types of MPFL reconstruction. One such technique, the diversion of a portion of the quadriceps tendon, has been described in the previous chapter. Hemiquad tendon transfer was first described by Steensen et al.[28] They harvested the medial and anterior one-third of the quadriceps tendon and redirect this detached tendon to the femur, securing it there with a tenodesis screw (Fig. 17.1A). Similar to the quadriceps diversion technique, various other pedicled graft techniques have been described in the literature. Steiner et al.[29] describe isolating the distal adductor group and redirecting it to the patella to reconstruct the MPFL. Furthermore, surgeons can also redirect a portion of the patellar tendon from the tibial tubercle to medial femoral condyle to recreate the path of the MPFL (Fig. 17.1B).

A free hamstring graft can also be used to reconstruct the MPFL, and there are a variety of methods to secure the graft currently used in practice. Although some surgeons prefer to use either the MCL of the knee or the adductor group as a pulley or site of fixation,[30,31] many prefer to create sockets or tunnels within the medial femoral condyle and patella to secure the free graft[32,33] (Fig. 17.1C,D). Hamstring autograft using the MCL as a pulley was described by Deie et al.[31] The authors detach the semitendinosus proximally and leave the distal insertion intact, then use a slit in the MCL as a pulley, finally attaching the graft to the patella to recreate the MPFL.[31] Similarly, Gomes[30] described a technique that takes advantage of the adductor's proximity to the native MPFL insertion on the femur and uses this attachment as a pulley for a gracilis or semitendinosus graft (Fig. 17.1E).

AUTHORS' PREFERRED TECHNIQUE

Graft Harvest

The semitendinosus is our preferred autograft choice. In some of the larger patients, the gracilis is of adequate size. In an isolated MPFL reconstruction, when not combined with a TTO, the semitendinosus is harvested from a transverse posteromedial incision, as it is cosmetically preferable to the anteromedial harvest (Fig. 17.2).

Once the tendon is identified, the open tendon harvester is placed around the tendon and sent proximally (Fig. 17.3).

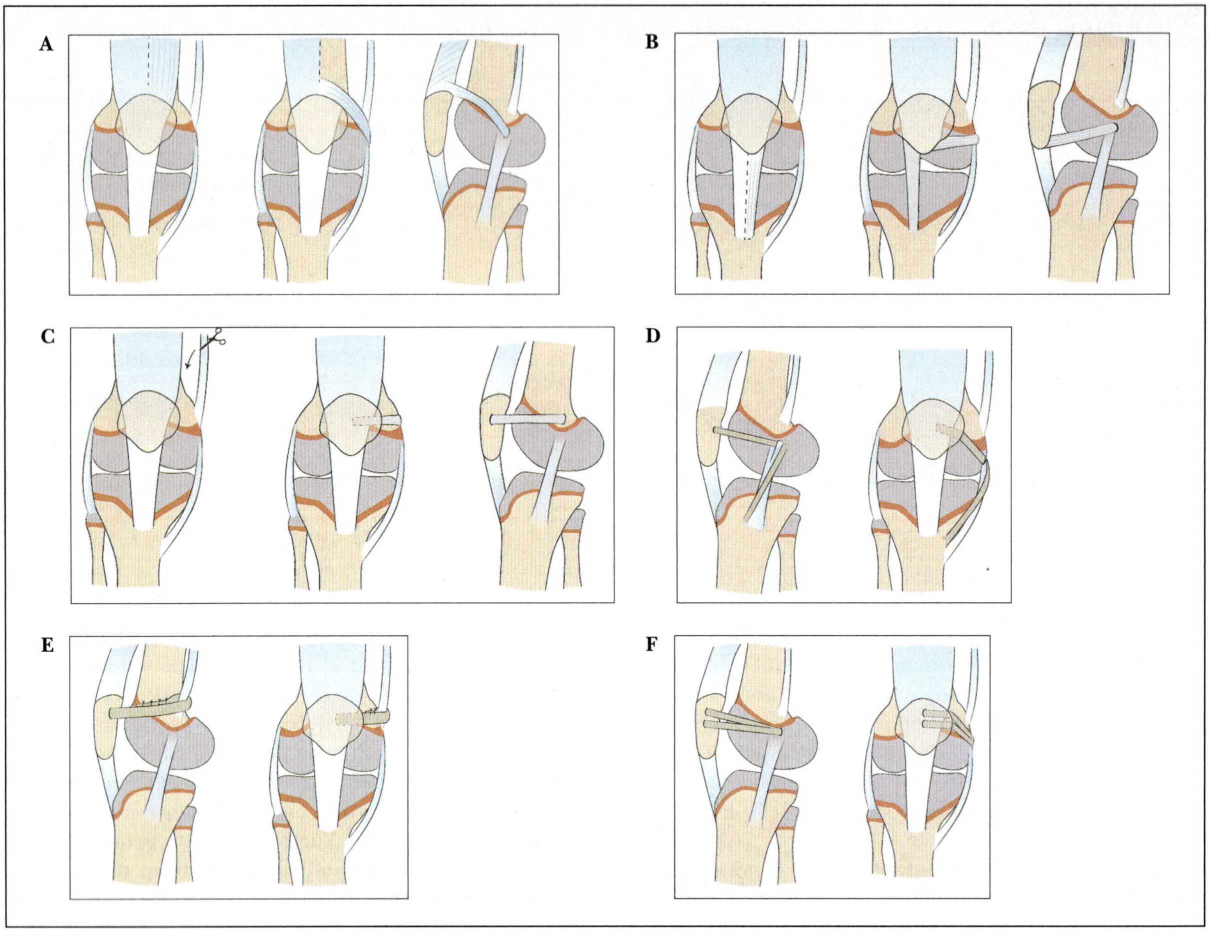

Figure 17.1. Various techniques of MPFL reconstruction. **A.** Hemiquadriceps tendon transfer. **B.** Hemipatellar tendon transfer. **C.** Adductor tendon pedicle graft. **D.** Hamstring graft using MCL as pulley. **E.** Hamstring graft using adductor tendon as a pulley. **F.** Double-bundle hamstring allograft using patellar and femoral sockets. (We would like to acknowledge and thank Cynthia Conklin for her illustration.)

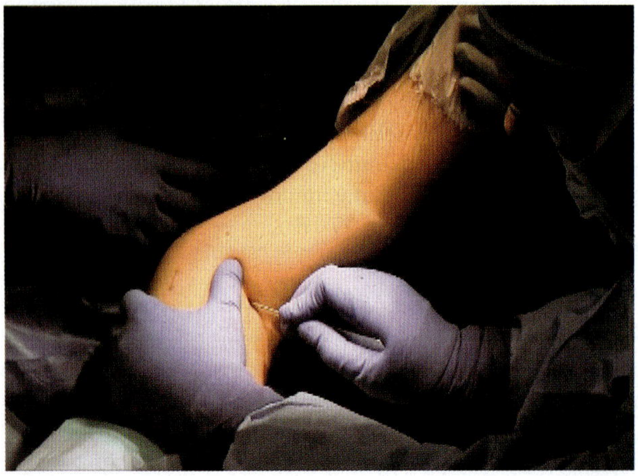

Figure 17.2. Posterior medial incision used to harvest hamstring tendon.

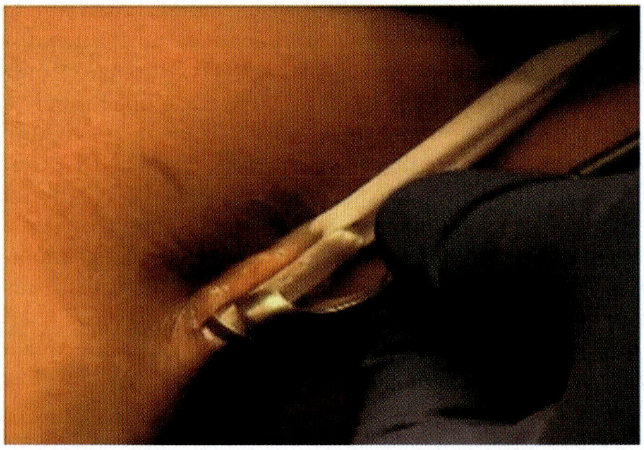

Figure 17.3. Insertion of the open hamstring harvester over the semitendinosus from the posteromedial incision.

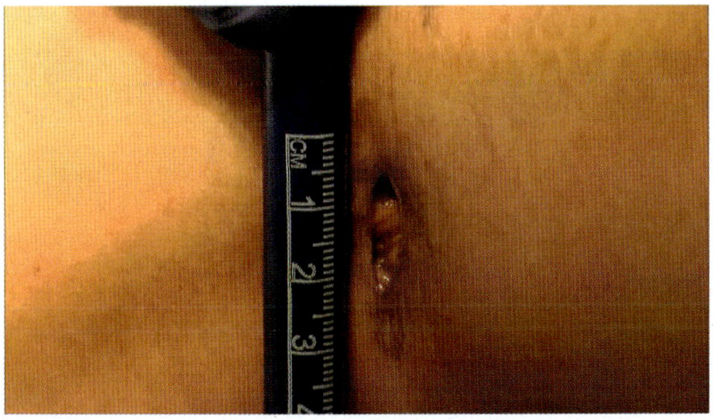

Figure 17.4. Size of posteromedial incision used to harvest hamstring graft.

The tendon is isolated at the musculotendinous junction. Then, a closed tendon harvester is inserted distally, crosses the tibial crest to the tendon's insertion, and then harvested. Approximately 200 mm of tendon length is needed for this technique in most pediatric patients. The final length of this incision is seen in Figure 17.4.

Graft Preparation

The semitendinosus is usually greater than 20 cm in length and therefore adequate for a double-bundle reconstruction. Single-bundle reconstruction is occasionally used in small children.

The graft is prepared such that there is 15 to 20 mm of tendon within each of the sockets. Most patients will have 5 to 6 cm between the femoral and patellar sockets. To meet these requirements, the doubled hamstring graft should measure approximately 90 mm on average, allowing for 15 to 20 mm of graft for placement within the patella and femoral sockets, respectively, and 50 to 60 mm between as the reconstructed MPFL. A modified Krackow stitch is placed along 15 to 20 mm of each limb of the graft to control the two ends (Fig. 17.5).

Femoral Socket

The femoral socket is ideally placed inferior to the adductor tubercle and superior to the origin of the MCL. On an AP radiograph, the socket rests distal to the physis. On the lateral view, the socket should be in line with a line drawn along the posterior cortex of the diaphysis of the femur (Fig. 17.6). A guide wire is inserted into the site and directed distally to the distal femoral physis so that the socket does not traverse the physis. Correct placement of the guide wire is confirmed using anteroposterior (AP) and lateral fluoroscopy. The size of the socket depends on the size of the patient, but generally, a 5.5-mm drill is used to create a socket length of 15 to 20 mm. The doubled end of the graft is inserted into the femoral socket and secured with a 6-0 tenodesis screw.

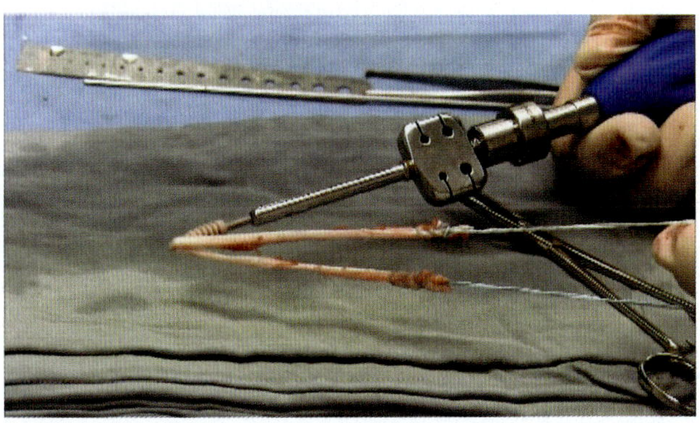

Figure 17.5. Free hamstring graft after preparation with Krackow stitch and load onto tenodesis screw.

Patellar Sockets

Next, attention is turned toward the patella. A 2-cm incision is made over the medial superior border of the patella.

Two short sockets are reamed in the superior half of the patella (Fig. 17.7). Again, the size of the sockets varies by patient size, but in general, a 4 to 5 mm reamer is used to create two sockets about 15 mm deep. It is important to note that at this step, the sockets do not cross the patella.

Securing the Graft

Next, the dissection is carried down to the most superficial layer of the knee and the retinaculum is incised. The retinaculum is tagged at this stage to help identify the correct layer for the graft placement. Then the second and third layers of the knee are separated with Mayo scissors, opening the potential space for the MPFL graft.

Then, two passing stitches are passed through this space. Each passing stitch grabs one of the two limbs of the graft, which is now secured in the medial femoral socket. Once the limbs traverse the native course of the MPFL in the second layer of the knee, they can be accessed from the patellar incision. Attention is then turned to graft sizing.

The graft length is adjusted based on the patellar stability as assessed at 30 degrees of knee flexion. Adjusting the length of the graft to instill an appropriate checkrein for the patella throughout knee range of motion is a crucial step in the procedure. Creating a graft that is too short can cause overloading of the medial facet and even limit knee range of motion.

Once appropriate length is confirmed, the shortened patella limbs of the graft are then typically secured into the patellar sockets with 4.75-mm peek swivel locks. In very young patients with small a patella or hamstring graft, a single socket at the patella is used.

Figure 17.8 demonstrates a patient 1 year following MPFL construction.

REHABILITATION

Postoperatively, the knee is placed in a brace locked in extension. Patients are allowed to weight bear as tolerated, and they generally use crutches until swelling subsides. Early range of motion and strengthening are encouraged, particularly quadriceps strengthening. They spend one night in the hospital, start continuous passive motion and are evaluated by physical therapy in house. They may ambulate without the brace once the quadriceps strength returns to 4/5.

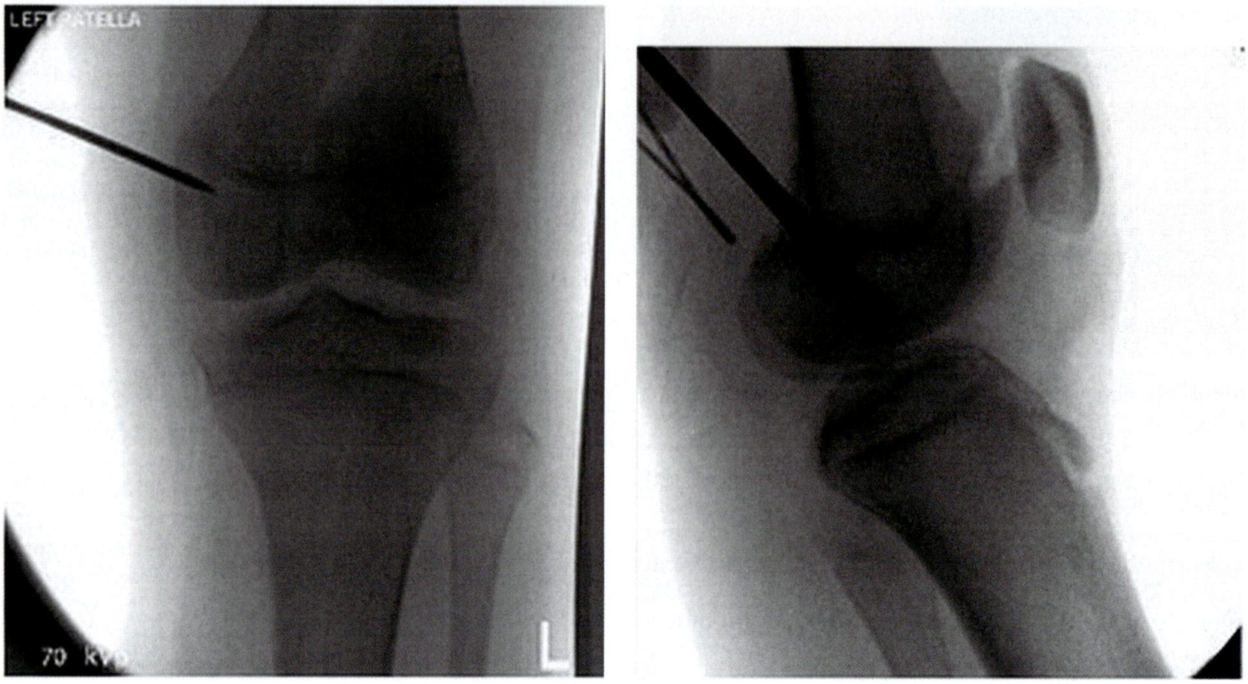

A B

Figure 17.6. **A.** AP plain radiograph is used intraoperatively to identify correct location of femoral socket on medial femoral condyle. The appropriate starting point, where the aperture of the socket should be placed, is distal to the distal femoral physis and proximal to the medial epicondyle. **B.** A true lateral radiograph demonstrating appropriate placement of medial femoral bone socket. The point of interest is not the tip of the guide wire but where the reamer meets the bone, which should be in line with the posterior diaphyseal cortex.

OUTCOMES

Although there are many surgeons who have reported outcomes of MPFL reconstruction in adults, the data is limited in isolated MPFL reconstruction in children and adolescence. Fernandez et al.[34] published a series of 30 patients with an average follow-up of 38 months. He reported excellent results in 90% of his patients based on the Larsen and Lauridsen score. Schöttle et al.[35] reported on 15 cases of double-bundle hamstring MPFL reconstruction and found that 5 of 15 (33%) had persistent patellar apprehension or a recurrent dislocation but an increase in Kujala score from 55 to 85.7. This study also tracked radiologic outcomes and found a decrease in patellar tilt from 11.3 to 9.2 degrees.[35] Another study reviewing radiologic outcomes after MPFL reconstruction noted that patella alta improved following MPFL reconstruction.[36]

The major complications reported in patients who underwent MPFL reconstruction include recurrent instability, stiffness,

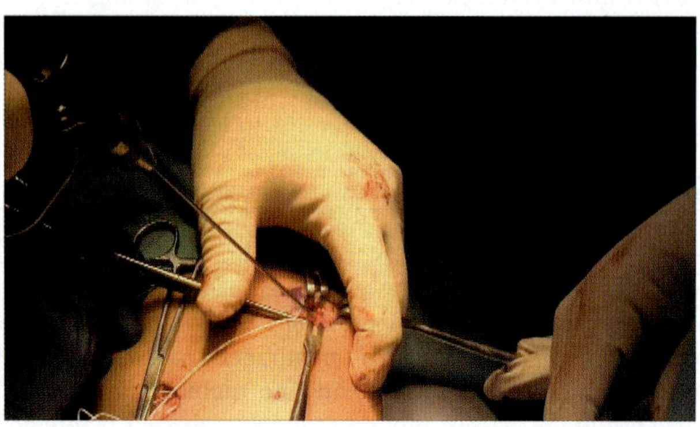

Figure 17.7. Drilling of two patellar bone sockets. These are made in the superior half of the patella.

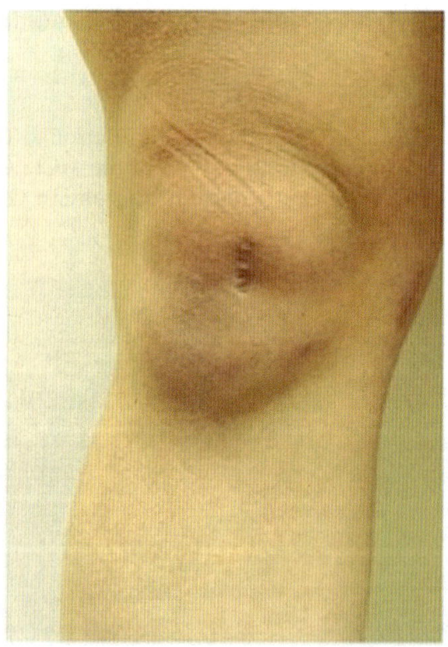

Figure 17.8. Picture of a patient's knee 1 year postoperatively following an MPFL reconstruction.

decreased range of motion and patellar fracture through the socket or tunnels.[32,37] Correct socket placement, particularly of the femoral socket and sizing the graft with the knee in 30 degrees of flexion, can avoid two of the most common complications: recurrent instability from too slack of a graft and decreased range of motion from a graft placed with excessive tension.

Proximal misplacement of the socket from its anatomic insertion on the femur by just 0.5 mm creates a lateral tilt moment on the patella, as opposed to the normal medial tilt moment in a native knee.[38] Another cadaveric study found that malposition of the femoral attachment by 5 mm proximally or distally created nonisometric length changes in the MPFL graft.[2] Both studies concluded that malpositioning of the femoral socket or tunnel had the potential for increasing contact pressure between the medial femoral condyle and the medial facet of the patella as well as loss of knee joint range of motion and graft failure.[2,38]

In addition to correct socket or tunnel positioning, securing the graft with the appropriate amount of tension is also now known to be critical to avoiding complications. In a cadaveric study, tensioning the MPFL graft at 10 N or more resulted in increased medial joint contact pressures and increased medial patellar tilting.[39]

Various studies have reported on complications of MPFL reconstruction in the adult population, but to date, just one study has evaluated complications specifically in a younger population.[32] Parikh et al.[32] reported their results of 179 knees with a complication rate of 16.2%, including eight patients who had recurrent lateral patellar instability, eight patients who experienced restricted knee flexion at follow-up, and six patients who had patellar fractures. The authors attributed the high rate of patellar fractures in their cohort to long oblique tunnels that traversed the patella and subsequently adapted a technique using just one 3.5-mm medial tunnel.[32] We feel that our technique of using patellar sockets in skeletally immature patients allows us to still use two fixation points while lowering the risk of fracture by not entirely traversing the patella.

CASE

A 12-year-old female presented to our clinic 1 month after dislocating her right patella while playing soccer. On physical examination, she had a trace knee effusion, increased lateral laxity of her right kneecap compared to her left, and mild quadriceps atrophy. She had full range of motion of the knee and no evidence of obligatory dislocation or subluxation of the patella. Her first set of plain films were done 1 month after the event and, aside from a mild patella alta, were unremarkable. The MRI at that time showed a near-complete detachment of the MPFL from the patella as well as osseous impaction injuries of the lateral femoral condyle and the medial patellar facet seen on the fat-suppressed sagittal image (Fig. 17.9A) as well as the cartilage-sensitive axial cuts (Fig 17.9B). Her TT-TG distance as measured on MRI was within normal range for her age (12 mm).

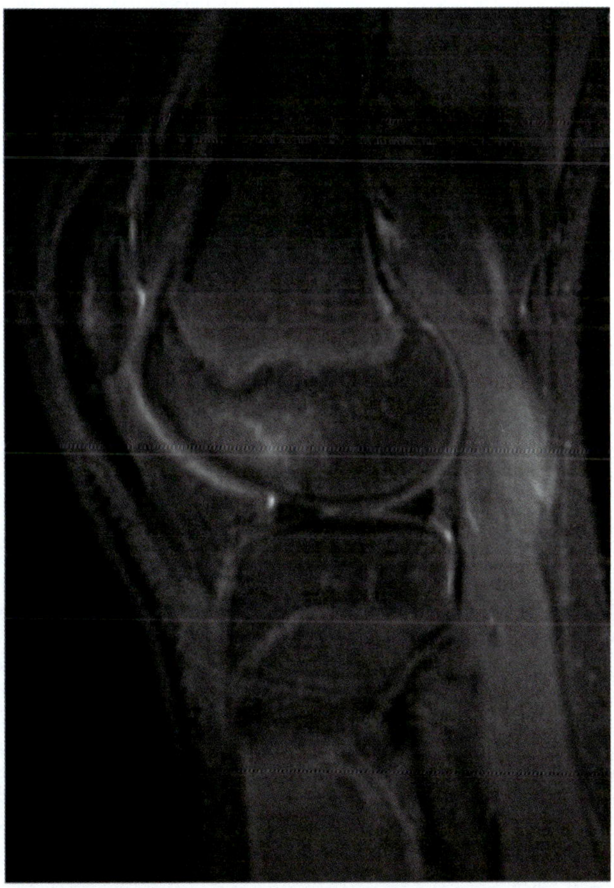

A

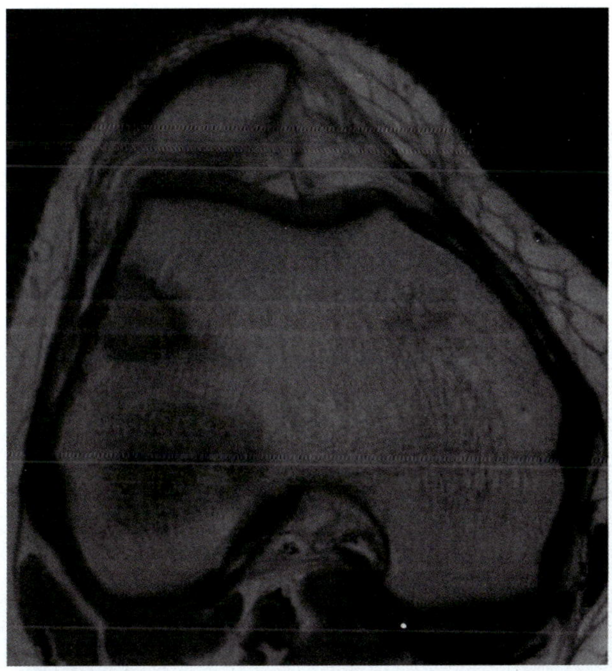

B

Figure 17.9. **A.** Lateral MRI STIR sequence demonstrating edema pattern on lateral femoral condyle. This pattern confirms recent patellar dislocation. **B.** Axial moderate echo time (TE) image demonstrates osteochondral lesion of lateral femoral condyle from impaction injury.

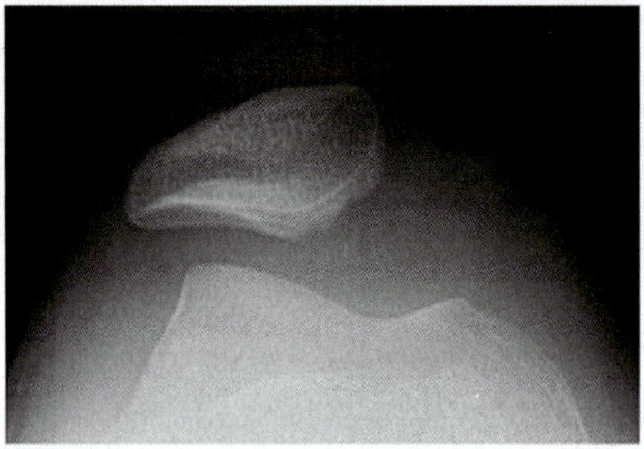

Figure 17.10. Merchant view of knee demonstrating loose body in the joint, likely cartilage loss from medial facet of the patella.

Given that this was her first dislocation and had no risk factors other than mild patella alta, she was prescribed 1 month of physical therapy focusing on knee, hip, and core strengthening.

She was asymptomatic for the next 2 years but presented again to our clinic when she was 14 years old after a second acute patellar dislocation. This time, she fell down a staircase which resulted in a recurrent patellar dislocation. She had a large right knee effusion and was limited in range of motion to flexion of 60 degrees. On Merchant view, she had a new 1-cm linear ossific fragment in the anterior joint space, likely an osteochondral lesion originating from the medial patellar facet (Fig. 17.10) as well as right patella lateral subluxation.

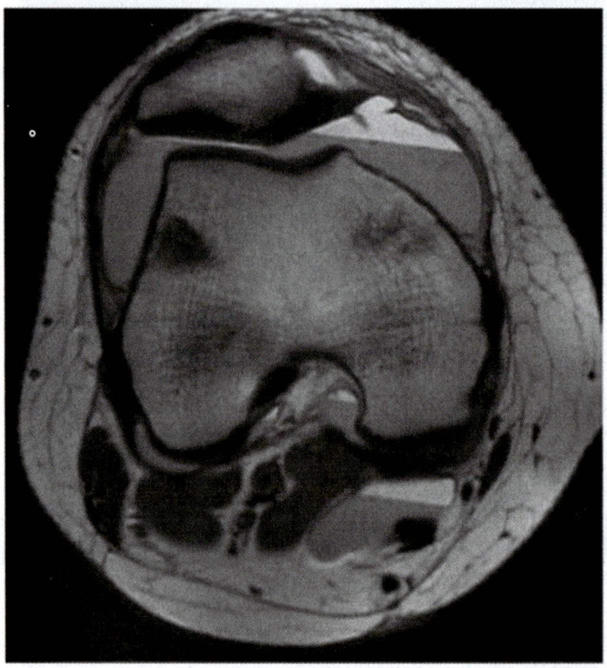

Figure 17.11. Cartilage-sensitive MRI axial image depicting a large knee hemarthrosis, an attenuated MPFL, and a further reimpaction of the inferomedial border of the patella with corresponding chondral damage.

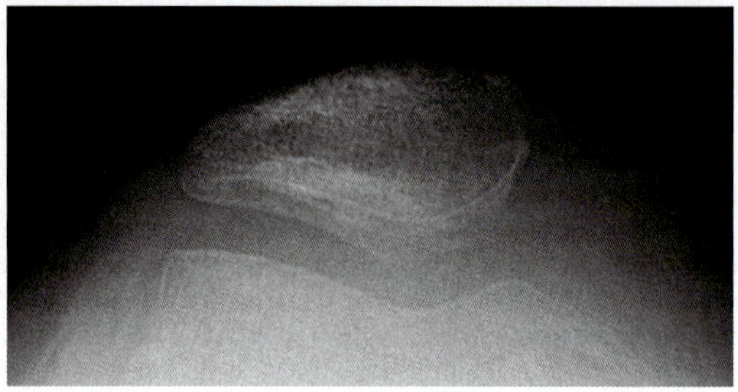

Figure 17.12. Merchant view radiograph taken 1 month postoperatively.

An MRI was obtained, demonstrating the large knee hemarthrosis, an attenuated MPFL, as well as further reimpaction of the inferomedial border of the patella with chondral damage (Fig. 17.11).

She underwent diagnostic knee arthroscopy, removal of a small and fragmented osteochondral loose body, and MPFL reconstruction 1 week after this recurrence using our autologous hamstring double-bundle technique. Figure 17.12 demonstrates an eccentrically reduced patella within the trochlear groove postoperatively.

REFERENCES

1. Beck P, Brown NA, Greis PE, et al. Patellofemoral contact pressures and lateral patellar translation after medial patellofemoral ligament reconstruction. *Am J Sports Med.* 2007;35(9):1557–1563.
2. Stephen JM, Lumpaopong P, Deehan DJ, et al. The medial patellofemoral ligament: location of femoral attachment and length change patterns resulting from anatomic and nonanatomic attachments. *Am J Sports Med.* 2012;40(8):1871–1879.
3. Amis AA, Firer P, Mountney J, et al. Anatomy and biomechanics of the medial patellofemoral ligament. *Knee.* 2003;10(3):215–220.
4. Petri M, von Falck C, Broese M, et al. Influence of rupture patterns of the medial patellofemoral ligament (MPFL) on the outcome after operative treatment of traumatic patellar dislocation. *Knee Surg Sports Traumatol Arthrosc.* 2013;21(3):683–689.
5. Seeley M, Bowman KF, Walsh C, et al. Magnetic resonance imaging of acute patellar dislocation in children: patterns of injury and risk factors for recurrence. *J Pediatr Orthop.* 2012;32(2):145–155.
6. Zaidi A, Babyn P, Astori I, et al. MRI of traumatic patellar dislocation in children. *Pediatr Radiol.* 2006;36(11):1163–1170.
7. Kepler CK, Bogner EA, Hammoud S, et al. Zone of injury of the medial patellofemoral ligament after acute patellar dislocation in children and adolescents. *Am J Sports Med.* 2011;39(7):1444–1449.
8. Weber-Spickschen TS, Spang J, Kohn L, et al. The relationship between trochlear dysplasia and medial patellofemoral ligament rupture location after patellar dislocation: an MRI evaluation. *Knee.* 2011;18(3):185–188.
9. Sanders TG, Morrison WB, Singleton BA, et al. Medial patellofemoral ligament injury following acute transient dislocation of the patella: MR findings with surgical correlation in 14 patients. *J Comput Assist Tomogr.* 2001;25(6):957–962.
10. Sallay PI, Poggi J, Speer KP, et al. Acute dislocation of the patella. A correlative pathoanatomic study. *Am J Sports Med.* 1996;24(1):52–60.
11. Warren LF, Marshall JL. The supporting structures and layers on the medial side of the knee: an anatomical analysis. *J Bone Joint Surg Am.* 1979;61(1):56–62.

12. Kang HJ, Wang F, Chen BC, et al. Functional bundles of the medial patellofemoral ligament. *Knee Surg Sports Traumatol Arthrosc.* 2010;18(11):1511–1516.
13. Mochizuki T, Nimura A, Tateishi T, et al. Anatomic study of the attachment of the medial patellofemoral ligament and its characteristic relationships to the vastus intermedius. *Knee Surg Sports Traumatol Arthrosc.* 2013;21(2):305–310.
14. Schöttle PB, Schmeling A, Rosenstiel N, et al. Radiographic landmarks for femoral tunnel placement in medial patellofemoral ligament reconstruction. *Am J Sports Med.* 2007;35(5):801–804.
15. Nikku R, Nietosvaara Y, Aalto K, et al. Operative treatment of primary patellar dislocation does not improve medium-term outcome: a 7-year follow-up report and risk analysis of 127 randomized patients. *Acta Orthop.* 2005;76(5):699–704.
16. Camp CL, Krych AJ, Dahm DL, et al. Medial patellofemoral ligament repair for recurrent patellar dislocation. *Am J Sports Med.* 2010;38(11):2248–2254.
17. Weeks K III, Fabricant PD, Ladenhauf HN, et al. Surgical options for patellar stabilization in the skeletally immature patient. *Sports Med Arthrosc.* 2012;20(3):194–202.
18. Nelitz M, Dornacher D, Dreyhaupt J, et al. The relation of the distal femoral physis and the medial patellofemoral ligament. *Knee Surg Sports Traumatol Arthrosc.* 2011;19(12):2067–2071.
19. Nietosvaara Y, Paukku R, Palmu S, et al. Acute patellar dislocation in children and adolescents. Surgical technique. *J Bone Joint Surg Am.* 2009;91(suppl 2, pt 1):139–145.
20. Cofield RH, Bryan RS. Acute dislocation of the patella: results of conservative treatment. *J Trauma.* 1977;17(7):526–531.
21. Hawkins RJ, Bell RH, Anisette G. Acute patellar dislocations. The natural history. *Am J Sports Med.* 1986;14(2):117–120.
22. Palmu S, Kallio PE, Donell ST, et al. Acute patellar dislocation in children and adolescents: a randomized clinical trial. *J Bone Joint Surg Am.* 2008;90(3):463–470.
23. Sillanpää PJ, Mäenpää HM. First-time patellar dislocation: surgery or conservative treatment? *Sports Med Arthrosc.* 2012;20(3):128–135.
24. Lewallen LW, McIntosh AL, Dahm DL. Predictors of recurrent instability after acute patellofemoral dislocation in pediatric and adolescent patients. *Am J Sports Med.* 2013;41(3):575–581.
25. Sillanpää PJ, Mäenpää HM, Mattila VM, et al. Arthroscopic surgery for primary traumatic patellar dislocation: a prospective, nonrandomized study comparing patients treated with and without acute arthroscopic stabilization with a median 7-year follow-up. *Am J Sports Med.* 2008;36(12):2301–2309.
26. Guerrero P, Li X, Patel K, et al. Medial patellofemoral ligament injury patterns and associated pathology in lateral patella dislocation: an MRI study. *Sports Med Arthrosc Rehabil Ther Technol.* 2009;1(1):17.
27. Dickens AJ, Morrell NT, Doering A, et al. Tibial tubercle trochlear groove distance: defining normal in a pediatric population. *J Bone Joint Surg Am.* 2014;96(4):318–324.
28. Steensen RN, Dopirak RM, Maurus PB. A simple technique for reconstruction of the medial patellofemoral ligament using a quadriceps tendon graft. *Arthroscopy.* 2005;21(3):365–370.
29. Steiner TM, Torga-Spak R, Teitge RA. Medial patellofemoral ligament reconstruction in patients with lateral patellar instability and trochlear dysplasia. *Am J Sports Med.* 2006;34(8):1254–1261.
30. Gomes JE. Comparison between a static and a dynamic technique for medial patellofemoral ligament reconstruction. *Arthroscopy.* 2008;24(4):430–435.
31. Deie M, Ochi M, Sumen Y, et al. Reconstruction of the medial patellofemoral ligament for the treatment of habitual or recurrent dislocation of the patella in children. *J Bone Joint Surg Br.* 2003;85(6):887–890.
32. Parikh SN, Nathan ST, Wall EJ, et al. Complications of medial patellofemoral ligament reconstruction in young patients. *Am J Sports Med.* 2013;41(5):1030–1038.
33. Ladenhauf HN, Berkes MB, Green DW. Medial patellofemoral ligament reconstruction using hamstring autograft in children and adolescents. *Arthrosc Tech.* 2013;2(2):e151–e154.
34. Fernandez E, Sala D, Castejon M. Reconstruction of the medial patellofemoral ligament for patellar instability using a semitendinosus autograft. *Acta Orthop Belg.* 2005;71(3):303–308.
35. Schöttle PB, Fucentese SF, Romero J. Clinical and radiological outcome of medial patellofemoral ligament reconstruction with a semitendinosus autograft for patella instability. *Knee Surg Sports Traumatol Arthrosc.* 2005;13(7):516–521.
36. Lykissas MG, Li T, Eismann EA, et al. Does medial patellofemoral ligament reconstruction decrease patellar height? A preliminary report. *J Pediatr Orthop.* 2014;34(1):78–85.
37. Singhal R, Rogers S, Charalambous CP. Double-bundle medial patellofemoral ligament reconstruction with hamstring tendon autograft and mediolateral patellar tunnel fixation: a meta-analysis of outcomes and complications. *Bone Joint J.* 2013;95-B(7):900–905.
38. Elias JJ, Cosgarea AJ. Technical errors during medial patellofemoral ligament reconstruction could overload medial patellofemoral cartilage: a computational analysis. *Am J Sports Med.* 2006;34(9):1478–1485.
39. Stephen JM, Kaider D, Lumpaopong P, et al. The effect of femoral tunnel position and graft tension on patellar contact mechanics and kinematics after medial patellofemoral ligament reconstruction. *Am J Sports Med.* 2014;42(2):364–372.

CHAPTER

18

Jeffrey J. Nepple
Scott J. Luhmann

Medial Patellar Tendon Transfer with Proximal Realignment

INTRODUCTION

The treatment of patellar instability in skeletally immature patients can be challenging. Patients presenting at a young age often have more severe underlying malalignment (i.e., trochlear dysplasia) that typically leads to the development of symptoms prior to skeletal maturity. Although soft tissue procedures (medial patellofemoral ligament reconstruction or proximal realignment) may be appropriate in some patients, many patients with developmental patellar dislocations have significant bony abnormalities (i.e., lateralized tibial tubercle) that are not addressed with soft tissue procedures alone. Alternative procedures in these patients include nonanatomic reconstructions such as the Roux-Goldthwait procedure and Galeazzi procedure. In our experience, the results of these procedures have not been reliable. Given the lack of reliable treatment options in patients with underlying bony malalignment, skeletally immature patients are frequently counseled to wait until skeletal maturity for definitive treatment (tibial tubercle osteotomy). Particularly in the young child with significant growth remaining, worsening of trochlear dysplasia and patellar instability often occur and can result in abnormalities that are difficult (if not impossible) to correct at skeletal maturity.

Medial patellar tendon transfer with proximal realignment (Fig. 18.1) has been used at our institution for over 30 years in children with congenital or developmental patellar dislocations and significant underlying bony malalignment. Gordon and Schoenecker[1] initially described our institution's early experience with this procedure. Transection of the patellar tendon with medial transfer and reattachment allows for near-anatomic reconstruction of underlying malalignment. In the child with significant growth remaining, restoring proper patellofemoral stability may contribute to favorable trochlear remodeling. For the surgeon without experience in this technique, transection of the patellar tendon is intimidating due to the potential concern for healing. In the extensive experience with this procedure at our institution, long leg cast immobilization postoperatively results in reliable healing without significant issues with arthrofibrosis in this population. In this chapter, we describe our surgical technique for medial patellar tendon transfer with proximal realignment.

TREATMENT

Skeletally immature patients with patellar dislocations require a thorough evaluation to understand the role that various factors play in their presentation. Medial patellar tendon transfer has been generally used in females younger than 11 years of age or male patients younger than 12 years of age. However, most patients undergoing the procedure are 10 years of age or younger. Patients generally present with a history of chronic patellar dislocations and subluxations and are often able to demonstrate a dislocatable patella on clinical exam. Significant patellofemoral crepitus is extremely rare in this population due to the degree of soft tissue laxity present. Clinical assessment of the patient's Q angle is generally abnormal. Additionally, assessment of standing lower extremity alignment (mechanical axis) and femoral/tibial rotational profile is important in this population.

Radiographic evaluation with anteroposterior (AP), lateral, notch, and Merchant views is used to assess for patellofemoral tracking as well as any other pathology. The Merchant view commonly demonstrates significant lateral subluxation (or even dislocation) of the patella in these patients. Additionally, some degree of trochlear dysplasia is commonly noted on Merchant and lateral radiographic projections. Patella alta is commonly noted as well. Three-dimensional imaging can be useful to characterize the underlying anatomy including measurement of the tibial tubercle–trochlear groove (TT-TG) distance.

AUTHORS' PREFERRED TECHNIQUE

Surgery is performed supine with a bump under the ipsilateral hip. A nonsterile tourniquet is placed prior to sterile prep of the surgical limb. Standard preoperative antibiotic prophylaxis is used. After exsanguination of the leg, the tourniquet is inflated. A midline incision from the level of the superior pole of the patella to 3 cm below the tibial tubercle is used (Fig. 18.2). Circumferential skin flaps are raised at the level of the retinaculum (Fig. 18.3). We have not routinely used arthroscopy in this young patient population, unless clinical evaluation

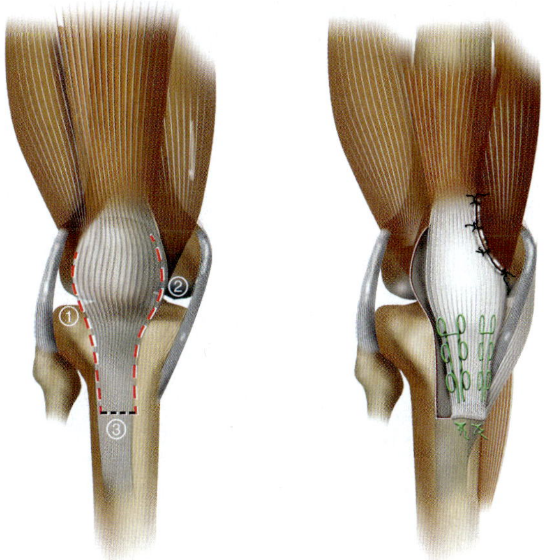

Figure 18.1. **A.** Diagram demonstrating localization of (1) lateral release, (2) incision from VMO advancement, and (3) medial patellar tendon transfer. **B.** Diagram demonstrating completed (1) lateral release, (2) VMO advancement, and (3) medial patellar tendon transfer.

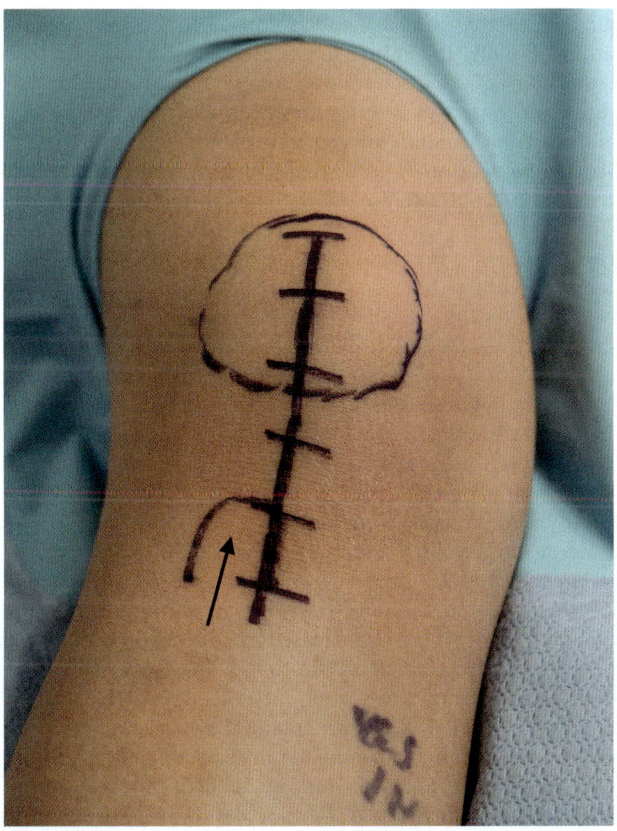

Figure 18.2. Midline incision extending from superior border to approximately 3 cm distal to the tibial tubercle. Note the typically lateralized tibial tubercle location in this patient population.

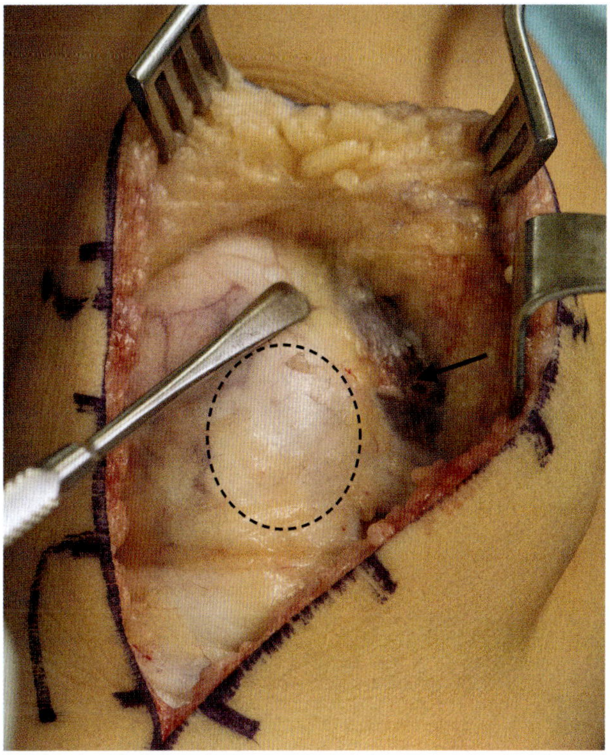

Figure 18.3. Exposure proceeds to raise large medial and lateral skin flaps at level of retinaculum and VMO (*arrow*). The patellar position is demonstrated with *dotted line.*

suggests underlying chondromalacia or loose body. We have found intra-articular pathology to be relatively uncommon in this patient population.

Proximal Realignment

Initial dissection for the proximal realignment is performed next. The lateral retinacular release is performed 1 cm lateral to the patella. Care is taken to identify the extrasynovial plane at the beginning of this dissection. This plane can then be followed proximally to the level of the superolateral patella and distally through the fat pad to the level of the tibial tubercle to complete the release. Care should be taken to avoid injury to the periosteum and physis in the distal aspect of the release. The lateral release is initially carried to the superior aspect of the patella, but frequently, an anomalous contracted band of vastus lateralis insertion on the patella is present deep to the initial dissection (Fig. 18.4). Failure to identify this band will result in persistent lateral maltracking.

Attention is then turned to the medial retinacular incision performed in preparation for vastus medialis obliquus (VMO) advancement. Similar to the lateral release, the extrasynovial plane is identified. The incision is performed approximately 1 cm medial to the distal half of the patella and extended along the medial border of the tendon. Above the midpoint of the patella, the release is taken across the VMO insertion, with care taken to leave a 5- to 7-mm cuff of tissue for subsequent repair. The release is extended approximately 2 cm into the quadriceps tendon to allow for adequate mobility for the

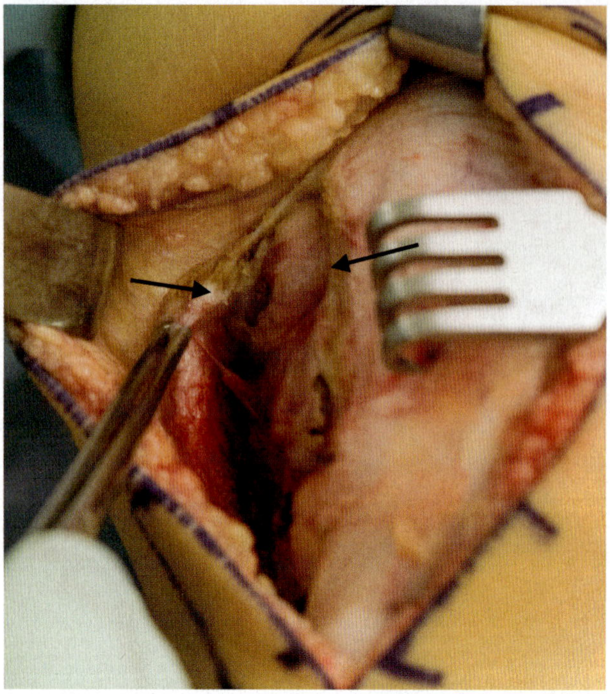

Figure 18.4. Lateral release is performed from superolateral aspect of patella to the lateral insertion of patellar tendon. Dissection is initially performed in extrasynovial plane. Frequently, additional release of contracted bands of vastus lateralis and/or contracted synovium is required to achieve proper balance. *Arrows* demonstrate completed lateral release.

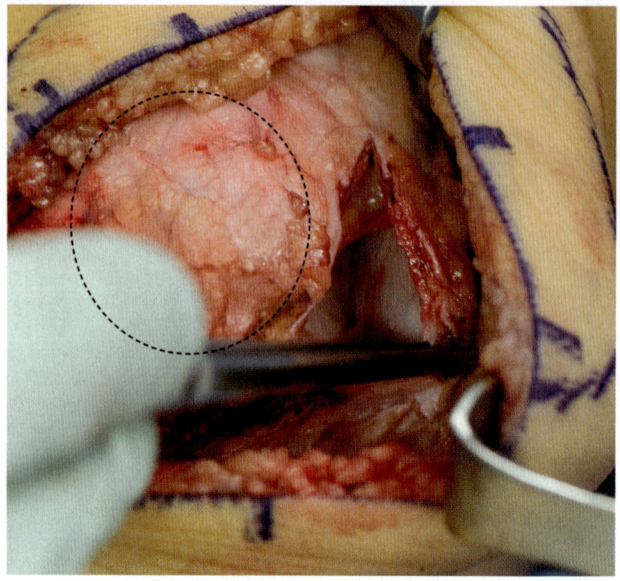

Figure 18.5. Medial release is performed (in similar fashion to lateral release) in preparation for VMO advancement. An adequate cuff of tissue is maintained on VMO flap to allow reattachment (patellar position shown with *dotted lines*). Note the extension of release extends slightly into quadriceps tendon to allow advancement.

VMO advancement (Fig. 18.5). The plane deep to the VMO is bluntly dissected to allow good mobility of the VMO for lateral advancement. The VMO advancement is not performed at this point but instead as the final step in the procedure after medial patellar tendon transfer.

Medial Patellar Tendon Transfer

The insertion of the patellar tendon onto the cartilaginous tibial tubercle is now identified. A curved clamp is passed behind the distal patellar tendon to confirm its bony attachment site (Fig. 18.6A). The patellar tendon insertion is then sharply transected with a fresh no. 15 blade. The tendon is transected with the scalpel oriented at a 45-degree angle proximally to maximize the length of the patellar tendon tissue and avoid damage to the underlying cartilaginous tibial tubercle (Fig. 18.6B). Further dissection posterior to the tendon is avoided to preserve its blood supply.

The patellar tendon is then medially transferred between 50% and 100% of its width depending on the underlying severity of patellar instability. A medial transfer of 50% of the patellar tendon width is most commonly performed. However, in cases of congenital or syndromic patellar dislocations, a translation of at least 100% is needed to normalize patellar mechanics. The location of the new patellar tendon insertion is identified and cleared of soft tissue.

The patellar tendon is secured to bone with two no. 2 FiberWire sutures. The lateral suture is started distally within the distal stump of the patellar tendon, usually at its midpoint, and exits at the cut edge (Fig. 18.7A). It then grasps the lateral half of the patellar tendon with a Krackow-type suture pattern. Finally, the suture is passed again through the most medial edge of the distal tendon stump at the tibial tubercle in the central aspect of the new insertion footprint. The second suture is then similarly placed to secure the medial aspect of the patellar tendon. The medial suture is frequently secured through both periosteum and the insertion of the pes tendons (Fig. 18.7B). Patellar tracking can be estimated at this point prior to securing the patellar tendon transfer. The sutures are then sequentially tied (Fig. 18.8).

At this point, patellar tracking should be thoroughly assessed. Knee flexion to 90 degrees should be present with stability of the patellar tendon insertion. The knee is evaluated through extension and flexion to assess patellar tracking. The patella should track centrally without the need for digital pressure, even prior to VMO advancement. If persistent lateral maltracking is present, the completeness of the lateral release should be reevaluated to determine if any abnormal tethering of the vastus lateralis was initially missed. Additionally, the vastus lateralis muscle can be bluntly dissected off of the posterior intermuscular septum to remove any additional abnormal lateral tethering. If further release is required, the vastus lateralis is sequentially released in 5- to 10-mm intervals at a 45-degree angle toward the midline. After each release, patellar tracking is again reevaluated. If persistent lateral maltracking is present, consideration for further medial transfer of the patellar tendon at the tibial tubercle distally may be needed. In severe cases of congenital or syndromic dislocation, excessive tension of the extensor mechanisms may prevent normalization of patellar tracking. The medial and lateral proximal releases can then be connected and a V-Y lengthening of the extensor mechanism can be performed, although this is fairly uncommon.

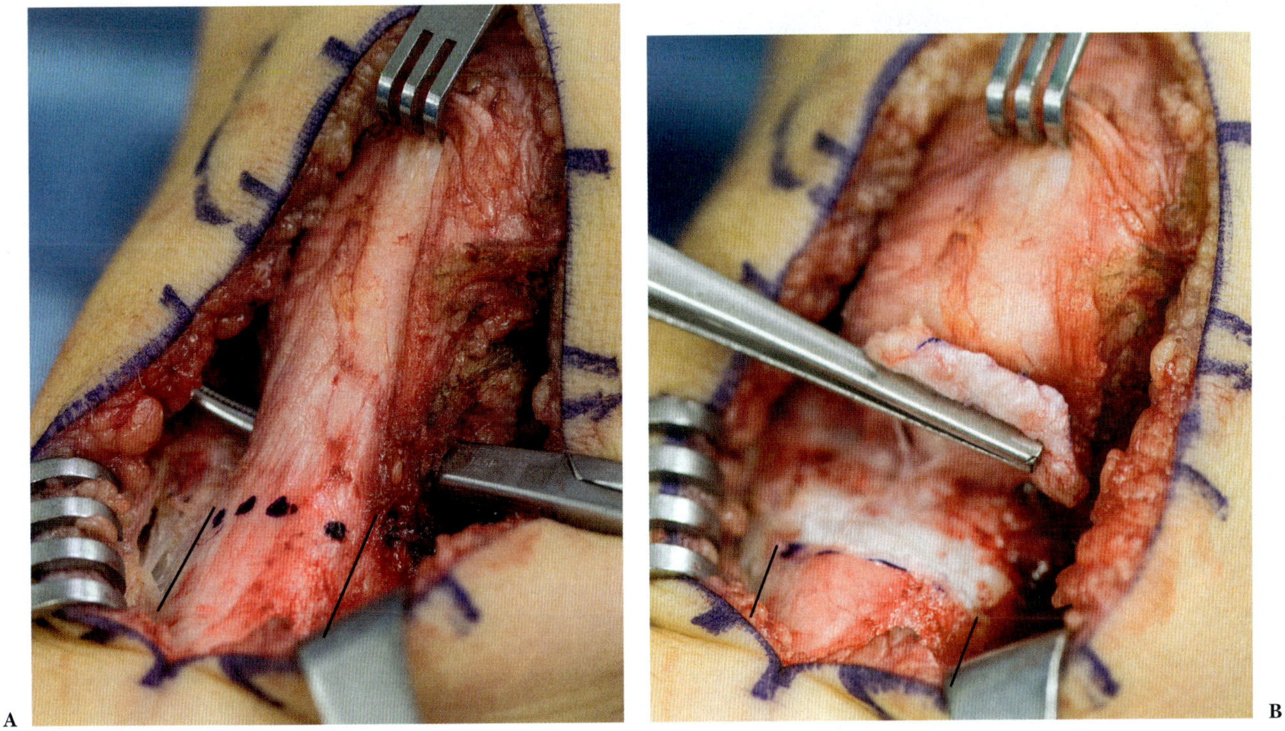

Figure 18.6. **A.** The insertion of patellar tendon to tibial tubercle is localized with the aid of a clamp passed beneath the tendon. Site of patellar tendon transection is localized with marker. **B.** Patellar tendon insertion is transected, with care not to injure the underlying cartilaginous tibial tubercle. Further dissection of fat pad from undersurface of patellar tendon is avoided to maintain vascular supply.

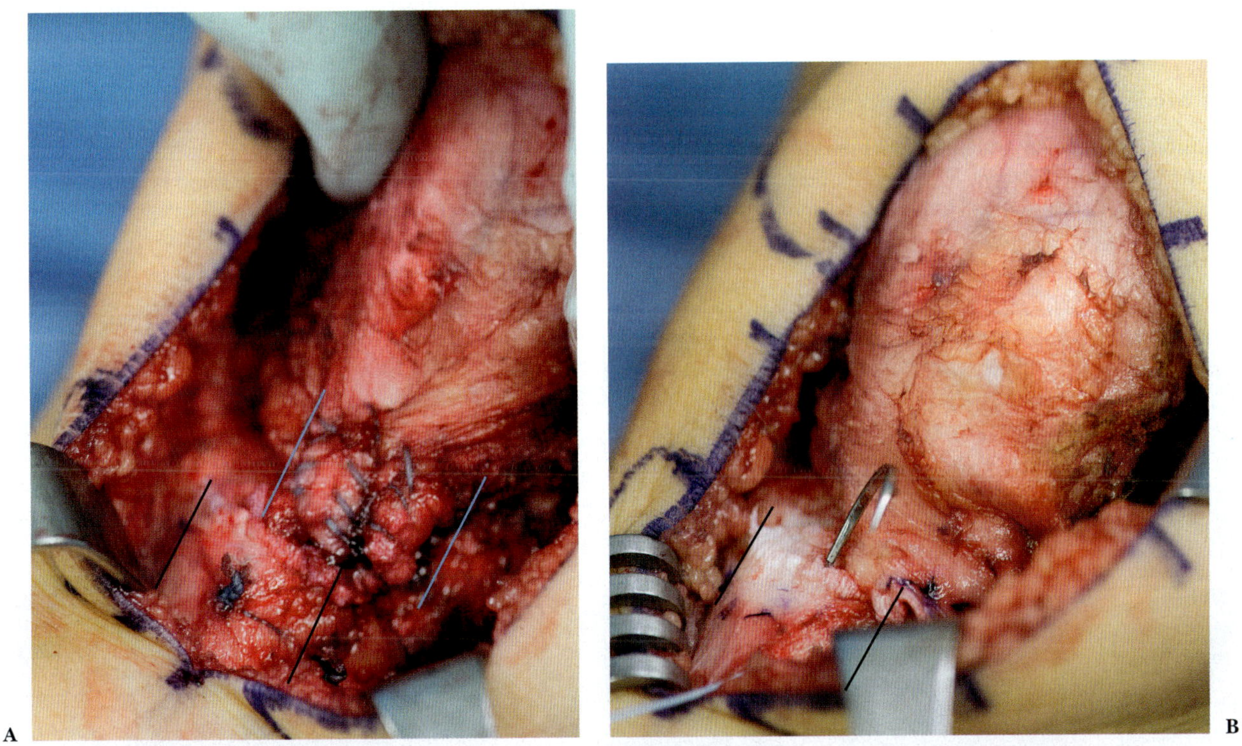

Figure 18.7. **A.** Patellar tendon insertion is medialized 50% to 100% of width of patellar tendon insertion (50% shown here). Two no. 2 FiberWire sutures are used to reattach the tendon. Initial suture is passed distal to proximal at the midpoint of the distal patellar tendon attachment on the tibial tubercle at the site of reattachment. **B.** The suture is then passed in the lateral half of the tendon with a Krackow-type stitch and a final pass through the most medial edge of the distal patellar tendon attachment on the tibial tubercle. A second suture is similarly passed in the medial half of the patellar tendon and secured distally into periosteum and the pes anserine insertion. Note the medial and lateral edges of native patellar tendon insertion are labeled by *vertical lines*.

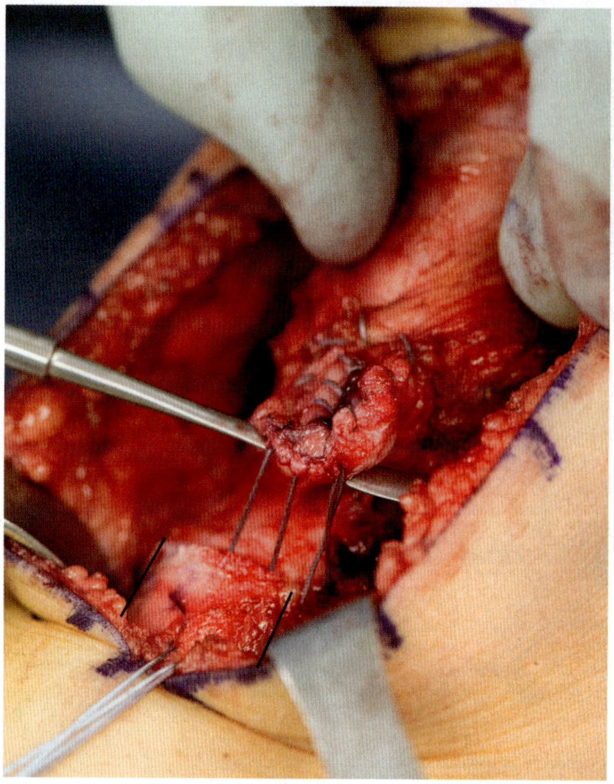

Figure 18.8. Completed medial patellar tendon transfer demonstrating medial transfer 50% the width of the patellar tendon insertion. Patellar tracking should be reassessed and 90 degrees of knee flexion achieved without difficulty.

Vastus Medialis Obliquus Advancement

Once satisfactory patellar tracking is achieved, the VMO advancement is then performed. The distal aspect of the VMO is grasped with an atraumatic clamp. The tension of the VMO is evaluated in flexion and extension to estimate the amount of VMO advancement. In severe cases, the VMO may require advancement to the midaspect of the dorsal patella. The VMO advancement is secured with three or four no. 1 Ethibond sutures placed through the dorsal periosteum of the patella (Fig. 18.9A). All sutures are sequentially placed in a horizontal mattress configuration and then tied with tension maintained on the other sutures (Fig. 18.9B). The VMO advancement is then further secured with no. 1 Vicryl sutures placed between previously placed Ethibond sutures. Final confirmation of appropriate patellar tracking without excessive tension at 90 degrees of flexion is performed.

The wound is then copiously irrigated with normal saline. Layered closure is performed with subcutaneous 2-0 clear polydioxanone (PDS) and subcuticular 4-0 Monocryl suture. A sterile dressing is applied, and the tourniquet is deflated.

POSTOPERATIVE REHABILITATION

Postoperatively, the leg is placed in a long leg cast or hinged knee brace locked in extension. In younger children, a long leg cast may be used to ensure compliance. The knee remains in extension for 4 weeks, followed by gradual increases in passive range of motion with a goal of 90 degrees of flexion by 8 weeks postoperatively. Active knee extension and quadriceps strengthening are initiated at 6 weeks postoperatively. Patients begin to bear weight with the brace locked in extension at 4 weeks postoperatively. The hinged knee brace is weaned at 3 months postoperatively.

Figure 18.9 illustrates a typical case of medial patellar tendon transfer in a 7-year-old female. Preoperative radiographs demonstrate significant lateral subluxation of the patella in a skeletally immature patient (Fig. 18.10A). The patient was treated with medial transfer of the patellar tendon as described here. Postoperative radiographs (Fig. 18.10B) demonstrate excellent reduction of the patella with some improvement in the underlying trochlear dysplasia.

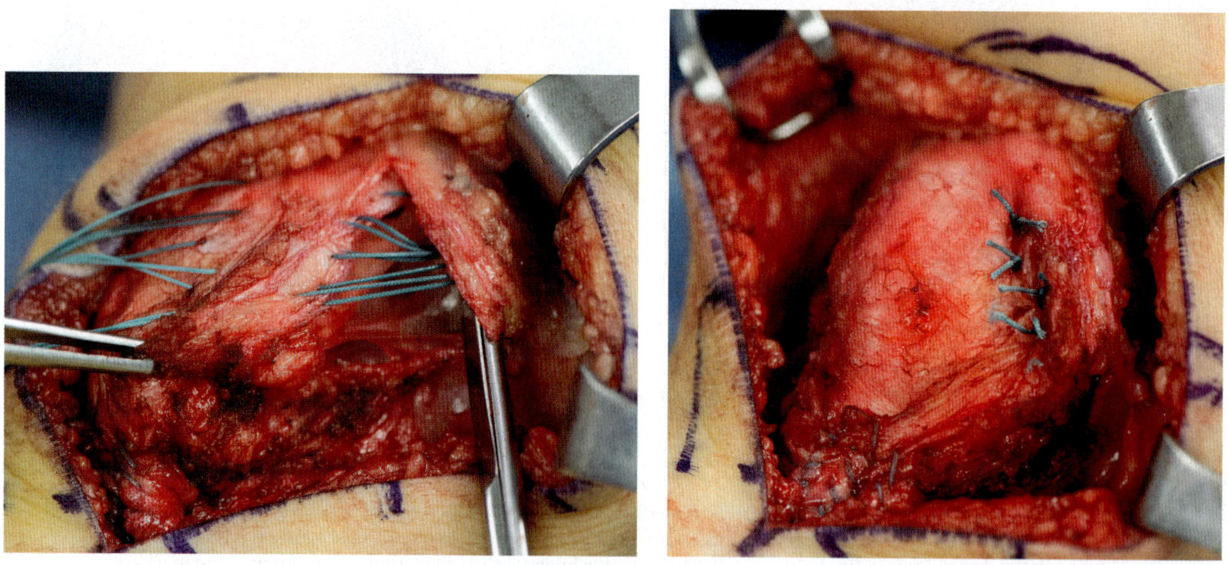

A B

Figure 18.9. **A.** Four no. 2 Ethibond sutures are used for VMO advancement. Sutures are sequentially passed in a horizontal mattress fashion through to the dorsal periosteum of the patella and then into the VMO. In severe cases, the VMO may need to be advanced significantly across the patella. **B.** Appearance of completed VMO advancement.

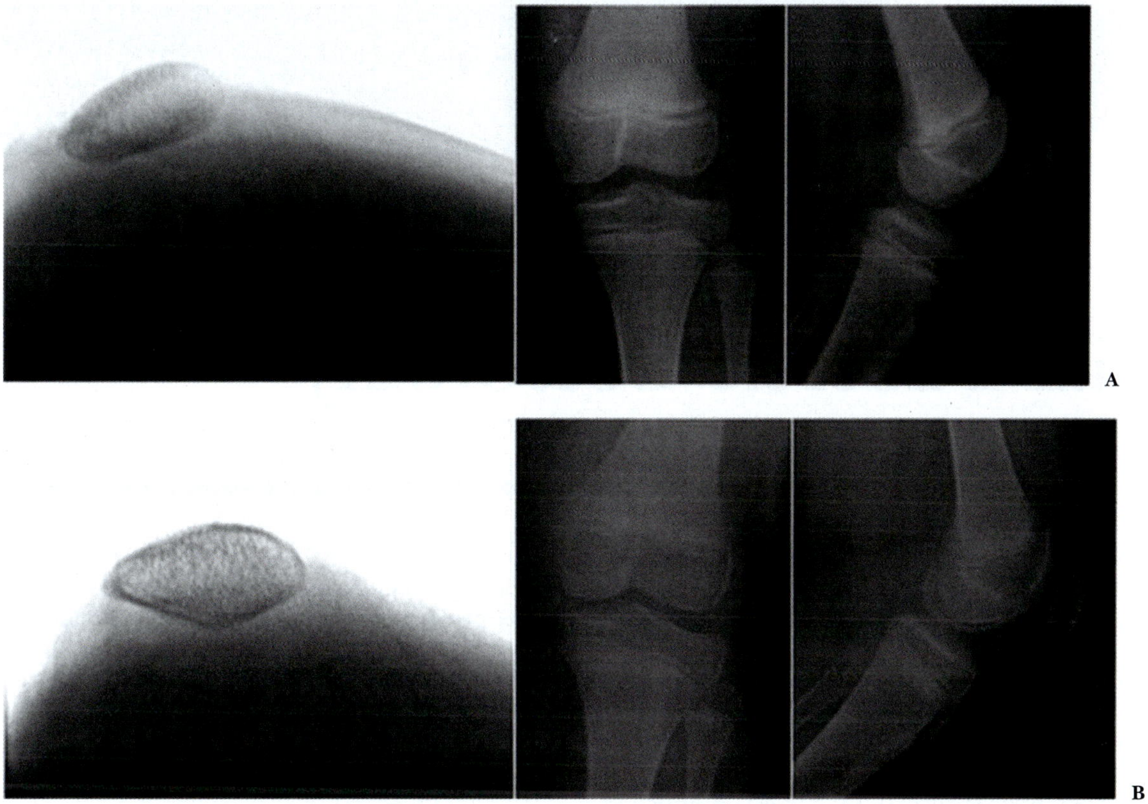

Figure 18.10. Case example. A 7-year-old female with chronic dislocations of left patella. **A.** Preoperative Merchant, AP, and lateral radiographs demonstrate lateral subluxation of patella. **B.** Postoperative radiographs 6 months after medial patellar tendon transfer with proximal realignment demonstrate improved patellofemoral alignment.

In our experience, this procedure offers a very reliable means of correcting significant underlying patellofemoral malalignment in skeletally immature patients. Rates of recurrent patellar instability are low after this procedure. Full quadriceps strength without extensor lag is routinely obtained. Using our postoperative protocol, we have not experienced significant difficulties with range of motion in this young patient population.

REFERENCE

1. Gordon JE, Schoenecker PL. Surgical treatment of congenital dislocation of the patella. *J Pediatr Orthop.* 1999;19(2):260–264.

CHAPTER

19

Brian Grawe
Jacqueline Munch
Beth Shubin Stein

Technique: Distal Realignment Tibial Tubercle Osteotomy

INTRODUCTION

Instability of the patellofemoral joint is a relatively common and often a challenging condition to treat in the pediatric and adolescent patient population.[1,2] A population-based study by Nietosvaara and colleagues[3] has demonstrated the annual incidence rate of acute patellar dislocation to be 0.04% (43 in 100,000) in those younger than 16 years of age. A myriad of potential risk factors have been implicated as precipitating etiologic features for both initial and recurrent patellofemoral instability, with some studies estimating the risk of recurrence, after a primary patellar dislocation event, to be as high as 49% to 69%.[4,5] The risk factors for recurrent lateral patellar instability can be defined as either demographic or anatomic. Female gender, sports participation, and a personal or family history of instability are important demographic variables. Anatomic risk factors of patellar instability include patella alta, an increased Q angle, generalized ligamentous laxity, vastus medialis weakness, and excessive pes/planus/subtalar joint pronation.[5] More recent work has demonstrated skeletal immaturity and trochlear dysplasia to be significant risk factors in terms of predictors of failure after initial nonoperative management.[5] From a conceptual point of view, pediatric and adolescent patients can be grouped into four distinct classes: syndromic, obligatory, fixed lateral, and traumatic.[2] The latter faction can be further subdivided into first time or recurrent, and it is this traumatic group that the subsequent chapter concentrates its attention.

Maintenance of a stable concentric reduction must be the principal goal of treating any dislocation of the patellofemoral joint, as the potential long-term sequelae of instability include knee pain, decreased activity level, recurrent instability/dislocation, chondral injury, and subsequent patellofemoral arthritis.[6] The traditional nonoperative approach of closed reduction, joint immobilization, and subsequent rehabilitation, although appropriate for a first-time dislocator, does not always consistently eliminate the risk of recurrence. Frequently, patients require surgical intervention if they go on to sustain a second instability event in order to prevent continued recurrence. Although controversy still exists regarding the indications, timing, and type of procedure to be performed for pediatric and adolescent patients with patellofemoral instability, a tailored surgical plan must be devised that accounts for history, age, status of physes, degree or presence of chondral injury, osseous alignment, and soft tissue injury.[7] The purpose of this chapter is to review the indications and surgical technique associated with distal osseous realignment surgery for pediatric and adolescent patients with patellofemoral instability. This chapter focuses on the authors' preferred method of treatment for tibial tubercle osteotomy (TTO).

TREATMENT

Indications

The presence of an unstable osteochondral lesion is generally the most accepted absolute indication for immediate surgery after a first-time acute patellar dislocation. Most authors would agree that symptomatic recurrent patellofemoral instability is a surgical problem that must be addressed with proximal, distal, or combined realignment. The decision to transfer the tibial tubercle, in patients with recurrent patellar dislocation, is based on a thorough clinical and radiographic assessment of the patient's anatomy. Although there is a paucity of evidence surrounding the radiographic parameters associated with TTO, many authors will use specific thresholds based on measurements that assess for both the height of the patella and presence of excessive lateral position of the tuberosity in relation to the trochlear groove. The presence and degree of cartilage wear and trochlear dysplasia must be noted on preoperative imaging studies as well, as these factors can ultimately affect joint stability and any proposed surgical plan.[8] Taken in concert with a thorough clinical history and physical examination, these radiographic parameters can be used to determine the amount and plane (anterior, medial, or distal) of correction needed to effectively obtain a stable and pain-free patellofemoral joint after tibial tubercle transfer.

Patellar height is best assessed via a true lateral radiograph of the patellofemoral joint. Alternatively, sagittal slices through the joint, as seen on magnetic resonance imaging (MRI) or computed tomography (CT), can also be used to measure vertical height of the patella. Various methods and ratios have been devised by a variety of authors to evaluate patellar height that include the Blumensaat method, the Insall-Salvati index, the Blackburne-Peel index, and the Caton-Deschamps index (CD index). The CD index is generally accepted as the most accurate diagnostic measurement as well as the most germane index regarding assessing patellar height before and after transfer. This ratio consists of plotting the distance between the inferior edge of the patellar joint surface and the anterosuperior angle of the tibia against the intra-articular length of the patella. It relies on identifiable and reproducible anatomic landmarks, is less dependent on knee flexion angles, and should be therapeutically altered after transfer of the tubercle.[9] A normal CD index is typically defined as 1, with the values of less than 0.8 and greater than 1.2 being considered pathology great enough to warrant surgical correction.[7]

Quantitatively, the amount of lateral displacement of the tibial tubercle can be measured in one of two ways and must be defined on advanced axial imaging studies (CT or MRI). The conventional and most accepted method involves measuring the linear distance between the tibial tubercle and the trochlear groove on superimposed axial imaging, Dejour's so called tibial tubercle–trochlear groove (TT-TG) distance.[8] A second and more novel method, which similarly involves measuring known anatomic landmarks on superimposed images, is called the *tibial tubercle–posterior cruciate ligament* (TT-PCL).[10] The TT-PCL measures the distance between the tibial tubercle and the posterior cruciate ligament and, secondary to its limited use in the literature, will not be discussed in this chapter. Careful measurement of the TT-TG can be accomplished by taking advantage of the roman arch of the trochlear groove and either the most proximal or distal portion of the tubercle. A linear distance is then measured between two lines that are perpendicular to posterior femoral condyle and pass through the middle of trochlear groove and the tibial tubercle, respectively.[11] Numerous authors have published on the measurement's reliability and acceptable correlation between CT and MRI.[12] However, there is limited data regarding normal values for TT-TG distance, and a cutoff magnitude of greater than 20 mm is generally regarded as the lower threshold of normal prior to medialization of the tibial tubercle.

The concept of trochlear dysplasia, as originally classified by Dejour and colleagues,[13] can be assessed on the lateral radiograph and will not be discussed in detail, as it is outside of the scope of this chapter. It must be recognized that the crux of this pathology lies within a flattened or convex geometrical shape of the trochlear and can portend a higher risk of recurrent patellofemoral instability.

Contraindications

There are a few important contraindications to TTO which are also germane to pediatric and adolescent patients with recurrent patellar instability. Principally, the presence of an open tibial tubercle apophysis is a contraindication to any distal osseous realignment procedure. The theoretical risk of premature physeal disruption/closure and possible subsequent genu recurvatum deformity are the primary concern for surgeons treating patients with a patent apophysis and concomitant patellofemoral instability. Admittedly, the literature is scarce in terms of this reported complication, and as a result, there is no steadfast age of remaining growth that can be considered an absolute cutoff for TTO consideration. Most of the trepidation, surrounding osteotomy in the skeletal immature patient, results from the knowledge garnered from orthopedic surgeons who have treated the recurvatum sequelae associated with traumatic fractures of the tibial tuberosity.[14] A comprehensive understanding of the physeal anatomy about the knee is imperative when treating pediatric and adolescent patellofemoral instability, and in the case of a pathologically abnormal patellar height or TT-TG distances, alternative procedures such as the Roux-Goldthwait, Galeazzi, Nietosvaara technique, or distal patellar tendon transfer can be used to correct the aforementioned malalignment parameters.[2] We prefer to stage these patients, addressing all soft tissue incompetencies while the patient is skeletally immature, and perform a final TTO after skeletal maturity is achieved. It must be noted that apophyseal closure of the tibial tuberosity usually commences at ages 15 and 17 years for females and males, respectively.[15]

Other relative contraindications also exist and essentially follow the general principles of any other lower extremity surgery. These contraindications include, but are not limited to, infection, open wound near the operative site, and active medical comorbidities that preclude surgical intervention.

Operative

Numerous techniques and methods for TTO have been developed, since Roux's first description of tuberosity transfer in 1888,[16] and nuances exist that can make each surgeon's specific approach different. Furthermore, a whole industry has arisen with different manufacturing companies developing cutting guides and systems to aid in surgical accuracy and efficiency. The tubercle can be transferred in multiple directions, and the vector that is chosen depends on the pathology that needs to be addressed. Medialization and distalization are the two directions that are most commonly discussed when addressing patellar instability. Anterior and posterior transfers, the so-called *Maquet and Hauser procedures,* will not be discussed in this chapter, as the former is employed for relief of patellar overload and the latter is of historic interest only.

The anteromedialization (AMZ) or Fulkerson[17] procedure is an extremely versatile transfer, as the degree of anterior and medial movement of the tubercle can be titrated by the slope of the tibial cut, and this concept will be further discussed in the "Authors' Preferred Treatment" section of the chapter. An additional and important advantage to the oblique cut that is made during the AMZ procedure is the broader base of bone that is taken with the shingle, thus enabling improved healing while still allowing for a tibial cut entry point that is relatively anterior. In the face of patellofemoral instability, it must be noted that the medialization portion of the procedure is what provides improved stability of the joint and is what will be primarily discussed in the remainder of the chapter. Careful preoperative evaluation must assess the absence of disease in the proximal and medial cartilage of the patella, as these areas will see increased load after medialization. Indications for medial transfer of the tubercle include a TT-TG that is greater than 20 mm or for those individuals with a TT-TG of greater than 15 mm with recurrent instability and failure of a previous soft tissue procedure. Distal transfer of the tuberosity is indicated in those patients with recurrent patellofemoral instability and patella alta, as determined by a CD index greater than 1.3.

AUTHORS' PREFERRED TREATMENT

Evaluation

Indicating a pediatric or adolescent patient for a TTO requires meticulous preoperative planning coupled with a thorough discussion regarding risks and benefits of the proposed procedure with the patient and the family. A detailed history including age and mechanism of injury of the first dislocation, as well as number and frequency of any subsequent dislocations or subluxations, should also be noted. The degree of trauma that each episode occurred with is also important; frequently, dislocations will begin to occur more easily with less trauma. In addition to the patient's history of dislocations, it is also important to inquire about any family history of patellar instability. The treating surgeon must also be aware of any previous therapeutic interventions, both conservative and surgical.

Physical examination begins by assessing for the presence or absence of generalized ligamentous laxity, measured by the Beighton criteria.[18] In this patient population, it is also very important to check for any overt signs of a significant collagen disorder (Marfan syndrome or Ehlers-Danlos syndrome) or skeletal dysplasia, as these disorders can affect other organ systems as well. A global assessment of the knee must be undertaken, including appraisal of standing alignment (to rule out pathologic genu valgum) and the presence of any soft tissue injuries. The presence of a "J sign" is always evaluated for, as this is indicative of inappropriate tracking of the patella within the trochlear. Palpable crepitus with open chain knee extension is an important sign that suggests potential cartilage damage from the previous dislocation, and this finding warrants an MRI to further evaluate the patellofemoral articular surfaces. Assessment regarding the integrity of the medial patellofemoral ligament (MPFL) on both physical examination and advanced imaging is an integral part of the initial patient evaluation. Our preferred technique for evaluation of the MPFL on physical examination is accomplished with the quadrant method, whereby one hand stabilizes the femur and the other hand laterally subluxes the midbody of the patella with the knee in full extension. Subluxation laterally into the fourth quadrant (medial border of the patella able to sit flush with the lateral portion of the lateral femoral condyle) indicates incompetency of the MPFL, with frank instability of the patellofemoral joint. We also question the patient whether or not there is any apprehension when performing this maneuver and, most importantly, assess the quality of the end point during lateral translation. Evaluating for lateral retinacular tightness is important during preoperative planning for a TTO. To assess for lateral tightness, we prefer to hold the patella reduced within the trochlear with attempted eversion of the lateral patellar facet while the knee is in full extension. Pathologic tightness is ultimately diagnosed if the lateral facet cannot be everted to the neutral position.

Our preferred radiologic assessment of the knee includes both plain radiographs and an MRI of the affected knee. The radiographic series that we obtain in the clinic includes an anteroposterior (AP) and lateral view of knee, along with an axial view of the patellofemoral joint. Our preferred axial view is a true Merchant view obtained at 30 degrees of flexion; it is important to avoid excess flexion when obtaining this view. We do not routinely obtain long-leg standing x-rays unless there is clinical concern for pathologic genu valgum. The AP view allows us to assess for any associated lesions of the tibiofemoral compartment, along with the patency of the distal femoral and proximal tibial physes. The lateral view of the knee allows us to assess for patella alta with measurement of the CD index and allows us to assess for degree of trochlear dysplasia (supratrochlear spur or crossing sign). Importantly, the lateral view of the knee allows us to check the status of apophysis on the tibial tubercle, as we believe a TTO is contraindicated in those patients with an open apophysis of the tibial tubercle. By obtaining an axial view of the patellofemoral joint, we can better objectify the presence of any lateral-sided tightness or lateral displacement of the patella. The axial view allows for assessment of congruence, tilt, and any possible subluxation of the patella. The axial view also allows for assessment of overall joint space of the patella in relation to the trochlear, and narrowing in either facet (or early osteophytes) indicates some degree of cartilage loss.

All patients being considered for a TTO get MRI as part of their preoperative workup. We believe that an MRI offers several advantages over a CT; most importantly, it offers a reduction of radiation exposure in this younger population. An MRI can demonstrate a loose body if present and allow for a thorough inspection of all cartilaginous surfaces, including the exact location and grade of any patellar chondral defects. Importantly, MRI allows for evaluation of the MPFL from its origin, between the adductor tubercle and the epicondyle, to its insertion on the medial patella. An MRI can definitively demonstrate the degree and location of injury to this important ligament, which is the so-called essential lesion seen in patellar dislocations. We also use the MRI to confirm the CD index and measure the TT-TG. A CD index of 1.3 is used as the threshold for whether or not we distalize the shingle during the TTO procedure. The critical TT-TG distance we use for determination of whether or not the tubercle should be moved medially is 20 mm or greater.

A complete workup, as listed earlier, is essential when evaluating any pediatric or adolescent patient with suspected instability of the patellofemoral joint. It must be noted that often, the diagnoses of patellar instability will be made in conjunction with other outstanding pathology of the knee. We routinely address all lesions at the time of surgery, which may include a lateral release for the treatment of retinacular tightness or MPFL reconstruction for traumatic or attritional injury that has led to MPFL incompetency. We also proceed with a cartilage restoration procedure of the patella or trochlear if Outerbridge grade IV[19] disease is noted on MRI or seen at the time of surgery. It has been our experience and the experience of others[20] that untreated lesions of the cartilage on the superior medial portion of the patella will ultimately lead to a poor surgical result after medial transfer of the tuberosity. A detailed discussion of the concomitant procedures that may need to be performed concomitantly with TTO is outside of the scope of this chapter, and the next section mainly focuses on our surgical technique for an isolated transfer of the tibial tubercle.

Surgical Technique

Setup for the procedure includes supine positioning on a flat table with a lateral post to aid with the valgus moment needed during knee arthroscopy of the medial compartment. A bump is placed under the affected hip (we prefer a 1 L saline IV bag) to eliminate any obligate external rotation of the extremity and allows for adequate visualization of the lateral tibia to protect the neurovascular bundle during surgery. A nonsterile thigh tourniquet is also placed on the patient's lower extremity and used to maintain hemostasis during the open portion of the procedure. At our institution, we prefer regional anesthesia with a spinal and conscious sedation. We believe that the avoidance of general anesthesia eliminates unnecessary risks in this younger patient population and provides a quicker perioperative recovery. We would recommend against the use of a femoral nerve block for postoperative pain control, as this type of neuraxial anesthesia may negatively affect postoperative quadriceps function.

Prior to commencement of the operation, we perform a thorough bilateral knee examination under anesthesia. This repeat examination allows us to confirm the overall range of motion, mobility of the patella (including integrity of the MPFL), and tightness of the lateral retinaculum and document any other associated ligamentous injuries. We also perform a knee arthroscopy on any patient we have indicated for a TTO. Performing a knee arthroscopy prior to transfer of the tubercle has many distinct diagnostic and therapeutic advantages. During the arthroscopic portion of the procedure, we are able to carefully evaluate the undersurface of the patella, note the location and severity of any articular lesions, and remove any loose bodies that may have resulted from the episodes of instability. If the patellar undersurface has sustained articular injury, we routinely perform a gentle débridement of any loose cartilage flaps. In those patients with grade IV cartilage lesions, we perform concomitant cartilage reconstruction (at this time, we prefer allograft juvenile particulate cartilage [Denovo, Zimmer Inc., Warsaw, IN]). The lateral portion of the patellofemoral joint is then evaluated for any overhang of the lateral facet in relation to the lateral trochlear, thus giving us the sense of whether or not the patella is centered. The knee is gently flexed off the side of the bed to document the temporal and spatial engagement of the patella within the trochlear. The tibiofemoral compartments, notch, and respective gutters are then evaluated in a standard fashion. Finally, we will perform the lateral release if on our examination under anesthesia the patella was unable to be everted to neutral, indicating an overtly tight retinaculum, then evaluate the tightness of the lateral retinaculum and perform a lateral release if indicated.

Topographical landmarks for the TTO are then marked out (Fig. 19.1), the limb is exsanguinated with the use of 4-in. Esmarch, and the tourniquet is inflated to 250 mm Hg. The incision is longitudinal and is laterally based off the edge of the tibial tuberosity if any degree of anteriorization is to be performed along with the medialization. If a straight medialization is planned, then the incision is centered over the tubercle. The optimal incisional length is 5 to 6 cm, beginning at the proximal portion of the tubercle, continuing distally. A lateral-based incision has the distinct advantage of preventing the patient from kneeling on his or her scar, and it must be noted that the steeper the cut, the more lateral one needs to be to gain complete access to the posterior tibia. Using sharp dissection, the incision it taken down to the periosteum of the tubercle and large skin flaps are then created. Blunt finger dissection (alternatively accomplished with a lap pad and a periosteal elevator) can often be very effective for atraumatic exposure of the skin flaps that must extend proximal to the insertion of the patellar tendon, distally below the tubercle, and in the mediolateral direction to allow for appropriate access to the

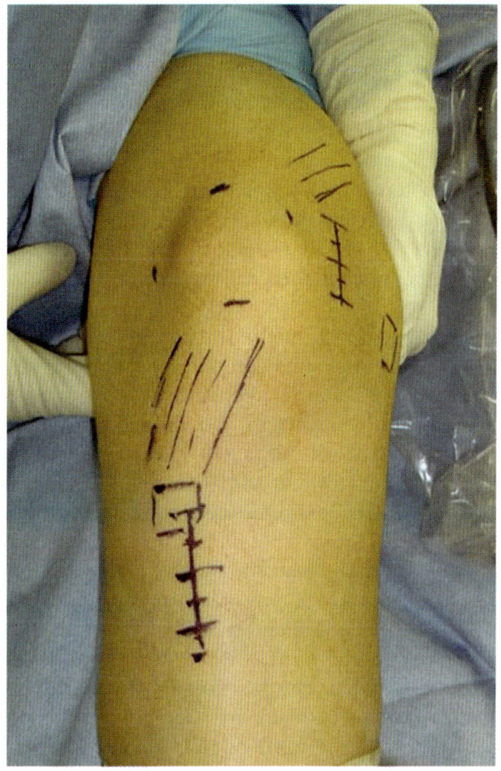

Figure 19.1. Demonstrates the overall topography of a patient with an excessive lateral tibial tubercle. Importantly, the incision for a TTO must be based on the lateral aspect of the tuberosity.

borders of the tibia. Developing large full-thickness skin flaps is a key to maintaining a small and cosmetic incision.

Next, we turn our attention to the inferior portion of the patellar tendon where it inserts into the superior portion of the tuberosity. Small capsulotomies are made on either side of the patellar tendon (Fig. 19.2). The medial and lateral borders

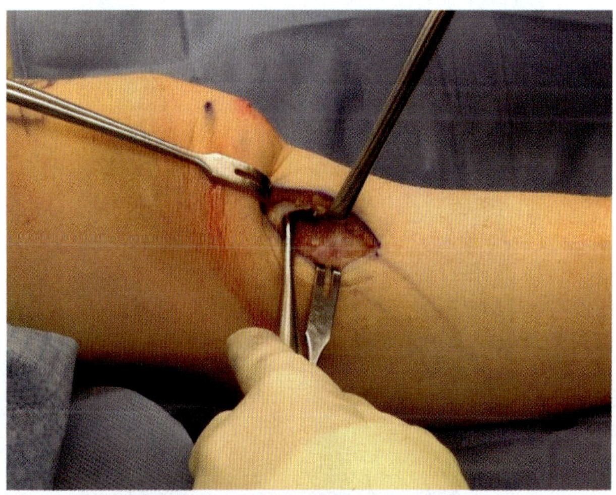

Figure 19.2. Shows the lateral capsulotomy that is necessary for complete mobilization of the distal portion of the patellar tendon. A periosteal elevator has been place transversely on the undersurface of the tendon, heading lateral to medial direction. A right-angle retractor has been placed under the tendon in retraction and tension during the mobilization process.

of the tendon must be free with scissor dissection, as eventually, this will need to be mobile for the transfer. Scissor dissection is then used to undermine the tendon, and a hemostat clamp is bluntly taken from lateral to medial to ensure complete mobility of the distal insertion of the tendon. Gently flexing the knee off the side of the table places the extensor mechanism on slight tension and greatly facilitates working around the borders of the distal patellar tendon attachment. Another pearl is to use a right-angle retractor under the tendon to allow for ventral retraction of the tendon during the undersurface dissection.

The length and width of the shingle are then marked out, and its borders are dissected with electrocautery. It is very important to maintain full-thickness periosteal tissue on the pedicle of the tuberosity and to not disrupt this important supply of vascular tissue that will ultimately facilitate osteotomy healing. Laterally, the anterior compartment must be atraumatically elevated off the tibia and safely retracted to protect the neurovascular structures. The shingle must be slightly wider than the patellar tendon and should be at least 5 cm in length (Fig. 19.3). Alternatively, if a distalization must also take place, the shingle can be made 6 cm in length, thus allowing for removal of the desired amount of distal bone to permit normalization of the CD index. On the proximal lateral border of the tibia, an oblique dissection in the superoanterior direction is carried out. This oblique connection is what allows for the connection cut between the tibial plateau and the tuberosity.

After careful exposure, two single-trocar 0.045-mm Kirschner wires (K-wires) are placed and serve as a template for the freehand cut. The K-wires are placed from the medial to lateral direction and should be angled in the anterior to posterior plane at either 30, 45, or 60 degrees, depending on the desired amount of anteriorization (if an anteriorization is being undertaken as an

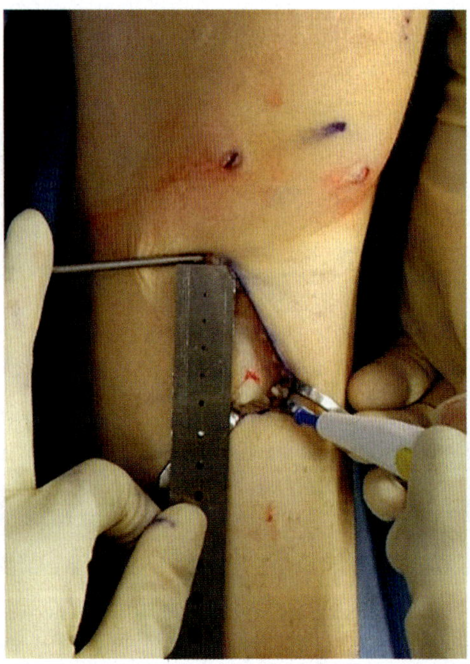

Figure 19.3. Demonstrates a rule which is used to mark out the overall length of the shingle; typically, at least 5 cm is used. Notice the overlying intact vascular periosteum.

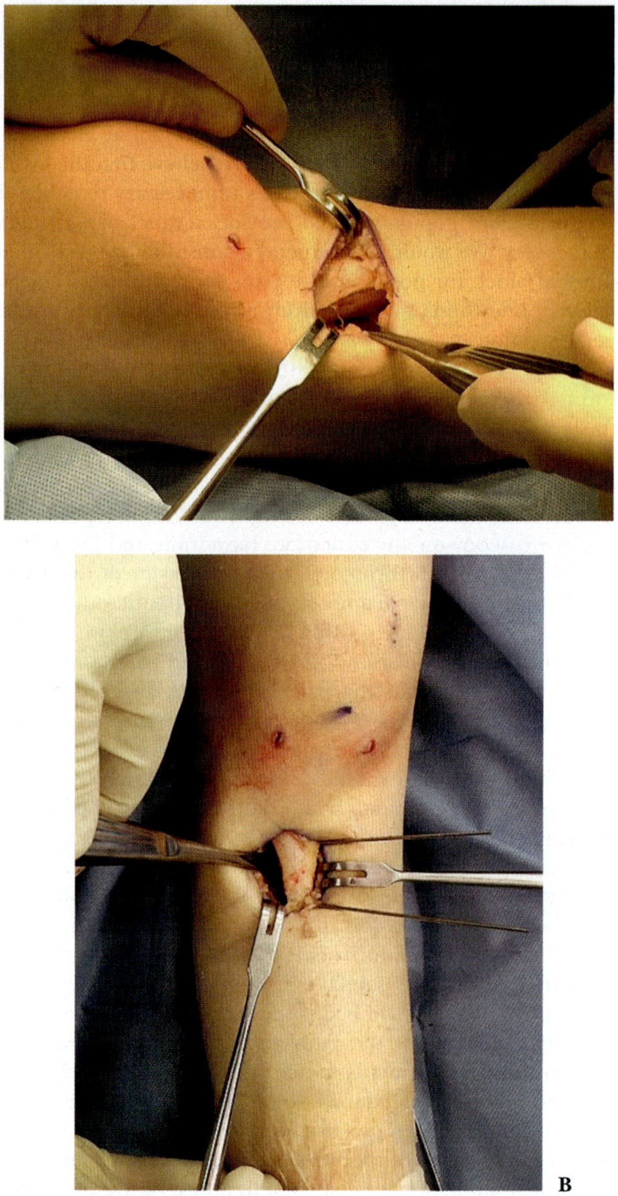

A

B

Figure 19.4. Demonstrates the shingle template prior to K-wire insertion **(A)** and shows the proximally and distally placed K-wires for cut templating/guidance purposes **(B)**. Notice that the K-wires are traversing in the medial to lateral direction and that a broad elevator is used to protect the anterior compartment musculature.

unloading portion of the osteotomy) (Fig. 19.4). If only coronal plane malalignment is being corrected with no anteriorization necessary, then the K-wires would be placed parallel to the floor to achieve a straight medialization. One K-wire is placed proximally and one is placed distally to help guide the osteotomy. A sagittal saw blade, 40 mm in size, is then used to cut the tibia. The cut is medially based and must progress in the anterior distal direction if AMZ is being performed. Broad periosteal elevators are placed on the posterior lateral border of the tibia and used for retraction of the anterior compartment and periosteum. Important pearls are to first score the bone medially to mark out the extent of the cut, to work in the proximal to distal direction, and to stay at the level of the previously placed K-wires and use

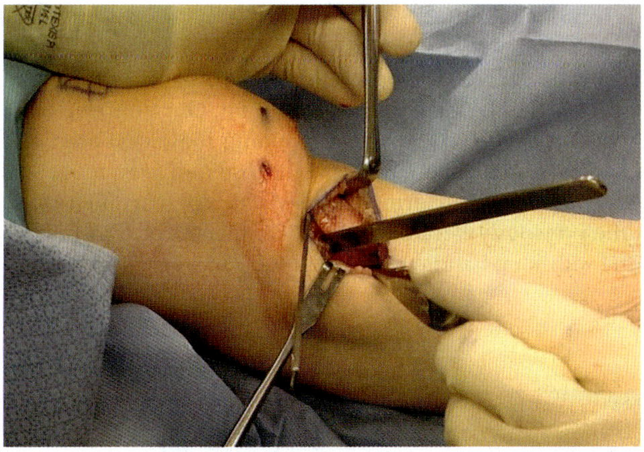

Figure 19.5. Demonstrates two thin flat osteotomes that are being used to complete the oblique portion of the proximal lateral osteotomy. This oblique cut connects the transverse cut just proximal to the patellar tendon insertion with the sagittal osteotomy or shingle.

their angle as saw guides. Next, we connect the dots to achieve a full-thickness cut with a straight 10-mm osteotome. A small 6-mm osteotome is used to make the transverse cut under the patellar tendon just proximal to its attachment on the anterior tibia (Fig. 19.5). A right-angle retractor is used during this portion of the case to elevate the tendon and avoid injury. At this point, we turn our attention to the oblique connection laterally, which is freed and completed with the use of a broad flat osteotome. The shingle should then be free to toggle, with its only remaining attachment site being distally based. If the shingle does not toggle, then any remaining medial, lateral, or proximal connections can be freed with an osteotome.

To free the distal portion of the tuberosity pedicle, a controlled greenstick fracture must be created. We accomplish this fracture with the use of a flat osteotome placed within the cut and then use controlled rotatory movements to crack the distal bone (while maintaining an intact periosteum). The osteotome must be placed as distal as possible within the cut to prevent fracture of the shingle more proximally than desired (Fig. 19.6). If we need to distalize the tuberosity, it is important that we preserve as much cancellous bone as possible and work the osteotome in the distal direction (with minimal rotatory movements). After the greenstick fracture is created, the tuberosity should be free to move en bloc with the extensor mechanism. The amount or degree of medialization should match the preoperative plan that appropriately corrects the TT-TG. We prefer to measure the amount of transfer with the width of an osteotome blade. The osteotome can then be left in situ to act as a shoe horn, during tuberosity fixation, so that no amount of correction is lost.

Once the tubercle is shifted, it must be fixed with two compression screws. We prefer to use a lag technique method to create good bony apposition at the osteotomy site. We first drill two 4.5-mm pilot holes at the center of the tubercle, taking great care to preserve an adequate bony bridge between screws. A 3.2-mm drill bit is then passed all the way through the distal 4.5-mm pilot holes into the posterior cortex and then left in place (unchucked from drill collet) to secure temporary fixation of the tuberosity (Fig. 19.7). Alternatively, this preliminary fixation can be achieved using a Steinmann

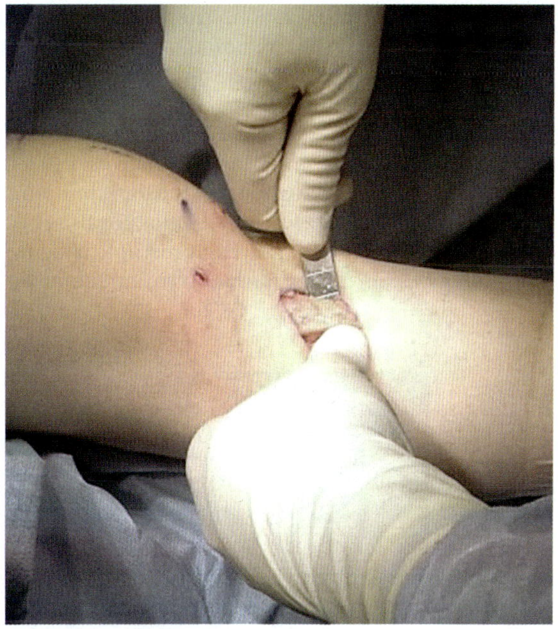

Figure 19.6. Shows the careful creation of a distally based greenstick fracture. A small flat osteotome is used and situated at the distal aspect of the cut to provide an improved lever arm. Controlled anteriorization with medial translation and rotation is used to create crack.

pin placed at a nonscrew portion of the bone to hold the shingle in place while the knee is placed through a full range of motion to check alignment. A second 3.2-mm drill bit is then placed through the proximal 4.5-mm anterior hole and drilled through the posterior cortex, and a fully threaded compression

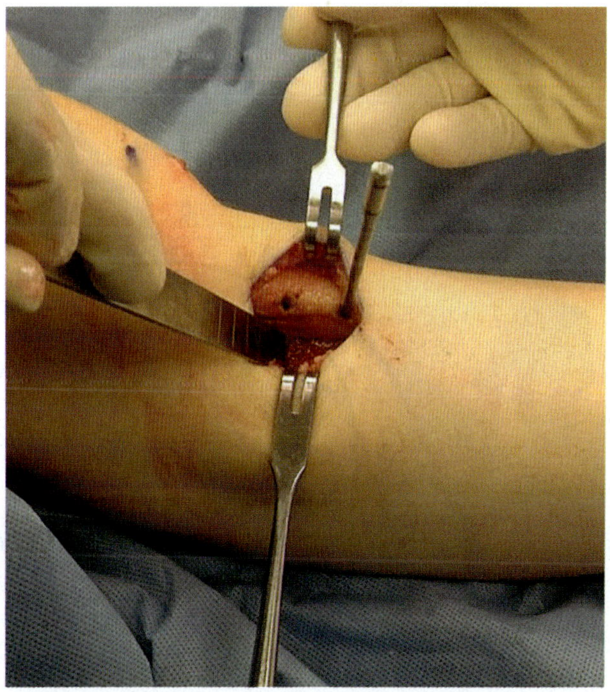

Figure 19.7. Demonstrates a 12-mm osteotome being used to measure and control the amount of correction and also shows a free 3.2-mm drill bit being used to temporarily secure the transferred tubercle prior to screw fixation.

screw is used for bicortical fixation. The preliminary fixation that was placed distally is then removed, and the 3.2-mm drill bit is drilled through the posterior cortex of the distal hole in a divergent fashion to the proximal screw and a second 4.5-mm fully threaded cortical screw is placed (Fig. 19.8). It must be noted that proximally, the bone can be relatively cancellous, and one should not expect as good of a bite or screw purchase that is felt with the distal screw. Screw lengths are also checked, after placement, with intraoperative fluoroscopic imaging.

Final points before closure include two important details. We routinely remove the proximal medial bone with a small rongeur that is now overhanging on the tibia, as it is usually a sharp edge that can be prominent and palpable to the patient in an area that has little subcutaneous fat. Our final step before a meticulous layered closure (including loose reapposition of the anterior compartment to the periosteum, preventing a cosmetic rent) is to perform a prophylactic compartment release of the previously elevated anterior compartment. The release is done with long-handle tissue dissection scissors.

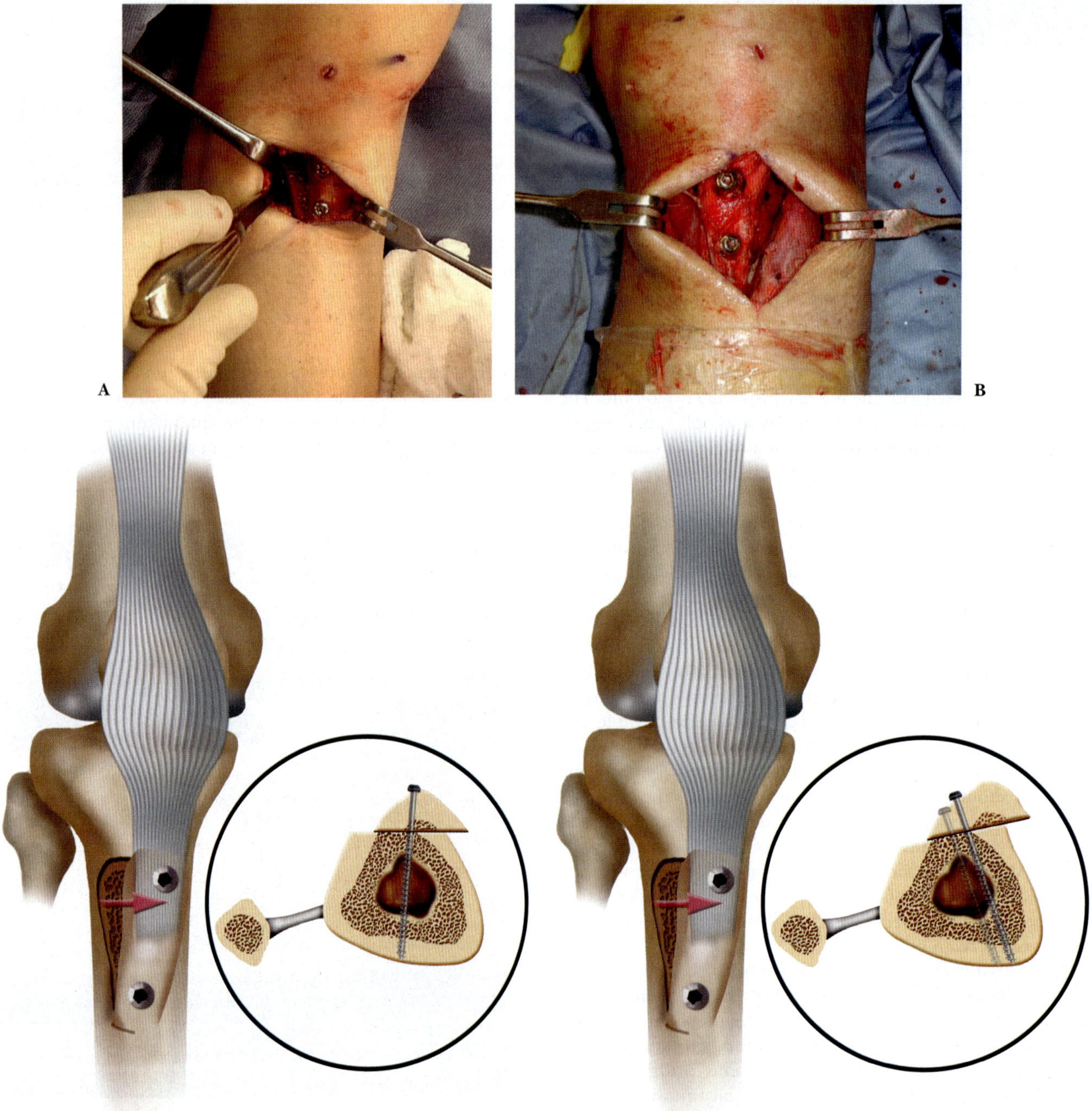

A B C D

Figure 19.8. **A,B.** Demonstrate a final pictorial representation of the TTO procedure. Notice broad cancellous base that allows for optimal healing. **C,D.** A schema demonstrating a medialization cut and an oblique cut (AMZ), highlighting the amount of correction that can be gained.

Rehabilitation

The immediate postoperative rehabilitation protocol that we prefer uses a hinged brace locked in extension. We also prefer the use of a continuous passive motion (CPM) machine. CPM parameters are initiated at 0 to 30 degrees and then advanced from 0 to 60 degrees as tolerated in the immediate perioperative period. The affected extremity is to remain strict non–weight bearing, and anecdotally, we often use a bone stimulator to aid in healing of the osteotomy site. An extended discussion of specific rehabilitation strategies and protocols is reserved for a later chapter.

Complications/Pearls on Avoiding

Various complications are associated with a TTO procedure that include delayed wound healing, skin necrosis, infection, tibia and/or tibial tuberosity fracture, delayed or nonunion of the osteotomy site, and hardware irritation necessitating later removal. Soft tissue healing and skin-related problems are generally attributed to overanteriorization of the tubercle, which is typically not a problem when transferring the tubercle for instability purposes. To facilitate healing of the osteotomy, we maintain weight-bearing restrictions for a minimum of 6 weeks and will often prescribe a bone stimulator. Fortunately, the rate of nonunion is rare after interfragmentary compression fixation, with an incidence of 3.7%.[21] Compartment syndrome and arthrofibrosis are two other devastating complications that can occur after TTO. We recommend a prophylactic compartment release of the anterior compartment and early range of motion to avoid these potential pitfalls.

REFERENCES

1. Dejour H, Walch G, Nove-Josserand, et al. Factors of patellar instability: an anatomic radiographic study. *Knee Surg Sports Traumatol Arthrosc.* 1994;2:19–26.
2. Weeks KD, Fabricant PD, Ladenhauf HN, et al. Surgical options for patellar stabilization in the skeletally immature patient. *Sports Med Arthrosc.* 2012;20:194–202.
3. Nietosvaara Y, Aalto K, Kallio PE. Acute patellar dislocation in children: incidence and associated osteochondral fractures. *J Pediatr Orthop.* 1994;14:513–515.
4. Fithian DC, Paxton EW, Stone ML, et al. Epidemiology and natural history of acute patellar dislocation. *Am J Sports Med.* 2004;32: 1114–11121.
5. Lewallen LW, McIntosh AL, Dahm D. Predictors of recurrent instability after acute patellofemoral dislocation in pediatric and adolescent patients. *Am J Sports Med.* 2013;41:575–581.
6. Stefancin JJ, Parker RD. First-time traumatic patellar dislocation: a systematic review. *Clin Orthop Relat Res.* 2007;455:93–101.
7. Sherman SL, Erickson BJ, Cvetanovich GJ, et al. Tibial tubercle osteotomy: indications, techniques, and outcomes. *Am J Sports Med.* 2013;42(8):2006–2017.
8. Dejour H, Walch G, Nove-Josserand L, et al. Factors of patellar instability: an anatomic radiographic study. *Knee Surg Sports Traumatol Arthrosc.* 1994;2:19–26.
9. Caton JH, Dejour D. Tibial tubercle osteotomy in patello-femoral instability and in patellar height abnormality. *Int Orthop.* 2010;34: 305–309.
10. Seitlinger G, Scheurecker G, Högler R, et al. Tibial tubercle-posterior cruciate ligament distance: a new measurement to define the position of the tibial tubercle in patients with patellar dislocation. *Am J Sports Med.* 2012;40:1119–1125.
11. Feller JA. Distal realignment (tibial tuberosity transfer). *Sports Med Arthrosc.* 2012;20:152–161.
12. Schoettle PB, Zanetti M, Seifert B, et al. The tibial tuberosity-trochlear groove distance; a comparative study between CT and MRI scanning. *Knee.* 2006;13:26–31.
13. Dejour H, Walch G, Neyret P, et al. Dysplasia of the femoral trochlear. *Rev Chir Orthop Reparatrice Appar Mot.* 1990;76:45–54.
14. Roy SP, Nag K. Simultaneous bilateral tibial tuberosity avulsion fractures in adolescence: case report and review of 60 years of literature. *Injury.* 2013;44:1953–1955.
15. Georgiou G, Dimitrakopoulou A, Siapkara A, et al. Simultaneous bilateral tibial tubercle avulsion fracture in an adolescent: a case report and review of the literature. *Knee.* 2007;15:147–149.
16. Dejour D, Le Coultre B. Osteotomies in patello-femoral instabilities. *Sports Med Arthrosc.* 2007;15:39–46.
17. Fulkerson JP. Anteromedialization of the tibial tuberosity for patellofemoral malalignment. *Clin Orthop Relat Res.* 1983;(177):176–181.
18. Beighton PH, Solomon L, Soskoline CL. Articular mobility in an African population. *Ann Rheum Dis.* 1973;32:413–417.
19. Outerbridge RE. The etiology of chondromalacia patellae. *J Bone Joint Surg Br.* 1961;43-B:752–757.
20. Pidoriano AJ, Weinstein RN, Buuck DA, et al. Correlation of patellar articular lesions with results from anteromedial tibial tubercle transfer. *Am J Sports Med.* 1997;25:533–537.
21. Farr J, Schepsis A, Cole B, et al. Anteromedialization: review and technique. *J Knee Surg.* 2007;20:120–128.

CHAPTER

20

Theresa A. Chiaia
Sarah M. Baker

Rehabilitation following Patellar Instability

INTRODUCTION

Patellar dislocation is a common injury found in children and adolescents, accounting for 2% to 3% of all knee injuries.[1] Four clinical categories of patellar instability for the pediatric and adolescent population have been described to conceptualize pathology: posttraumatic, syndromic, obligatory, and fixed.[2] Traumatic dislocations are the most common and are then further categorized as first-time or recurrent dislocators.

There are many variables that can affect the course of postoperative rehabilitation such as the nature of the injury (traumatic or atraumatic), concomitant injuries and/or procedures, the level of dysfunction (development of compensatory patterns), the chronicity of the dysfunction, the degree of pathology, the age of the patient, and the surgical procedure. Predisposing factors must be recognized: prior history of dislocation, genetic, ligamentous laxity, skeletal dysplasias, collagen disorders, muscular imbalances, and/or faulty movement strategies.

The medial patellofemoral ligament (MPFL), a discrete component of the medial retinaculum, guides the patella to properly engage the trochlea during early knee flexion. MPFL reconstruction (MPFLR) uses allograft or autograft tissue tensioned to balance the patella within the trochlear groove—it is a soft tissue procedure which requires 12 weeks of healing (Fig. 20.1A).

A tibial tubercle transfer (TTT) is a bone procedure—an osteotomy of the tibial tubercle (Fig. 20.1B). Due to the more extensive pathology and more invasive nature of a distal realignment, or TTT, the patient will have restricted weight bearing. Once the bone has healed and patients are fully weight bearing and functioning pain free, their progression is criterion-based and individualized, much like the patient with an MPFLR. These patients are about 6 weeks behind those status post isolated MPFLR in the earlier stages due to the restricted weight bearing. This will delay the introduction of postural stability, neuromuscular (NM) control, quadriceps strengthening, and, obviously, gait training.

The following guidelines and time frames are based on an isolated MPFLR. Please note the different time frames for an MPFL (Appendix 1) versus a TTT (Appendix 2). The presence of underlying or concomitant pathology will lengthen the rehabilitation process for these patients.

PREOPERATIVE PHASE

Build a Foundation

The individual can work toward building a foundation of muscular balance prior to surgery. Emphasis will be on the core, the pelvis, hips, and quadriceps and can include postural retraining, soft tissue lengthening, progressive strengthening, and NM control. With chronic dislocators, this is achieved with a home exercise program (HEP) and/or working with a performance coach. In the case of the acute traumatic dislocator, the goal of physical therapy (PT) is to prepare the knee for surgery: control effusion, regain quadriceps function, regain full ROM, and normalize gait.

Set Realistic Expectations

Prepare the patient for the road ahead. The course of rehabilitation, with emphasis on progression of function, is discussed with the patient. If a patient is not seen preoperatively, this should be done at the initial evaluation postoperatively.

Patients tend to be more compliant and less frustrated when they understand what to expect. Realistic expectations are outlined regarding ambulation/crutches, brace, pain, activity modification, exercise progression, function, PT visits, and the patient's goals. Ballpark time frames are discussed in the context of criterion-based progression.

Gait/Ambulation

The first inquiries we hear from the patient are related to crutches and the brace: When will I be off crutches? How long will I have to wear this brace? In the athletic individual, the first question is when can I play again?

Following MPFLR, the patient will be weight bearing as tolerated (WBAT) with the brace locked in extension for the initial 4 to 6 weeks. After 2 to 3 weeks, the patient may be ambulating without crutches as long as the knee is tolerating the load. This is determined by the absence of active swelling, well-controlled pain, return of quadriceps contraction, and progression of range of motion (ROM). With progression of quadriceps strength and NM control at the knee, the brace

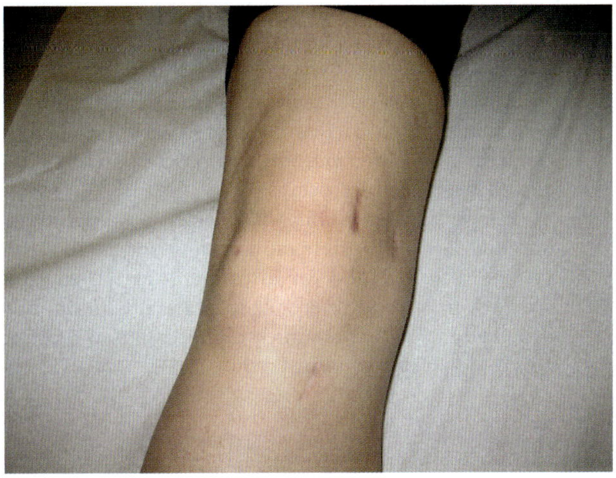

A

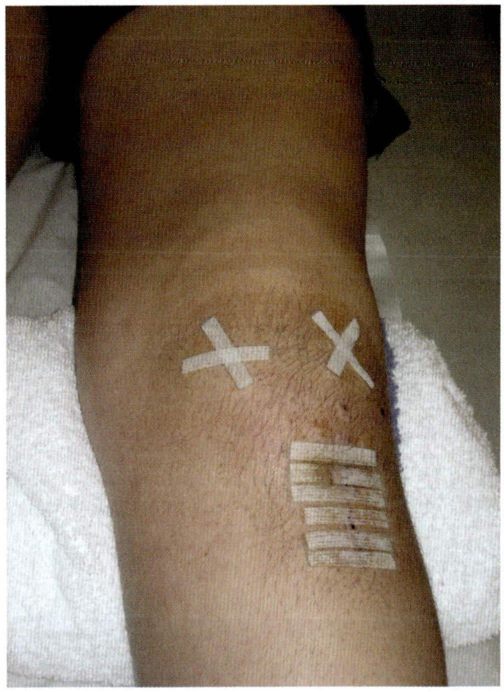

B

Figure 20.1. **A.** Medial patellofemoral ligament reconstruction incision. **B.** Tibial tubercle transfer incision.

will be unlocked from 0 to 60 degrees at a minimum depending on the available ROM (with increased knee flexion ROM, the brace will be opened to a greater degree); however, the patient will be returned to crutches WBAT when the brace is unlocked to help foster a normal gait pattern. Always confirm weight bearing and ROM restrictions with the surgeon because they might change based on graft choice and/or surgeon preference.

Following TTT, the patient will be non–weight bearing or toe-touch weight bearing (TTWB)—depending on the surgeon's preference—with the brace locked in extension for the initial 6 weeks. Radiographs at 6 weeks will guide the progression of weight bearing with crutches and the brace locked in extension over the course of the next 2 to 3 weeks (equals 8 weeks postoperatively). The progression of weight bearing will be guided by the surgeon. The knee's tolerance to weight bearing is monitored. During weeks 9 and 10, the patient ambulates full weight bearing (FWB) with the brace locked in extension, devoid of an assistive device. Crutches are reintroduced when the brace is unlocked at week 11 and are used WBAT until the patient demonstrates the ability to achieve full knee extension at heel strike and tolerate adequate knee flexion and weight bearing during the loading response.

Cryotherapy

The patient is encouraged to continue to use cryotherapy throughout the rehabilitation process as the level of activity continues to change.

Activity Modification

The patient's activity level will be guided by the knee's tolerance, not the patient's tolerance, to activity. This is determined by pain, swelling, ROM progression, and quadriceps function.

Therapy Visits

How many times a week do I have to come to therapy? PT visits must be managed. In this school-age population, use all resources available to the patient: the school athletic trainer, the school nurse, and school equipment.

Therapeutic Exercise

Exercise is discussed as it relates to functional progression and activity level. Progression will be based on the return of muscle balance and strategy of movement. Emphasis is on quality of movement: movement strategy, alignment, symmetry, and control.

PHASE I: PROTECTION PHASE (WEEKS 0 TO 6)

The stage is set for the rehabilitation process in this initial 6 weeks. Postoperative treatment includes a home-based program of a continuous passive motion (CPM) machine, quadriceps setting with neuromuscular electrical stimulation (NMES), and cryotherapy. Following TTT, a bone stimulator will be added to the home program. The goals of controlling pain and effusion, minimizing quadriceps inhibition, regaining knee ROM, and patellar mobility are interrelated. The patient is seen once during this phase at 3 to 4 weeks for an ROM check and progression of the HEP to include ROM in the seated position, quadriceps setting, straight-leg raise (SLR) series as tolerated—pain-free SLR in supine (with brace or without brace), hip abduction in side lying or prone, and hip extension in prone; heel raises (MPFLR) or plantarflexion with resistance bands (TTT); and gastrocnemius stretching. If ROM is less than 90 degrees, then formal PT is continued. If ROM is 90 degrees with a good end feel, then the patient continues with a home-based program until the 6-week mark.

Cryotherapy

Even minimal quadriceps effusion has been shown to inhibit quadriceps function. After dextrose saline was injected at 50 mm Hg into nonpathologic knees, quadriceps peak torque, muscle fiber conduction velocity, and root mean square of electromyography (EMG) signals of the vastus medialis were significantly decreased. After 20 minutes of ice application, quadriceps torque and muscle fiber conduction velocity significantly increased as compared to controls.[3] Joint effusion can lead to increased pain and decreased ROM, so it is imperative that patients use cryotherapy immediately and often postoperatively.

Gait/Ambulation

The patient is in a brace locked in extension with an appropriate assistive device: WBAT following MPFLR and NWB following TTT.

Therapeutic Exercise

Balance and Proprioception

Weight shifting onto the operative side can be introduced with the brace locked in extension for the MPFLR patient.

Strength

Quadriceps: NMES is used for quadriceps reeducation to abate loss of quadriceps strength and control. Most research with NMES has been done with patients after ACL reconstruction but the same benefits are observed clinically.[4]

Patients are instructed in quad sets over a towel roll both with and without NMES. The use of the towel roll provides tactile feedback and minimizes fat pad irritation. The goal is to do a pain-free SLR with no lag by the end of this phase. When that is accomplished, they have demonstrated enough quad control to ambulate with brace unlocked.

Proximal and Distal: Evaluation-based gluteal strengthening is initiated. The patient can begin NWB hip strengthening including abduction while standing on the contralateral leg, then progress to side-lying hip abduction against gravity.[5] Distal strengthening is initiated to address weaknesses and prepare for push-off.

Range of Motion

The MPFL tightens in early to midflexion and then slackens during deeper flexion after 60 degrees.[6,7] A CPM is used 2 to 3 hours per day or 6 to 8 hours with a concomitant cartilage procedure. If a joint is immobilized too long, there will be a loss of ground substance and dehydration in the extracellular matrix, leading to approximation of the fibers.[8,9] This approximation causes friction and the formation of adhesions. Active and passive ROM at the knee joint will reverse damaging effects of immobilization by stimulating collagen synthesis and optimizing the alignment of healing tissues.

Patients begin seated at the edge of the plinth for active–assistive range of motion (AAROM) into knee flexion. They then use the contralateral leg for passive knee extension to avoid open chain knee extension early on with quadriceps weakness and especially with cartilage injury. Communication with the surgeon is imperative in this phase if knee flexion is not progressing.

A loss of passive extension is not often seen, but full extension must be maintained via gastrocnemius and hamstring stretching and intermittent heel prop so an antalgic gait on a flexed knee does not occur.

Passive patellar mobility is assessed postoperatively to make sure there is appropriate mobility and end point. The quadrant system[10] can be used for assessment, as the contralateral leg may not be a good reference if bilateral hypermobility is present. Patients will sometimes demonstrate apprehension with this due to a history of instability.

Precautions

Patellar mobilization in the lateral direction is avoided in this early phase to allow for healing; however, it is evaluated by the physical therapist to get a sense of its end point. Be cautious not to load the knee with slight knee flexion, as this is the ROM that the MPFL is most vulnerable because there is no bony stability offered by the trochlea. Following TTT, the patient must obey the restricted weight bearing because this is a bony procedure and complications are related to fixation and possible fracture through the osteotomy or screw holes.

Troubleshooting

In the first few visits, get a sense of the progression of knee flexion ROM to avoid postoperative stiffness. Reasons for stiffness after MPFLR include chondral injuries, femoral tunnel malpositioning, improper graft tensioning, excessive pain, or noncompliance with PT.[11,12]

PHASE II: GAIT PHASE (MEDIAL PATELLOFEMORAL LIGAMENT RECONSTRUCTION: WEEKS 7 TO 10; TIBIAL TUBERCLE TRANSFER: WEEKS 7 TO 12)

The goal is to foster a normalized gait pattern. The hallmark of this phase is NM control, alignment, and postural stability in single limb stance.

Control Symptoms

Monitoring the knee for active swelling and pain with resultant loss of motion and quadriceps function is necessary, as the patient's activity level usually increases during this phase. Staying within his or her envelope of function is continually reinforced.

Standing Posture

Postural retraining with a neutral pelvis with sternal lift and soft knees with symmetrical weight bearing is reinforced throughout the day. (A simple reminder of postural checks when "texting" with friends.) Weight bearing through one hip only is discouraged as is hanging on ligaments with recurvatum in double-limb weight bearing.

Gait/Ambulation

Gait training is performed with an assistive device, or on a hydro-treadmill (with adequate wound healing) or antigravity treadmill, if available. During this time, a normal gait pattern is emphasized:

- *Full knee extension at heel strike.* Without active knee extension ROM to 0 degree, the individual will not achieve full knee extension during heel strike and will walk with a bent knee gait. This will continually load the extensor mechanism and result in anterior knee pain.
- *Adequate knee flexion during loading response.* Inadequate NM/eccentric control at the knee and/or pain will not allow the knee to go from knee extension to slight knee flexion during the loading response, resulting in knee extension with sinking into the hip during the loading response. This will, in essence, make the stance leg longer and lead to hip adduction and lengthening of the abductors with resultant weakness (Fig. 20.2). This gait pattern is one of quad avoidance and is often present preoperatively. It will continue postoperatively if not addressed and is often present on the contralateral limb. Decreased shock absorption is a consequence which then leads to increased loading at the tibiofemoral joint and progressive deterioration.[13]

The individual will be weaned from the assistive device as eccentric quadriceps strength and NM control improve, thereby increasing the tolerance to load and normalizing gait. The assistive device also slows the patient down and encourages quality of gait while discouraging quick, unpredictable movements inherent in this population. In an urban setting or school environment, the assistive device also provides a sign to others to go around. The individual may be allowed to ambulate without an assistive device in a controlled setting such as at home.

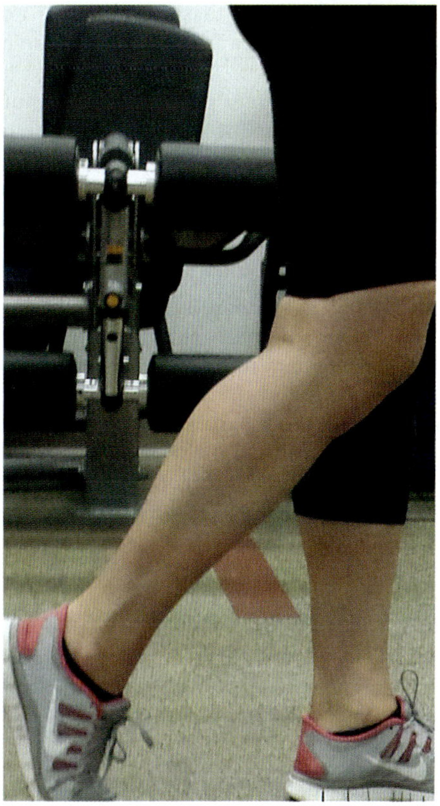

Figure 20.3. Release of the knee at heel off to initiate swing phase. Length of two joint hip flexors is required.

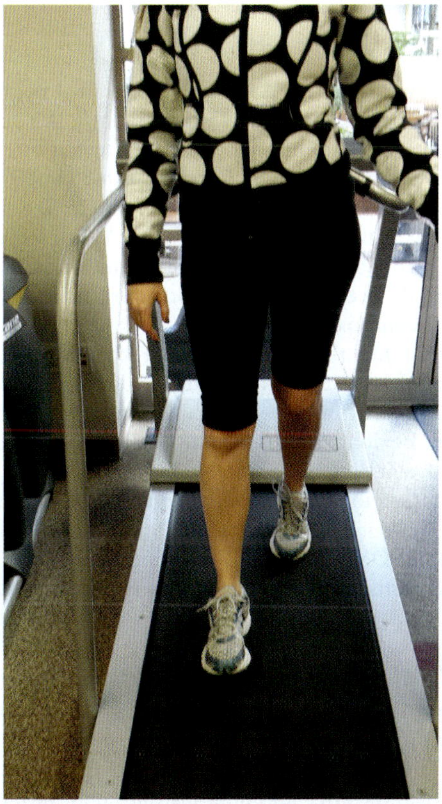

Figure 20.2. Poor NM/eccentric control during the loading response results in hip adduction.

Therapeutic exercise can be used to break down the gait cycle. Release of the knee at heel off (to initiate swing phase) (Fig. 20.3) and weight shift (retrostepping or forward stepping) onto involved limb with a soft knee (stance) are practiced.

Therapeutic Exercise

Neuromuscular Control and Proprioception

Reestablishing NM control at the knee joint is an important piece of the rehabilitation process and is required for full functional recovery. The objective of NM training is to improve the nervous system's ability to generate fast and optimal muscle firing patterns and thus increase dynamic joint stability and decrease joint forces.[22] This training can enhance the patient's awareness of peripheral sensations and thus process these signals into more coordinated motor strategies. It is required during daily life and sports-specific activities. Balance training with double-limb support is introduced in the sagittal plane on a balance board, rocker board, or commercial balance system. With good alignment and NM control, single limb stance is performed on a level surface. The rehabilitation specialist must watch for quality and ensure that the patient is not working in genu recurvatum but has a "soft knee" with the quadriceps engaged (Fig. 20.4).

Water is a good medium to practice this until full weight is tolerated on land. With enhanced NM control, the patient can hopefully protect the joint from further injury.[23]

The MPFL seems to resist lateral patellar subluxation most near knee extension, and it has been shown that proprioception is of great importance to protect the joint against extreme flexion and extension movements. Enhanced proprioception will help decrease stress on a newly reconstructed MPFL near full knee extension when it is relied on the most.[24] It is important to consider the patient population you are working with and their preoperative status. Jerosch and Prymka[24] showed that patients with posttraumatic recurrent patellar dislocation had highly significant deterioration in the proprioception of the injured knee joint. Compared to controls, these patients also had a worse position sense in their uninjured contralateral leg. Because they often already have a deficit, it is even more important to train this system postoperatively.

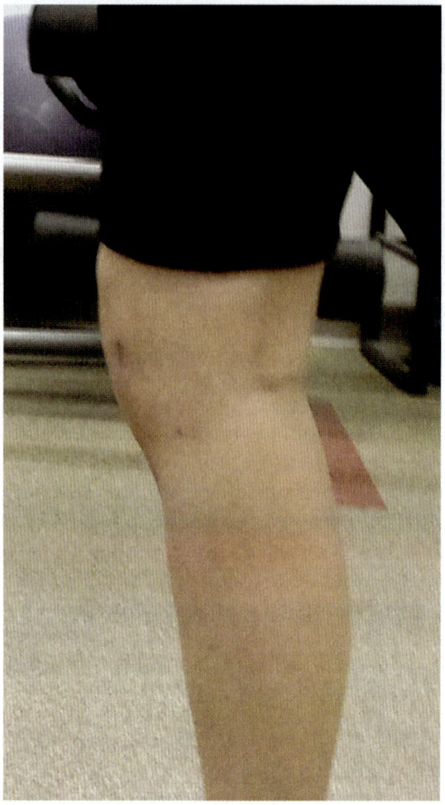

Figure 20.4. Single limb stance requires alignment + neuromuscular control + stability. This demonstrates NM control which is important for normal loading response.

Strength

Quality of movement is emphasized with functional strength training.

Quadriceps: Quadriceps strengthening is essential and must be performed in a pain-free arc of motion. Understanding the biomechanics of the patellofemoral joint, patellofemoral joint stress, joint reaction forces, contact areas, and, if present, the location of cartilage lesion will aid exercise prescription.[16–18] Closed-chain quadriceps strengthening, such as leg press, is introduced at latter phase 1/early phase 2 (MPFLR) with adequate ROM and quadriceps function. The weight lifted is a delicate balance between stimulating the quadriceps muscle and not overloading the patellofemoral joint. In an effort to compensate for weakness and/or pain, a number of compensations may be observed: hip hike to open up the knee angle to decrease patellofemoral stress and high or deep foot placement on the leg press or the step, respectively, to increase use of posterior musculature (the knee is extended through the action of the hip extensors instead of the quadriceps).

Proximal: *Proximal strengthening* continues to progress with emphasis on the gluteus maximus, gluteus medius, and abdominals to control limb alignment.[19] Non–weight-bearing hip extension with knee flexion can be performed in prone, quadruped, or bent over the side of the table until bridging and other weight-bearing exercises are tolerated. To preferentially train the gluteals while minimizing contribution from tensor fascia lata, the clamshell, side steps, unilateral bridge, and quadruped hip extension are used.[20] The Sahrmann[21] deep abdominal progression can be introduced along with planks. All exercises when performed correctly should engage the core. The authors believe that Sahrmann level 3 is important for athletes to achieve.

Range of Motion/Flexibility

Progression of ROM is without limits. At 60-degree knee flexion, the patella is fully engaged in the groove and the MPFL is at its maximum length. As quadriceps control is gained, and knee flexion ROM increases to approximately 125 degrees, the patient can begin supine wall slides and a stair stretch. Short crank cycle ergometry can be initiated with 80 to 90 degrees of knee flexion. As knee flexion increases to 115 degrees, a standard upright stationary bike is tolerated.[14] With increased ability on the standard stationary bike, the individual is instructed to consistently pedal at 80 revolutions per minute (RPMs) to control the compressive forces.

Two joint hip flexor length must be addressed because 60 degrees of knee flexion with hip extension is required for limb advancement in gait.[15] Initially, the patient can perform active knee flexion with the hip in neutral extension in prone and then in standing to begin to achieve this.

Mobility of the patella is monitored for postoperative complications such as medial subluxation, lateral subluxation, knee flexion ROM as a result of scarring, overtightening of the medial restraints, and/or an overzealous lateral release.

Precautions

Proprioceptive training in the coronal or transverse plane is introduced in this phase to respect the healing process. Soft tissue healing is a 12-week process. If the patient lacks adequate NM control at the knee and demonstrates poor hip/pelvic control, the healing graft will be at risk before the patella is engaged in the trochlea.

PHASE III: STRENGTHENING (MEDIAL PATELLOFEMORAL LIGAMENT RECONSTRUCTION: WEEKS 11 TO 18+; TIBIAL TUBERCLE TRANSFER: WEEKS 13 TO 24+)

Be Patient! Explore the Cause!

This phase presents an opportunity to assess the biomechanical issues unique to that individual which may have put him or her at risk for injury and/or pain. The patella is most unstable near full extension and during early flexion, relying on soft tissue restraints, lower extremity alignment, and bony geometry for stability. MPFL function becomes more critical when soft tissue imbalances, muscular imbalances, lack of NM control, structural abnormalities, and/or limb malalignment are present. Predisposing factors that play a role in patellofemoral joint stress and contribute to patellar instability are addressed. Local as well as proximal and distal factors contribute to dynamic alignment of the lower extremity. The focus is now on the individual presentation of that patient as it relates to the surgical procedure and not just on the surgical procedure. The return of muscle balance, in particular quadriceps function in this phase, will ultimately dictate the length of the rehabilitation process.

Gait/Ambulation

Normalization of gait on level surfaces and stairs is the goal.

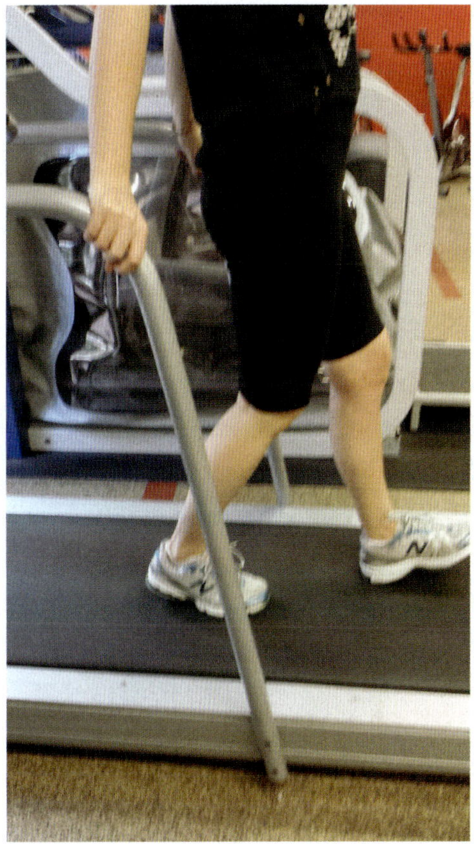

Figure 20.5. Retro treadmill (RTM). Retrostepping with controlled heel descent is used to achieve NM/eccentric control at the knee.

Therapeutic Exercise

Balance and Proprioception

As stated earlier, patellar dislocation causes a decrease in knee joint proprioception. Decreased position sense could be the cause of injury as well as the result of injury. Numerous authors have shown the presence of mechanoreceptors in structures responsible for patella stability.[24] NM control can be further challenged with ambulating backward (Fig. 20.5) on a treadmill, which has been found to help facilitate quadriceps control during midstance and dynamic balance.[25,26] Multiple planes (beginning with frontal plane and progressing to transverse plane) and unstable surfaces can be added. Alignment and stability in single limb stance on a level surface are the prerequisites. A general rule of thumb for progressive proprioception training is to decrease the base of support and increase surface difficulty. Patients can progress from double leg to single leg, stable surface to unstable surface, uniplanar directional challenges to multiplanar challenges, static to dynamic to reactive, and eyes open to eyes closed. Various commercial products are available to help challenge balance in all directions.

Strengthening

Quadriceps: Stay the course. Return of quadriceps function depends on many previously described variables and time frames can vary. Concomitant procedures, in particular cartilage procedures, will guide exercise selection. The location of the lesion and subjective complaints must be taken into account. Squatting is introduced in a pain-free arc of motion with enough strength to perform symmetrically and pain-free. The author's preferred method is stand to sit in a chair (Fig. 20.6). A foam cushion is added so the individual works in the available range (based on pain, strength, symmetry). A ball can be used if it supplements the free squat. It is not functional if the feet are forward and the patient is leaning on the ball. Close attention is paid to symptoms, movement strategy, symmetry, and alignment. In the sagittal plane, there should be a balanced hip and knee strategy to decrease potential patellofemoral joint overload.[27] Often, patients need instruction to initiate the movement with their hips instead of their knees and to sit back into hip flexion with a natural trunk inclination to achieve this.

Leg press can progress from double leg to single leg eccentric to prepare for forward step-up (FSU) and forward step-downs (FSDs). As the individual demonstrates the ability to ascend a 6-in step without compensations, the elliptical trainer can be added. Improved eccentric quadriceps control is demonstrated with FSD.[28] Note that peak patellofemoral joint stress is 20% greater during the FSD exercise as a result of increased patellofemoral joint reaction forces. A higher knee extensor moment and increased knee flexion angle contribute to this.[29] Knee flexion during the FSD is performed with the hip extended—requiring appropriate length of the two joint hip flexors. Perform this exercise when it is pain-free, without compensatory strategies, and on a height that meets the patient's functional level. In the frontal and transverse planes, it is important to monitor FSU and FSD to ensure that the knee does not fall into a functional valgus with femoral internal rotation and adduction or demonstrate a contralateral hip drop (Fig. 20.7).

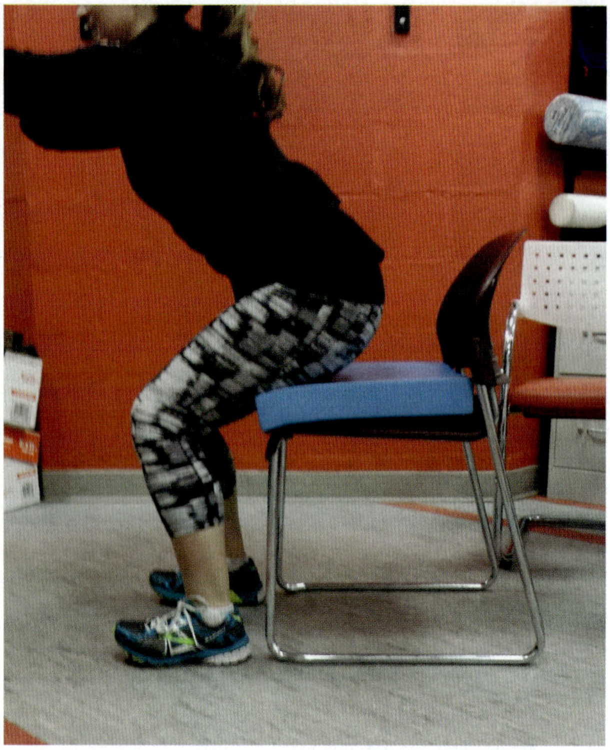

Figure 20.6. The squat is practiced with stand to sit in a chair. A cushion is added to work within the patient's functional ability: pain-free and good form.

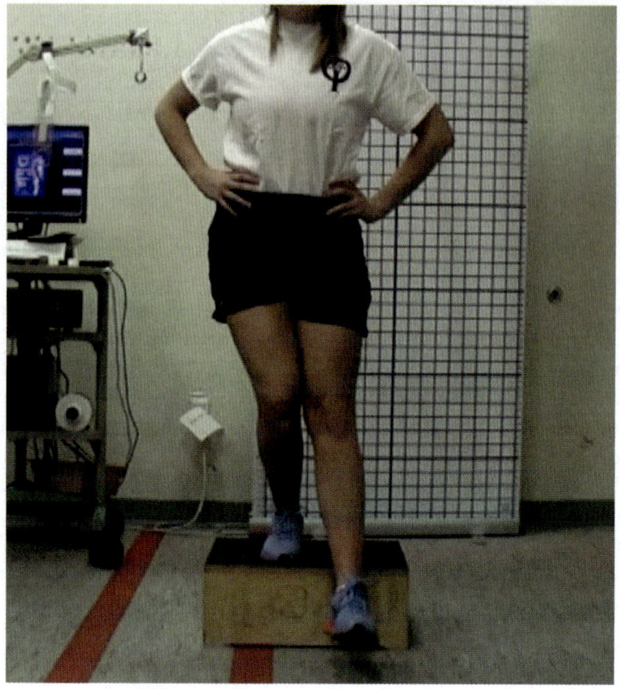

Figure 20.7. Functional valgus during the FSD can occur because of pain, structural limitations, soft tissue limitations, decreased hip stability, and/or quadriceps weakness.

This is a common movement pattern that may be present with pain, structural or soft tissue limitations, decreased hip stability, and/or quadriceps weakness. One can also see poor control (eccentric drop) as a result of quadriceps weakness and/or pain. A mirror for visual feedback is very helpful.

Proximal: *Proximal and distal strengthening* continues and is now progressed in the weight-bearing position. Bolgla and Uhl[5] found weight-bearing exercises such as closed-chain hip abduction and pelvic drop apply greater external torque on the hip and require greater gluteus medius EMG activity. They are also more functional and appropriate for patients as they are fully weight bearing. Distefano et al.[19] found single-leg squat and single limb deadlift exercises were prime gluteus maximus activators. Other options include side steps versus resistance band, hip clocks, and windmills for total lower extremity strengthening with a focus on gluteal strengthening because there is growing evidence in the literature linking poor gluteal strength and pelvic control with patellofemoral pain.[30] Findings by both Powers et al.[31] and Souza et al.[32] suggest that control of femoral internal rotation can help restore normal patellofemoral joint mechanics.[30]

Range of Motion/Flexibility

ROM/flexibility proximal and distal to the knee is evaluated and addressed. Foam rolling with the addition of horizontal release and active ROM can be effective. Continue to assess two joint hip flexors length as well as address limitations in ankle mobility (especially dorsiflexion) and triceps surae length. Decreased dorsiflexion at the talocrural joint can contribute to functional valgus by causing increased pronation as the motion comes from the subtalar joint.

Progression of Functional Training

Demonstration of adequate eccentric quadriceps and gluteal strength and endurance in order to maintain good single limb alignment and stability will allow the individual to initiate more dynamic activities such as running (intervals) and plyometrics (bilateral jumps up).

Precautions

This can be a long phase especially in this population who does not have a foundation of strength prior to injury. Ignoring quality of movement and criteria-based progression will lead to movement compensations, pain, ups and downs in rehabilitation, frustration, and ultimately delay of functional progression.

PHASE IV: ADVANCED STRENGTHENING AND FUNCTION (MEDIAL PATELLOFEMORAL LIGAMENT RECONSTRUCTION: WEEKS 19 TO 24; TIBIAL TUBERCLE TRANSFER: TIME FRAME IS APPROXIMATELY 8 WEEKS)

Cardiovascular Fitness

It can be achieved with cross-training. Changing one variable at a time and with a 10% increase are guidelines that allow the individual to progress safely. Cycling with high RPMs initially, with manipulation of resistance and time, helps keep compressive forces low.

Plyometrics

Plyometrics can progress to squat jump, jumping rope, then to jumping down. Jumping progresses from vertical jumping and landing to horizontal jumping and landing. The athlete progresses to single-limb jumping with adequate strength and movement strategies. This is a prerequisite for deceleration training.

PHASE V: RETURN TO PLAY (MEDIAL PATELLOFEMORAL LIGAMENT RECONSTRUCTION: WEEKS 25 TO 30+; TIBIAL TUBERCLE TRANSFER: AT 36 TO 52 WEEKS)

Return to play following MPFLR or TTT occurs at approximately 6 to 9 months or 12 months postoperative, respectively.

A patient must present with a lack of pain and apprehension with sport-specific movements to meet the demands of his or her particular sport. Qualitative and quantitative measures are used to safely return the patient to play.[33] Sport-specific actions and drills should be completed easily, pain-free, and with confidence in a safe and controlled environment such as the clinic before an athlete returns to the field. He or she must have the ability to demonstrate functional movements such as deceleration with running, the ability to change direction with running, control, and alignment with takeoff and landing in double-leg and single-leg jumps. A patient should attain at least 85% limb symmetry in a single-leg hop test or crossover hop test. Dynamic assessment tools such as the Star Excursion Balance Test[34] can be used in conjunction with patient-reported outcome measures (PROMs) such as the Kujala[35] or Knee Injury and Osteoarthritis Outcome Score (KOOS).[36] Although these measurements are quantitative in nature, continue to assess for quality of movement. At this point in the rehabilitation process, the athlete is often already transferred to a trainer or coach, especially if insurance has limited visits. For a successful transition to the field, it is important to communicate with all providers and the referring surgeon about the athlete's readiness to return to play. Once back, the athlete should continue a maintenance program focused on flexibility; soft tissue balance; NM control; and quadriceps, core, and gluteal strengthening to maintain good functional alignment and decrease stress on recently repaired structures.

Appendix 1

HOSPITAL
FOR
SPECIAL
SURGERY

Sports Rehabilitation & Performance Center
Medial Patellofemoral Ligament Reconstruction Guidelines© *

The following MPFL guidelines were developed by the Sports Rehabilitation and Performance Center team at Hospital for Special Surgery. Progression is based on healing constraints, functional progression specific to the patient. Phases and time frames are designed to give the clinician a general sense of progression. Acute versus chronic, as well as, concomitant procedures such as cartilage procedure, lateral release, tibial tubercle transfer will alter the guideline.

Follow physician's modifications as prescribed

Phase I: Protection Phase (Weeks 0–6)

GOALS:

- Independence in home therapeutic exercise (HEP) program
- Promote healing
- Control post-operative pain/swelling
- Prevent quadriceps inhibition: fair to good quadriceps contraction
- Straight leg raise (SLR) without lag, pain-free
- ROM: 0° KE to ≥90° KF
- Independent ambulation WBAT with brace locked in extension, and appropriate assistive device on level surfaces and stairs

Emphasize
- Ambulation with brace locked in extension
- Improving quadriceps contraction
- Controlling pain/effusion
- Compliance with home instructions: cold therapy unit, CPM, quadriceps re-education with estim unit

PRECAUTIONS:

- Ambulation without brace
- Lateralization of patella
- AA-AROM KE, especially with significant quad atrophy, and articular cartilage injury
- Symptom provocation: quadriceps shut down, joint effusion, active inflammation
- KF ROM as per surgeon's guidelines

TREATMENT RECOMMENDATIONS:

- Emphasize patient compliance to HEP and weight bearing precautions/progression
  - WBAT with brace locked in extension with appropriate assistive device on level surfaces and stairs
  - Cryotherapy: home cold therapy unit
  - **C**ontinuous **P**assive **M**otion: 2–3 hours/day; with cartilage procedure = 6–8 hours/day
  - Electrical stimulation for quadriceps re-education: quadriceps sets with towel roll under knee
- Sitting knee ROM exercise: AAROM KF, PROM KE
- Quad set with towel roll under knee
- Hip progressive resisted exercises: pain-free SLR with brace if lag is present
- Distal strengthening (PF)
- Flexibility exercises (hamstrings, gastrocnemius)

MINIMUM CRITERIA FOR ADVANCEMENT TO NEXT PHASE:

- Fair to good quadriceps contraction
- Good patellar mobility in medial direction
- ROM: 0° knee extension to ≥90° knee flexion
- 0/10 pain at rest
- Able to SLR pain-free without quadriceps lag

* Developed by the HSS Rehabilitation Department Sports Rehabilitation and Performance Center
525 East 71st Street Belaire Building, Ground Floor Tel: 212.606.1005 Fax: 212.774.2089

Page 1 of 5

HOSPITAL FOR SPECIAL SURGERY

Phase II: Gait Phase (weeks 7–10)

GOALS:

- Independence in HEP, as instructed
- Control pain, inflammation, effusion
- Promote healing
- ROM 0° KE-110° KF (8 weeks), 120° (10 weeks) to full ROM
- Good patella mobility
- Good quad contraction
- Normalize gait with brace and assistive device, prn
- Postural stability, alignment and N-M control in single limb stance
- 0/10 pain with ADLs, therapeutic exercise: Recognize pain-free arc of motion

Emphasize

- Symptom control with ADLs, therex
- Minimizing knee effusion
- Normal gait pattern
- Postural stability, alignment, neuro-muscular (N-M) control during stance

PRECAUTIONS:

- Sign and symptom provocation: pain, inflammation, quadriceps shut down, joint effusion
- Concomitant procedures: TTT, articular cartilage procedure
- Lateralization of the patella
- Pathological gait pattern (quadriceps avoidance; bent knee)
- Arc of motion during exercise

TREATMENT RECOMMENDATIONS:

- HEP: advance as tolerated. Continue phase I exercises, as appropriate
- Patient education: Activity modification, progression of gait training, cryotherapy
- Patellar mobilization, MD directed
- ROM exercises:
  - Sitting PROM to AAROM KE in a pain-free arc of motion (no cartilage injury) to AAROM KF
  - KF: sitting progressing to stair ROM, supine wall ROM as tolerated (~125°KF in sitting, quad control)
- Gait training: heel toe gait pattern with brace open to 90° or functional brace and assistive device [with adequate quad control (SLR without a lag, ability to achieve terminal knee extension) and knee ROM] to ensure normal loading response; hydro–treadmill (adequate wound healing) or anti gravity treadmill. Low grade elevation or retro-walking to encourage N-M control with KF during loading response
- Quadriceps strengthening: progress pain-free arc of motion, close chain preferred
  - Continue with Estim, biofeedback, quad sets, submaximal multi angle isometrics, as needed
  - Leg press: monitor arc of motion (bilateral, eccentric)
  - Initiate forward step up (FSU) progression, 6″ step with adequate strength
- Bicycle: progressing from short crank to standard crank as ROM allows (115° KF in sitting), 80 RPMs
- Flexibility exercises - evaluation-based: AROM KF with hip extension in standing
- Advance proximal strength and core training: (i.e. hip extension with knee flexion, side planks, bridge)
- Hydrotherapy for gait, single limb alignment and stability, proximal strengthening
- Initiate balance and proprioceptive training: double limb support on progressively challenging surfaces to single limb support on level surface only with demonstration of good alignment, stability and N-M control

MINIMUM CRITERIA FOR ADVANCEMENT:

- ROM 0° KE → 115° KF
- Normal gait pattern
- Good patella mobility
- Postural stability, alignment and N-M control in single limb stance
- 0/10 pain with ADLs and therapeutic exercise
- Independent HEP

HOSPITAL
FOR
SPECIAL
SURGERY

PHASE III: STRENGTHENING (WEEKS 11–18+)

Emphasize

- Normal gait
- Identifying and addressing muscle/soft tissue imbalances
- Neuromuscular control
- Functional progression
- Quality of movement

GOALS:

- Independent HEP
- Control pain, effusion and inflammation
- 0/10 pain with ADLs, therapeutic exercise
- ROM: WNLs, 130° (12 weeks)
- Normalize gait on level surfaces and stairs
- Address imbalances
- Core stability: Single leg bridge = 30 s, Sahrmann ≥ level 3
- Good single limb dynamic balance
- Eccentric quadriceps and pelvic control with 6″/8″ FSD
- Initiate running program, plyometrics (bilateral)
- Symmetry, quality, alignment during selected movement patterns: squat, jump in place

PRECAUTIONS:

- Sign and symptom provocation: pain, and active inflammation/effusion, quadriceps shutdown
- Gait deviations
- "Too much, too soon" progression
- Disregarding quality of movement

TREATMENT RECOMMENDATIONS:

- HEP, as instructed
- Educate patient: Activity modification, individualized, and cryotherapy
- Quadriceps strengthening: progress as tolerated, monitor arc of motion, closed chain preferred
  - FSU progression: 6″ step progressing to 8″ step (dependent on patient height)
  - Eccentric leg press progressing to:
  - Forward step down (FSD) progression: 6″ step progressing to 8″ step (dependent on patient height)
  - Squat progression: chair squats, (use ball if necessary with buttocks moving under ball), to free squats
- ROM exercises:
  - (AA) ROM KE (monitor arc of motion) to AAROM KF in sitting to supine wall slides to stair stretch
- Gait training to emphasize heel-toe gait pattern with emphasis on loading response
- Advance proximal strength through functional activities (bridging progression, hip extension with KF, clock, RDL, windmill, lawn mower) and core training (planks, side planks, Sahrmann progression)
- Balance progression with postural alignment and N-M control (static to dynamic, introduce different planes of motion, challenging surfaces)
- Address muscle imbalances – evaluation-based: (i.e. 2 joint hip flexor length)
- Cross training: elliptical trainer initiated with good strength/quality during 6″ FSU, bicycle (80 RPMs), swimming (crawl, back stroke)
- Initiate running program (late phase): with eccentric quadriceps control during 8″ FSD and MD clearance
  - 30 second interval initially
- Initiate plyometric program with MD clearance and evidence of good eccentric quadriceps control
  - Vertical jumping progression: Jump up to jump in place

CRITERIA FOR ADVANCEMENT:

- ROM WNLs
- No pain or swelling
- Normalize gait
- Ability to demonstrate alignment, control, stability in single limb stance during dynamic activities
- Core stability: Single leg bridge = 30 s, Sahrmann ≥ level 3
- Able to ascend 6″/8″ step with good control
- Able to descend 6″/8″ step with good control, and alignment
- Symmetry, quality, alignment during selected movement patterns
- Independence in a home exercise program

* Developed by the HSS Rehabilitation Department Sports Rehabilitation and Performance Center
525 East 71st Street Belaire Building, Ground Floor Tel: 212.606.1005 Fax: 212.774.2089

HOSPITAL FOR SPECIAL SURGERY

Phase IV: Advanced Strengthening and Function (weeks 19–24)

Emphasize
- Quality of movement
- Functional progression

GOALS:

- Lack of pain, apprehension with sport specific movements
- Maximize strength and flexibility as to meet demands of individual's sport activity
- Ability to demonstrate strategy, symmetry, quality, control and alignment during selected movement patterns: squat, jump (vertical and horizontal), single leg squat
- Isokinetic test: 180°/sec and 300°/sec 85% limb symmetry index (LSI)
- Cardiovascular fitness to meet demands of sport

PRECAUTIONS:

- Pain with therapeutic exercise & functional activities
- Inadequate strength, functional strength, ROM, flexibility, fitness when returning to sport

TREATMENT RECOMMENDATIONS:

- Continue to advance LE strengthening, flexibility, dynamic single limb stability & agility programs
- Continue to address muscle imbalances – evaluation-based
- Advance core stability
- Cross training
- Advance plyometric program with MD clearance and evidence of good eccentric quadriceps control
  - Vertical jumping progression: Jump down
  - Horizontal jumping progression: Broad jump, single leg landings
  - Progress running program
  - Cutting, deceleration, change of direction with MD clearance and dynamic single limb stability

CRITERIA FOR ADVANCEMENT:

- Isokinetic test at 180°/sec and 300°/sec: 85% limb symmetry index (LSI)
- Demonstrate symmetry, quality, alignment during selected movement patterns
- Medical clearance by surgeon for return to play progression
- Lack of apprehension with sport specific movements
- Flexibility to meet demands of sport

* Developed by the HSS Rehabilitation Department Sports Rehabilitation and Performance Center
525 East 71st Street Belaire Building, Ground Floor Tel: 212.606.1005 Fax: 212.774.2089

HOSPITAL
FOR
SPECIAL
SURGERY

PHASE V: RETURN TO PLAY (WEEKS 25–30)

GOALS:

- Lack of pain, apprehension with sport specific movements
- Maximize strength and flexibility as to meet demands of individual's sport activity
- Ability to decelerate with good control, and alignment on single limb
- Isokinetic test: 180°/sec and 300°/sec 85% limb symmetry index (LSI)
- Cardiovascular fitness to meet demands of sport
- Hop Test ≥ 85% limb symmetry

PRECAUTIONS:

- Pain with therapeutic exercise & functional activities
- Inadequate strength, functional strength, ROM, flexibility, fitness when returning to sport

TREATMENT RECOMMENDATIONS:

- Continue to advance LE strengthening, flexibility, dynamic single limb stability, core stability & agility
- Advance plyometric program: with MD clearance
    - Horizontal jumping progression: Broad jump to Hop to opposite to Single leg hop
- Advance cutting, deceleration training
- Progress cardiovascular fitness to meet demands of sport

CRITERIA FOR DISCHARGE:

- Isokinetic test: 180°/sec and 300°/sec 85% limb symmetry index (LSI)
- Ability to decelerate with good control, and alignment on single limb
- Medical clearance by surgeon for return to play
- Hop Test ≥ 85% limb symmetry
- Lack of apprehension with sport specific movements
- Flexibility to meet demands of sport
- Independence with gym program for maintenance and progression of therapeutic exercise program
- Demonstrate quality of movement with required sports specific activities

* Developed by the HSS Rehabilitation Department Sports Rehabilitation and Performance Center
525 East 71st Street Belaire Building, Ground Floor Tel: 212.606.1005 Fax: 212.774.2089

Appendix 2

HOSPITAL FOR **SPECIAL SURGERY**

Sports Rehabilitation & Performance Center
Tibial Tubercle Transfer Guidelines© *

The following TTT guidelines were developed by the Sports Rehabilitation and Performance Center team at Hospital for Special Surgery. Progression is both criteria-based and patient specific. Phases and time frames are designed to give the clinician a general sense of progression. Concomitant procedures such as cartilage procedure, lateral release, medial patellofemoral ligament repair/reconstruction, as well as chronicity of condition will alter the guideline.

Follow physician's modifications as prescribed

PHASE I: PROTECTION PHASE (WEEKS 0–6)

GOALS:

- Independence in home therapeutic exercise (HEP) program
- Promote healing
- Control post-operative pain/swelling
- Prevent quadriceps inhibition: fair quadriceps contraction
- Straight leg raise (SLR) without lag, pain-free
- ROM: 0° KE to ≥90° KF
- Independent ambulation NWB with crutches and brace locked in extension, on level surfaces and stairs

Emphasize

- Non weight bearing status
- Improving quadriceps contraction
- Controlling pain/effusion
- PROM KE
- Compliance with home instructions: cold therapy unit, CPM, bone stimulator, quad re-ed with estim unit

PRECAUTIONS:

- Weight bearing status
- Avoid AA-AROM KE
- Symptom provocation: quadriceps shut down, joint effusion, active inflammation
- KF ROM as per surgeon's guidelines

TREATMENT RECOMMENDATIONS:

- Emphasize patient compliance to HEP and weight bearing precautions/progression
    - NWB with brace locked in extension with crutches on level surfaces and stairs
    - Cryotherapy: home cold therapy unit
    - **C**ontinuous **P**assive **M**otion: 3–4 hours/day; with cartilage procedure: 6–8 hours/day
    - Bone stimulator: 20 minutes/day (2–3×)
    - Electrical stimulation for quadriceps re-education: towel roll under knee
- Sitting knee ROM exercise: A/AAROM KF, PROM for KE
- Quad set with towel roll under knee
- Patella mobilization as per MD guidelines
- Hip progressive resisted exercises: pain-free SLR with brace until no lag
- Distal strengthening (elastic band for triceps surae)
- Flexibility exercises (hamstrings, gastrocnemius)

MINIMUM CRITERIA FOR ADVANCEMENT TO NEXT PHASE:

- Radiographic evidence of adequate healing, and clearance from surgeon
- Fair quadriceps contraction
- Good patellar mobility
- ROM: 0° knee extension to ≥90° KF
- 0/10 pain at rest
- Able to SLR pain-free without quadriceps lag

* Developed by the HSS Rehabilitation Department Sports Rehabilitation and Performance Center
525 East 71st Street Belaire Building, Ground Floor Tel: 212.606.1005 Fax: 212.774.2089

HOSPITAL
FOR
SPECIAL
SURGERY

Phase II: Gait Phase (weeks 7–12)

Emphasize

- Symptom control with ADLs, therex
- Minimizing knee effusion
- Normal gait pattern
- Postural stability, alignment, n-m control in single limb stance

GOALS:

- Independence in HEP, as instructed
- Control pain, inflammation, effusion
- Promote healing
- ROM 0° KE-110° KF (8 wks.), 130°KF (12 wks.) to full ROM
- Good patella mobility
- Good quadriceps contraction
- Normalize gait without an assistive device
- 0/10 pain with ADLs, therapeutic exercise: Establish pain-free arc of motion
- Weight bearing progression as per surgeon's guidelines based on radiographic evidence of healing

PRECAUTIONS:

- Sign and symptom provocation: pain, inflammation, quadriceps shut down, joint effusion
- Cartilage procedure
- Progression of weight bearing as per surgeon's prescription
- Pathological gait pattern (quadriceps avoidance; bent knee)
- Pain-free arc of motion during exercise

TREATMENT RECOMMENDATIONS:

- HEP: advance as tolerated. Continue phase I exercises, as appropriate
- Patient education: Activity modification, progression of gait training, cryotherapy
- Patellar mobilization, as per surgeon's guidelines
- ROM exercises:
  - Sitting PROM - AAROM KE in a pain free arc of motion, (no cartilage injury) to AROM - AAROM KF
  - KF: sitting progressing to supine wall ROM, as tol (~125°KF in sitting, quadriceps control, pain-free)
- Gait training: wks 7–8 =WBing progression, MD directed with crutches and brace locked in extension. Wks 9–10: WBAT with brace locked in extension without an assistive device. Wks 11–12: normalize gait pattern with brace open or functional brace and assistive device to ensure KF during loading response; hydro–treadmill (adequate wound healing) or anti-gravity treadmill. Retro-walking to encourage n-m control with KF during loading response
- Quadriceps strengthening progression in pain-free arc of motion (esp. w/ known cartilage injury/procedure)
  - Continue with Estim, biofeedback, submaximal multi angle isometrics
  - Leg press: monitor arc of motion (bilateral, eccentric in latter phase)
- Bicycle: progressing from short crank to standard crank as ROM allows (115° KF in sitting), 80 RPMs
- Flexibility exercises - evaluation-based: AROM KF with hip extension in standing
- Advance proximal strengthening and core: (i.e. hip extension with knee flexion, side planks, bridge)
- Hydrotherapy for gait, single limb alignment and stability, strengthening
- Initiate balance and proprioceptive training: double limb support on progressively challenging surfaces to single limb support on level surface only with demonstration of good alignment, stability and n-m control

MINIMUM CRITERIA FOR ADVANCEMENT:

- ROM 0° KE → 130° KF
- Normal gait pattern without assistive device
- Good patella mobility
- Postural stability, alignment and neuromuscular control in single limb stance
- 0/10 pain with ADLs and therapeutic exercise
- Independent HEP

* Developed by the HSS Rehabilitation Department Sports Rehabilitation and Performance Center
525 East 71st Street Belaire Building, Ground Floor Tel: 212.606.1005 Fax: 212.774.2089

HOSPITAL FOR SPECIAL SURGERY

Phase III: Strengthening (weeks 13–24+)

GOALS:

- Independent HEP
- Patient education
- Control pain, effusion and inflammation
- 0/10 pain with ADLs, therapeutic exercise
- ROM: WNLs
- Normalize gait on level surfaces and stairs
- Good single limb dynamic balance
- Good eccentric quadriceps control
- Pelvic control during step down

Emphasize

- Normal gait
- Identifying and addressing muscle/soft tissue imbalances
- Neuromuscular control
- Functional progression
- Quality of movement

PRECAUTIONS:

- Sign and symptom provocation: pain, and active inflammation/ effusion, quadriceps shutdown
- Gait deviations
  "Too much, too soon" progression
- Overloading the joint
- Disregarding quality of movement

TREATMENT RECOMMENDATIONS:

- HEP, as instructed
- Educate patient: Activity modification, individualized, and cryotherapy
- Quadriceps strengthening: progress as tol, monitor arc of motion, closed chain preferred
  - Forward Step Up (FSU) progression: pain-free, 6″ step progressing to 8″ step (patient height dependent)
  - Eccentric leg press progressing to:
  - Forward step down (FSD) progression: 6″ step progressing to 8″ step (dependent on patient height)
  - Squat progression: chair squats, [ball squats if necessary (with buttocks moving under ball)], to free squats
- ROM exercises:
  - (AA)ROM KE (monitor arc of motion) to AAROM KF in sitting and supine wall slides to stair stretch
- Gait training to emphasize heel-toe gait pattern with emphasis on loading response
  - Treadmill: utilize small grade elevation (%) to encourage loading response
  - Retro-walking for neuromuscular control during loading response
- Advance proximal strength through functional activities: (bridging progression, hip extension with KF, clock, RDL, windmill, lawnmower) and core training (planks, side planks, Sahrmann progression)
- Balance progression with postural alignment and N-M control (static to dynamic, introduce different planes of motion)
- Address muscle imbalances – evaluation-based: (i.e. 2 joint hip flexor length)
- Cross training: elliptical trainer initiated with good strength/quality during 6″ FSU, bicycle (80 RPMs), swimming (crawl, back stroke)

CRITERIA FOR ADVANCEMENT:

- ROM WNLs
- No pain or swelling
- Normalize gait
- Ability to demonstrate alignment, control, stability in single limb stance during dynamic activities
- Core stability: Single leg bridge = 30s, Sahrmann ≥ level 3
- Able to ascend 6″/8″ step with good control, and alignment
- Able to descend 6″/8″ step with good control, and alignment
- Symmetry, quality, alignment during selected movement patterns
- Independence in a home exercise program

* Developed by the HSS Rehabilitation Department Sports Rehabilitation and Performance Center
525 East 71st Street Belaire Building, Ground Floor Tel: 212.606.1005 Fax: 212.774.2089

HOSPITAL FOR SPECIAL SURGERY

Phase IV: Advanced Strengthening and Function (~8 weeks duration)

GOALS:

- Control pain with sport specific movements
- 0/10 pain with ADLs, therapeutic exercise
- Strength and flexibility to meet demands of sport
- Isokinetic test: 180°/sec and 300°/sec 85% limb symmetry index (LSI)
- Ability to demonstrate movement strategy, symmetry, quality, control and alignment during selected movement patterns: squat, jump (vertical and horizontal), single leg squat
- Good single limb dynamic balance
- Cardiovascular fitness to meet demands of sport

PRECAUTIONS:

- Pain with therapeutic exercise & functional activities
- Inadequate strength, functional strength, ROM, flexibility, for progression

TREATMENT RECOMMENDATIONS:

- Continue to advance LE strengthening, flexibility, dynamic single limb stability & agility
- Continue to address muscle imbalances – evaluation-based
- Advance core stability
- Cross training
- Initiate plyometric program: with MD clearance and evidence of good eccentric quadriceps control
    - Vertical jumping progression: Jump up progressing to Jump in place progressing to Jump down
- Initiate running program: with evidence of eccentric quadriceps control during 8″ FSD and MD clearance
    - Start with 30 second intervals

CRITERIA FOR ADVANCEMENT:

- Good single limb dynamic balance
- Isokinetic test at 180°/sec and 300°/sec: 85% limb symmetry index (LSI)
- Medical clearance by surgeon for return to play progression
- Demonstrate symmetrical, quality, alignment during selected movement patterns
- Cardiovascular fitness, flexibility to meet demands of sport
- Independence with gym program for progression of therapeutic exercise program

* Developed by the HSS Rehabilitation Department Sports Rehabilitation and Performance Center
525 East 71st Street Belaire Building, Ground Floor Tel: 212.606.1005 Fax: 212.774.2089

HOSPITAL FOR SPECIAL SURGERY

Phase V: Return to Play (~8 weeks duration; 36–52 weeks)

GOALS:

- Lack of pain, apprehension with sport specific movements
- Maximize strength and flexibility as to meet demands of individual's sport activity
- Ability to decelerate with good control, and alignment on single limb
- Symmetry, quality, alignment during selected movement patterns
- Ability to demonstrate hip strategy, alignment, and control, with take-off and landing
- Isokinetic test: 180°/sec and 300°/sec 85% limb symmetry index (LSI)
- Cardiovascular fitness to meet demands of sport

PRECAUTIONS:

- Pain with therapeutic exercise & functional activities
- Inadequate strength, functional strength, ROM, flexibility, fitness when returning to sport

TREATMENT RECOMMENDATIONS:

- Continue to advance LE strengthening, flexibility, dynamic single limb stability, core stability & agility
- Advance plyometric program: with MD clearance
    - Horizontal jumping progression: Broad jump to Hop to opposite to Single leg hop
- Advance cutting, deceleration training
- Progress cardiovascular fitness to meet demands of sport

CRITERIA FOR DISCHARGE:

- Isokinetic test: 180°/sec and 300°/sec 85% limb symmetry index (LSI)
- Ability to decelerate with good control, and alignment on single limb
- Medical clearance by surgeon for return to play
- Hop Test ≥ 85% limb symmetry
- Lack of apprehension with sport specific movements
- Flexibility to meet demands of sport
- Independence with gym program for maintenance and progression of therapeutic exercise program
- Demonstrate quality of movement with required sports specific activities

* Developed by the HSS Rehabilitation Department Sports Rehabilitation and Performance Center
525 East 71st Street Belaire Building, Ground Floor Tel: 212.606.1005 Fax: 212.774.2089

REFERENCES

1. Stefancin JJ, Parker RD. First-time traumatic patellar dislocation: a systematic review. *Clin Orthop Relat Res.* 2007;455:93–101.
2. Weeks KD III, Fabricant PD, Ladenhauf HN, et al. Surgical options for patellar stabilization in the skeletally immature patient. *Sports Med Arthrosc.* 2012;20(3):194–202.
3. Rice D, McNair PJ, Dalbeth N. Effects of cryotherapy on arthrogenic muscle inhibition using an experimental model of knee swelling. *Arthritis Rheum.* 2009;61(1):78–83.
4. Fitzgerald GK, Piva SR, Irrgang JJ. A modified neuromuscular electrical stimulation protocol for quadriceps strength training following anterior cruciate ligament reconstruction. *J Orthop Sports Phys Ther.* 2003;33(9):492–501.
5. Bolgla LA, Uhl TL. Electromyographic analysis of hip rehabilitation exercises in a group of healthy subjects. *J Orthop Sports Phys Ther.* 2005;35(8):487–494.
6. Yoo YS, Chang HG, Seo YJ, et al. Changes in the length of the medial patellofemoral ligament: an in vivo analysis using 3-dimensional computed tomography. *Am J Sports Med.* 2012;40(9):2142–2148.
7. Higuchi T, Arai Y, Takamiya H, et al. An analysis of the medial patellofemoral ligament length change pattern using open-MRI. *Knee Surg Sports Traumatol Arthrosc.* 2010;18(11):1470–1475.
8. Vailas AC, Tipton CM, Matthes RC, et al. Physical activity and its influence on the repair process of medial collateral ligaments. *Connect Tissue Res.* 1981;9(1):25–31.
9. Noyes FR. Functional properties of knee ligaments and alterations induced by immobilization: a correlative biomechanical and histological study in primates. *Clin Orthop Relat Res.* 1977;123:210–242.
10. Manske RC, Stovak M. Preoperative and postsurgical musculoskeletal examination of the knee. In: Manske RC, ed. *Postsurgical Orthopedic Sports Rehabilitation: Knee and Shoulder.* St. Louis, MO: Mosby; 2006:31–52.
11. Shah JN, Howard JS, Flanigan DC, et al. A systematic review of complications and failures associated with medial patellofemoral ligament reconstruction for recurrent patellar dislocation. *Am J Sports Med.* 2012;40(8):1916–1923.
12. Parikh SN, Nathan ST, Wall EJ, et al. Complications of medial patellofemoral ligament reconstruction in young patients. *Am J Sports Med.* 2013;41(5):1030–1038.
13. Powers CM, Heino JG, Rao S, et al. The influence of patellofemoral pain on lower limb loading during gait. *Clin Biomech.* 1999; 14(10):722–728.
14. Schwartz RE, Asnis PD, Cavanaugh JT, et al. Short crank cycle ergometry. *J Orthop Sports Phys Ther.* 1991;13(2):95–100.
15. Perry J. *Gait Analysis: Normal and Pathological Function.* New York, NY: McGraw-Hill; 1992.
16. Goodfellow J, Hungerford DS, Zindel M. Patello-femoral joint mechanics and pathology: functional anatomy of the patello-femoral joint. *J Bone Joint Surg Br.* 1976;58(3):287–290.
17. Hungerford DS, Lennox DW. Rehabilitation of the knee in disorders of the patellofemoral joint: relevant biomechanics. *Orthop Clin North Am.* 1983;14(2):397–402.
18. Steinkamp LA, Dillingham MF, Markel MD, et al. Biomechanical considerations in patellofemoral joint rehabilitation. *Am J Sports Med.* 1993;21(3):438–444.
19. Distefano LJ, Blackburn JT, Marshall SW, et al. Gluteal muscle activation during common therapeutic exercises. *J Orthop Sports Phys Ther.* 2009;39(7):532–540.
20. Selkowitz DM, Beneck GJ, Powers CM. Which exercises target the gluteal muscles while minimizing activation of the tensor fascia lata? Electromyographic assessment using fine-wire electrodes. *J Orthop Sports Phys Ther.* 2013;43(2):54–64.
21. Sahrmann SA. *Diagnosis and the Treatment of Movement Impairment Syndromes.* St. Louis, MO: Mosby; 2002.
22. Risberg MA, Mørk M, Jenssen HK, et al. Design and implementation of a neuromuscular training program following anterior cruciate ligament reconstruction. *J Orthop Sports Phys Ther.* 2001;31(11):620–631.
23. Pendidikan F. A development of neuromuscular control exercise protocol of the knee with patellofemoral pain syndrome: a concept paper. *J Edupres.* 2011;1:55–64.
24. Jerosch J, Prymka M. Knee joint proprioception in patients with posttraumatic recurrent patella dislocation. *Knee Surg Sports Traumatol Arthrosc.* 1996;4(1):14–18.
25. Flynn TW, Soutas-Little RW. Mechanical power and muscle action during forward and backward running. *J Orthop Sports Phys Ther.* 1993;17(2):108–112.
26. Flynn TW, Soutas-Little RW. Patellofemoral joint compressive forces in forward and backward running. *J Orthop Sports Phys Ther.* 1995;21(5):277–282.
27. Monson J, Arendt EA. Rehabilitative protocols for select patellofemoral procedures and nonoperative management schemes. *Sports Med Arthrosc.* 2012;20(3):136–144.
28. Cavanaugh JT, Stump TJ. Forward step down test. *J Orthop Sports Phys Ther.* 2000;30(1):A–46.
29. Chinkulprasert C, Vachalathiti R, Powers CM. Patellofemoral joint forces and stress during forward step-up, lateral step-up, and forward step-down exercises. *J Orthop Sports Phys Ther.* 2011;41(4):241–248.
30. Powers CM. Clinical commentary: the influence of abnormal hip mechanics on knee injury: a biomechanical perspective. *J Orthop Sports Phys Ther.* 2010;40(2):42–51.
31. Powers CM, Ward SR, Fredericson M, et al. Patellofemoral kinematics during weight-bearing and non-weight-bearing knee extension in persons with lateral subluxation of the patella: a preliminary study. *J Orthop Sports Phys Ther.* 2003;33(11):677–685.
32. Souza RB, Draper CE, Fredericson M, et al. Femur rotation and patellofemoral joint kinematics: a weight-bearing magnetic resonance imaging analysis. *J Orthop Sports Phys Ther.* 2010;40(5):277–285.
33. Engelen-van Melick N, van Cingel RE, Tijssen MP, et al. Assessment of functional performance after anterior cruciate ligament reconstruction: a systematic review of measurement procedures. *Knee Surg Sports Traumatol Arthrosc.* 2013;21(4):869–879.
34. Gribble PA, Hertel J, Plisky P. Using the Star Excursion Balance Test to assess dynamic postural-control deficits and outcomes in lower extremity injury: a literature and systematic review. *J Athl Train.* 2012;47(3):339–357.
35. Paxton EW, Fithian DC, Stone ML, et al. The reliability and validity of knee-specific and general health instruments in assessing acute patellar dislocation outcomes. *Am J Sports Med.* 2003;31(4):487–492.
36. Roos EM, Roos HP, Lohmander LS, et al. Knee Injury and Osteoarthritis Outcome Score (KOOS)—development of a self-administered outcome measure. *J Orthop Sports Phys Ther.* 1998;28(2):88–96.

SECTION

3

Osteochondritis Dissecans

Eric W. Edmonds
Henry G. Chambers

CHAPTER 21

Osteochondritis Dissecans: Overview, Epidemiology, Etiology, Classification, Assessment

INTRODUCTION

Although loose bodies within a joint were first described by Paget,[1] König later suggested three methods by which loose bodies could be created: (1) direct trauma with acute fracture, (2) minimal trauma that develops into osteonecrosis and subsequent fragmentation, or (3) no trauma with spontaneous fragmentation. The latter variety he coined osteochondritis dissecans (OCD).[2,3] Although it should be pointed out that the exact pathophysiology remains unknown, it is agreed that OCD is likely an acquired lesion of subchondral bone.

Beyond this characterization, it is less clear. There are degrees of osseous resorption, collapse, and sequestrum formation with possible involvement of the articular cartilage through delamination unrelated to an acute osteochondral fracture of normal cartilage (Fig. 21.1).[4,5] This understanding of the end point of the disease process has led to many etiologies of OCD being postulated (particularly concerning the knee) including trauma,[6,7] inflammation,[2,8] genetics,[9] vascular abnormalities,[10,11] and constitutional factors.[12] However, the etiology remains unknown, even though our veterinary medicine colleagues have made some leaps in understanding over recent years.[13,14]

Historically, there has been a distinction between juvenile-onset OCD and adult-onset OCD. Many surgeons have suggested that skeletally immature patients (juvenile onset) have a better prognosis that has been inconsistently defined in the literature as either radiographic healing or merely resolution of pain.[4,5,9,11,12,15] Despite the lack of an open physis at the time of diagnosis in an adult OCD, however, many authors suggest that the only true difference between juvenile- and adult-onset OCD is purely a reflection of patient age at the time of diagnosis.

A recent definition of human OCD lesions, proposed by the Research in Osteochondritis of the Knee (ROCK) study group, highlights the fact that these are (1) focal, (2) idiopathic, (3) involve subchondral bone, and (4) risk instability and disruption of articular cartilage with potential long-term consequences, such as premature osteoarthritis.[16] This definition is the summary of epidemiology, etiology, classification, and assessment of OCD.

EPIDEMIOLOGY

There are only three true epidemiology papers regarding knee OCD.[10,17,18] The first was performed by Marsden and Wiernik[18] in a review of 18,405 radiographs at a military hospital. They found an incidence of symptomatic OCD of 2.3% of the radiographs and an overall incidence (including incidental discovery) of 4% OCD in their cohort.

A classic study by Linden[10] in 1977 from Malmo, Sweden demonstrated an incidence of 29 per 100,000 boys and 19 per 100,000 girls. More importantly, after he reviewed radiographs and obtained follow-up with many of these patients 33 years later, he discovered that there was an "accumulated risk of roentgenographic gonarthrosis in patients who have had osteochondritis dissecans." If he assumed the risk of arthritis to be 0% at the start of life, this was unchanged at age 40 years with an OCD; but the risk increased to 70% at age 48 years and continued to increase to 95% at 70 years of age. However, in those initially discovered with juvenile-onset OCD, he could not directly correlate any pathology such as gonarthritis with their OCD directly.

The only other study was published in 2014 and included a review of just over 1 million children aged 2 to 19 years within a closed health system.[17] These authors found 192 children with 206 OCD lesions of the knee. The majority (64%) of the lesions involved the medial femoral condyle, and the overall incidence seen in the cohort was 18.1 per 100,000 boys and 3.9 per 100,000 girls. The incidence of knee OCD varied by ethnicity: non-Hispanic white was 10.3 per 100,000 overall (17.3 and 3.0 per 100,000 for boys and girls, respectively), non-Hispanic black was 10.3 per 100,000 overall (17.3 and 3.0 per 100,000 for boys and girls, respectively), Hispanic was 8.6 per

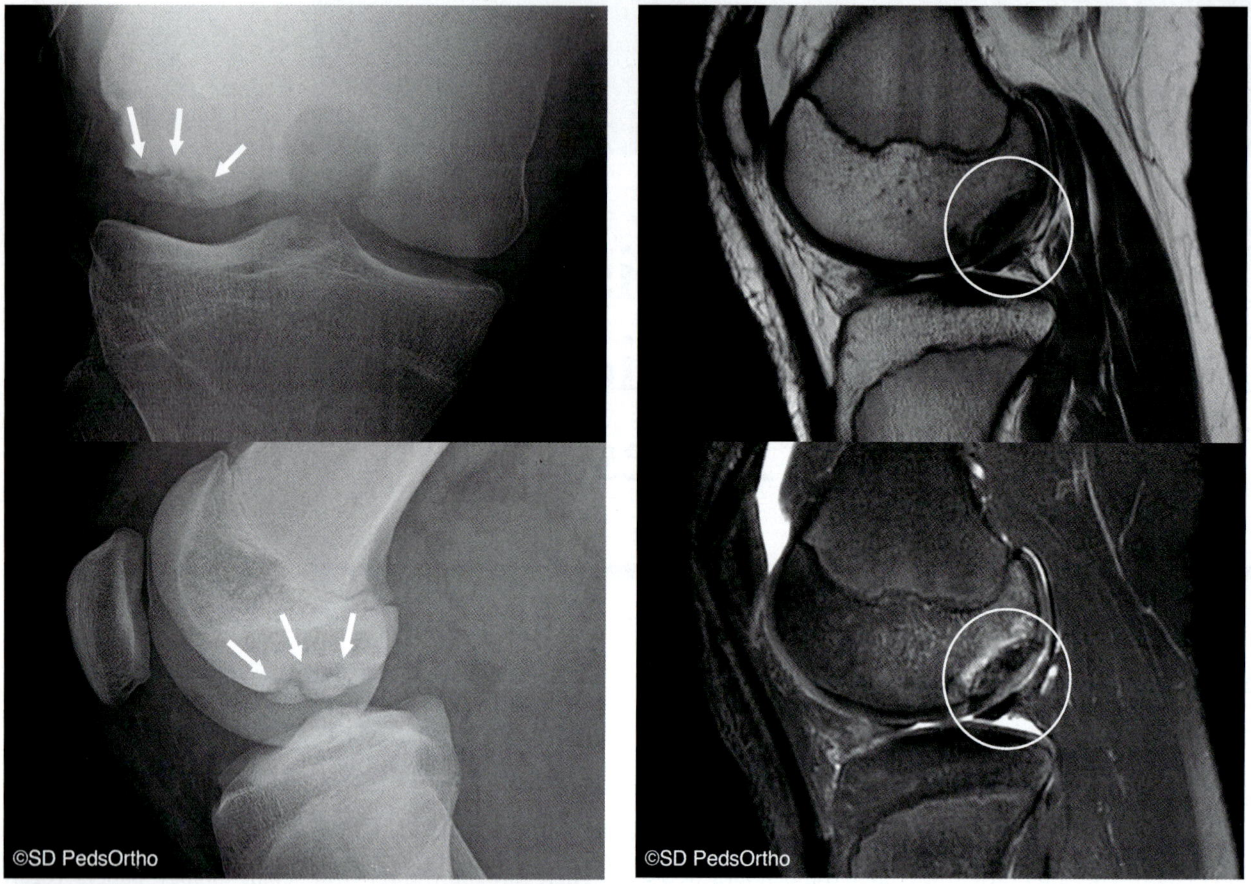

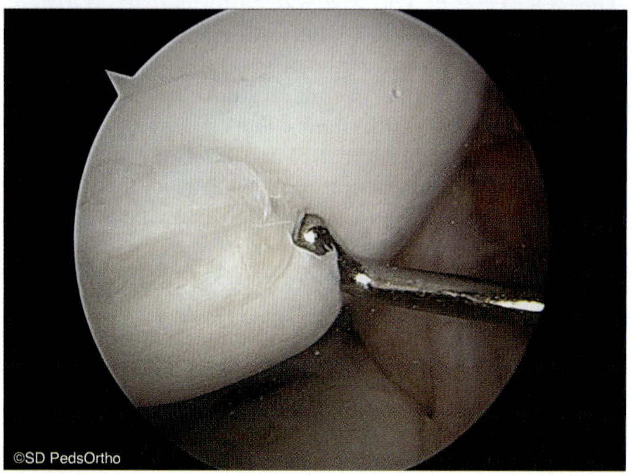

Figure 21.1. Clinical example of 13-year-old girl soccer player who presented with anterior knee pain that was insidious in onset. **A.** Radiographs at the initial visit demonstrating the OCD lesion (*arrows*). **B.** MRI evidence of the lesion (*within circles*). **C.** Arthroscopic appearance of the lesion on the lateral femoral condyle, evidence of disrupted cartilage with probing.

100,000 overall (14.3 and 2.8 per 100,000 for boys and girls, respectively), and Asian was 4.7 per 100,000 overall (9.1 and 0.0 per 100,000 for boys and girls, respectively). These authors performed multivariable logistic regression analysis that revealed a 3.3-fold increased risk of OCD of the knee in children aged 12 to 19 years compared with those aged 6 to 11 years. Moreover, boys had 3.8 times greater risk of OCD than girls.

Finally, there is the discrete possibility that knee OCD may occur in both knees. In the literature, there is a relatively wide range of bilaterality noted with about a 3% to 30% chance of discovering it in both knees by x-ray.[5,18–23]

ETIOLOGY

No definitive etiology has yet been determined for the origin of knee OCD. There are, of course, many hypotheses that have been presented and tested primarily via ex vivo histology. The potential etiologies include inflammation, spontaneous osteonecrosis and vascular deficiency, genetic predisposition, and repetitive trauma. Each of these will be discussed.

As suggested by the name "osteochondritis," the first description in 1888 by König,[2] by definition was atraumatic and it was postulated to be a result of inflammation. However, histologic studies have not supported this etiology[7,24]; instead, these works appear to highlight findings of necrosis within the OCD lesions rather than inflammation.

Based on their histology findings, Green and Banks[12,19] proposed that ischemia was the primary etiology, and Milgram,[22] identifying revascularization in partially detached OCD lesion, further promoted this concept of poor vascularity. Yet, Yonetani and colleagues[25] found no evidence of necrosis on biopsies. Uozumi and colleagues[26] discovered a discrete absence of subchondral bone in many of their biopsy samples and, in those who had an osseous component present, only two demonstrated no viable osteocytes. The difference between the first two studies and the second two is state of the OCD lesion prior to biopsy. When the lesion was unstable (or even a loose body) at the time of biopsy, then necrosis was found by microscopic evaluation. However, if the lesion was fully intact and in situ, then there was less definitive evidence for avascular necrosis.

Another hypothesis of the etiology is familial inheritance of OCD lesions. A mild form of skeletal dysplasia with associated short stature has even been proposed.[9,23,27–29] Two different authors, via different family tree assessments, have identified what they believe to be an autosomal dominant inheritance pattern.[9,28] In contrast, Petrie[30] reported on a radiographic examination of first-degree relatives of those patients with known OCD and discovered only 1.2% with OCD themselves. This suggests that the majority of knee OCD does not follow a predictable inheritance pattern. However, it does not exclude the possibility that genetics may still play a role in OCD etiology.

Whether the aforementioned etiologies are primary or secondary remains a question unto itself, and the concept of repetitive microtrauma is another distinct possibility. For example, despite the original description by König, there could be a significant traumatic event leading to avascular necrosis or there could be repetitive traumatic events that progressively develop vascular disruption. In 1933, Fairbanks[31] proposed traumatic contact between the lateral aspect of the medial femoral condyle and the tibial spine; yet, this theory would only explain OCD lesions on the lateral aspect of the medial femoral condyle. However, the idea of repetitive trauma still holds our attention for the other locations of OCD as well. Aichroth[6] demonstrated that 60% of the patients with knee OCD in his cohort were involved in high-level, competitive sports. Moreover, Linden[11] showed an association between the incidence of OCD and the increased involvement in organized sports in Sweden between 1965 and 1974. A large multicenter study conducted by the European Pediatric Orthopaedic Society demonstrated that nearly 55% of those with OCD were regularly active in sports or performed "strenuous athletic activity."[20] Evidence to support repetitive trauma as an etiology for OCD is mostly conjecture and circumstantial at best.

Perhaps abnormal pressure on the cartilage anlage is a better way of describing "microtrauma," as several studies have noted associations between lateral femoral condyle OCD lesions and discoid menisci.[32–34] Moreover, there is an apparent association with poor mechanical axis alignment and the presence of knee OCD.[35] In fact, the association between alignment shifts and location of OCD development was predictive, with varus malalignment predicting medial OCD lesions and valgus malalignment predicting lateral OCD lesions.[35] These findings suggest that aberrant mechanical pressure on the condyles may be an etiology to the formation of OCD (at least in the knee).

Perhaps the unifying theory can be found in the work by our veterinary colleagues on horse and pig comparative models. They believe that the OCD lesions in these animals originate within the cartilage anlage of the subchondral bone.[13,14] They have actually been able to create an animal model for OCD by description of the cartilage canals (which is the blood supply to the epiphyseal anlage cartilage). This further hints toward a possible traumatic injury that disrupts the blood supply. They also suggest modifying the term *osteochondritis* to *osteochondrosis* given the complete lack of inflammation being seen as a possible etiology. Furthermore, they would include the modifier "dissecans" when the articular cartilage becomes involved but recommend using the terms *latens* when there is only necrosis of the anlage cartilage or *manifesta* in the presence of focal failure of enchondral ossification to differentiate the timing of discovery. In other words, these authors believe that by the time this pathologic process becomes clinically evident in the knee, it has already evolved through all three stages and is in the final necrotic form of OCD (Fig. 21.2).

This concept is not new to human physicians, but the concept of disrupted cartilage canals is novel to the previous hypothesis of Ribbing[36] in 1937. His thesis was presented in a 107-page supplement to the journal *Acta Radiologica* discussing abnormalities of endochondral ossification of the epiphysis. His hypothesis was then further modified by Barrie[7,24] to further define possible etiologies of OCD formation via epiphyseal secondary growth. Basically, at an index event, there is an insult (single or repetitive) to the endochondral epiphyseal growth plate or perhaps to the cartilage canals just deep to subchondral bone. With skeletal development, the uninjured region of endochondral epiphyseal ossification continues to ossify unhindered, creating an ever enlarging OCD central to the normal growth.

Although the concepts of disrupted cartilage canals or endochondral epiphyseal growth plates are appealing etiologies, there remains a gap in the explanation regarding how and why these structures become injured in the first place. All children are quite active, jumping, playing, running, and falling. So why do some develop an OCD and some do not develop an OCD? This question is yet to be answered.

CLASSIFICATION

The simplest form of knee OCD classification is that set forth by Hefti and colleagues[20] that merely describes location of the OCD. The most common site of OCD is the lateral aspect of the medial femoral condyle (51% involvement), with other sites being involved with less frequency: 19% central medial femoral condyle, 17% lateral femoral condyle, 7% medial side of the medial femoral condyle, and 7% patella. It may be important to note that irregular ossification centers of the distal femoral condyle tend to be found more posteriorly on the condyle (although they can be anywhere on the condyle) and are associated with younger age. Cahill[12] wrote a review of OCD and identified multiple other authors who have similarly classified knee OCD by location, but he makes no mention of classifying the lesions in any other method (stability, outcomes, etc.).

De Smet and colleagues[37] took things to the next level and classified the OCD either stable or unstable and correlated their

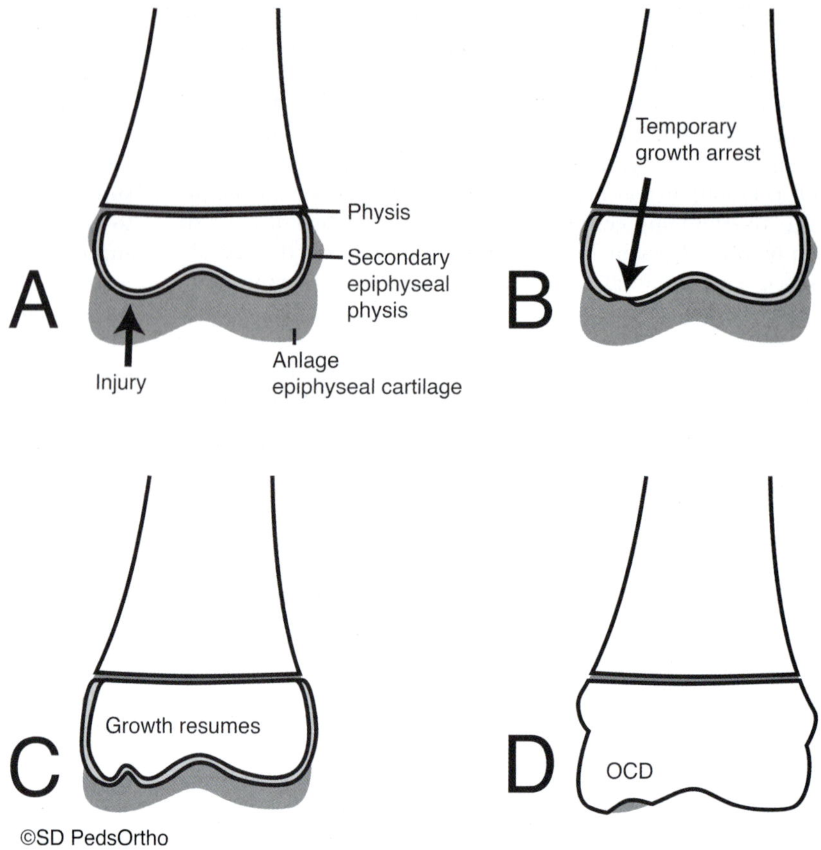

Figure 21.2. Line drawing demonstrating the possible course of temporary cessation of epiphyseal growth and its potential relation to OCD development. **A.** An insult occurs such as vascular injury, disruption of cartilage canal, and microtrauma. **B.** Epiphyseal physeal growth arrest occurs but intact part continues to ossify the anlage cartilage. **C.** Growth resumes throughout (but delayed at location of insult). **D.** The insulted physis does not fully recover and an OCD forms.

magnetic resonance imaging (MRI) findings with arthroscopic findings. They reported that a high signal interface between the OCD lesion and the normal femoral bone was indicative of instability by arthroscopy. This same author then later improved his assessment by MRI and added three other signs of instability that are discussed in the following text (Fig. 21.3).[38]

The arthroscopic classification of OCD lesions is the gold standard in understanding the lesion, yet even here, we do not have associated outcomes. Guhl[39] was the first to set an arthroscopy classification and it has been used as a template for other authors: (1) intact lesions, (2) lesions showing signs of early separation,(3) partially detached lesions, and (4) crater with

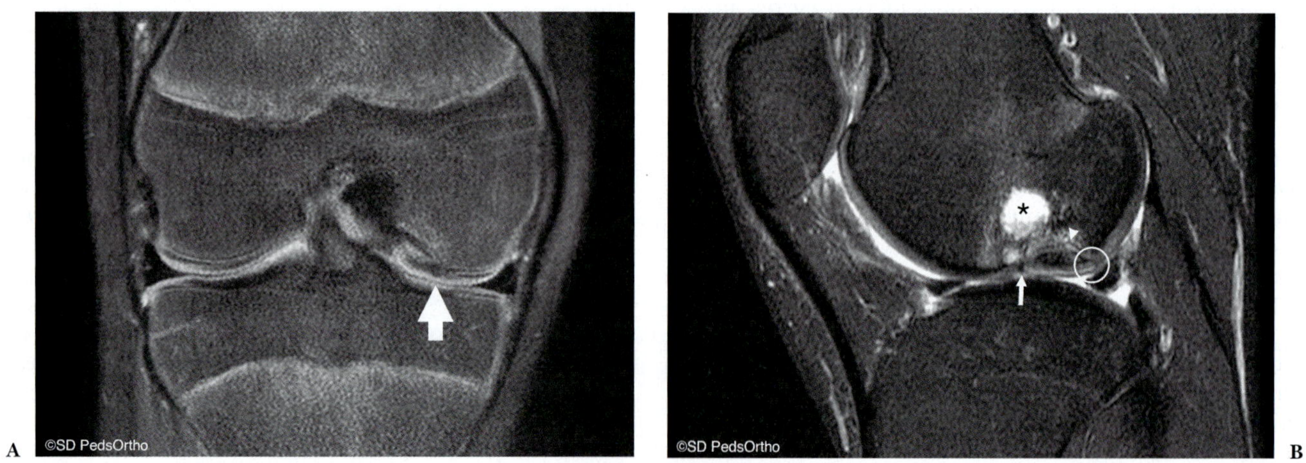

Figure 21.3. MRI classification of OCD lesions, discerning stable from unstable lesions. **A.** A stable OCD lesion confirmed by arthroscopy, note the completely intact appearance of the articular cartilage (*broad arrow*). **B.** An unstable lesion with the following criteria: high signal line beneath the lesion (*arrowhead*), a focal defect in the articular cartilage (*arrow*), a fracture of the articular cartilage (*circle*), and the presence of subchondral cyst (*asterisk*).

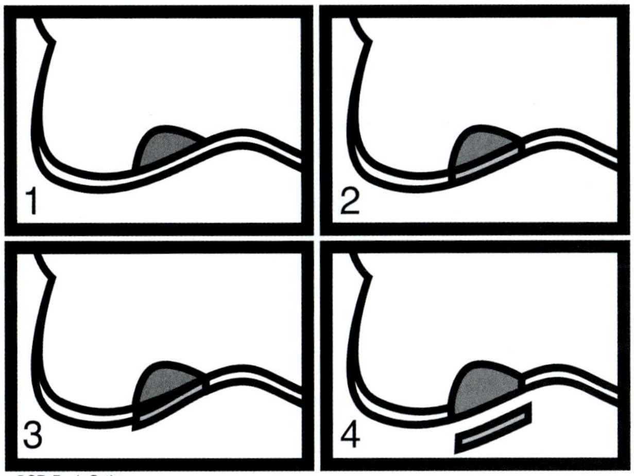

Figure 21.4. The Guhl classification of OCD lesions, an arthroscopic assessment to delineate the severity of the lesion: (*1*) intact cartilage, (*2*) demarcated OCD otherwise intact, (*3*) partial displacement, (*4*) completely displaced loose OCD.

loose bodies (salvageable or unsalvageable) (Fig. 21.4). To this point, no correlation with outcomes has been made.

ASSESSMENT

Most authors[20,40] suggest that treatment for knee OCD should be based on skeletal maturity and lesion stability. A number of classification systems mentioned earlier includes these two principles.[12,37–39] Therefore, it is important to identify OCD, identify skeletal maturity, and identify OCD stability.

Children with OCD may have two different presentations, either the OCD is an incidental radiographic findings or it may be thought to be the cause of their symptoms.[41,42] Cahill and Ahten[43] reported that 80% of the children had mild pain and limp for a mean of 14 months prior to presentation—suggesting that the symptoms associated with knee OCD may not differ greatly from idiopathic adolescent knee pain. However, there may be substantial symptoms associated with the OCD lesion, such as mechanical symptoms of locking and popping. Effusion is present in less than 20% at presentation.[20] Wilson[53] described a test on physical examination to diagnose OCD: The knee is flexed to 90 degrees, the tibia is externally rotated, and the knee is gradually extended to 30 degrees of flexion. A positive test is characterized by pain over the anteromedial aspect of the knee as the knee is extended to 30 degrees with relief of pain with internal rotation of the tibia. Anatomically, this maneuver is believed to cause impingement of the tibial spine on the lateral aspect of the medial femoral condyle (and therefore would only be positive on those particular OCD lesions). The Wilson test is of limited diagnostic value with a reported positive test in only 16% of knees with radiographically proven OCD lesions.[20]

The diagnosis of OCD is truly dependent on imaging rather than history or physical examination. Especially considering that many OCD lesions may be asymptomatic until separation or dislodgment occurs resulting in significant effusion and pain—this is considered a late finding in the treatment of these lesions. Most lesions can be identified by plain radiographs and will usually not be missed as long as four views are obtained, including anteroposterior (AP), lateral, tunnel (notch), and Merchant (sunrise) views. To date, there is no historical literature assessing the sensitivity or specificity of radiographs to identify OCD lesions, and the American Academy of Orthopaedic Surgeons (AAOS) clinical pathway guideline task force recommended that there was only limited evidence to support obtaining initial plain radiographs in the assessment of knee OCD (and inconclusive evidence to obtain contralateral films at initial evaluation).[40] In the assessment of children with an OCD lesion, it appears to be clinically acceptable to obtain contralateral films to evaluate for bilateral involvement, given the high rate of bilateral involvement seen in past studies.[45,46]

Often, MRI is the next step in the assessment of the OCD, looking for instability of the lesion as well as better defining the size and extent of the pathologic changes. MRI can also be helpful in distinguishing irregular centers of ossification from OCD, and some authors have suggested that the improved outcomes seen in juvenile OCD may be related to an incorrect diagnosis of OCD. However, once again, the AAOS clinical guidelines task force found limited evidence for obtaining initial MRI for evaluation and inconclusive evidence for using MRI in subsequent follow-up evaluation.[40] MRI characteristics consistent with irregular ossification includes low signal intensity of the lesion bone being similar to the surrounding subchondral bone and high signal demarcation being equal to the surrounding articular cartilage.[48] The characteristics of OCD are varied, but there are a few findings to note: There is often surrounding bone marrow edema, there is a sclerotic rim of bone demarcating the lesion ± high signal intensity layer highlighting the demarcation, there may or may not be bone within the progeny fragment, there may be cyst-like formations along the demarcation, and there could be articular cartilage disruption.

Radiographic assessment should be obtained at intervals depending on the treatment being rendered but should be continued until there is a clear demonstration of lesion resolution because symptoms are not trustworthy guides in the stability of the lesion. If the lesion exhibits any radiographic signs of worsening (enlargement or increased sclerotic border), or the lesion fails to resolve as the child grows, then not only is a diagnosis of OCD appropriate over irregular ossification but also a change in intervention may be warranted. The definition of healing by plain film or MRI is not well defined. The various definitions usually try to take into account the conversion of cartilaginous lesion to osseous density, or some percentage of that process, whereas others define healing by resolution, or resorption, of the sclerotic margin.[49] Unfortunately, some authors still define healing as the resolution of symptoms regardless of any radiographic changes.[44,47] No one, as yet, correlated radiographic findings with healing because healing has not yet been defined.

There is some agreement regarding the definition of an unstable OCD lesion: either fractured cartilage or separation of the underlying subchondral bone.[50] This distinction, stable versus unstable, is important because it can often dictate the treatment and prognosis. In general, stable lesions are believed to have better outcomes and stable OCD lesions may be considered for nonoperative management, whereas unstable lesions are better treated with surgical intervention.[20,40] There are[37,38] four criteria (on T2 weighted magnetic resonance [MR] images) that correlate with instability when compared with arthroscopy findings: (1) a high signal line beneath the lesion,

(2) a focal defect in the articular cartilage, (3) a fracture of the articular cartilage, and (4) the presence of subchondral cysts. The presence of a high T2 signal line between the lesion and the remainder of the normal bone was the most predictive factor for instability in a mixed age cohort of patients, but Yoshida et al.[34] evaluated a skeletally immature cohort with this same high T2 signal line separating the lesion and he found no correlation. However, he reported that this line could not predict stability because the majority of the juvenile OCD lesions healed.

Another study[51] suggested that if the criteria for instability included both the high T2 signal separating the lesion and a breach of the articular cartilage on T1 weighted images, then the accuracy in predicting instability shifted from 45% to 85%. Kijowski and colleagues[52] examined the aforementioned criteria of MRI stability and applied it to predicting arthroscopic instability (defined as cartilage disruption or motion of the overlaying cartilage at the OCD) and found that all four criteria (together) had 100% sensitivity and 100% specificity for instability in adult OCD and 100% sensitivity but only 11% specificity for juvenile OCD lesions.

REFERENCES

1. Paget J. On the production of some of the loose bodies in joints. *St Bartholomew's Hosp Rep.* 1870;6:1–4.
2. König F. Ueber freie korper in den gelenken. *Dtsch Z Chir.* 1887;27:90–109.
3. Freifberg AH, Woolley PG. Osteochondritis dissecans: concerning its nature and relation to formation of joint mice. *J Bone Joint Surg Am.* 1910;8:477–494.
4. Crawford DC, Safran MR. Osteochondritis dissecans of the knee. *J Am Acad Orthop Surg.* 2006;14:90–100.
5. Kocher MS, Tucker R, Ganley TJ, et al. Management of osteochondritis dissecans of the knee: current concepts review. *Am J Sports Med.* 2006;34:1181–1191.
6. Aichroth P. Osteochondritis dissecans of the knee. A clinical survey. *J Bone Joint Surg Br.* 1971;53:440–447.
7. Barrie HJ. Hypothesis—a diagram of the form and origin of loose bodies in osteochondritis dissecans. *J Rheumatol.* 1984;11:512–513.
8. Schenck RC Jr, Goodnight JM. Osteochondritis dissecans. *J Bone Joint Surg Am.* 1996;78:439–456.
9. Mubarak SJ, Carroll NC. Familial osteochondritis dissecans of the knee. *Clin Orthop Relat Res.* 1979;(140):131–136.
10. Linden B. Osteochondritis dissecans of the femoral condyles: a long-term follow-up study. *J Bone Joint Surg Am.* 1977;59:769–776.
11. Linden B. The incidence of osteochondritis dissecans in the condyles of the femur. *Acta Orthop Scand.* 1976;47:664–667.
12. Cahill BR. Osteochondritis dissecans of the knee: treatment of juvenile and adult forms. *J Am Acad Orthop Surg.* 1995;3:237–247.
13. Olstad K, Hendrickson EH, Carlson CS, et al. Transection of vessels in epiphyseal cartilage canals leads to osteochondrosis and osteochondrosis dissecans in the femoro-patellar joint of foals; a potential model of juvenile osteochondritis dissecans. *Osteoarthritis Cartilage.* 2013;21(5):730–738.
14. Ytrehus B, Carlson CS, Ekman S. Etiology and pathogenesis of osteochondrosis. *Vet Pathol.* 2007;44(4):429–448.
15. Bradley J, Dandy DJ. Osteochondritis dissecans and other lesions of the femoral condyles. *J Bone Joint Surg Br.* 1989;71:518–522.
16. Edmonds EW, Shea KG. Osteochondritis dissecans: editorial comment. *Clin Orthop Relat Res.* 2013;471(4):1105–1106.
17. Kessler JI, Nikizad H, Shea KG, et al. The demographics and epidemiology of osteochondritis dissecans of the knee in children and adolescents. *Am J Sports Med.* 2014;42(2):320–326.
18. Marsden C, Wiernik G. The incidence of osteochondritis dissecans. *J R Army Med Corps.* 1956;102(2):124–130.
19. Green WT, Banks HH. Osteochondritis dissecans in children. *J Bone Joint Surg Am.* 1953;35:26–47; passim.
20. Hefti F, Beguiristain J, Krauspe R, et al. Osteochondritis dissecans: a multicenter study of the European Pediatric Orthopedic Society. *J Pediatr Orthop B.* 1999;8:231–245.
21. Hughston JC, Hergenroeder PT, Courtenay BG. Osteochondritis dissecans of the femoral condyles. *J Bone Joint Surg Am.* 1984;66:1340–1348.
22. Milgram JW. Radiological and pathological manifestations of osteochondritis dissecans of the distal femur. A study of 50 cases. *Radiology.* 1978;126:305–311.
23. Mubarak SJ, Carroll NC. Juvenile osteochondritis dissecans of the knee: etiology. *Clin Orthop Relat Res.* 1981;(157):200–211.
24. Barrie HJ. Hypertrophy and laminar calcification of cartilage in loose bodies as probable evidence of an ossification abnormality. *J Pathol.* 1980;132:161–168.
25. Yonetani Y, Nakamura N, Natsuume T, et al. Histological evaluation of juvenile osteochondritis dissecans of the knee: a case series. *Knee Surg Sports Traumatol Arthrosc.* 2010;18:723–730.
26. Uozumi H, Sugita T, Aizawa T, et al. Histologic findings and possible causes of osteochondritis dissecans of the knee. *Am J Sports Med.* 2009;37:2003–2008.
27. Kozlowski K, Middleton R. Familial osteochondritis dissecans: a dysplasia of articular cartilage? *Skeletal Radiol.* 1985;13:207–210.
28. Phillips HO, Grubb SA. Familial multiple osteochondritis dissecans. Report of a kindred. *J Bone Joint Surg Am.* 1985;67:155–156.
29. Wright RW, McLean M, Matava MJ, et al. Osteochondritis dissecans of the knee: long-term results of excision of the fragment. *Clin Orthop Relat Res.* 2004;(424):239–243.
30. Petrie PW. Aetiology of osteochondritis dissecans. Failure to establish a familial background. *J Bone Joint Surg Br.* 1977;59:366–367.
31. Fairbanks H. Osteochondritis dissecans. *Br J Surg.* 1933;21:67–82.
32. Mitsuoka T, Shino K, Hamada M, et al. Osteochondritis dissecans of the lateral femoral condyle of the knee joint. *Arthroscopy.* 1999;15:20–26.
33. Stanitski CL, Bee J. Juvenile osteochondritis dissecans of the lateral femoral condyle after lateral discoid meniscal surgery. *Am J Sports Med.* 2004;32:797–801.
34. Yoshida S, Ikata T, Takai H, et al. Osteochondritis dissecans of the femoral condyle in the growth stage. *Clin Orthop Relat Res.* 1998;(346):162–170.
35. Jacobi M, Wahl P, Bouaicha S, et al. Association between mechanical axis of the leg and osteochondritis dissecans of the knee: radiographic study on 103 knees. *Am J Sports Med.* 2010;38:1425–1428.
36. Ribbing S. Studies on hereditary, multiple epiphyseal disorder. *Acta Radiol.* 1937;34:1–107.
37. De Smet AA, Fisher DR, Graf BK, et al. Osteochondritis dissecans of the knee: value of MR imaging in determining lesion stability and the presence of articular cartilage defects. *AJR Am J Roentgenol.* 1990;155:549–553.
38. De Smet AA, Ilahi OA, Graf BK. Reassessment of the MR criteria for stability of osteochondritis dissecans in the knee and ankle. *Skeletal Radiol.* 1996;25:159–163.
39. Guhl JF. Arthroscopic treatment of osteochondritis dissecans. *Clin Orthop Relat Res.* 1982;(167):65–74.
40. Chambers HG, Shea KG, Anderson AF, et al. American Academy of Orthopaedic Surgeons clinical practice guideline on: the diagnosis and treatment of osteochondritis dissecans. *J Bone Joint Surg Am.* 2012;94(14):1322–1324.
41. Glancy GL. Juvenile osteochondritis dissecans. *Am J Knee Surg.* 1999;12:120–124.
42. Kocher MS, Micheli LJ, Yaniv M, et al. Functional and radiographic outcome of juvenile osteochondritis dissecans of the knee treated with transarticular arthroscopic drilling. *Am J Sports Med.* 2001;29:562–566.

43. Cahill BR, Ahten SM. The three critical components in the conservative treatment of juvenile osteochondritis dissecans (JOCD). Physician, parent, and child. *Clin Sports Med.* 2001;20:287 298, vi.

44. Wall EJ, Vourazeris J, Myer GD, et al. The healing potential of stable juvenile osteochondritis dissecans knee lesions. *J Bone Joint Surg Am.* 2008;90:2655–2664.

45. Cahill BR, Phillips MR, Navarro R. The results of conservative management of juvenile osteochondritis dissecans using joint scintigraphy. A prospective study. *Am J Sports Med.* 1989;17:601–605; discussion 605–606.

46. Garrett JC. Fresh osteochondral allografts for treatment of articular defects in osteochondritis dissecans of the lateral femoral condyle in adults. *Clin Orthop Relat Res.* 1994;(303):33–37.

47. Gebarski K, Hernandez RJ. Stage-I osteochondritis dissecans versus normal variants of ossification in the knee in children. *Pediatr Radiol.* 2005;35:880–886.

48. Nawata K, Teshima R, Morio Y, et al. Anomalies of ossification in the posterolateral femoral condyle: assessment by MRI. *Pediatr Radiol.* 1999,29.781–784.

49. Edmonds EW, Albright J, Bastrom T, et al. Outcomes of extra-articular, intra-epiphyseal drilling for osteochondritis dissecans of the knee. *J Pediatr Orthop.* 2010;30:870–878.

50. Wall E, Von Stein D. Juvenile osteochondritis dissecans. *Orthop Clin North Am.* 2003;34:341–353.

51. O'Connor MA, Palaniappan M, Khan N, et al. Osteochondritis dissecans of the knee in children. A comparison of MRI and arthroscopic findings. *J Bone Joint Surg Br.* 2002;84:258–262.

52. Kijowski R, Blankenbaker DG, Shinki K, et al. Juvenile versus adult osteochondritis dissecans of the knee: appropriate MR imaging criteria for instability. *Radiology.* 2008;248:571–578.

53. Wilson JN. A diagnostic sign in osteochondritis dissecans of the knee. *J Bone Joint Surg Am.* 1967;49:477–480.

CHAPTER

22

Samir K. Trehan
Benton E. Heyworth

Transarticular Drilling of Osteochondritis Dissecans

INTRODUCTION

Osteochondritis dissecans (OCD) is a pathologic process affecting subchondral bone and the adjacent articular cartilage, which can advance to osteochondral fragment instability and loose body formation.[1] The pathophysiologic basis for the condition has not been definitively established but, in most cases is felt to involve impaired vascular supply and/or healing response in a focal area of subchondral bone. The knee is the most commonly affected joint in the body, with the medial femoral condyle being most frequently affected location in the knee. Although described in adults, OCD most commonly affects skeletally immature patients (which has traditionally been referred to as *juvenile OCD*, a term most authors now do not favor), which generally have a better prognosis than OCD in adults.

Presenting symptoms of OCD are variable but may include limp, knee pain, mechanical symptoms such as clicking or locking, and/or effusion. Obtaining standard anteroposterior (AP) (Fig. 22.1) and lateral knee radiographs, with the addition of a tunnel or notch view, to allow for better assessment of the commonly affected posterior aspect of the condyle represents the primary initial diagnostic step. However, magnetic resonance imaging (MRI) has emerged as the gold standard for classifying OCD lesions as either stable (Fig. 22.2A,B) or unstable, a distinction that dictates the approach to treatment. Stable lesions are generally characterized by an intact articular cartilage surface overlying the subchondral bone lesion. This chapter focuses on the most commonly used technique of surgical treatment for stable juvenile OCD lesions transarticular drilling.

TREATMENT

Indications

Patients with stable OCD lesions of the knee and open physes should be initially managed nonoperatively. Conservative modalities may range from simple activity modification (i.e., avoiding offending activities such as running, competitive sports, or impact activities) to protected weight bearing with crutches, bracing, and/or immobilization. Although the traditional approach of immobilization through casting is rarely pursued today, use of a locked hinged knee brace or knee immobilizer may be a reasonable substitute. Alternatively, valgus unloader bracing has the advantage of allowing knee motion while still decreasing loads on the affected medial femoral condyle. Incomplete, transient, or lack of radiographic or MRI-based healing after approximately 3 to 6 months of nonoperative treatment is generally an indication for surgical intervention.[2]

OPERATIVE

Drilling of the OCD lesion is considered the gold standard of surgical treatment of stable OCD in skeletally immature knees. Drilling is thought to disrupt the sclerotic margin of the lesion and consequently promote healing via growth factors released from healthy underlying cancellous bone. There are two primary methods of drilling knee OCD lesions: transarticular (or retrograde) and retroarticular (also referred to as *anterograde*).

Transarticular drilling involves perforation of the articular cartilage under direct visualization of the OCD lesion, whereas retroarticular drilling through the affected condyle spares the articular cartilage and used intraoperative fluoroscopy to perforate the OCD from the backside of the lesion. Theoretical advantages of the transarticular drilling technique include relative technical simplicity and direct visualization and assessment of the OCD lesion and K-wire entry sites during drilling (Fig. 22.3). Consequently, drilling passes can be optimally spaced relative to the lesion's borders and relative to each other (Fig. 22.4). Finally, intraoperative fluoroscopy is rarely required to localize lesion (in contrast to retroarticular drilling). The theoretical disadvantage of transarticular drilling is the direct articular surface perforation and uncertain long-term implications of these perforations. Also, from a practical standpoint, far posterior condylar lesions may be difficult to access from transarticular approach due to required knee hyperflexion.

Although high-quality studies comparing transarticular and retroarticular drilling are lacking, a recent systematic review concluded no difference in patient outcomes or radiographic healing for skeletally immature patients with stable knee OCD lesions treated with these techniques. In total, 12 studies were

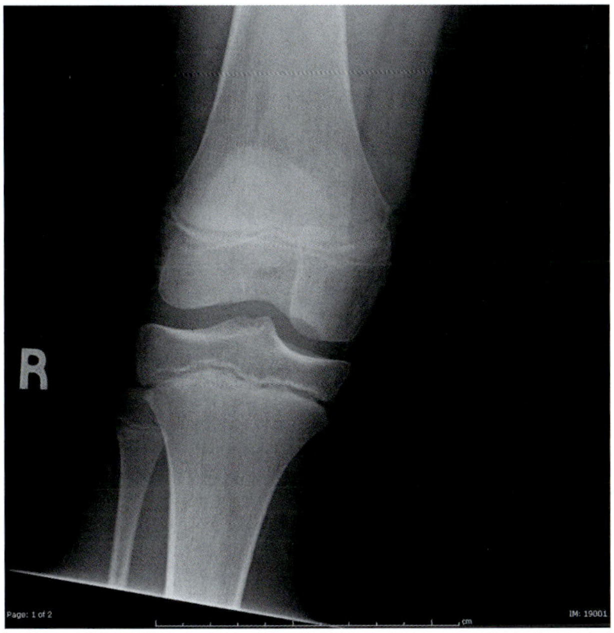

Figure 22.1. Standard AP knee radiograph demonstrating OCD lesion on the lateral aspect of the medial femoral condyle of a 12-year-old athlete with open physes.

included which demonstrated a 91% radiographic healing rate in average of 4.5 months for transarticular drilling versus 86% in average of 5.6 months for retroarticular drilling with no differences in clinical response.[3]

A summary of the currently published literature on transarticular drilling in isolation for the treatment of juvenile knee OCD lesions is summarized in Table 22.1.[4–9] Across all studies, there is agreement on the indications for drilling, in that almost every patient had a stable OCD lesion which had failed at least 3 months of nonoperative management. The clinical and radiographic outcomes reported are excellent overall. Significant variability exists in terms of intraoperative drilling technique and postoperative rehabilitation.

AUTHORS' PREFERRED TREATMENT

Surgical Technique

The patient is positioned supine on operating room table with a nonsterile thigh tourniquet. Standard anterolateral and anteromedial knee arthroscopic portals are established and a diagnostic arthroscopy is performed. The OCD lesion is then assessed for size and stability. The latter is especially important, given that in rare instances, a "stable" lesion may have progressed since the time of last imaging that may alter operative plan. Drilling is performed with either a 0.062- or 0.045-in K-wire. We prefer to use the smaller sized K-wire to minimize disruption of the articular cartilage. The K-wire is directed perpendicular to the chondral surface and advanced with a power wire driver to an appropriate depth through the affected subchondral bone. Withdrawal of the wire from the articular surface may occasionally be followed by visualization of fat bubbles and/or bone marrow bleeding, indicating adequate perforation into the deeper healthy cancellous bone. Although injury to the distal femoral physis is a concern with overpenetration during drilling, this can be avoided by measuring the distance from the articular surface to the physis on preoperative MRI and ensuring penetration no deeper than the shorted distance. However, we are not aware of any published cases detailing this complication. In order to successfully access the lesion and appropriately orient the K-wire perpendicular to the chondral surface, the wire may need to be introduced percutaneously

A

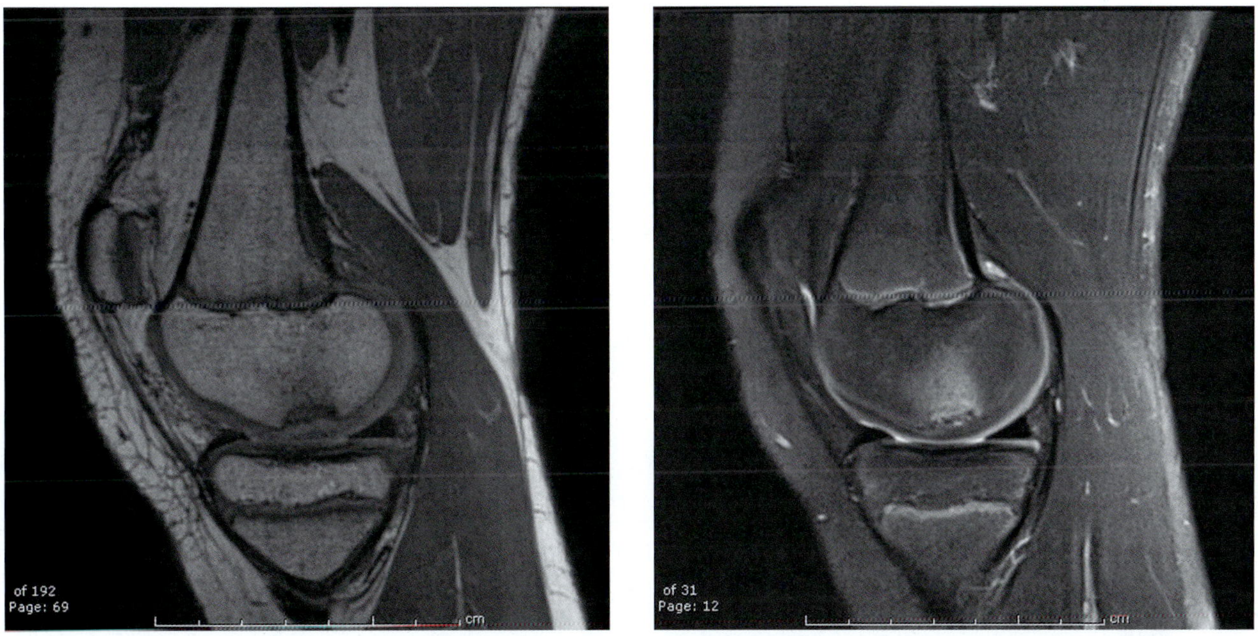

B

Figure 22.2. MRI with both T1 weighted **(A)** and T2 weighted **(B)** sagittal sequences demonstrating a stable OCD lesion with no signs of instability (e.g., chondral breach, fissure, or articular incongruity) but significant surrounding bone marrow edema.

TABLE 22.1 Details of Published Studies Assessing Transarticular Drilling of OCD

			Preoperative			*Operative Technique*			*Postoperative*				
Author (Year)	*No. of Patients (No. of Lesions)*	*Average Age at Surgery (y)*	*Lesion Location*	*Lesion Characteristic*	*Average Nonoperative Treatment Duration*	*Portals*	*Drill Diameter (mm)*	*No. of Perforations*	*WB Status*	*Mean Follow-up (y)*	*No. of Lesions Healed on X-ray*	*Average Time to Healing*	*Patient Outcome*
Bradley and Dandy (1989)	10 (11)	12.9	MFC	—	At least 6 mo	—	1.5	At least 6 holes	WBAT	2.7	10 (91%)	—	Resolution of pain in 9 (out of 11) patients
Aglietti et al. (1994)	14 (16)	12.8	MFC	Stage 1 ("normal articular cartilage")	16 mo	AM, AL, transpatellar	2	3–4 holes per sq cm (3 bone perforations per cartilage hole)	Protected WB × 1 mo	4.7	16 (100%)	4.9 mo	Resolution of pain in all patients
Anderson et al. (1997)	17 (20)	13.5	15 MFC, 5 LFC	19 grade 1, 1 grade 3 (Ewing & Voto)	At least 3 mo	AM, AL	0.62 (with Jacobs drill chuck)	Multiple ("uniformly cover lesion")	TTWB × 6 wk	5	18 (90%)	4.4 mo	IKDC: 14 NL, 4 NN, 1 ab, 1 sev ab Hughston: 15 excellent, 4 good, 1 poor
Kocher et al. (2001)	23 (30)	12.3	MFC	Grade 1 (Ewing & Voto)	6 mo	—	1.6	6–10 (depend on size)	NWB × 1 mo	3.9	30 (100%)	4.4 mo	Lysholm score: 58 → 93
Louisia et al. (2003)	? (17)	13.8	MFC	16 grade 1, 1 grade 2	22 mo	—	1.5 or 2	4–6 holes (with 4–5 perforations per hole)	NWB × 2 mo	11.8	12 (71%)	—	Hughston: 12 excellent, 2 good, 1 fair, 2 poor (2 required reoperation for "fragment excision")
Cepero et al. (2005)	48 (48)	12.6	86.6% MFC	"Intact lesions with soft articular cartilage"	3.4 mo	—	—	"Multiple"	PWB crutches	3.25	All?	6.6 mo	44 excellent, 3 good, 1 poor (required reoperation for "fragment extraction")

MFC, medial femoral condyle; AM, anteromedial; AL, anterolateral; LFC, lateral femoral condyle; WB, weight bearing; WBAT, weight bearing as tolerating; TTWB, toe touch weight bearing; IKDC, International Knee Documentation Committee; NL, normal; NN, nearly normal; ab, abnormal; sev ab, severely abnormal; NWB, non weight bearing; PWB, partial weight bearing.

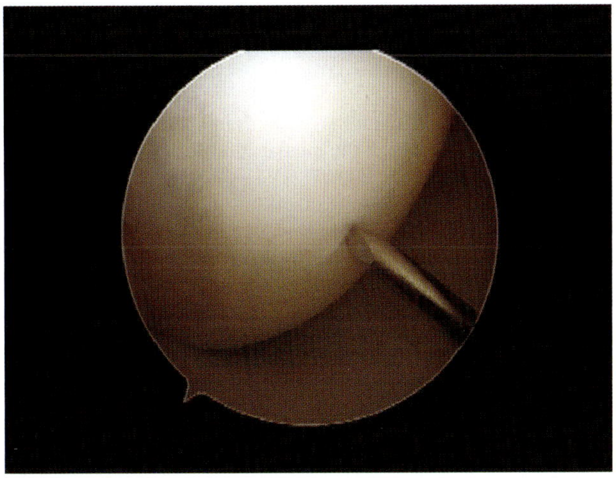

Figure 22.3. Direct arthroscopic visualization of a small K-wire (0.045 in) aligned perpendicularly to the chondral surface of the medial femoral condyle of a right knee, immediately prior to a transarticular drilling pass.

at several sites and knee position may need to be adjusted in varying degrees of flexion. The number and distribution of drilling passes varies considerably in the literature. Depending on lesion size, we will generally use 6 to 10 drilling passes with articular cartilage perforations being evenly distributed and separated by at least several millimeters so as not to promote lesion instability.[10]

Rehabilitation

The optimal approach to postoperative rehabilitation after OCD drilling is not well established in the literature. The authors' preference is to protect weight bearing with crutches for 6 weeks while performing non–weight-bearing knee range of motion exercises to optimize the healing environment for the subchondral bone while minimizing chance of lesion progression or instability. Range of motion is pursued as early as possible postoperatively. Postoperative radiographs are obtained at follow-up visits every 6 to 12 weeks to assess healing, which is characterized by progressive decrease in the sclerotic margin of the lesion and increase in the opacification of the prior lucency (Fig. 22.5). Return to sport is dictated by both clinical and radiographic improvement. Specifically, significant subchondral bone healing on radiographs or MRI, as well as resolution of pain, effusion, and any quadriceps or hamstring weakness, should be observed prior to allowing return to athletics. These criteria are especially important for patients planning to return to sports requiring cutting, pivoting, and impact activities. Finally, patients are followed for at least 1 year after return to play to ensure continued symptomatic improvement and no radiographic evidence of lesion progression.

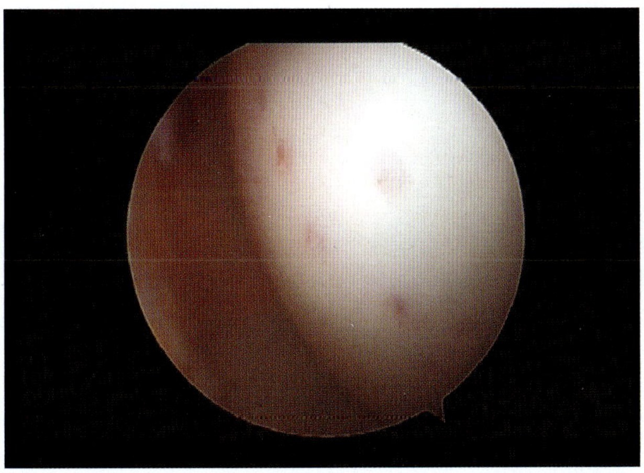

Figure 22.4. The articular surface of a medial femoral condyle in a left knee following multiple, evenly spaced passes of a 0.045-in K-wire.

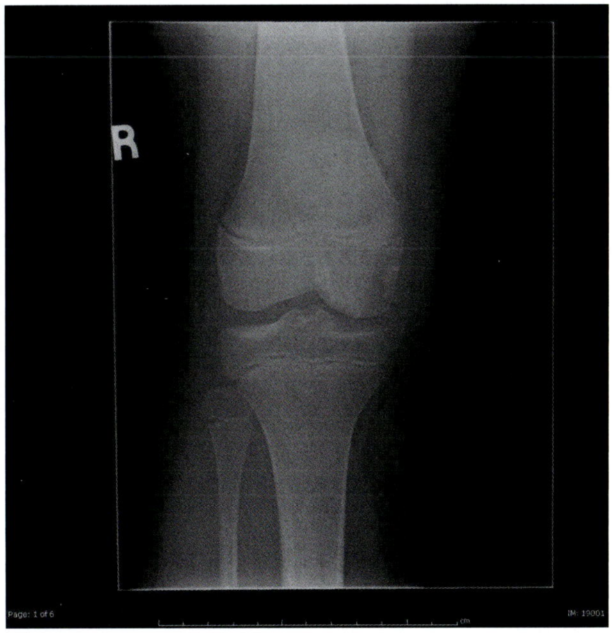

Figure 22.5. Postoperative AP radiograph obtained 2.5 months following transarticular drilling of OCD lesion previously shown in Figure 22.1, now demonstrating less distinct margins and increased opacification of the lesion, suggestive of interval healing.

Complications/Pearls on Avoiding

Complication rates for this procedure are very low with no reported complications in the case series referenced in Table 22.1. Theoretical intraoperative considerations include keeping the drill perpendicular to the chondral surface with each drill pass to avoid iatrogenic injury as well as having fluoroscopy available intraoperatively in case lesion margins cannot be ascertained from probe-based palpation. Postoperatively, patients can develop stiffness, which is why we favor immediate postoperative range of motion as opposed to immobilization in a cast, for example.

REFERENCES

1. Hughston JC, Hergenroeder PT, Courtenay BG. Osteochondritis dissecans of the femoral condyles. *J Bone Joint Surg Am.* 1984;66(9):1340–1348.
2. Kocher MS, Tucker R, Ganley TJ, et al. Management of osteochondritis dissecans of the knee: current concepts review. *Am J Sports Med.* 2006;34(7):1181–1191.

3. Gunton MJ, Carey JL, Shaw CR, et al. Drilling juvenile osteochondritis dissecans: retro- or transarticular? *Clin Orthop Relat Res.* 2013;471(4):1144–1151.
4. Aglietti P, Buzzi R, Bassi PB, et al. Arthroscopic drilling in juvenile osteochondritis dissecans of the medial femoral condyle. *Arthroscopy.* 1994;10(3):286–291.
5. Anderson AF, Richards DB, Pagnani MJ, et al. Antegrade drilling for osteochondritis dissecans of the knee. *Arthroscopy.* 1997; 13(3):319–324.
6. Cepero S, Ullot R, Sastre S. Osteochondritis of the femoral condyles in children and adolescents: our experience over the last 28 years. *J Pediatr Orthop B.* 2005;14(1):24–29.
7. Kocher MS, Micheli LJ, Yaniv M, et al. Functional and radiographic outcome of juvenile osteochondritis dissecans of the knee treated with transarticular arthroscopic drilling. *Am J Sports Med.* 2001;29(5):562–566.
8. Louisia S, Beaufils P, Katabi M, et al. Transchondral drilling for osteochondritis dissecans of the medial condyle of the knee. *Knee Surg Sports Traumatol Arthrosc.* 2003;11(1):33–39.
9. Bradley J, Dandy DJ. Results of drilling osteochondritis dissecans before skeletal maturity. *J Bone Joint Surg Br.* 1989;71(4):642–644.
10. Heyworth BE, Edmonds EW, Murnaghan ML, et al. Drilling techniques for osteochondritis dissecans. *Clin Sports Med.* 2014;33(2): 305–312.

John D. Polousky

CHAPTER 23

Retroarticular Drilling of Osteochondritis Dissecans

INTRODUCTION

Surgical drilling of osteochondritis dissecans (OCD) lesions is a commonly performed treatment for stable lesions in skeletally immature patients. Drilling of OCD lesions is thought to facilitate healing by creating channels in the subchondral bone, which allow revascularization and, ultimately, bony union of the fragment.[1] Outcomes of retroarticular and transarticular drilling techniques have been reported by multiple authors to produce high rates of healing.[1,2] Transarticular drilling penetrates the articular cartilage to access the subchondral bone. Concerns with this technique have been the long-term consequences of perforating the articular cartilage. In contrast, retroarticular drilling allows perforation of the subchondral bone without violating the articular cartilage. Concerns with retroarticular drilling involve the need for intraoperative fluoroscopy and the potential for incomplete drilling because the lesion cannot be visualized directly. In a recent systematic review of the literature comparing transarticular drilling with retroarticular drilling, Gunton et al.[1] concluded that both techniques produced high rates of radiographic healing and comparable patient-oriented outcomes.

TREATMENT

Retroarticular drilling was first described in a case report by Lee and Mercurio[3] in 1981. Since then, multiple authors have reported retrospective case series of patients treated with similar technique. All series report generally good to excellent clinical outcomes and radiographic healing rates ranging from 83% to 100%.[4–8]

Indications

- Stable OCD
- Failure of nonoperative treatment
- Open physes

Contraindications

- Unstable OCD requiring fixation
- Unsalvageable OCD
- Closed physes

AUTHOR'S PREFERRED TREATMENT

Equipment

- Arthroscope
- 0.062-in Kirschner wires (K-wires)
- Micro Vector pin guide (Smith & Nephew, Memphis, TN) (Fig. 23.1A,B)
- C-arm fluoroscopy
- Radiolucent operating table

SURGICAL TECHNIQUE

1. The patient is positioned supine on the operating table. The leg of the bed is not dropped. This allows the surgeon to place K-wires under fluoroscopic guidance with the knee in an extended position in order to facilitate a good anteroposterior (AP) image of the lesion.
2. A standard arthroscopic examination of the knee is performed, with careful inspection of the chondral surface to confirm that the lesion is indeed stable. Care is taken to probe the area, ensuring that there are no fissures at the periphery of the lesion and that the articular cartilage overlying the lesion is in good condition. Often, the OCD is not readily visualized from the chondral surface and only found by subtle softening of the cartilage on gentle probing (Figs. 23.2 and 23.3).
3. Once the arthroscopic examination has confirmed that the lesion is appropriate for retroarticular drilling, the arthroscope is removed.
4. The knee is placed in full extension on the radiolucent table, and the C-arm is used to obtain an AP view of the knee joint visualizing the lesion. It is helpful for the C-arm to be positioned on the side opposite the surgeon. Note that this position will change based on whether the lesion is on the medial or lateral femoral condyle. For example, when drilling a medial lesion, the surgeon will find it easiest to stand on the medial side and have the C-arm come from the lateral side. This setup is reversed for lateral lesions.
5. After localizing the lesion and the physis, a K-wire is placed percutaneously at the medial or lateral edge of the epiphysis

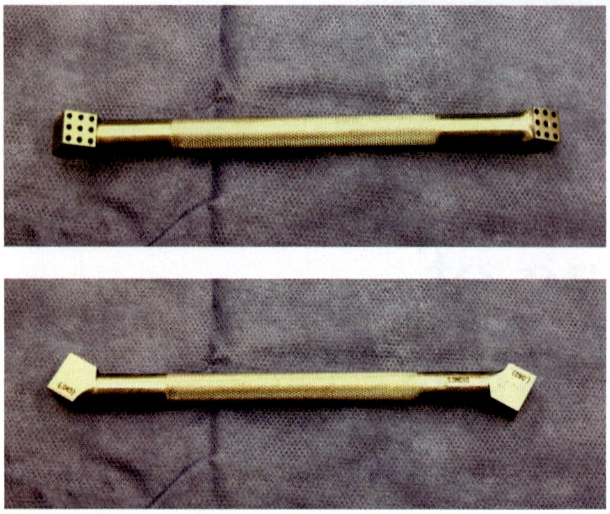

A

B

Figure 23.1. **A,B.** Smith & Nephew Micro Vector pin guide.

directed toward the center of the lesion. The pin driver is used to drill the pin to the center of the lesion. Care is taken not to advance the pin through the articular cartilage. Note that generally, the surgeon can detect a slight increase in resistance while drilling as the wire passes through the sclerotic rim of the lesion.

6. The position of the wire is checked on both the AP and lateral images to confirm its position in or near the lesion.
7. Once the surgeon is satisfied with the position of the initial pin, a small longitudinal incision is made proximal and distal to the K-wire (1 to 2 cm). Making a small incision serves two purposes: (1) The pin guide can be placed directly against the bone, allowing for more accurate K-wire placement, and (2) the incision prevents multiple perforations in the skin by the wire, which can cause tattooing from the heat created by the spinning K-wire (Fig. 23.4).

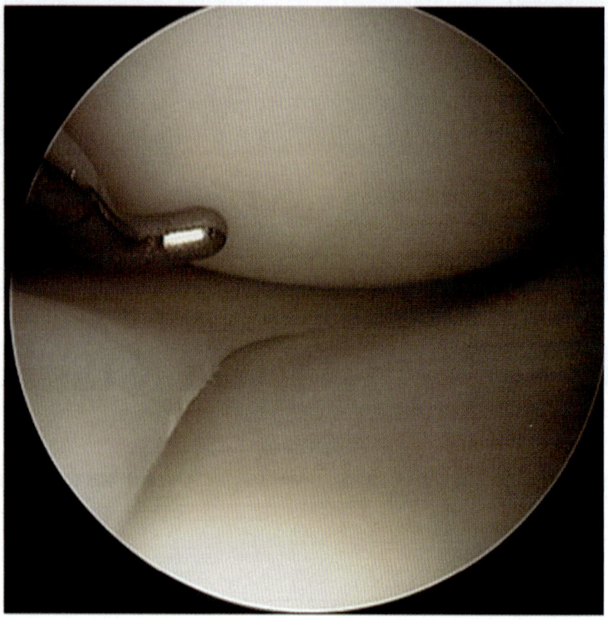

Figure 23.2. Arthroscopic examination of a stable-appearing lesion. Note that the lesion is not grossly visible. The surgeon can localize the lesion by gently probing for areas of subtle softening on the articular surface.

8. The pin guide is then placed over the initial wire and seated on the femur. Multiple K-wires are then drilled into the lesion through the guide while checking the position periodically on AP and lateral images. The pin guide can be shifted over a single reference wire to ensure that the entirety of the lesion is drilled (Fig. 23.5A,B).

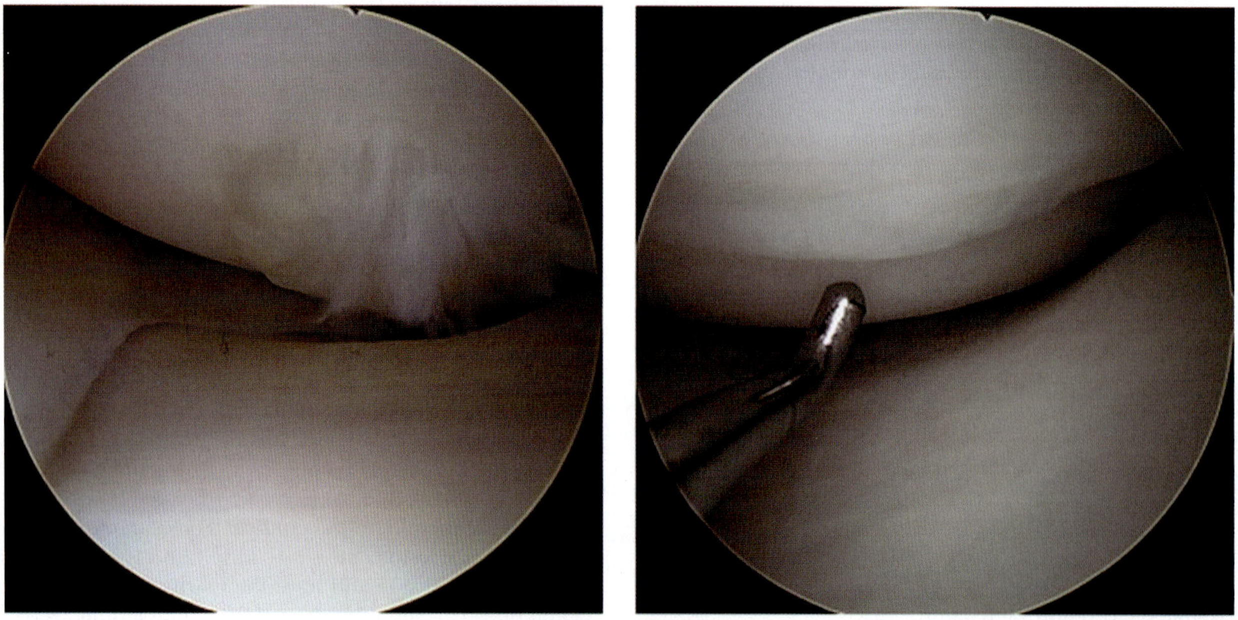

A

B

Figure 23.3. **A,B.** Arthroscopic appearance of an unstable lesion. Note the circumferential fissure. This is not an appropriate lesion for retroarticular drilling alone.

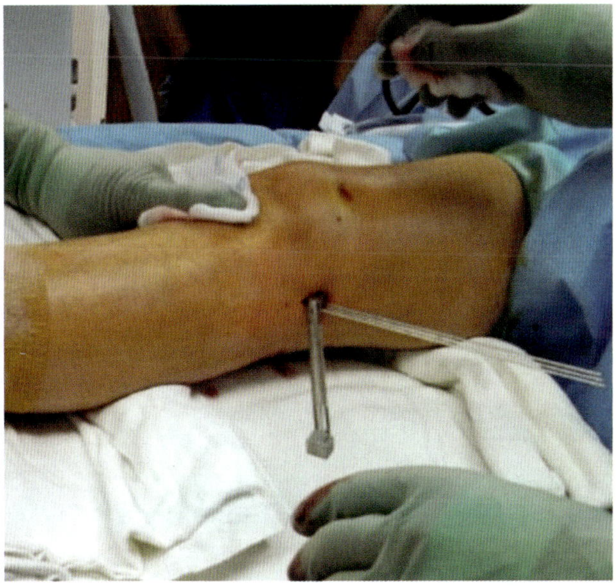

Figure 23.4. A small incision is made over the epicondyle to facilitate guide placement and pin passage.

9. Once the surgeon has confirmed that the lesion has been completely drilled, the K-wires are removed and the incision is irrigated and closed.

Aftercare

Following surgery, patients are allowed toe-touch weight bearing and unlimited range of motion for 6 weeks. During that time, they perform physical therapy, working on range of motion and non–weight-bearing strengthening of the quadriceps, hamstrings, and hips. At 6 weeks postoperative, patients transition to weight bearing as tolerated without impact activities, such as running and jumping, for an additional 6 weeks. Radiographs are taken at 6 weeks to assess healing. At 12 weeks, radiographs are taken again. If patients demonstrate both radiographic and clinical improvement, they are allowed to gradually return to full activities as long as they remain symptom-free (Fig. 23.6A,B).

Complications

Surgical complications with arthroscopic drilling are fortunately quite rare. Multiple authors have reported that they did not have complications with retroarticular drilling in their series.[1] Certainly, retroarticular drilling involves the general risks associated with any type of surgery. The most common problem following any sort of drilling procedure is that the lesion fails to heal. Lesions that fail to heal with drilling are candidates for other procedures described in other chapters in this text. The surgeon can likely maximize the potential for healing by ensuring that the lesion is completely drilled and that the lesions drilled are appropriately selected. Any significant deterioration of the cartilage at the rim of the lesion should prompt the surgeon to question the stability of the lesion and perhaps consider more aggressive procedures with fixation and bone grafting.

Clinically, there are patients who are symptom-free following drilling but fail to completely heal radiographically. In a recent series, Boughanem et al.[9] demonstrated that 2 of 34 lesions remained radiographically stable at a mean follow-up of 4 years but did not completely resolve and yet did not have a poor clinical outcome. Therefore, it does not appear that complete radiographic healing is a prerequisite for a favorable clinical outcome. The author prefers to allow these patients return to full activities as long as they remain asymptomatic. The patients are then followed radiographically every 6 to 12 months.

A

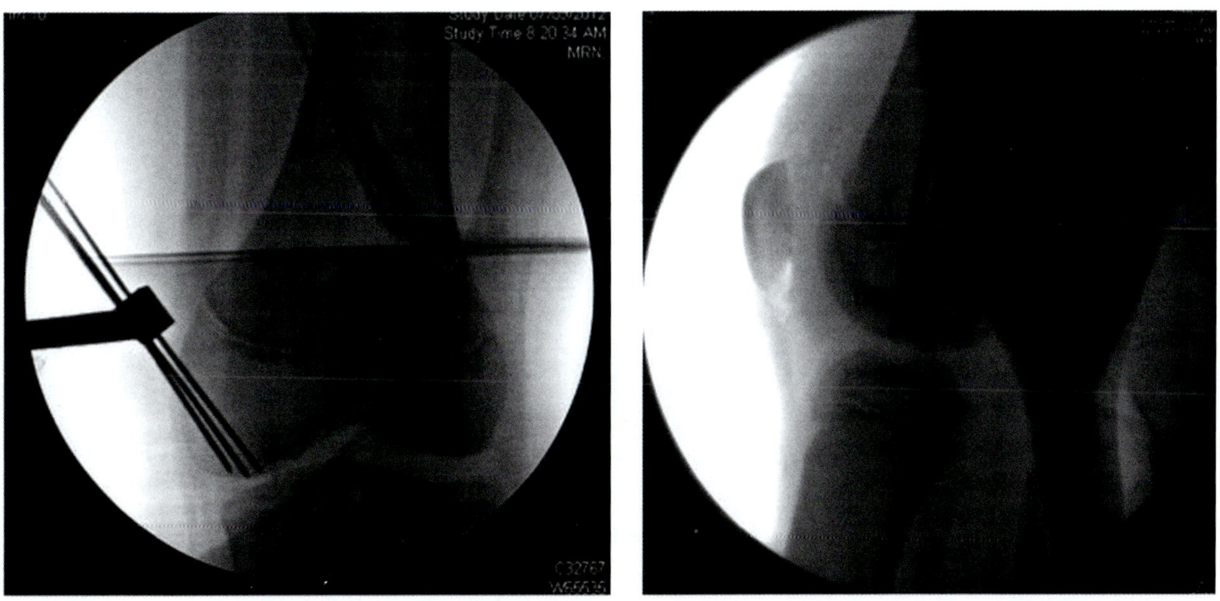

B

Figure 23.5. **A,B.** AP and lateral fluoroscopic images of pin placement.

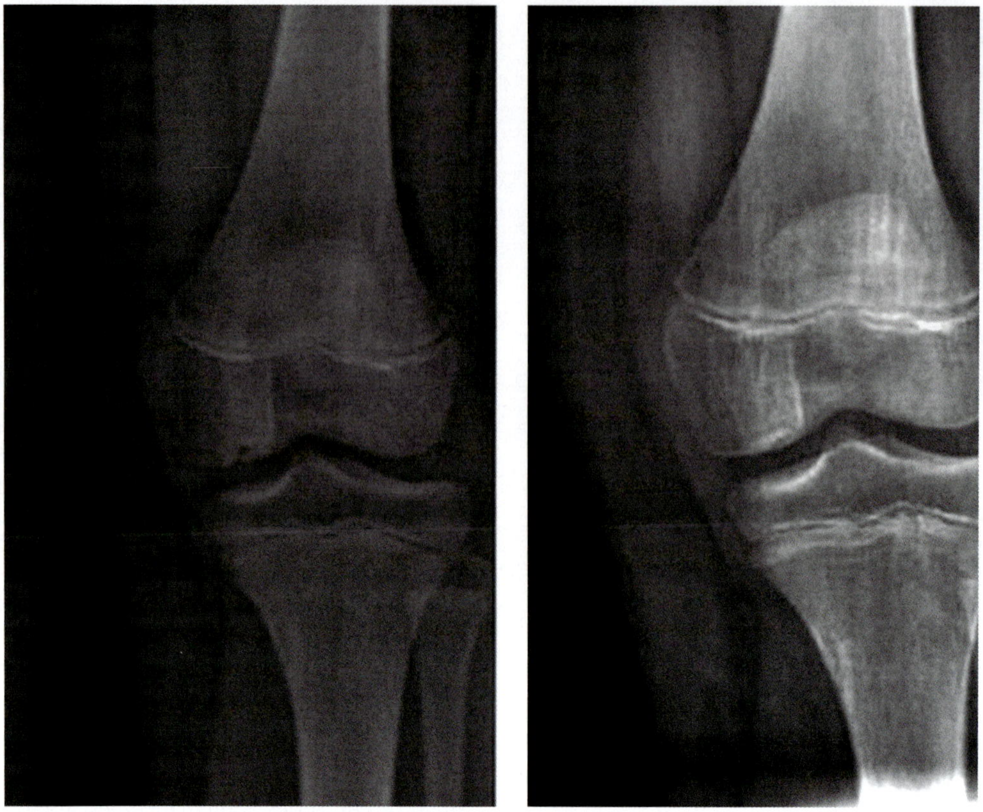

A B

Figure 23.6. A,B. Pre- and postoperative radiographs of a stable OCD that demonstrated both clinical and radiographic healing following retroarticular drilling.

REFERENCES

1. Gunton MJ, Carey JL, Shaw CR, et al. Drilling juvenile osteochondritis dissecans: retro- or transarticular? *Clin Orthop Relat Res.* 2013;471(4):1144–1151.
2. Heyworth BE, Edmonds EW, Murnaghan ML, et al. Drilling techniques for osteochondritis dissecans. *Clin Sports Med.* 2014;33(2):305–312.
3. Lee CK, Mercurio C. Operative treatment of osteochondritis dissecans in situ by retrograde drilling and cancellous bone graft: a preliminary report. *Clin Orthop Relat Res.* 1981;(158):129–126.
4. Kawasaki K, Uchio Y, Adachi N, et al. Drilling from the intercondylar area for treatment of osteochondritis dissecans of the knee joint. *Knee.* 2003;10(3):257–263.
5. Donaldson LD, Wojtys EM. Extraarticular drilling for stable osteochondritis dissecans in the skeletally immature knee. *J Pediatr Orthop.* 2008;28(8):831–835.
6. Adachi N, Deie M, Nakamae A, et al. Functional and radiographic outcome of stable juvenile osteochondritis dissecans of the knee treated with retroarticular drilling without bone grafting. *Arthroscopy.* 2009;25(2):145–152.
7. Edmonds EW, Albright J, Bastrom T, et al. Outcomes of extra-articular, intra-epiphyseal drilling for osteochondritis dissecans of the knee. *J Pediatr Orthop.* 2010;30(8):870–878.
8. Ojala R, Kerimaa P, Lakovaara M, et al. MRI-guided percutaneous retrograde drilling of osteochondritis dissecans of the knee. *Skeletal Radiol.* 2011;40(6):765–770.
9. Boughanem J, Riaz R, Patel RM, et al. Functional and radiographic outcomes of juvenile osteochondritis dissecans of the knee treated with extra-articular retrograde drilling. *Am J Sports Med.* 2011;39(10):2212–2217.

Davietta C. Butty
Adam B. Yanke
Brian J. Cole

CHAPTER

24

Open Reduction Internal Fixation Metal Compression Techniques for Juvenile Osteochondritis Dissecans

INTRODUCTION

The hallmark of osteochondritis dissecans (OCD) is pathologic destruction of the subchondral bone with secondary changes to the overlying articular cartilage. These changes can lead to pain, instability, and early-onset arthritis. The true etiology is not well understood; however, it has been proposed that the following are contributing factors: repetitive microtrauma, vascular insufficiency,[1] genetic predisposition, ossification abnormalities, and endocrine dysfunction. OCD lesions are most common in the knee but can also occur in the wrist, elbow, and ankle. In the knee, the lateral aspect of the medial femoral condyle is the most common lesion location, followed by the lateral femoral condyle and patellofemoral joint. The prevalence of OCD lesions is 15 to 29 per 100,000 individuals, with an average age of onset ranging from 11.3 to 13.4 years.[2] Males are 2 to 3.8 times as likely to have an OCD compared to females, and bilateral lesions are present in 12% to 30% of cases.[3–5] Moreover, ethnic and demographic data demonstrates that blacks have the highest odds ratio of OCD in the knee compared to other ethnicities.[5] The overall incidence of OCD lesions is increasing in addition to the incidence of OCD in females, a trend which some attribute to earlier participation in more competitive sports.[2,6] Adult OCD lesions are mainly juvenile lesions that become symptomatic after the closure of the physis and therefore present in adulthood.[7] This delineation is important, as the treatment of OCD lesions depends greatly on the ability of the host to heal the lesion. Therefore, treatment of juvenile lesions with open physes varies greatly from those in patients with closed physes, as 50% of stable juvenile OCD lesions will heal on their own within 10 to 18 months.[8] Concerns for the early development of arthritis and its associated morbidity provide the impetus for early operative treatment in symptomatic unstable lesions.[9]

HISTORY AND PHYSICAL EXAM

Because the incidence of OCD lesions has been reported to be 0.015% to 0.03% in asymptomatic patients, making an accurate diagnosis is critical.[10] It is important to elicit from the patient how long the symptoms have been present and determine if prior treatments have been offered, including specific amounts of time spent with protected weight bearing or relative rest from higher impact activities. Longer duration of symptoms may manifest itself in quadriceps atrophy at the time of exam. The signs and symptoms of a patient with a juvenile OCD lesion are often very sensitive but nonspecific. Typical findings include knee pain, swelling after activity, and, occasionally, mechanical symptoms such as catching and locking. However, the presence of mechanical symptoms is suggestive of and potentially pathognomonic for the presence of a loose body or unstable osteochondral fragment.[6]

On physical exam, the examiner may observe an antalgic gait, and the patient may be tender to palpation over the anteromedial knee if the lesion is in the classic location of the distal medial femoral condyle. Although the "Wilson" test (internal rotation of the tibia while extending the knee against resistance)[11] has been described for these lesions, it is not very reliable.[6,10,12] The examiner may differentiate an OCD lesion from meniscal pathology by noting more tenderness at the femoral condyle than the joint line itself. Although physical exam is important for confirming objective signs of intra-articular pathology, imaging is the keystone for determining surgical treatment.

IMAGING

Initial evaluation of the patient with a suspected OCD lesion should include standard radiographs of the knee with bilateral anteroposterior (AP) and lateral weight bearing, Merchant (axial), and Rosenberg (posteroanterior at 45-degree flexion) views.[10,13] Tunnel and skyline views may also be beneficial.[14] These views allow for an assessment of physeal status and lesion size, location, sclerosis, fragmentation, and displacement.[10,13] Magnetic resonance imaging (MRI) is also used to evaluate lesions and has recently been referred to as the *gold standard*[15] to further delineate the lesion. The most crucial

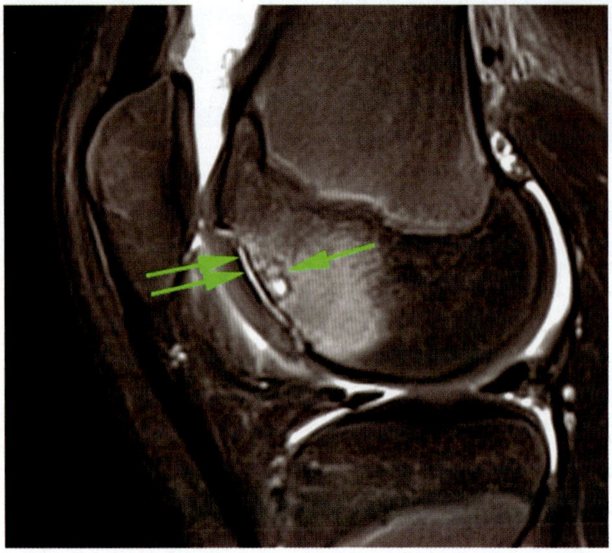

Figure 24.1. Skeletally immature patient with OCD lesion to the trochlea with high signal intensity deep to the lesion (*double arrow*) and cystic changes with bone marrow edema as well (*single arrow*).

portion of the MRI is determining the presence of signal deep to the lesion, indicating instability (Fig. 24.1). The De Smet MRI criteria are the most prevalent classification system used[16]:

1. A thin line of high signal intensity measuring 5 mm or more in length at the interface between the OCD lesion and the underlying bone
2. A discrete, round area of homogeneous high signal intensity 5 mm or more in diameter beneath the lesion
3. A focal defect with a width of 5 mm or more in the articular surface of the lesion
4. A high signal intensity line traversing the articular cartilage and subchondral bone plate into the lesion

TREATMENT

The goal of any treatment is to reduce pain and improve function of the knee. Surgical decisions are based on a number of factors including clinical symptoms; patient age; physeal maturity; and lesion stability, location, and size.[17]

Nonoperative Treatment

Currently, there is no role for treatment of an incidental juvenile OCD lesion. Most juvenile OCD lesions respond well to activity modification and limited weight bearing when stable. Nonoperative management consists of anti-inflammatory medications, relative rest, and protected weight bearing for 6 to 8 weeks. After this time, if the patient is symptom-free, a gradual return to sports and other high-impact activities takes place over another 6 to 8 weeks. Immobilization is controversial, as this can lead to stiffness and contradicts the initial work done by Salter et al.[10,18] Immobilization for a period of greater than 16 weeks can lead to stiffness, cartilage degeneration, muscle atrophy, and poor healing[10,19] and should be avoided. In a multicenter review by Hefti et al.,[4] young patients treated nonoperatively had better results when they had lesions less than 2 cm^2, had no signs of infection, and no effusion at the time of diagnosis. Classic location on the medial femoral condyle was also associated with higher healing rates,[2] whereas larger lesions and those on the lateral femoral condyle had lower healing rates.[20] Healing rates for skeletally immature patients with nonoperative treatment range from 50% to 94% at 10 to 18 months.[21]

Operative Treatment

Surgical management of juvenile OCD lesions is indicated for patients with detached or unstable lesions or patients who fail a conservative course of treatment.[2,10] There are a number of palliative, reparative, restorative, and reconstructive surgical procedures used to treat OCD lesions, depending on lesion characteristics and patient activity (Fig. 24.2). There is no consensus on which surgical procedure yields the best outcomes. A systematic review of surgical procedures for juvenile OCD lesions showed that radiographic and clinical improvements at short-, mid-, and long-term follow-up were lower for fragment excision than for drilling, microfracture, autologous chondrocyte implantation (ACI), osteochondral autograft/allograft, and fragment fixation.[22] There was no difference in expected outcomes between the other procedures. Some authors conversely report success with fragment excision.[15] The one option that remains the gold standard is repairing the native fragment in situ whenever possible. The reparative strategy of open reduction and internal fixation (ORIF) technique with metal compression screw fixation is ideal if the fragment conformation allows and will be discussed here.

Open Reduction and Internal Fixation with Metal Compression Screws

Conceptually, unstable OCD lesions are biologically similar to a fracture nonunion, and to that extent, the same biomechanical principles apply related to enabling biology and adhering to the basic principles of osteosynthesis. As such, the goals of internal fixation of an unstable OCD lesion are to reapproximate the articular cartilage surfaces, promote vascular perfusion of the defect, and provide compressive force to aid in osseous integration, such that the fragment is effectively incorporated into the surrounding subchondral bone and articular cartilage.[19,23]

TECHNIQUE

Patient Positioning and Setup

The patient should be positioned supine on the operating table, typically with the leg of the bed lowered and the thigh placed in a leg holder. This position allows for hyperflexion of the knee. However, if a patellar or trochlear lesion is present, open treatment is preferred and requires an arthrotomy. In this setting, the operating table can remain flat and no leg holder is needed. Diagnostic arthroscopy is always performed first to remove loose bodies and determine lesion stability, size, and ability to place a compression screw. Importantly, if

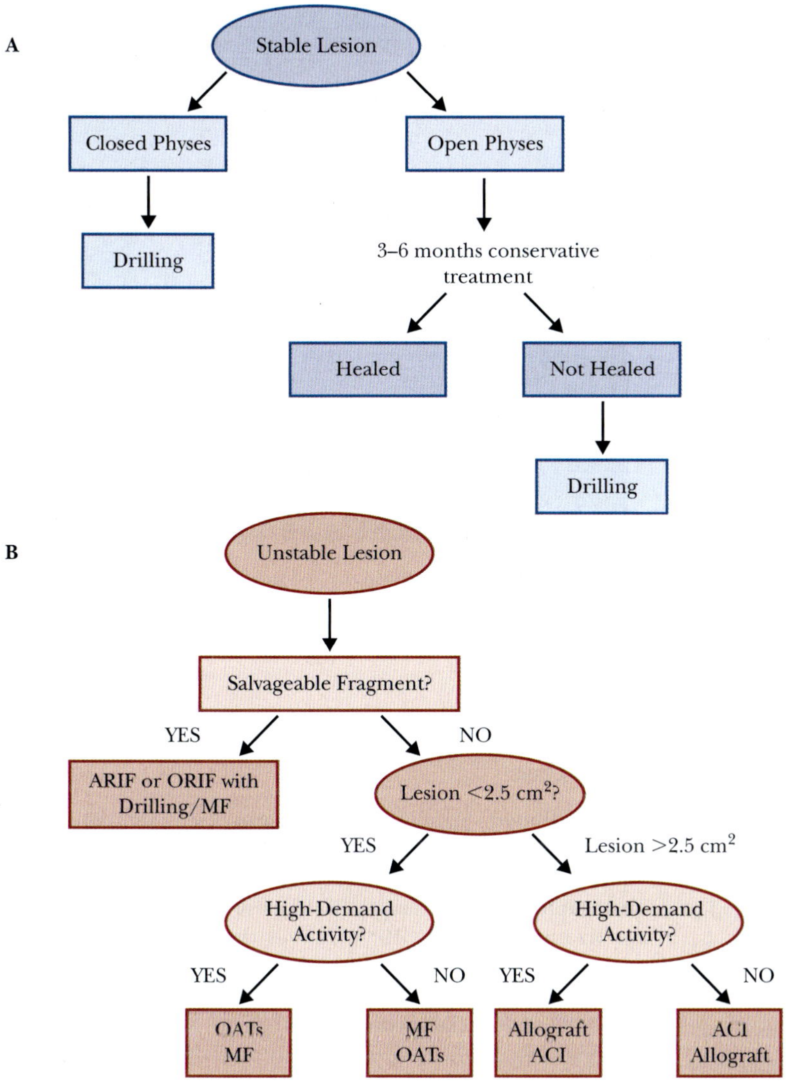

Figure 24.2. Treatment algorithm for OCD of the knee. *ARIF,* arthroscopic reduction internal fixation; *ORIF,* open reduction internal fixation; *MF,* microfracture; *OATs,* osteochondral autograft/allograft transplant; *ACI,* autologous chondrocyte implantation.

the patient has evidence of an unstable lesion on imaging, the clinician must be appropriately aggressive with probing during arthroscopy, as symptomatic lesions may go untreated. Portals are placed in the typical anteromedial and anterolateral positions; however, a spinal needle can be used to establish an accessory portal used for fixation.

Defect Preparation

A probe or elevator can be used to elevate the fragment from its bed and assess for the quantity and quality of the bone on the backside of the fragment (Fig. 24.3). Ideally, a small hinge is left intact, keeping the fragment in the vicinity and preventing free rotation. Using an arthroscopic shaver, any remaining soft tissue at the interface is removed and débrided until bone is encountered. Bleeding can be stimulated from the lesion bed using microfracture awls, Kirschner wires (K-wire), or a drill. Turning off the inflow temporarily with mildly increased outflow should demonstrate egress of bone marrow elements. If unstable edges that will likely not remain viable are present, the combination of a basket and no. 11 blade scalpel is used to débride the edge of the defect.

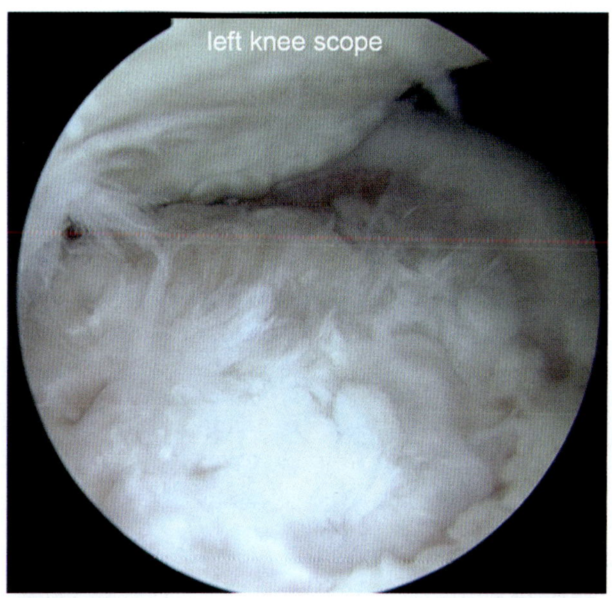

Figure 24.3. Arthroscopic evaluation demonstrates minimal cartilage available on this OCD fragment but enough required for fixation.

Fragment Reduction and Fixation

Once the débridement of the defect site is complete, the fragment can be provisionally reduced with an arthroscopic probe. Occasionally, there are cystic changes or attritional bone loss that may benefit from local bone grafting. If required, an osteochondral autograft harvesting tube can be used to obtain small amounts of cancellous autograft from the intercondylar notch or lateral trochlear edge similar to obtaining a donor plug used in an osteochondral autograft/allograft transplant (OATs) procedure. The procedure can still be performed entirely arthroscopically or through a small arthrotomy if need be.

Typically, the surgeon should plan for the number of screws required for fixation, which is ideally a minimum of two to neutralize rotational forces. As the authors prefer the use of cannulated metal screws, placement of K-wires should be located where the screw will ultimately be placed. The K-wires are commonly placed through an accessory portal that is determined by initially triangulating with a spinal needle placed percutaneously to optimize a portal, allowing perpendicular access to the lesion surface. The authors prefer small-diameter, differentially pitched screws which have the following qualities: headless, cannulated, self-drilling, and variable pitch to allow for compression. First, one to two 0.045-in guide wires are placed into the lesion and defect. A depth gauge can be used to measure the length of the screw needed, which should be within 2 mm of the posterior cortex and typically 2 mm shorter than what is measured (allows for compression). Using a cannulated profile drill over the K-wire can aid in screw placement in young patients with dense bone. The screw is introduced with a manual screwdriver until the head is recessed within the cartilage surface, typically at least two turns. A second screw is placed when possible in a similar fashion. If using two or more screws, avoid parallel placement and err on the side of divergent placement to increase stability. Because the screws will likely be removed, it is helpful to use screw lengths of at least 24 to 26 mm when possible to facilitate screw removal.

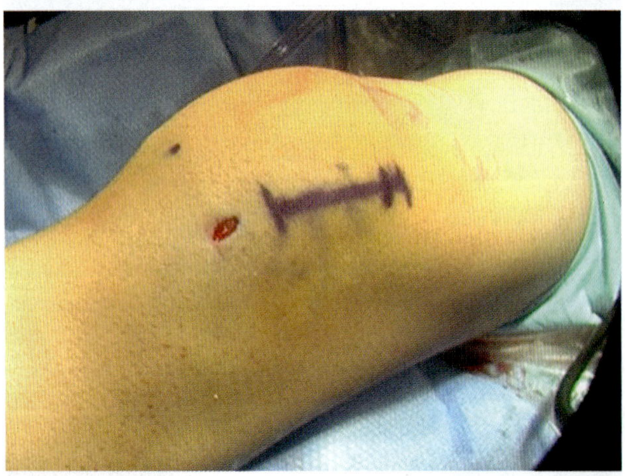

Figure 24.4. The mini-arthrotomy is marked out for open treatment of a trochlear OCD.

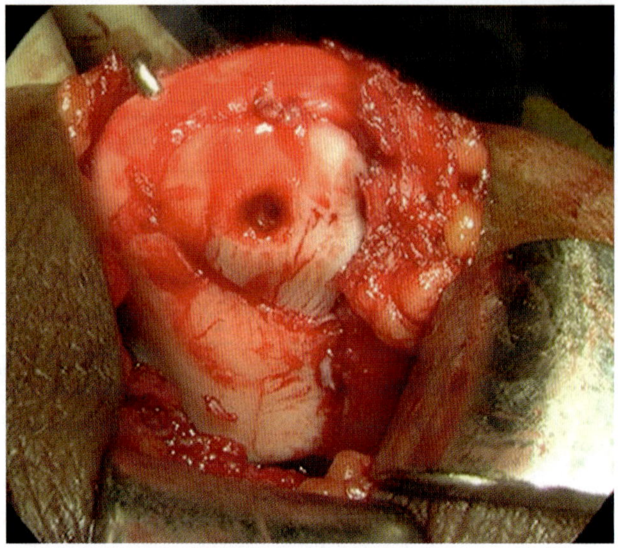

Figure 24.5. Open arthrotomy and patellar eversion for treatment of a patellar OCD.

CASES

Open Case

As mentioned, patellofemoral lesions (see Fig. 24.1) are often difficult to treat arthroscopically; therefore, the authors prefer the open approach. In this setting, the defect is first explored arthroscopically to ensure proper indications for fixation (see Fig. 24.3). This is then followed by a limited arthrotomy for trochlear lesions (Fig. 24.4) versus patellar eversion for patellar lesions (Fig. 24.5). The defect site is débrided and microfracture is performed, leading to a bleeding bed (Fig. 24.6). K-wires are then placed into the fragment

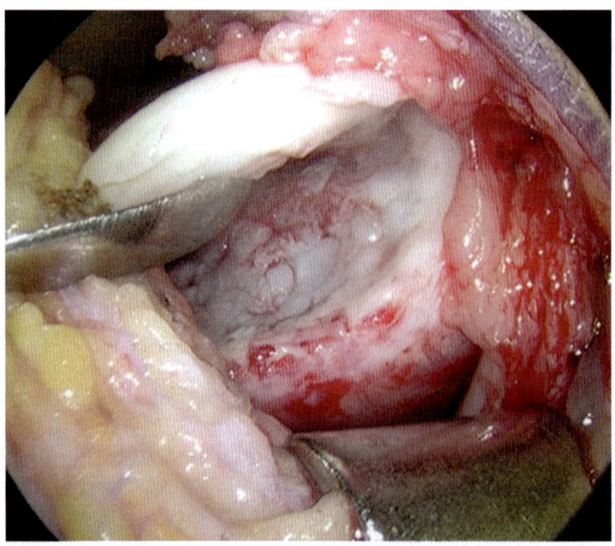

Figure 24.6. Débridement of the osseous bed, in this case with microfracture awls, aids in defect healing.

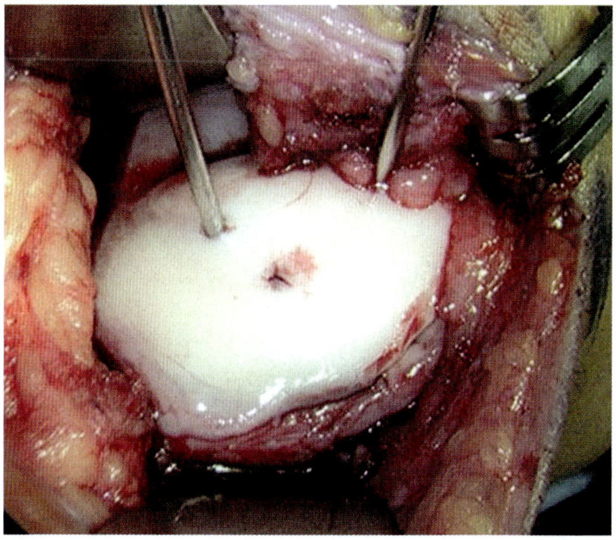

Figure 24.7. K-wire placement allows for provisional reduction and guidance of the cannulated screws.

for reduction (Fig. 24.7) followed by pilot drilling (Fig. 24.8) and screw placement (Fig. 24.9).

Arthroscopic Case

Patients with medial or lateral femoral condyle lesions can typically be treated arthroscopically with an accessory portal. In this case, the condylar lesion was probed and demonstrated to be unstable (Fig. 24.10) with a fibrous union (Fig. 24.11). This is then débrided with an arthroscopic shaver and curette (Fig. 24.12) followed by stimulation of marrow elements, in this case, with microfracture awls (Fig. 24.13). Spinal needle localization perpendicular to the fragment allows placement of the accessory portal (Fig. 24.14). As described, this is followed by placement of the K-wires, over-reaming, and screw insertion (Figs. 24.15 to 24.18).

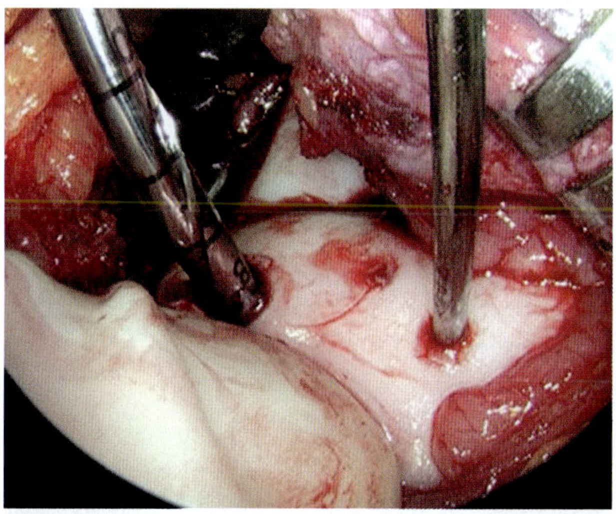

Figure 24.8. The pilot drill is used to over-ream the K-wire, and the surgeon's finger is used as an open reduction aid to prevent fragment rotation.

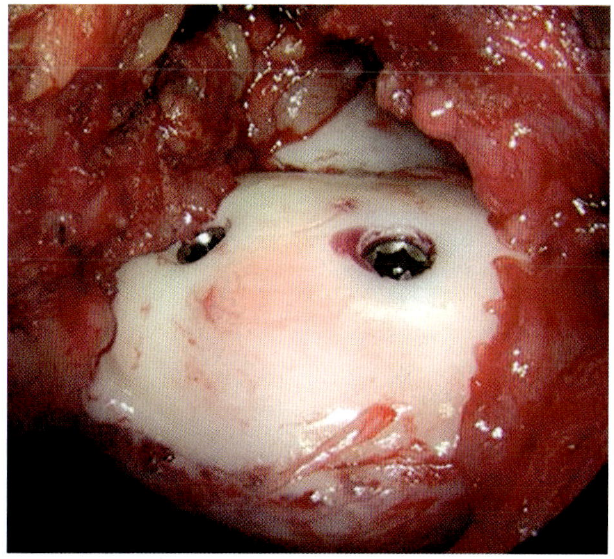

Figure 24.9. Metal cannulated screws are then placed over the K-wire. The screw should be placed at least two turns past the chondral surface.

Equipment Used

- Standard 30-degree arthroscope
- 3.5-mm arthroscopic shaver and curettes
- Arthroscopic probe
- Microfracture awls, K-wire and driver, or drill device
- Acutrak Mini Screws (or equivalent)
- Osteochondral autograft harvesting tubes

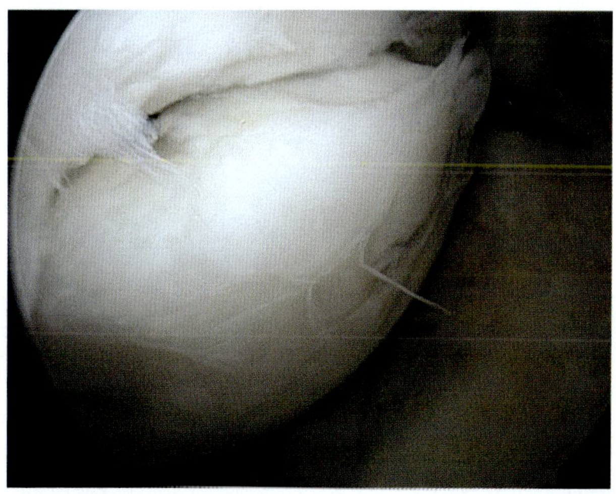

Figure 24.10. Arthroscopic probing of the condylar defect demonstrated its instability.

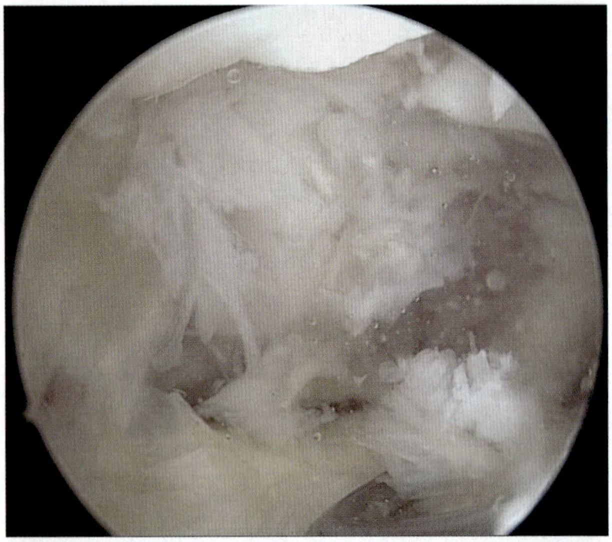

Figure 24.11. Evaluation of the defect demonstrates an appropriate osseous fragment for fixation and soft tissue fibrous union at the bed.

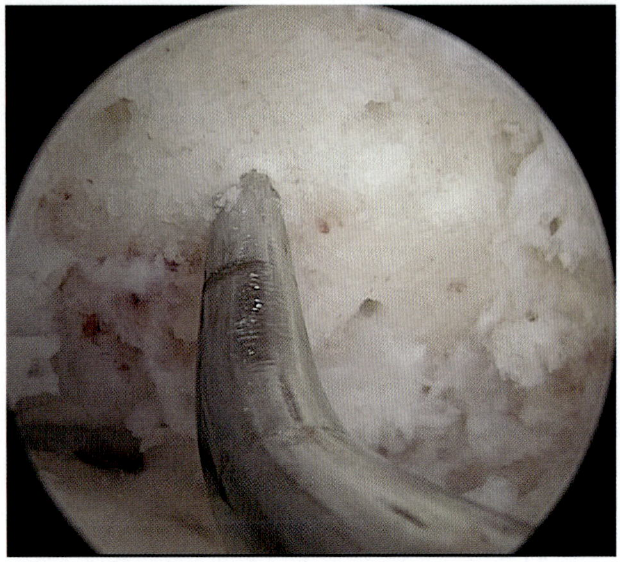

Figure 24.13. Microfracture of the defect site to gain access to the marrow elements.

Postoperative Rehabilitation

The goals of postoperative rehabilitation are to restore range of motion, strength, and overall function of the knee. Our approach begins with effective pain management and early knee mobilization through the use of a continuous passive motion (CPM) machine beginning on the first postoperative day. The patient is instructed to use the CPM machine for 6 to 8 hours each day. Initially, the knee is ranged from 0 to 30 degrees and is advanced as tolerated to 0 to 120 degrees by 6 weeks postoperatively. Strength training exercises during this time are low impact and focus on straight-leg raises and quadriceps strengthening. Patients may heel-touch or partial weight bear as tolerated for the first 8 weeks. Hardware is typically removed at the 8th- to 10th-week postoperative mark during a second-look arthroscopic and radiographic assessment of the healing progress. We recommend abstaining from high-impact activities for 8 to 12 weeks following the second-look arthroscopy to ensure proper fragment union. The primary reason to remove

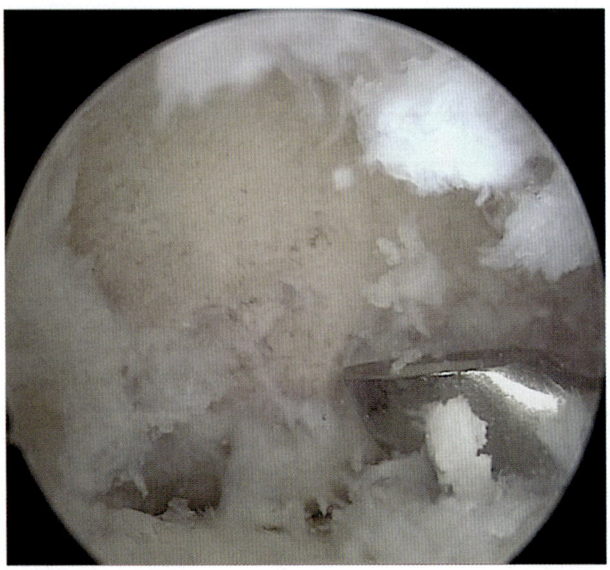

Figure 24.12. Arthroscopic débridement of the OCD bed with curette and shaver.

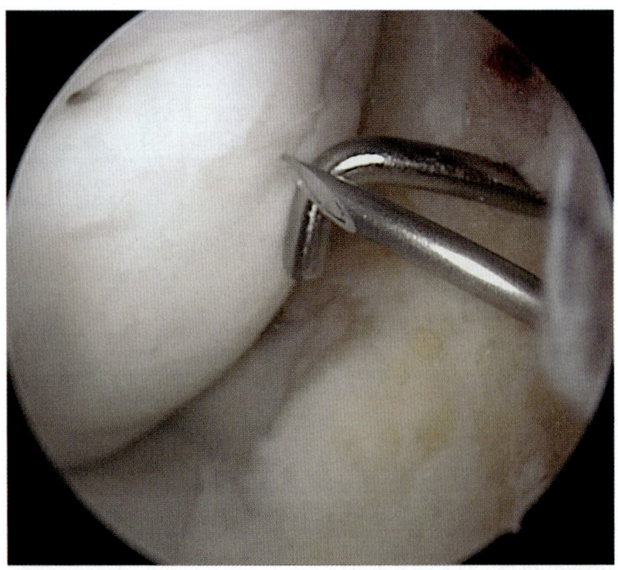

Figure 24.14. Spinal needle accessory portal localization to allow for perpendicular access.

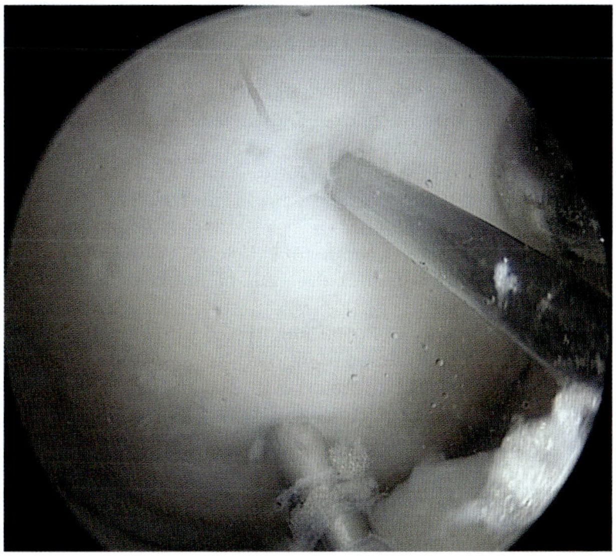

Figure 24.15. Arthroscopic K-wire placement for fragment reduction and cannulated screw placement.

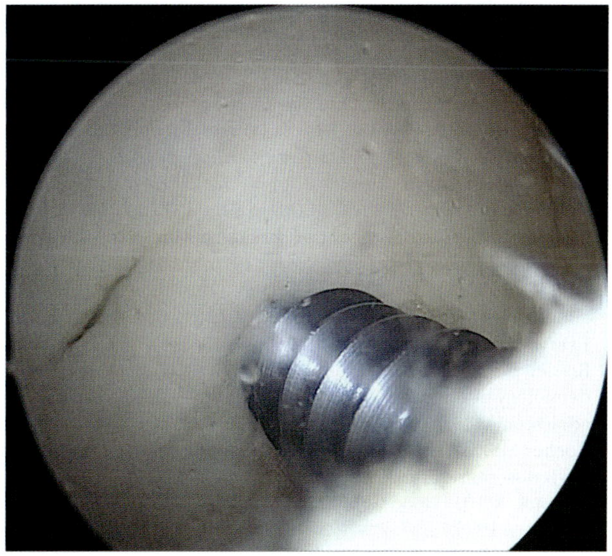

Figure 24.17. Cannulated screw placement over the K-wire.

the screws is because, if patients still have pain postoperatively, the second look allows verification and potential débridement of nonhealed portions of the lesion. In addition, the fragment can settle in the defect bed, and if this occurs, the screw heads can become prominent, affecting the opposing articular surface.

Complications

Complications can arise from fixing the OCD fragment with the screws proud relative to the surrounding articular cartilage surface instead of recessing them in the articular cartilage surface. Proud screws can cause erosion of the opposing cartilage and cause continued pain and discomfort for the patient. Aside from being proud, hardware can also break, causing pain with possible mechanical symptoms from loose bodies.[17] Additionally, complications can include fragment instability from poor fixation or fragment nonunion as well as from inaccurate fragment reduction.[24] Synovitis is also a potential complication from hardware reactions.

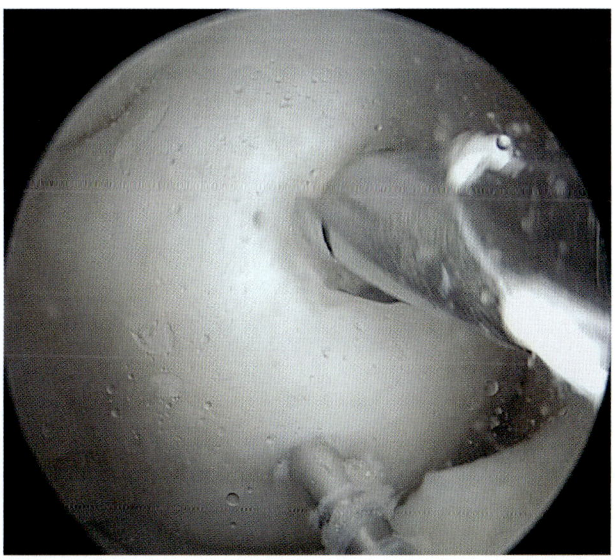

Figure 24.16. Over-reaming the K-wire for screw placement.

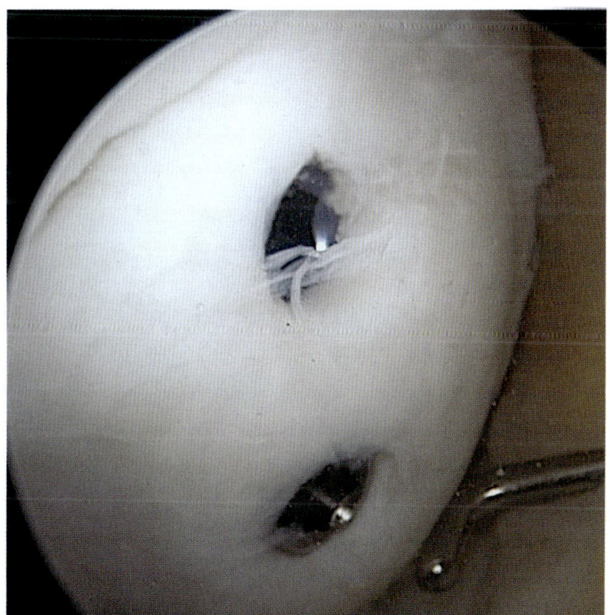

Figure 24.18. Final construct in place with two cannulated screws recessed from the articular cartilage surface.

REFERENCES

1. Olstad K, Hendrickson EH, Carlson CS, et al. Transection of vessels in epiphyseal cartilage canals leads to osteochondrosis dissecans in the femoro-patellar joint of foals; a potential model of juvenile osteochondritis dissecans. *Osteoarthritis Cartilage.* 2013;21(5):730–738.
2. Cahill BR. Osteochondritis dissecans of the knee: treatment of juvenile and adult forms. *J Am Acad Orthop Surg.* 1995;3:237–247.
3. Lindén B. The incidence of osteochondritis dissecans in the condyles of the femur. *Acta Orthop Scand.* 1976;47:664–667.
4. Hefti F, Beguiristain J, Krauspe R, et al. Osteochondritis dissecans: a multicenter study of the European Pediatric Orthopedic Society. *J Pediatr Orthop B.* 1999;8(4):231–245.
5. Kessler JI, Nikizad H, Shea KG, et al. The demographics and epidemiology of osteochondritis dissecans of the knee in children and adolescents. *Am J Sports Med.* 2014;42:320–326.
6. Kocher MS, Tucker R, Ganley TJ, et al. Management of osteochondritis dissecans of the knee. *Am J Sports Med.* 2006;34(7):1181–1191.
7. Schenck RC Jr, Goodnight JM. Osteochondritis dissecans. *J Bone Joint Surg.* 1996;78(3):439–456.
8. Cahill BR, Berg BC. 99m-Technetium phosphate compound joint scintigraphy in the management of juvenile osteochondritis dissecans of the femoral condyles. *Am J Sports Med.* 1983;11:329–335.
9. Twyman RS, Desai K, Aichroth PM. Osteochondritis dissecans of the knee: a long-term study. *J Bone Joint Surg.* 1991;73(3):461–464.
10. Erickson BJ, Chalmers PN, Yanke AB, et al. Surgical management of osteochondritis dissecans of the knee. *Curr Rev Musculoskelet Med.* 2013;6(2):102–114.
11. Wilson JN. A diagnostic sign in osteochondritis dissecans of the knee. *J Bone Joint Surg Am.* 1967;49(3):477–480.
12. Conrad JM, Stanitski CL. Osteochondritis dissecans: Wilson's sign revisited. *Am J Sports Med.* 2003;31(5):777–778.
13. Allen CR, Safran MR. Surgical treatment of osteochondritis dissecans of the knee. In: Elattrache NS, ed. *Surgical Techniques in Sports Medicine.* Philadelphia, PA: Lippincott Williams & Wilkins; 2007:534–543.
14. Nakagawa T, Kurosawa H, Ikeda H, et al. Internal fixation for osteochondritis dissecans of the knee. *Knee Surg Sports Traumatol Arthrosc.* 2005;13:317–322.
15. Pascual-Garrido C, Moran CJ, Green DW, et al. Osteochondritis dissecans of the knee in children and adolescents. *Curr Opin Pediatr.* 2013;25(1):46–51.
16. De Smet AA, Ilahi OA, Graf BK. Reassessment of the MR criteria for stability of osteochondritis dissecans in the knee and ankle. *Skelet Radiol.* 1996;25(2):159–163.
17. Pascual-Garrido D, McNickle AG, Cole BJ. Surgical treatment options for osteochondritis dissecans of the knee. *Sports Health.* 2009;1(4):326–334.
18. Salter RB, Simmonds DF, Malcolm BW, et al. The biological effect of continuous passive motion on the healing of full-thickness defects in articular cartilage. An experimental investigation in the rabbit. *J Bone Joint Surg Am.* 1980;62(8):1232–1251.
19. Harada Y, Tomita N, Nakajima M, et al. Effect of low loading and joint immobilization for spontaneous repair of osteochondral defect in the knees of weightless (tail suspension) rats. *J Orthop Sci.* 2005;10(5):508–514.
20. Webb JE, Lewallen LW, Christophersen C, et al. Clinical outcome of internal fixation of unstable juvenile osteochondritis dissecans lesions of the knee. *Orthopedics.* 2013;36(11):e1444–e1449.
21. Cahill Br, Phillips MR, Navarro R. The results of conservative management of juvenile osteochondritis dissecans using joint scintigraphy. A prospective study. *Am J Sports Med.* 1989;17:601–605.
22. Trinh TQ, Harris JD, Flanigan DC. Surgical management of juvenile osteochondritis dissecans of the knee. *Knee Surg Sports Traumatol Arthrosc.* 2012;20:2419–2429.
23. Gomoll AH, Flik KR, Hayden JK, et al. Internal fixation of unstable Cahill type-2C osteochondritis dissecans lesions of the knee in adolescent patients. *Orthopedics.* 2007;30(6):487–490.
24. Camp CL, Krych AJ, Stuart MJ. Arthroscopic preparation and internal fixation of an unstable osteochondritis dissecans lesion of the knee. *Arthrosc Tech.* 2013;2(4):e461–e465.

Jonathan D. Haskel
Tyler J. Uppstrom
Daniel W. Green

CHAPTER 25

Bioabsorbable Fixation of Symptomatic Juvenile Osteochondritis Dissecans Lesions in Children and Adolescents

GENERAL PRINCIPLES IN JUVENILE OSTEOCHONDRITIS DISSECANS MANAGEMENT

For large lesions and unstable lesions that are partially or completely detached, internal fixation is indicated to stabilize the fragment(s). Stabilization with internal fixation promotes vascular perfusion of the osteochondral lesion and stimulates bony healing through the application of a compressive force.[1,2] Internal fixation of juvenile osteochondritis dissecans (JOCD) lesions has historically been performed using metallic hardware. However, recent innovations in fixation have led to the development of a number of types of bioabsorbable implants.

A recent study by Adachi et al.[3] retrospectively evaluated the outcomes of 33 unstable JOCD lesions that underwent fixation using bioabsorbable pins. The authors found that after an average of 2.4 months, 32 of the 33 lesions had healed, as evidenced by plain radiographs.[3] Additionally, in this study, no complications with bioabsorbable fixation instrumentation such as infection, synovitis, or inflammation were evident.

Another study conducted by Dines et al.[4] evaluated the efficacy of bioabsorbable nails composed of poly(L-lactic acid) (PLLA) for internal fixation of JOCD lesions in nine patients. The mean postoperative Lysholm score was 94 and postoperative magnetic resonance imaging (MRI) analysis revealed that seven of the nine lesions had fully healed.

Abouassaly et al.[5] recently published a systematic review that compared the efficacy of the different surgical techniques aimed to treat JOCD lesions. Of the 516 lesions included in the analysis, 94.1% were deemed healed postoperatively in spite of the diversity of techniques employed by the various authors included in the study. We await long-term studies to further characterize the efficacy of bioabsorbable implants in pediatric patients as they skeletally mature.

ADVANTAGES AND DISADVANTAGES OF BIOABSORBABLE AND METALLIC FIXATION OF JUVENILE OSTEOCHONDRITIS DISSECANS LESIONS

Bioabsorbable implants for fixation of JOCD lesions have specific advantages over metallic fixation. Bioabsorbable fixation does not require harvesting healthy tissue, does not interfere with MRI imaging, and may be associated with a lower incidence of hardware prominence.[3] Darts and tacks are typically smaller than screws and therefore induce less damage to the articular cartilage while allowing for more points of fixation. Most importantly, the use of bioabsorbable implants does not require a second operation to remove hardware. The increasing popularity of bioabsorbable implants has also exposed important complications associated with their use. Namely, various studies have reported implant failure and development of a delayed local inflammatory synovitis weeks after implantation.[6] Additionally, most bioabsorbable implants employ a less significant compressive force compared to metallic screws.[3]

At the same time, metallic fixation is also associated with certain disadvantages. The most significant disadvantage is that metallic fixation demands removal of hardware, which can be especially upsetting for pediatric patients who are active in sports and recreation. Having to undergo a second procedure further delays the time for children to return to play and function. Furthermore, Guhl[7] reported that metallic implants are associated with pin breakage, loosening, and migration through the skin. Finally, metallic hardware prominence resulting in damage to the opposing joint surface or screw head breakage may require additional surgical intervention.

IMPLANT OPTIONS

The recent popularity of bioabsorbable fixation has spurred the development of numerous bioabsorbable implant options. The implants that are typically composed of PLLA alone include the SmartScrew, the SmartNail, the Bio-Compression Screw, and the Chondral Dart. However, other implants are copolymers between PLLA and PGA (polyglycolic acid). These include the ReUnite screw and the LactoNail. One study compared the compression forces and pullout strengths of four different bioabsorbable implants (SmartScrew, SmartNail, LactoNail, ReUnite Screw) for osteochondritis dissecans (OCD) lesion fixation using a synthetic bone model.[8] The authors found that the SmartScrew generated the greatest compression force as well as the greatest pullout strength compared to the other three implants. See Table 25.1 for a summary of the bioabsorbable implant options.

AUTHORS' PREFERRED TECHNIQUE: OPEN REDUCTION AND INTERNAL FIXATION USING BIOABSORBABLE FIXATION IMPLANTS

Diagnostic arthroscopy is performed to verify the size and quality of the lesion while simultaneously removing small loose bodies and debris within the joint. For hinged or partially detached lesions, a probe can be used to elevate the fragment, exposing the fragment–bed interface for assessment. An arthroscopic shaver is used to clean and débride any soft tissue on each surface until bone is encountered. For completely detached osteochondral lesions, attention is first directed toward débridement of the subchondral bed in which the lesion sits. Fibrous tissue within the bed is removed, and multiple drill holes are introduced into the sclerotic bed of bone using microfracture awls, K-wires, or drills to allow improved access to the subchondral blood supply for repair. Next, the fragment is débrided and fibrous tissue is removed. Frayed or incompetent edges and flaps are removed from the fragment and bed. It is important to inspect the fit of the fragment, given the size of the bed. If the bed is depressed, consider local bone autografting from the lateral trochlear edge or other bone graft sites such as the iliac crest. For the majority of completely detached cases, this procedure can be performed through a small arthrotomy. However, for most partially detached fragments, arthroscopic techniques can be used. For best visualization, we use both a 30- and 70-degree arthroscope.

The implant-introducing device is advanced into the joint and positioned onto the surface of the osteochondral fragment. When contact has been made, 1.5-mm K-wires are advanced through accessory portals into the joint and through the lesion to provide additional fixation of the fragment and ensure alignment of the implant-introducing tip. Next, a hole is drilled through the osteochondral lesion using a 1.5-mm drill. The SmartNail drill is advanced to the preferred depth when the desired depth marks on the drill align with the side holes near the handle.

A bioabsorbable SmartNail bone fixation implant is inserted into the rear of the handle. A piston is advanced into the rear of the handle until it reaches the silicon cover of the fixation implant. The piston is then tapped with a hammer until the piston reaches its preferred position. We typically use three to four 1.5-mm SmartNails for a 1 cm loose body.

The authors of this chapter prefer to treat each patient whom we feel is an appropriate candidate for surgical management of a JOCD lesion with biodegradable fixation implants. However, we prefer to always have metal interference screws accessible in the operating room during each JOCD case in the event that additional fixation of the osteochondral defect is desired.

POSTOPERATIVE MANAGEMENT OF JUVENILE OSTEOCHONDRITIS DISSECANS LESIONS

Patients are recommended non–weight bearing on crutches for at least 6 weeks while performing non–weight-bearing knee range-of-motion exercises to prevent postoperative stiffness. After 6 weeks, we typically recommend weight bearing as tolerated without running and jumping for an additional 6 weeks. Return to sports can commence after clinical and radiographic evidence of healing. Healing of the treated lesion is determined by evaluating the patient's plain radiographs and MRI at follow-up. Resolution of the radiolucent area on anteroposterior (AP) and lateral views of plain radiographs, as well as disappearance of the high-intensity signal around the lesion on MRI, indicate initiation of healing. Repeat arthroscopy is indicated if the patient is symptomatic or if any area of the lesion is incompletely healed on postoperative radiographs.

CASES

Case 1

An 11-year-old male presented with a painful JOCD lesion of his right medial femoral condyle (Fig. 25.1A). Arthroscopic assessment found the lesion to be unstable. Arthroscopic treatment included debridement of intervening fibrous tissue and fixation with multiple bioabsorbable SmartNails. At 5-months follow-up, MRI evaluation displayed significant signs of healing (Fig. 25.1B).

Case 2

A 16-year-old male presented with a JOCD lesion of his left medial femoral condyle (Fig. 25.2AB). He underwent arthroscopic debridement and internal fixation of the loose body with multiple bioabsorbable SmartNails. At 1-year post-op, the patient's distal femoral and proximal tibial physes were open, and his follow-up MR revealed good healing of the subchondral bone and overlying cartilage (Fig. 25.2CD).

TABLE 25.1 Bioabsorbable Fixation Implants for Juvenile Osteochondritis Dissecans

	Fixation	*Manufacturer*	*Composition*	*Sizes (mm)*	*Picture*
SmartScrew	Screw	Conmed Linvatec (Largo, FL)	PLLA	2.0 × 10–20 2.7 × 10–24 3.5 × 14–40	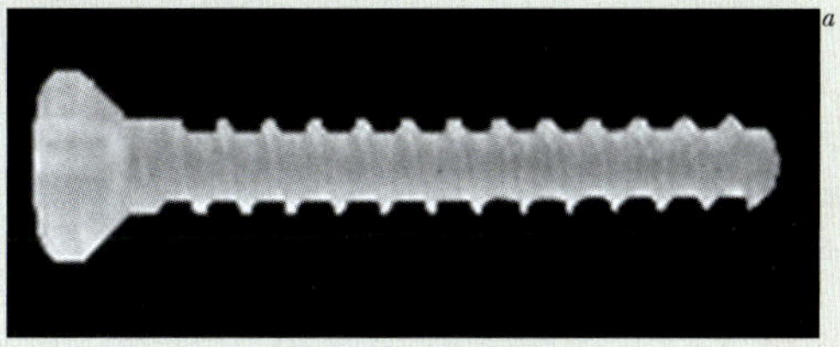 *a*
ReUnite	Screw	Arthrotek Biomet, Inc. (Warsaw, IN)	PGA/PLLA	2.0 × 5–17 2.5 × 5–27 2.8 × 11–33	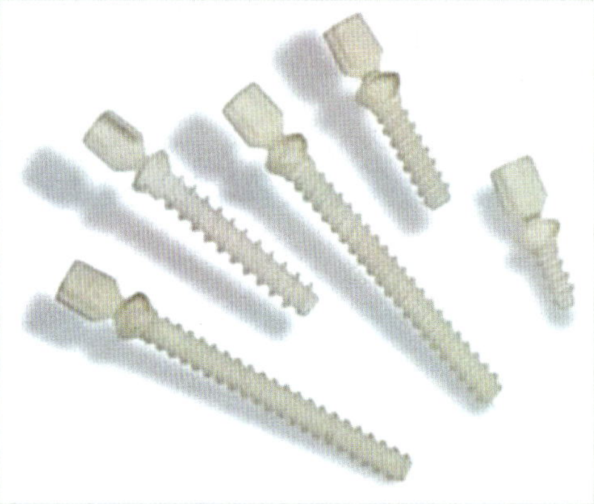 *b*
Bio-Compression Screw	Screw	Arthrex, Inc. (Naples, FL)	PLLA	2.7 × 16–26	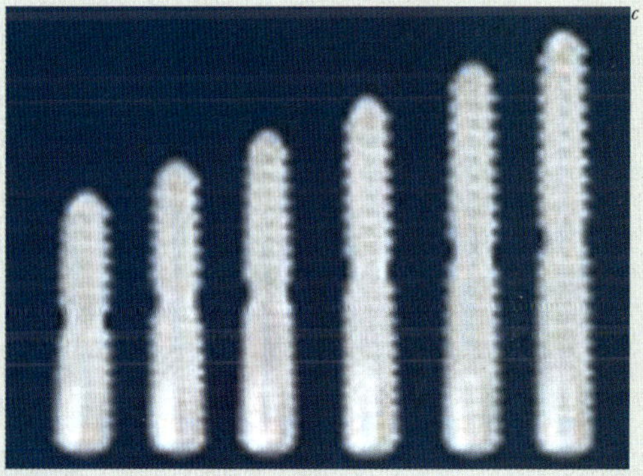 *c*
SmartNail	Nail	Conmed Linvatec (Largo, FL)	PLLA	1.5 × 16–25 2.4 × 16–45	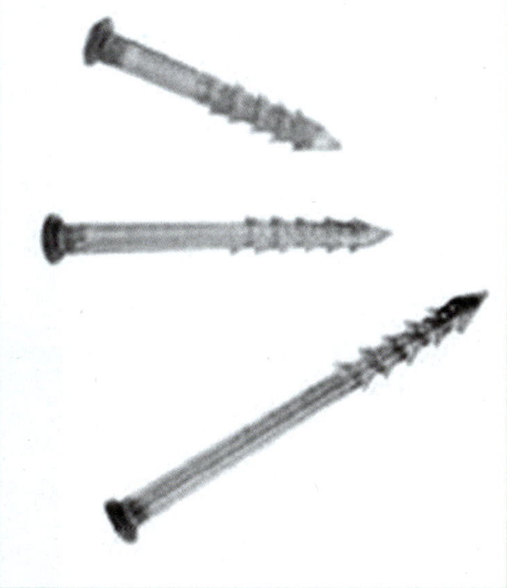 *d*

(continued)

TABLE 25.1 Bioabsorbable Fixation Implants for Juvenile Osteochondritis Dissecans *(continued)*

	Fixation	*Manufacturer*	*Composition*[a]	*Sizes (mm)*	*Picture*
LactoNail	Nail	Arthrotek Biomet, Inc. (Warsaw, IN)	PGA/PLLA	2.6 × 26	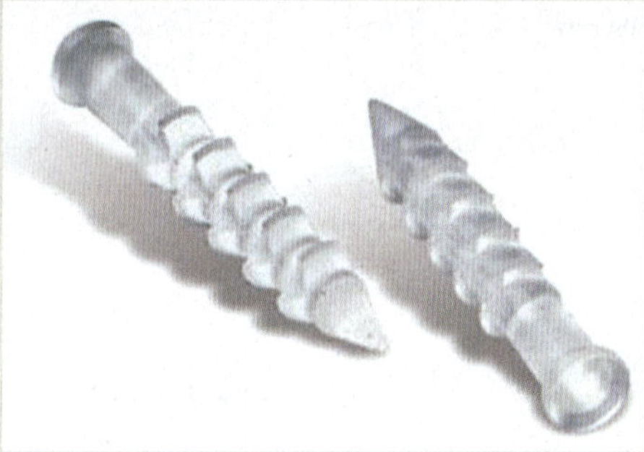 [e]
Chondral Dart	Pin	Arthrex, Inc. (Naples, FL)	PLLA	1.3 × 18	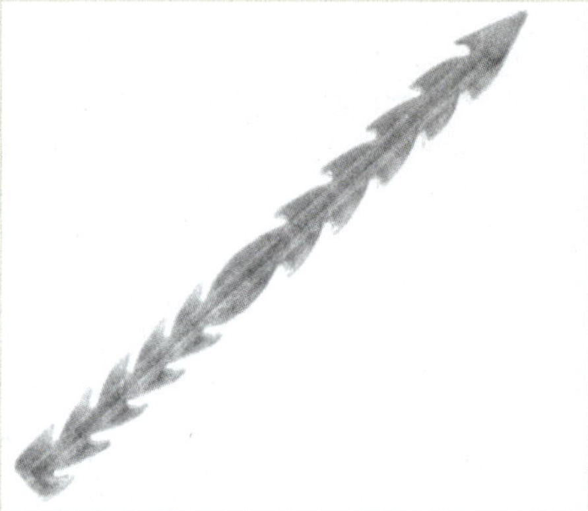 [f]

PLLA, poly(L-lactic acid); PGA/PLLA, copolymer; PGA, polyglycolic acid.
[a]Adapted from http://footandanklefixation.com/product/conmed-linvatec-smartscrew-ii/.
[b]Adapted from www.biomet.com/sportsmedicine/productDetail.cfm?category=30&product=96.
[c]Adapted from www.arthrex.com/foot-ankle/biocompression-screws.
[d]Adapted from www.conmed.com/products/fracture-fixation-smartnail.php.
[e]Adapted from www.biomet.com/sportsmedicine/productDetail.cfm?category=28&subCategory=24&product=64.
[f]Adapted from www.arthrex.com/knee/chondral-dart.

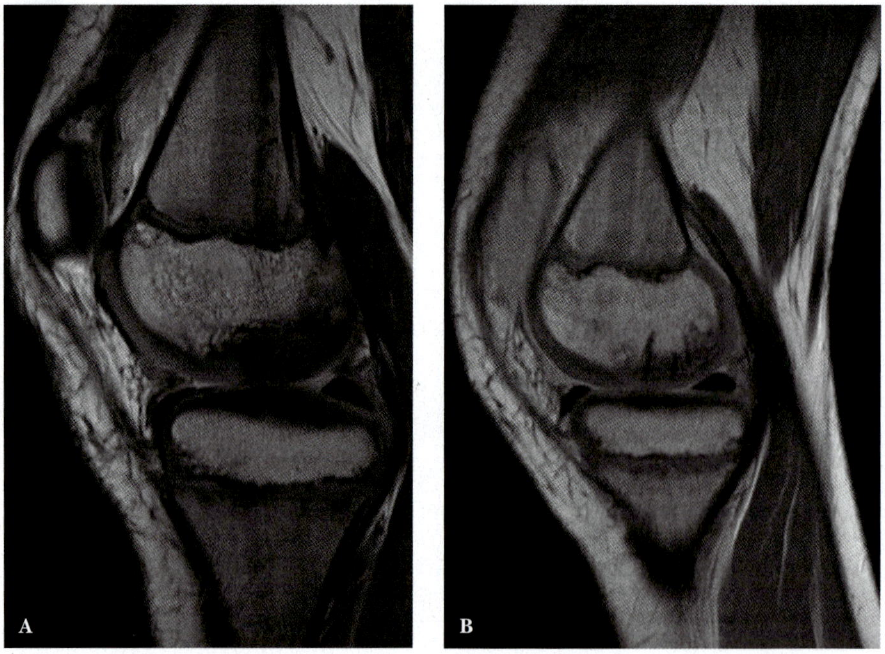

Figure 25.1. **A.** Pre-operative sagittal proton density MRI demonstrating JOCD lesion of the medial femoral condyle. **B.** 5-month post-operative sagittal proton density MRI showing healing of subchondral bone and overlying cartilage.

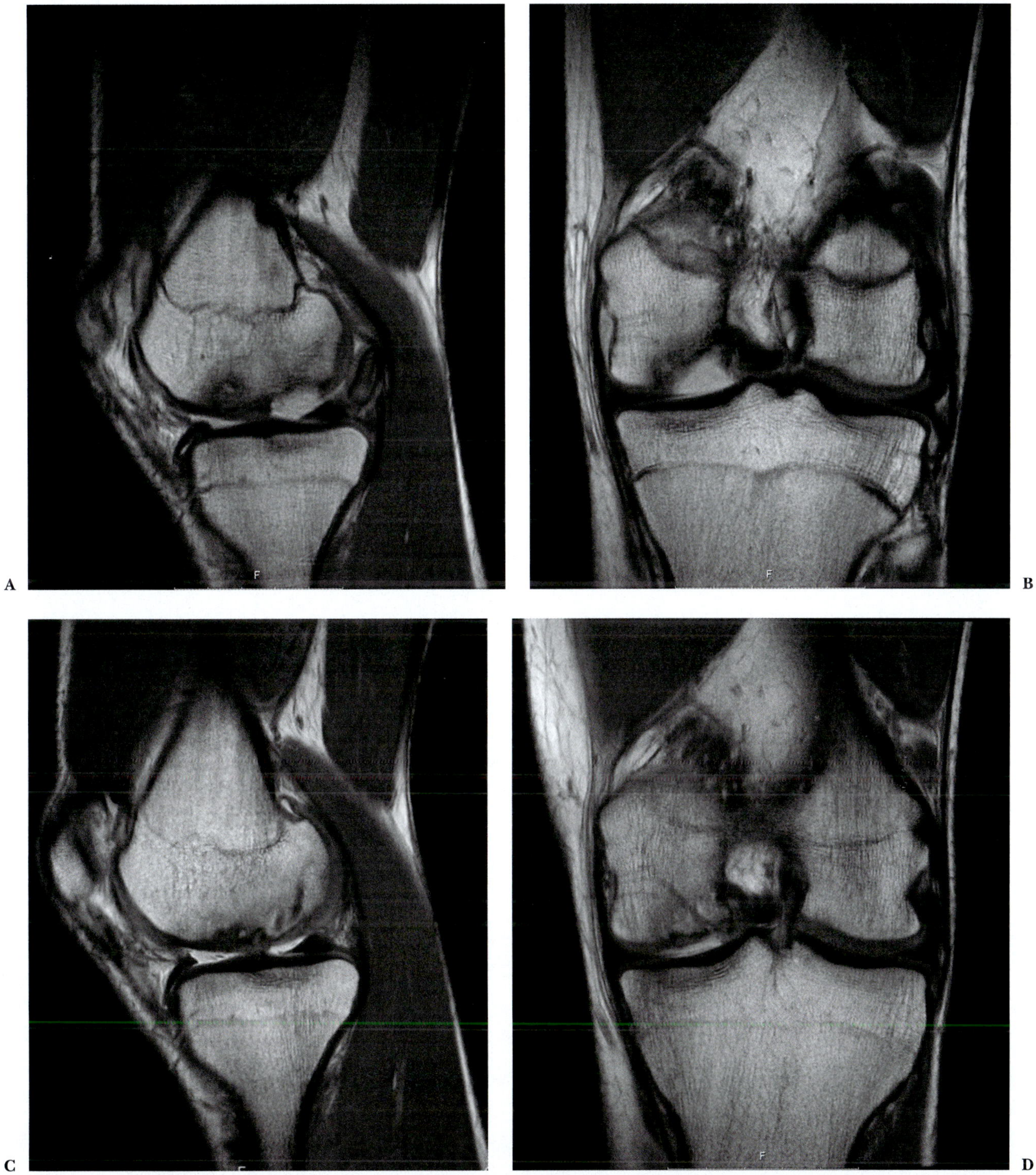

Figure 25.2. **A,B.** Pre-operative sagittal and coronal proton density MRI demonstrating JOCD lesion of the medial femoral condyle. **C,D.** 12-month post-operative sagittal and coronal proton density MRI showing healing of subchondral bone and overlying cartilage.

REFERENCES

1. Harada Y, Tomita N, Nakajima M, et al. Effect of low loading and joint immobilization for spontaneous repair of osteochondral defect in the knees of weightless (tail suspension) rats. *J Orthop Sci.* 2005;10(5):508–514.
2. Gomoll AH, Flik KR, Hayden JK, et al. Internal fixation of unstable Cahill Type-2C osteochondritis dissecans lesions of the knee in adolescent patients. *Orthopedics.* 2007;30(6):487–490.
3. Adachi N, Deie M, Nakamae A, et al. Functional and radiographic outcomes of unstable juvenile osteochondritis dissecans of the knee treated with lesion fixation using bioabsorbable pins. *J Pediatr Orthop.* 2015;35:82–88.
4. Dines JS, Fealy S, Potter HG, et al. Outcomes of osteochondral lesions of the knee repaired with a bioabsorbable device. *Arthroscopy.* 2008;24(1):62–68.
5. Abouassaly M, Peterson D, Salci L, et al. Surgical management of osteochondritis dissecans of the knee in the paediatric population: a systematic review addressing surgical techniques. *Knee Surg Sports Traumatol Arthrosc.* 2014;22(6):1216–1224.
6. Webb JE, Lewallen LW, Christopherson C, et al. Clinical outcome of internal fixation of unstable juvenile osteochondritis dissecans lesions of the knee. *Orthopedics.* 2013;36(11): e1444–e1449.
7. Guhl JF. Arthroscopic treatment of osteochondritis dissecans. *Clin Orthop Relat Res.* 1982;(167):65–74.
8. Nuzzo MS, Posner M, Warme WJ, et al. Compression force and pullout strength comparison of bioabsorbable implants for osteochondral lesion fixation. *Am J Orthop (Belle Mead NJ).* 2011;40(4): E61–E63.

Stephanie W. Mayer
Curtis D. VandenBerg
Jay C. Albright

CHAPTER 26

Osteochondral Autograft Transplantation/Allograft

INTRODUCTION

Although a large percentage of osteochondritis dissecans (OCD) lesions in the pediatric and adolescent population will heal and become asymptomatic with nonsurgical management, there remains a subset which do not heal and remain symptomatic. If the lesion is stable, primary fixation or drilling to promote revascularization are options for treatment.[1] Some lesions, however, will present as or become unstable, end-stage lesions with compromise of both the chondral surface and the subchondral bone.[2] This can present difficult clinical challenges because the age of these patients precludes arthroplasty options. Osteochondral autograft transplantation (OAT) and osteochondral allograft transplantation are options for treatment in this situation.[3–14]

Both of these involve replacement of the osseous and cartilaginous portions of the OCD lesion with an osteochondral plug harvested from a non–weight-bearing portion of the affected knee (OAT) or the appropriately matched portion of a cadaveric knee (osteochondral allograft transplantation). The premise of this type of treatment option is to transplant mature hyaline cartilage with viable chondrocytes and surrounding collagen matrix along with subchondral bone for a composite graft, which can provide structure and function.[15] The goal is to restore the weight-bearing cancellous and subchondral bone as well as the articular hyaline cartilage with a plug of the same size and contour. Only OAT and osteochondral allograft transplantation have the ability to restore all of these properties of the lesion.

OSTEOCHONDRAL AUTOGRAFT TRANSPLANTATION

Indications

The OAT procedure is an option for treatment of grade 3 or 4 (unstable) lesions of the medial or lateral femoral condyle or trochlea. Grade 3 lesions are nondisplaced but have a rim of T2 high signal circumscribing the lesion at the subchondral zone on magnetic resonance imaging (MRI), meaning that the lesion is unstable and joint fluid has tracked behind the chondral surface. Grade 4 lesions are also unstable and are either free pieces within the bed of the lesion or loose bodies within the joint. A single OAT plug is generally used if the defect is less than 2.5 cm^2 and is well contained on all sides by borders of healthy hyaline cartilage.[16] When the defect is larger than 9 to 10 mm^2 up to 4 cm^2, multiple osteochondral dowels can be harvested and placed into the defect adjacent to each other to fill as much of the defect as possible, termed *mosaicplasty*.[17,18] The edges of the donor OAT plug and the recipient lesion as well as between dowels in mosaicplasty heal with fibrocartilage, leading some authors to use allograft when a lesion will require multiple plugs to reduce the fibrocartilage healing and maximize the amount of articular cartilage present.[16] Contraindications to the OAT/mosaicplasty technique include a defect larger than 4 cm^2, lesions that are not well contained by surrounding articular cartilage, and kissing lesions or defects on two surfaces which are in contact during weight bearing.

Authors' Preferred Surgical Technique

We use the Arthrex (Naples, FL) OAT system including the single-use OAT set and OAT sizer/tamp instrumentation set. Description of the technique will be based on this system.

Preoperatively, the size of the lesion can be estimated (Fig. 26.1). However, the true size of the lesion and/or OAT plug(s) needed is often underestimated and cannot be fully determined until the lesion is débrided and prepared for implantation.[19] General anesthesia with a regional single-shot block of the femoral and sciatic nerve is performed by the anesthesia team. The operative limb is then examined under anesthesia for range of motion and ligamentous stability. Block to full range of motion under anesthesia suggests a large loose body within the knee. A nonsterile tourniquet is applied to the upper thigh and generally set to 250 mm Hg. After sterile preparation and draping, a standard diagnostic arthroscopy using two anterior portals with or without a superior outflow portal is performed. Following careful inspection of the joint for loose bodies, identifying the location of the OCD lesion, and defining any other intra-articular pathology, the surgeon can begin to prepare the bed of the lesion.

Any loose, fibrillated, or unstable full-thickness articular cartilage defect should be removed from the bed of the lesion

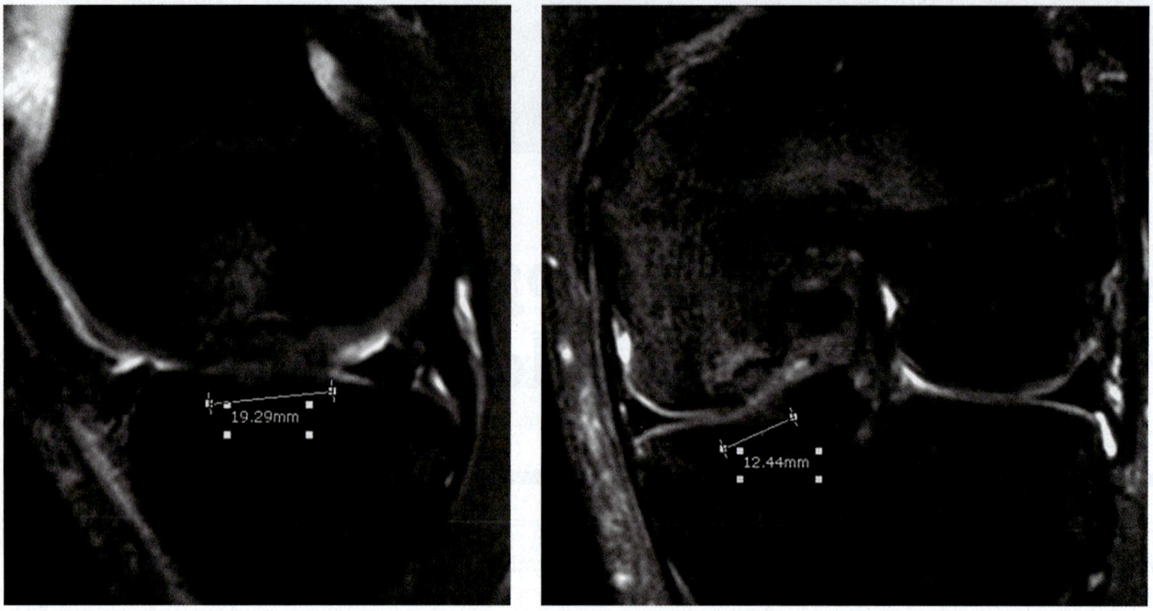

A B

Figure 26.1. **A.** Sagittal and **(B)** coronal sections of a T2 weighted MRI showing measurements of a 19.2 mm by 12.4 mm OCD lesion of the medial femoral condyle.

using a curette, ring curette, and motorized shaver (Fig. 26.2). Take care to remove large fragments of cartilage from the joint as they are removed from the lesion to prevent loose bodies. The edges of the lesion should be débrided to have vertical smooth walls to circumferentially contain the OAT plug(s) using a scalpel or small curette (Fig. 26.3). When the lesion is completely prepared, the total diameter can be sized with a plastic sizing tamp (Fig. 26.4). If multiple donor plugs will be needed, the surgeon can make an assessment of the appropriate number and sizes of plugs.

If the lesion is located in a more anterior or distal position on the femoral condyle, the remainder of the procedure may be performed arthroscopically. If the lesion is more posterior on the femoral condyle, an appropriate angle for harvesting the lesion and placing the plug may not be feasible, in which case an arthrotomy should be made. The decision for an arthroscopic or open technique is ultimately at the discretion of the surgeon. (Figures in this section depict the use of an arthrotomy for visualization and perspective in this text.) If an open incision is used, a longitudinal incision is made through the skin from the distal pole of the patella to the tibial plateau. The location of the skin incision can be midline or parapatellar on the side of the lesion at the discretion of the surgeon. Often, it is possible to plan the incisions to incorporate one of the initial anterior arthroscopy portals into the incision for a more cosmetic result. The subcutaneous tissue is divided in line

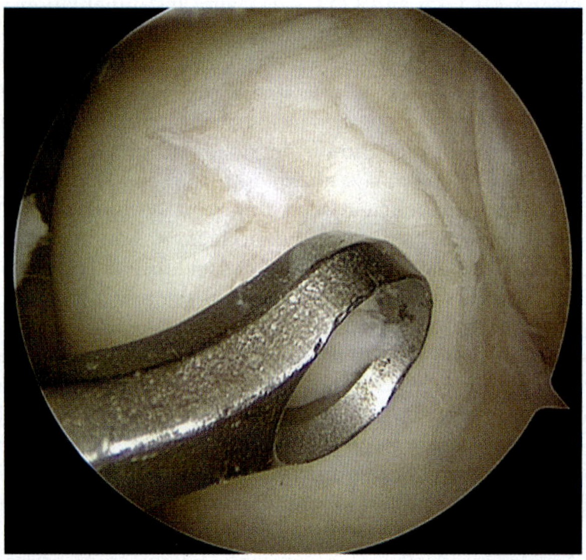

Figure 26.2. Débridement of an unstable chondral flap with a ring curette.

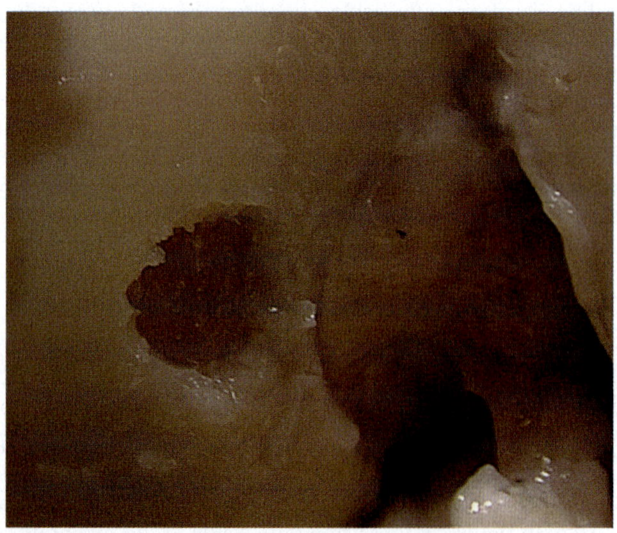

Figure 26.3. Medial femoral condyle OCD lesion following débridement to healthy subchondral bone. Note the lesion is contained by vertical borders of normal articular cartilage.

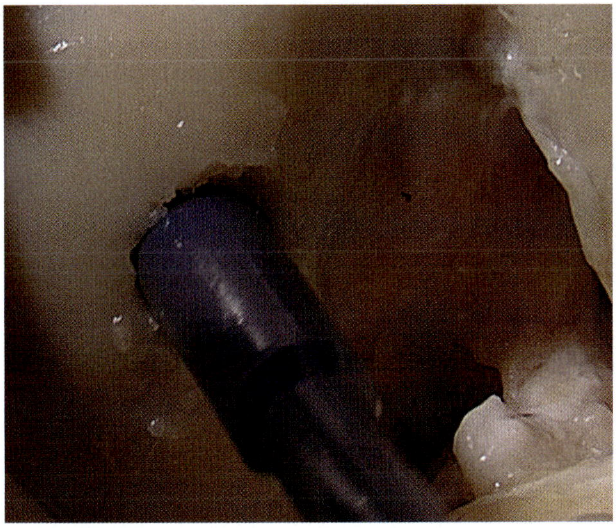

Figure 26.4. A sizer tamp is placed into the lesion for accurate sizing of the final defect after débridement.

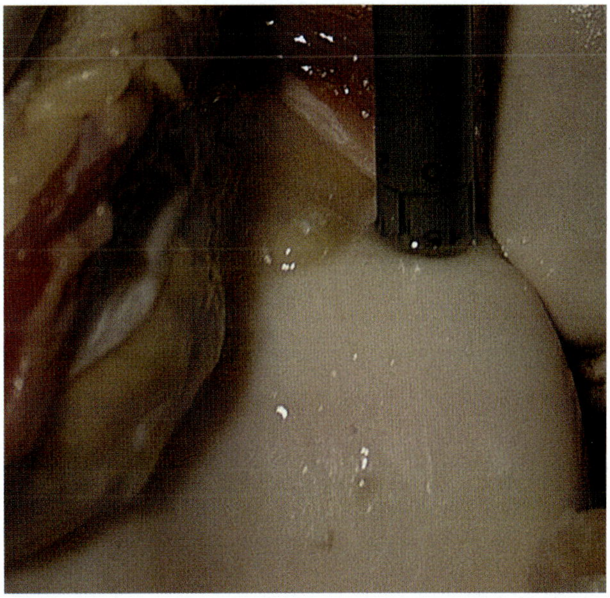

Figure 26.5. The donor graft harvester is inserted perpendicular to the articular surface down to a depth of 15 mm.

with this incision down to the paratenon of the patellar tendon. A medial or lateral parapatellar arthrotomy is made adjacent to the patellar tendon depending on the location of the lesion. The skin incision and/or arthrotomy may need to be extended for visualization and should be tailored to the location of the lesion and the comfort of the surgeon. Controlling flexion and extension of the knee is helpful in allowing for a smaller arthrotomy by bringing the lesion into view.

Should the previously described incision allow for access for the donor plug harvest, no further incision is needed. If not, a separate arthroscopy portal, open incision, or extension of the arthrotomy is made. The autograft osteochondral donor plugs are harvested from a non–weight-bearing portion of the femoral condyle. Options for locations of harvest include areas of the femur which are not major load-bearing areas such as the lateral supracondylar ridge, medial supracondylar ridge, posterior femoral condyle, lateral aspect of the lateral femoral condyle just above the sulcus terminalis, medial or lateral portions of the trochlea, and the superior aspect of the intercondylar notch. The size and contour of the recipient site should be taken into account when deciding where to harvest the plug. The distal medial aspect of the trochlea has been shown to have the least load-bearing area during range of motion followed by the intercondylar notch.[20] The same study found that the medial and lateral trochlea matched recipient sites on the femoral condyles well, and the central portion of the non–load-bearing trochlea in the notch matched trochlear lesions best.[20] Another consideration in the decision for a donor site in the skeletally immature population is the open physis. Harvest of the plug should be performed under fluoroscopic control and as far from the physis as possible to avoid inadvertent damage. The supracondylar ridge is the closest to the physis. The authors' preferred technique is to harvest the donor graft from the distal medial trochlea in skeletally immature patients to stay farther from the physis and in a non–load-bearing zone.

For implantation of a single OAT donor plug, the harvester size 1 mm larger than the size of the measured lesion is chosen so that upon seating of the donor plug, there will be a press fit. The harvester should be placed perpendicular to the articular surface and the angle should not be changed during harvesting. Using a mallet, the donor plug harvester is impacted to a depth of 15 mm using the numbered laser lines as a guide (Fig. 26.5). Without changing its angle, rotate the harvester clockwise 90 degrees twice and pull the device straight out of the lesion. It is recommended to harvest grafts perpendicular to the articular surface and without any levering during extraction to obtain the most anatomically suited graft for the recipient site.[21,22] Both arthroscopic and open techniques can yield an appropriate graft with attention to proper harvesting technique.[21,22] The donor plug will be withdrawn inside the harvester. The actual depth of donor plug that was taken can be measured inside the harvester device through the window and is then used to determine the depth of the recipient plug that will be removed. Leave the donor plug in place within the harvester until needed for implantation.

The recipient site harvester corresponding to the size of the lesion (1 mm smaller than the donor plug) is chosen and placed over the recipient defect perpendicular to the articular surface (Fig. 26.6). The recipient plug depth should be approximately 1 to 2 mm shallower than the donor plug length to avoid countersinking the donor plug. This harvester is then malleted in to this depth using the laser lines etched on the outside of the harvester as a guide. Similar to the harvest of the donor plug, take care not to change the angle of the device during this step. The harvester is again removed with two 90-degree clockwise turns and by pulling straight back on the device. The plug is removed and an alignment rod is inserted into the recipient site to recheck the depth and visualize the angle needed for insertion of the OAT donor plug.

To remove the donor plug, a plastic delivery tube is placed over the donor harvester. The core extruder is placed into the harvester and the donor plug is advanced until it is flush with the edge of the harvester. This complex is placed into the recipient site at the previously determined angle. The core extruder is then used to advance the OAT plug. The plug can

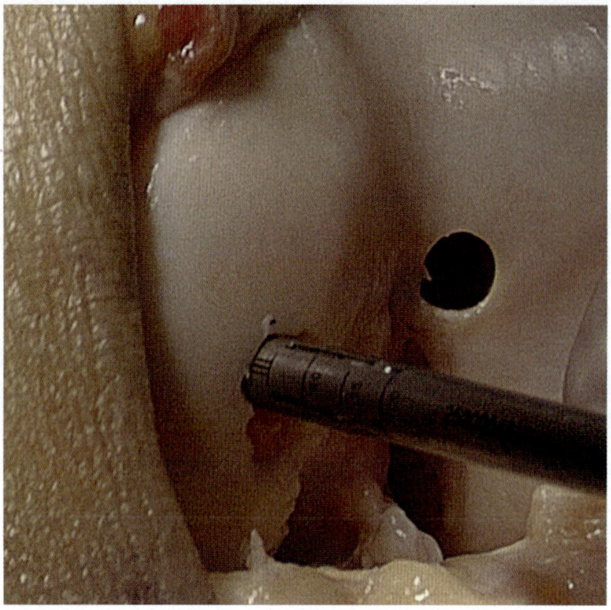

Figure 26.6. Completed donor plug harvest, in this case from the lateral distal trochlea/notch region, with donor plug region. The recipient lesion is being harvested using a harvester which is 1 mm smaller in diameter than the donor plug.

also be seated by removing it from the harvester with the core extruder, placing it over the recipient site at the appropriate angle and using a plastic tamp and mallet to tap the plug into position (Fig. 26.7). Grafts have been shown to incorporate best when they are press fit between 0 and 2 mm of being flush with the surrounding articular surface but not countersunk below the articular surface.[22] If impacting the osteochondral dowel, a larger number of less forceful blows has been shown to decrease damage to chondrocytes.[16,23] If using a mosaicplasty technique, following placement of the first graft, the steps are repeated for subsequent grafts (Fig. 26.8). Once the donor plug is inserted, the knee should be taken through a range of motion to ensure that there is no mechanical block to full motion and the graft is stable.

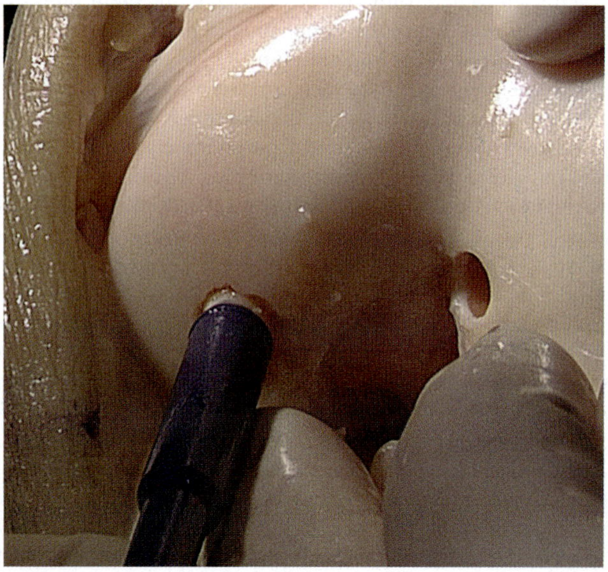

Figure 26.7. Donor plug being seated into the recipient lesion using the plastic tamp and mallet.

Postoperative Protocol and Rehabilitation

The limb is placed into a hinged knee brace locked in extension until the initial physical therapy visit within the first few days post op. For femoral condylar lesions, unrestricted passive range of motion is begun at the initial therapy session, followed by strengthening once full active range of motion is recovered. Touchdown weight bearing with crutches is permitted, in weight-bearing lesions, for the first 6 weeks, and at that time, a gradual return to full weight bearing is started. We require brace wear locked in extension during weight bearing until

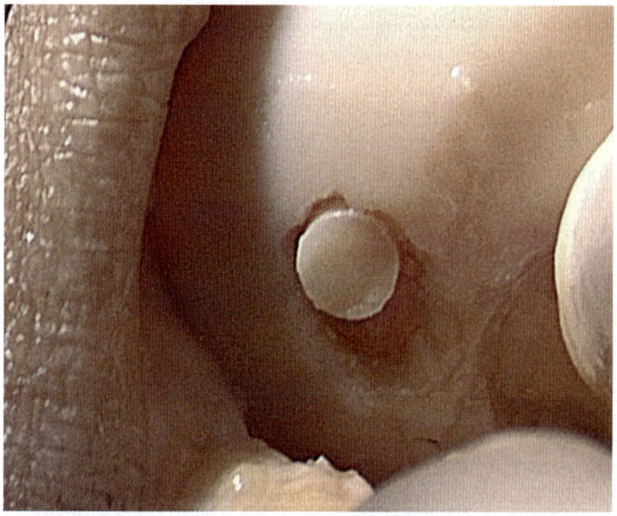

A

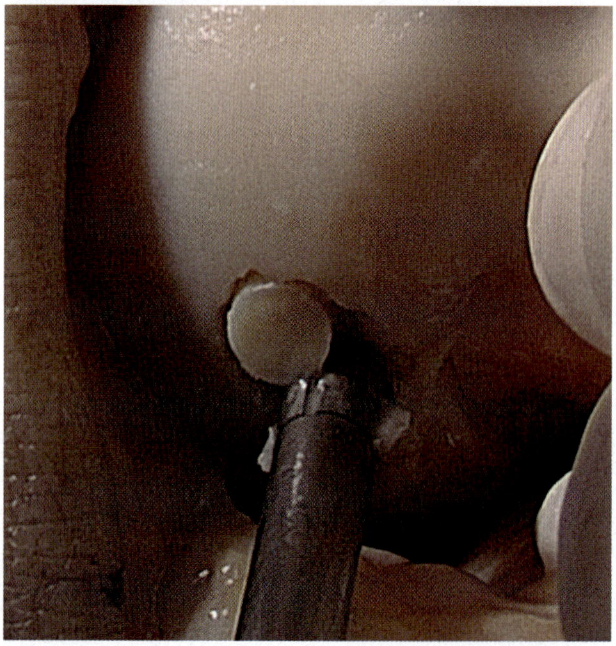

B

Figure 26.8. Mosaicplasty technique for large ovoid OCD lesion. **A.** Initial plug in place. **B.** Harvest of the second plug.

quadriceps strength and endurance is adequate to prevent falls. For patellar or trochlear lesions, full range of motion and full weight bearing is allowed with the brace locked in extension immediately as pain allows.

Outcomes

Short- and medium-term results of OAT in patients younger than the age of 18 years are encouraging. Gudas et al.[8] found that 84% of patients returned to their preinjury activity level between 9 and 14 months postoperatively, and 81% were still involved in sports at this level at an average of 4.2 years. All patients returned to their previous level of sports at an average of 5.7 months in another small series of patients who received both single plugs and mosaicplasty.[24] A variation of the traditional OAT technique using internal fixation of a portion of the OCD lesion with a small osteochondral autograft plug with[25,26] and without[27,28] augmentation of the defect with further OAT plugs has also been described with good short-term results.

OSTEOCHONDRAL ALLOGRAFT TRANSPLANTATION

The use of fresh osteochondral allograft transplantation in the knee was first reported in 1908.[29] Fresh osteochondral allograft transplantation involves the transplantation of mature hyaline cartilage containing viable chondrocytes that survive hypothermic storage while maintaining the metabolic activity of the chondrocytes and maintaining the integrity of the surrounding collagen matrix. The second portion of the osteochondral allograft is the osseous portion. The osseous portion of the graft differs from the hyaline cartilage component in that the osseous portion was originally vascularized tissue and its cells are not thought to survive transplantation. Rather, the osseous portion of the osteochondral graft functions like other types of bone graft in that it provides a scaffold for healing to the host through creeping substitution.[15,30] In the 1970s and 1980s, the use of fresh osteochondral allografts for posttraumatic reconstruction of the knee was popularized.[31–34] More recently, many authors have reported good to excellent short- and medium-term success using fresh osteochondral allografts for the treatment of OCD and focal chondral lesions in young, active patients.[5,6,10–12,35] Retrieval studies have shown successful graft incorporation up to 25 years after implantation and that histologic features associated with long-term osteochondral allograft survival include viable chondrocytes, functional preservation of matrix, and complete replacement of the bone graft with host bone.[33,36]

Indications

Debridement, microfracture, and OAT are often ineffective or impractical for lesions greater than 2 cm^2 to 2.5 cm^2. Osteochondral allograft transplantation is a single-stage surgical technique that is particularly useful in the setting of an OCD lesion with extensive subchondral edema or extensive bone loss that requires restoration.[15] Fresh osteochondral allografting for OCD has been used at some institutions as both a salvage procedure and as a primary treatment when the fragment could not be reinserted.[6]

Authors' Preferred Surgical Technique

The same anesthetic plan and surgical setup described in the OAT section is used.

Graft Acquisition and Storage

Osteochondral allograft tissue became commercially available in the late 1990s from tissue banks whose guidelines for sterile procurement and processing were established by the American Association of Tissue Banks, with oversight by the U.S. Food and Drug Administration. Donor tissue should be recovered from the cadaver specimen with 24 hours of expiration, and the age criterion for donors of fresh grafts is generally between 15 and 40 years. Chondrocyte viability directly correlates with the clinical success of osteochondral allograft transplantation. Osteochondral allograft storage methods (e.g., frozen, cryopreserved, fresh) have different effects of chondrocyte viability, immunogenicity, and time to transplantation. Among the available storage options, fresh osteochondral allografts have been shown to have the highest level of chondrocyte viability. Fresh osteochondral allografts stored hypothermically at 4°C, chondrocyte viability, and graft biomechanical properties begin to deteriorate at 14 days, and in general, the maximal recommended time from harvest to transplantation is 28 days. Tissue banks currently retain osteochondral allografts until microbiologic and serologic testing is complete, which often takes longer than 14 days. Donors are screened for HIV, hepatitis B surface and core antigens, hepatitis C antibodies, and syphilis, among others. Although the articular cartilage portion of an osteochondral graft elicits no humoral immune response, the subchondral bone and marrow components of the graft elicit a strong immune response, and for grafts larger than 10 cm^2, a systemic immune response can take place; however, pharmacologic immune suppression is unnecessary.[30,36–39]

Before the procedure, the donor and recipient are matched on the basis of size using standard anteroposterior radiographs of the recipient knee corrected for magnification, and the donor knee is measured directly by the tissue bank. MRI can also be useful in assessing defect size but, as stated previously, has been shown to underestimate the defect area by as much as 60%.[19] A match is considered acceptable if it is within 2 mm of the recipient condyle. There can be substantial variability in anatomy that is not always recognized on sizing measurements. In particular, in patients with OCD, the pathologically affected condyle typically is larger, wider, and flatter; therefore, a larger donor condyle generally should be used. In light of this, it is imperative that the surgeon inspect all tissue being considered for transplantation prior to undertaking the actual procedure.[6,30,36–38]

Types of Allograft Transplantation

Procedures are performed through a medial or lateral parapatellar arthrotomy. For small or solitary defects, a quadriceps-sparing mini-arthrotomy may be performed.

A solitary plug (dowel) technique is ideal when the defect is well-circumscribed in an easily accessible surface of the knee. The dowel technique requires a set of specialized reamers to achieve a press fit between the donor bone and recipient site. First, the diameter of the required graft is determined. A guide pin is placed through the center of the sizer with the sizer in

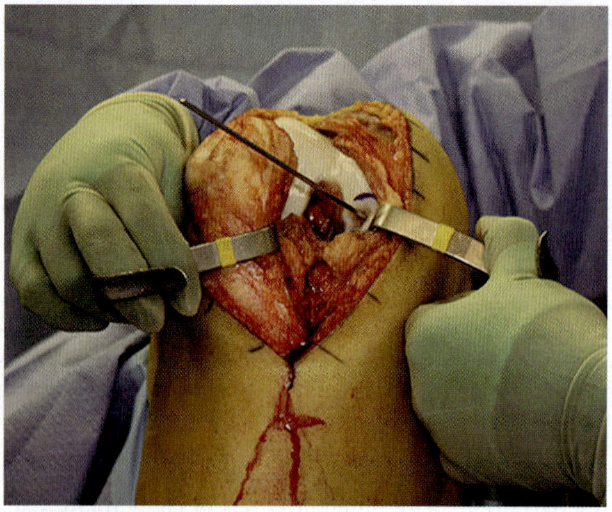

Figure 26.9. Solitary plug (dowel) technique. The guide pin is placed at the center of the lesion perpendicular to the articular surface. (Reproduced from Polousky JD, Albright J. Salvage techniques in osteochondritis dissecans. *Clin Sports Med.* 2014;33:321–333.)

even contact with the articular surface, which ensures that the trajectory of the guide pin is perpendicular to the articular surface (Fig. 26.9). The corresponding recipient site reamer is selected and the site is reamed over the guide pin until healthy, bleeding subchondral bone is encountered, generally 8 to 15 mm from the chondral surface. The 12 o'clock position is marked on the articular surface. Depth measurements are taken and recorded at the 3, 6, 9, and 12 o'clock positions. Attention is now turned to the donor condyle. The corresponding anatomic area is identified to match the contour of the recipient as closely as possible. A guide pin can be placed through the sizer to assist with maintaining a perpendicular trajectory with the reamer if necessary. Again, the cartilage of the donor is scored; the 12 o'clock position is marked on the graft, and it is cut with the dowel reamer. The graft is then removed from the donor condyle with a sagittal saw, taking care to preserve the appropriate depth (Fig. 26.10). When the dowel is free, it is trimmed to

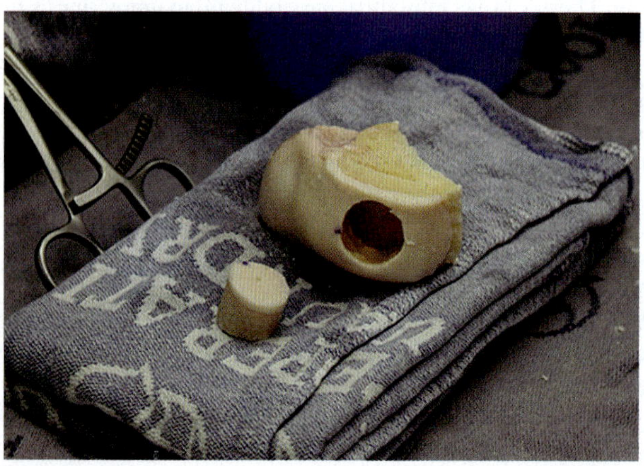

Figure 26.10. Graft harvested using the dowel reamer from allograft hemicondyle. (Reproduced from Polousky JD, Albright J. Salvage techniques in osteochondritis dissecans. *Clin Sports Med.* 2014;33:321–333.)

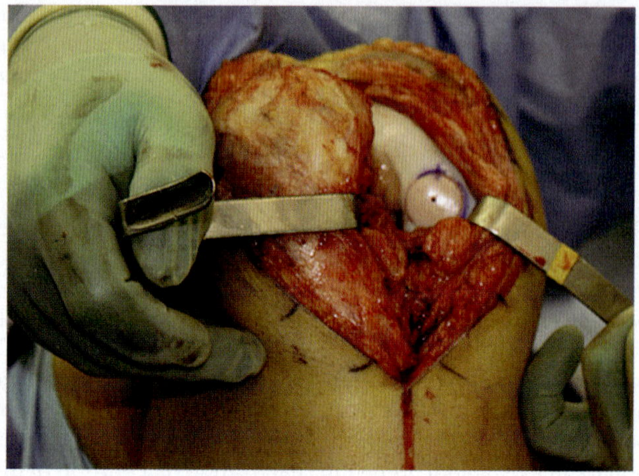

Figure 26.11. Allograft following placement into the lesion bed. (Reproduced from Polousky JD, Albright J. Salvage techniques in osteochondritis dissecans. *Clin Sports Med.* 2014;33:321–333.)

the appropriate depths at the marked clock positions. Pulsatile irrigation is used to remove marrow elements from the donor bone and the graft is placed. Generally, the diameter of the plug can be precisely matched to the size of the defect, providing complete coverage of the area and stable integration with the surrounding host bone and cartilage[2,39] (Fig. 26.11).

For large or multiple lesions, it is critical to visualize the entire zone of injury to ensure that no damaged cartilage remains and that the osteochondral allograft will have healthy recipient cartilage at the periphery of the lesion.

Using multiple grafts, the "snowman" technique allows for coverage of a larger area of condyle than solitary plugs alone, particularly when the length of the lesion (proximal to distal) is longer than the width (medial to lateral). The second graft is placed interdigitating with the first graft. Before reaming into the first graft, it is important for the surgeon to fix the graft temporarily with two small Kirschner wires to prevent displacement. Significant gaps between plugs must be avoided to prevent uneven cobblestoning, which may affect clinical outcome.

For larger asymmetrical lesions (e.g., whole patella/large trochlea) or for lesions in locations that are difficult to access (e.g., posterior femoral condyles), the shell technique is useful. Once the lesion is exposed, it is débrided to form a simple geometric shape. Approximately 2 to 3 mm of subchondral bone is removed from the recipient site to expose healthy host bone. Autogenous bone grafting may be performed for large, deep bony defects. Once the defect is sculpted into a simple shape with a smooth flat base, a template can be drawn noting the lengths of the sides and depth at each edge of the defect. The surface contour of the donor and recipient condyle is matched. Once the area of best fit is localized, the graft is cut using a small sagittal saw. Multiple trials and trimmings are usually needed to refine the fit of the graft. Once the appropriate fit is achieved with the graft either flush or slightly recessed, the graft is irrigated with pulsatile lavage and implanted. The graft is then secured with a combination of interference fit and small, absorbable, polydioxanone pins, and interfragmentary screws when needed.[2,39]

For all osteochondral allograft procedures, surgical techniques should include meticulous washing of marrow elements and minimizing the width of underlying transplanted bone (6 to 8 mm) to decrease the immune response. Additionally, because allograft bone heals by creeping substitution, it is beneficial to minimize the amount of bone transplanted, thus decreasing the amount of time necessary for replacement by host bone and full osseous graft incorporation. Copious irrigation during graft harvest can help to decrease thermal necrosis of donor chondrocytes. During graft impaction and insertion, chondrocyte injury and subsequent death can occur; thus, it is important to minimize the force of impaction. When possible, a press fit should be obtained. For contained allografts (i.e., plug and snowman techniques), fixation can be augmented with either bioabsorbable screws or chondral darts when necessary. Uncontained grafts (i.e., shell) require the use of low-profile interfragmentary screws for stable fixation.[39]

Postoperative Protocol and Rehabilitation

Postoperatively, patients are kept touchdown weight bearing for 6 to 12 weeks and slowly progressed to weight bearing as tolerated depending on the size of the allograft used and on radiographic evidence of healing. Weight-bearing status varies depending on lesion location, but the goal is to avoid placing shear or compressive stresses on the transplanted area. When satisfactory graft stability is achieved at the time of surgery, full and immediate range of motion is allowed. Some authors recommend limited knee flexion (<45 degrees) for the first 4 to 6 weeks in patients treated for patellar or trochlear lesions. If the osteochondral graft was placed only in the patellofemoral joint, patients are allowed to weight bear as tolerated immediately post op with the knee locked in full extension. Full return to sports-related activities is not allowed before 6 months, and all patients are followed until radiographic evidence of complete healing is demonstrated.[15,39]

Outcomes

Although published data on long-term results of osteochondral allograft transplantation for OCD is limited, in general, studies for this procedure for focal osteochondral lesions of the femoral condyles have demonstrated good to excellent outcomes in terms of graft survival and patient function. Recent literature on this subject primarily consists of small case series, and level I evidence is lacking. Existing studies have reported graft survival rates ranging from 84.5% to 100% at 5 years, 71% to 89% at 10 years, 74% to 76% at 15 years, and 66% at up to 20 years. Poor results have been reported with large (>10 cm^2), chronic lesions and when malalignment was uncorrected.[6,10,11,31,32,35,36] Outcomes following osteochondral allograft transplantation for patellofemoral lesions remain poor; one series reported graft survival rates of 43% at 5 years and 29% at 10 years postoperatively, and another study reported a graft survival rate of 75% after an average follow-up of 8 years.[40,41] Results of osteochondral allograft transplantation in an athletic population are limited. In a study of 43 athletes treated with osteochondral allograft transplantation in the knee, 38 (88%) had limited return to sport, and 34 (79%) returned to sport at the preinjury level. Patients older than 25 years of age and those with preoperative symptoms lasting longer than 12 months were less likely to return to sport.[10]

REFERENCES

1. Polousky JD. Juvenile osteochondritis dissecans. *Sports Med Arthrosc.* 2011;19:56–63.
2. Polousky JD, Albright J. Salvage techniques in osteochondritis dissecans. *Clin Sports Med.* 2014;33:321–333.
3. Abouassaly M, Peterson D, Salci L, et al. Surgical management of osteochondritis dissecans of the knee in the paediatric population: a systematic review addressing surgical techniques. *Knee Surg Sports Traumatol Arthrosc.* 2014;22(6):1216–1224.
4. Cahill BR. Osteochondritis dissecans of the knee: treatment of juvenile and adult forms. *J Am Acad Orthop Surg.* 1995;3:237–247.
5. Chahal J, Gross AE, Gross C, et al. Outcomes of osteochondral allograft transplantation in the knee. *Arthroscopy.* 2013;29:575–588.
6. Emmerson BC, Gortz S, Jamali AA, et al. Fresh osteochondral allografting in the treatment of osteochondritis dissecans of the femoral condyle. *Am J Sports Med.* 2007;35:907–914.
7. Gudas R, Kalesinskas RJ, Kimtys V, et al. A prospective randomized clinical study of mosaic osteochondral autologous transplantation versus microfracture for the treatment of osteochondral defects in the knee joint in young athletes. *Arthroscopy.* 2005;21:1066–1075.
8. Gudas R, Simonaityte R, Cekanauskas E, et al. A prospective, randomized clinical study of osteochondral autologous transplantation versus microfracture for the treatment of osteochondritis dissecans in the knee joint in children. *J Pediatr Orthop.* 2009;29:741–748.
9. Kocher MS, Tucker R, Ganley TJ, et al. Management of osteochondritis dissecans of the knee: current concepts review. *Am J Sports Med.* 2006;34:1181–1191.
10. Krych AJ, Harnly HW, Rodeo SA, et al. Activity levels are higher after osteochondral autograft transfer mosaicplasty than after microfracture for articular cartilage defects of the knee: a retrospective comparative study. *J Bone Joint Surg Am.* 2012;94:971–978.
11. LaPrade RF, Botker J, Herzog M, et al. Refrigerated osteoarticular allografts to treat articular cartilage defects of the femoral condyles. A prospective outcomes study. *J Bone Joint Surg Am.* 2009;91:805–811.
12. Lyon R, Nissen C, Liu XC, et al. Can fresh osteochondral allografts restore function in juveniles with osteochondritis dissecans of the knee? *Clin Orthop Relat Res.* 2013;471:1166–1173.
13. Pascual-Garrido C, Moran CJ, Green DW, et al. Osteochondritis dissecans of the knee in children and adolescents. *Curr Opin Pediatr.* 2013;25:46–51.
14. Robertson W, Kelly BT, Green DW. Osteochondritis dissecans of the knee in children. *Curr Opin Pediatr.* 2003;15:38–44.
15. Gortz S, Bugbee WD. Allografts in articular cartilage repair. *J Bone Joint Surg Am.* 2006;88:1374–1384.
16. Erickson BJ, Chalmers PN, Yanke AB, et al. Surgical management of osteochondritis dissecans of the knee. *Curr Rev Musculoskelet Med.* 2013;6:102–114.
17. Hangody L, Fules P. Autologous osteochondral mosaicplasty for the treatment of full-thickness defects of weight-bearing joints: ten years of experimental and clinical experience. *J Bone Joint Surg Am.* 2003;85-A(suppl 2):25–32.
18. Hangody L, Rathonyi GK, Duska Z, et al. Autologous osteochondral mosaicplasty. Surgical technique. *J Bone Joint Surg Am.* 2004;86-A(suppl 1):65–72.
19. Campbell AB, Knopp MV, Kolovich GP, et al. Preoperative MRI underestimates articular cartilage defect size compared with findings at arthroscopic knee surgery. *Am J Sports Med.* 2013;41:590–595.
20. Ahmad CS, Cohen ZA, Levine WN, et al. Biomechanical and topographic considerations for autologous osteochondral grafting in the knee. *Am J Sports Med.* 2001;29:201–206.
21. Epstein DM, Choung E, Ashraf I, et al. Comparison of mini-open versus arthroscopic harvesting of osteochondral autografts in the knee: a cadaveric study. *Arthroscopy.* 2012;28:1867–1872.
22. Pearce SG, Hurtig MB, Clarnette R, et al. An investigation of 2 techniques for optimizing joint surface congruency using multiple cylindrical osteochondral autografts. *Arthroscopy.* 2001;17:50–55.

23. Kang RW, Friel NA, Williams JM, et al. Effect of impaction sequence on osteochondral graft damage: the role of repeated and varying loads. *Am J Sports Med.* 2010;38:105–113.
24. Sasaki K, Matsumoto T, Matsushita T, et al. Osteochondral autograft transplantation for juvenile osteochondritis dissecans of the knee: a series of twelve cases. *Int Orthop.* 2012;36:2243–2248.
25. Miniaci A, Tytherleigh-Strong G. Fixation of unstable osteochondritis dissecans lesions of the knee using arthroscopic autogenous osteochondral grafting (mosaicplasty). *Arthroscopy.* 2007;23:845–851.
26. Miura K, Ishibashi Y, Tsuda E, et al. Results of arthroscopic fixation of osteochondritis dissecans lesion of the knee with cylindrical autogenous osteochondral plugs. *Am J Sports Med.* 2007;35:216–222.
27. Berlet GC, Mascia A, Miniaci A. Treatment of unstable osteochondritis dissecans lesions of the knee using autogenous osteochondral grafts (mosaicplasty). *Arthroscopy.* 1999;15:312–316.
28. Yoshizumi Y, Sugita T, Kawamata T, et al. Cylindrical osteochondral graft for osteochondritis dissecans of the knee: a report of three cases. *Am J Sports Med.* 2002;30:441–445.
29. Lexer E. The use of free osteoplasty together with trials on arthrodesis and joint transplantation. *Clin Orthop Relat Res.* 2008;466:1771–1776.
30. Gortz S, Bugbee WD. Fresh osteochondral allografts: graft processing and clinical applications. *J Knee Surg.* 2006;19:231–240.
31. Ghazavi MT, Stockley I, Yee G, et al. Reconstruction of massive bone defects with allograft in revision total knee arthroplasty. *J Bone Joint Surg Am.* 1997;79:17–25.
32. Gross AE, Shasha N, Aubin P. Long-term followup of the use of fresh osteochondral allografts for posttraumatic knee defects. *Clin Orthop Relat Res.* 2005;(435):79–87.
33. Gross AE, Kim W, Las Heras F, et al. Fresh osteochondral allografts for posttraumatic knee defects: long-term followup. *Clin Orthop Relat Res.* 2008;466:1863–1870.
34. McDermott AG, Langer F, Pritzker KP, et al. Fresh small-fragment osteochondral allografts. Long-term follow-up study on first 100 cases. *Clin Orthop Relat Res.* 1985;(197):96–102.
35. Levy YD, Gortz S, Pulido PA, et al. Do fresh osteochondral allografts successfully treat femoral condyle lesions? *Clin Orthop Relat Res.* 2013;471:231–237.
36. Williams SK, Amiel D, Ball ST, et al. Analysis of cartilage tissue on a cellular level in fresh osteochondral allograft retrievals. *Am J Sports Med.* 2007;35:2022–2032.
37. Williams RJ III, Dreese JC, Chen CT. Chondrocyte survival and material properties of hypothermically stored cartilage: an evaluation of tissue used for osteochondral allograft transplantation. *Am J Sports Med.* 2004;32:132–139.
38. Murphy RT, Pennock AT, Bugbee WD. Osteochondral allograft transplantation of the knee in the pediatric and adolescent population. *Am J Sports Med.* 2014;42:635–640.
39. Sherman SL, Garrity J, Bauer K, et al. Fresh osteochondral allograft transplantation for the knee: current concepts. *J Am Acad Orthop Surg.* 2014;22:121–133.
40. Torga Spak R, Teitge RA. Fresh osteochondral allografts for patellofemoral arthritis: long-term followup. *Clin Orthop Relat Res.* 2006;444:193–200.
41. Jamali AA, Emmerson BC, Chung C, et al. Fresh osteochondral allografts: results in the patellofemoral joint. *Clin Orthop Relat Res.* 2005;(437):176–185.

Ellie Ci-En Choi
Keng Lin Wong
James H.P. Hui

CHAPTER 27

Technique: Frontiers of Cartilage Restoration

INTRODUCTION

Articular cartilage is composed of hyaline cartilage and allows for low-friction movement of the joint. Traumatic mechanical destruction or progressive wear and tear can destroy the cartilage and cause symptoms such as pain, swelling, and decreased range of motion.

Athletes are known to be at higher risk for traumatic cartilage injuries due to the increased demands placed on the knee. A systematic review by Flanigan et al.[1] found the overall prevalence of full-thickness chondral defects in athletes to be 36%. These injuries can cause marked limitation of sporting activities and an inability to return to sports.[2] Osteochondritis dissecans (OCD) and chondromalacia patellae are two common conditions in adolescents affecting cartilage in the knee. OCD is a chronic condition in which a limited lesion of subchondral bone necrosis progresses toward the separation of a segment of articular cartilage and the underlying subchondral bone from the surrounding cancellous bone.[3] Chondromalacia patellae involve degeneration of articular cartilage of the posterior surface of the patella. In early stages, the cartilage becomes soft, and subsequently, fissures develop resulting in cartilaginous flakes and gradual erosion of cartilage down to the subchondral bone.[4]

Cartilage has a limited capacity for repair[5] and, when left untreated, can cause severe and progressive disability of the joint leading to osteoarthritis.[6] Therefore, early diagnosis and treatment of chondral defects not only facilitates a quicker return to sporting activity but also decreases the risk of developing osteoarthritis. Various procedures have been described in the literature for the treatment of cartilage injuries in adolescents, ranging from fixation, osteochondral allografts transfer system (OATS), marrow stimulation techniques, and, more recently, cell-based techniques.

Fixation of osteochondral lesions with screws, pins, and rods have been described to stabilize the fragment and retain a congruent articulation.[7,8] Autologous osteochondral transplant, in which a cylindrical osteochondral graft is taken from the femoral condyle and transplanted to the defect, is also well documented as a surgical treatment for chondral defects.[9,10]

Marrow stimulation techniques such as abrasion arthroplasty and microfracture are commonly used[11–13] to penetrate the subchondral bone, allowing the release of stem cells and growth factors from the bone marrow, thereby promoting cartilage repair. Steadman et al.[14] showed improved symptoms, function, and activity levels in football league players with full-thickness chondral defects treated with microfracture. However, marrow stimulation has been shown to stimulate growth of fibrocartilage, which is inferior to hyaline cartilage and does not have long-term benefits.[15–17]

Interest in cell-based therapy increased and developed in the 1990s with a landmark study by Brittberg et al.[18] In the study, 23 patients with full-thickness cartilage defects were treated with autologous chondrocyte implantation (ACI) and results showed regain of considerable knee function in patients with femoral defects at 3 years follow-up. Biopsies taken showed production of hyaline cartilage in 11 of 15 femoral transplants, which resembles normal articular cartilage and is superior to fibrocartilage.

Cell-based therapy broadly encompasses chondrocyte implantation and mesenchymal stem cell (MSC) implantation. It involves harvesting of chondrocytes or MSC, culturing them in the laboratory, and subsequently returning the cultured cells to the defect. In a study by Peterson et al.,[19] ACI for femoral or patellar cartilage defects was associated with durable function for as long as 11 years. Another prospective cohort study showed that ACI and microfracture had significantly better results at final follow-up (mean 7.5 years) as compared to microfracture alone in a group of high-level male soccer players.[20] At a 3 month posttransplantation arthroscopy, Brittberg et al.[18] found that transplants had the same macroscopic appearance as the surrounding cartilage. Bentley et al.[21] also reported that second-look arthroscopy at 1 year demonstrated excellent or good functional outcomes in 82% after ACI using the Cincinnati Rating System and Stanmore Functional Rating System.

Apart from harvesting chondrocytes, MSCs can also be harvested for in vitro culture from various tissues such as bone marrow[22,23] and adipose tissue.[24] Their easy availability makes harvesting simpler and reduces the problem of donor site morbidity that is a concern in ACI.

Two studies in a rabbit model and human population have demonstrated that human bone marrow is a better source of MSCs with better chondrogenic capacity than adipose tissue.[25,26]

Bone marrow–derived mesenchymal stem cells (BMSCs) have been shown to differentiate into chondrocytes as early as 2 weeks posttransplantation[27] and resulted in significant arthroscopic[28] and clinical improvement[29] in patients with chondral defects. Comparisons have been made clinically between ACI and autologous BMSC implantation. In an observation cohort study led by Nejadnik et al.,[30] 72 matched patients (lesion and age) underwent cartilage repair using chondrocytes or BMSCs. Both groups had significant improvements in the quality of life after cartilage repair (physical and mental components of the Short Form-36 questionnaire included in the International Cartilage Repair Society [ICRS] package). There was no difference in clinical outcome except that BMSCs were better for physical role functioning, with a greater improvement over time. The study showed BMSCs to be as effective as chondrocytes while avoiding the disadvantages associated with chondrocyte implantation such as donor site morbidity from the sacrifice of healthy cartilage, pain from the site of harvest of the periosteal patch, and risks and costs of a second surgery.

BMSCs, once harvested and cultured, can be delivered into the knee joint via two general approaches: open and intra-articular. In the open technique, cultured cells may be implanted directly into the defect, or via a suitable matrix or scaffold such as collagen or fibrin, seeded with chondroprogenitor cells and signalling substances. However, these methods are invasive, requiring a second surgery for transplantation, and none has shown to be superior to the rest.[31]

To reduce the need for a second surgery, a novel technique of administering MSCs via intra-articular injections was developed and published by McIlwraith et al.[28] in an equine model. Improvements were seen in both arthroscopic and immunohistologic examination after the administration of intra-articular BMSCs and hyaluronic acid (HA) with microfracture when compared with HA and microfracture alone.

A study led by Lee et al.[32] in a porcine model showed that the outcomes of intra-articular injections of autologous BMSCs and HA were comparable with an open technique using BMSCs implanted beneath a sutured periosteal patch over the defect. The authors' present technique translates this intra-articular injection method to human patients to restore cartilage defects in the knee.

PATIENT SELECTION/INDICATIONS/CONTRAINDICATIONS

For adolescent patients with OCD, the indications for surgery are pain, locking, and instability. Contraindications include early osteoarthritic changes, inflammatory diseases such as rheumatoid arthritis, previous trauma or infection to the growth plate, and underlying tibial femoral malalignment. In the authors' study on cell-based therapy in patellar OCD,[33] patients with ICRS grade 3 or 4 patellar OCD diagnosed clinically and radiographically were included.

PREOPERATIVE INVESTIGATIONS

A detailed clinical evaluation is carried out by the orthopedic surgeon to assess the clinical condition of the affected knee. Preoperative plain radiographs of the knee including anteroposterior, lateral, intercondylar, and skyline views are taken. Further imaging such as computed tomography (CT) and magnetic resonance imaging (MRI) are performed to further delineate the anatomy and pathology.

PATIENT SETUP AND SURGICAL TECHNIQUE

Various surgical procedures can be done in conjunction with stem cell therapy to improve the efficacy and outcomes of treatment.

Patients with associated patellar tilt and/or subluxation may undergo concomitant distal realignment or lateral release surgery. Microfracture as a form of marrow stimulation can be performed, as described by Steadman et al.,[34] where specially designed awls are used to make perforations into the subchondral bone plate at interval spacing of 3 to 4 mm (Fig. 27.1). For arthroscopy, patients are positioned supine with side support on the lateral aspect of the hip on the operating side. Incisions made for arthroscopic access to the knee are of the standard medial and lateral arthroscopic portals. Surgery is performed under general anesthesia and tourniquet control.

PREPARATION OF BONE MARROW–DERIVED MESENCHYMAL STEM CELLS TECHNIQUE

Harvesting

Autologous MSCs are harvested from the bone marrow of the iliac crest. This may be done under local or general anesthesia in the operating theatre and is done in the same setting as any concomitant surgery such as microfracture or realignment.

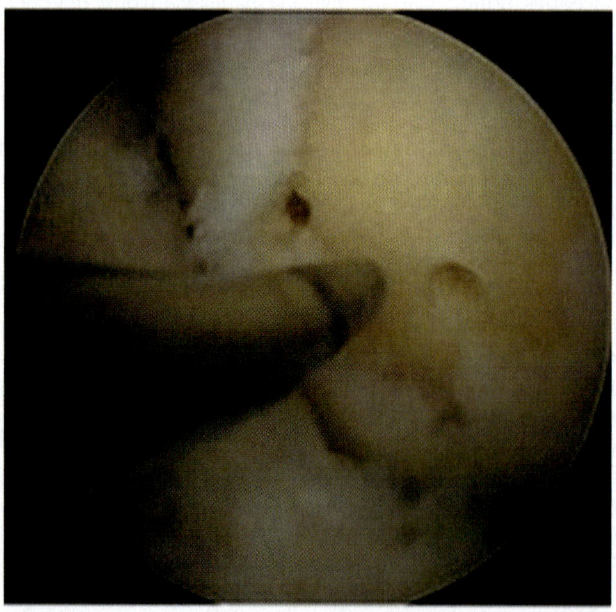

Figure 27.1. Microfracture technique via arthroscopy.

A stab incision is made over the anterior iliac crest and 60 mL of marrow is aspirated using a Jamshidi needle into a heparinized tube (Fig. 27.2). The bone marrow aspirate is processed within 60 minutes. Seventy milliliters of uncoagulated whole blood is also collected from which autologous serum is prepared and stored at −20°C.

Culture

Culture of autologous MSCs from the harvested bone marrow is carried out in a class B clean room environment. Marrow aspirate contains a mixture of different red blood cells, platelets, and leukocytes. MSC and MSC precursors compose only less than 0.05% of low-density mononuclear cells,[35] and thus the purpose of culture is to generate MSCs of sufficient concentration (Fig. 27.3).

The heparinized bone marrow aspirate is mixed with a one-fifth volume of 6% (w/v) dextran (molecular weight 100,000) (Sigma-Aldrich, St. Louis, MO) and left standing at room temperature for 30 minutes to eliminate erythrocytes. The remain-

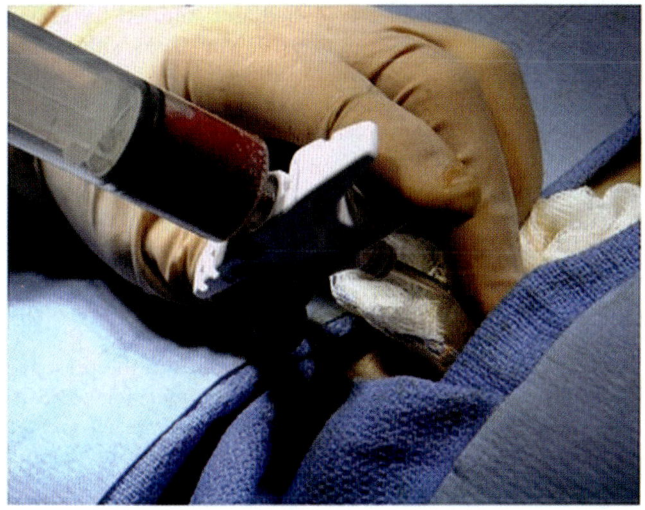

Figure 27.2. Bone marrow harvesting via iliac crest.

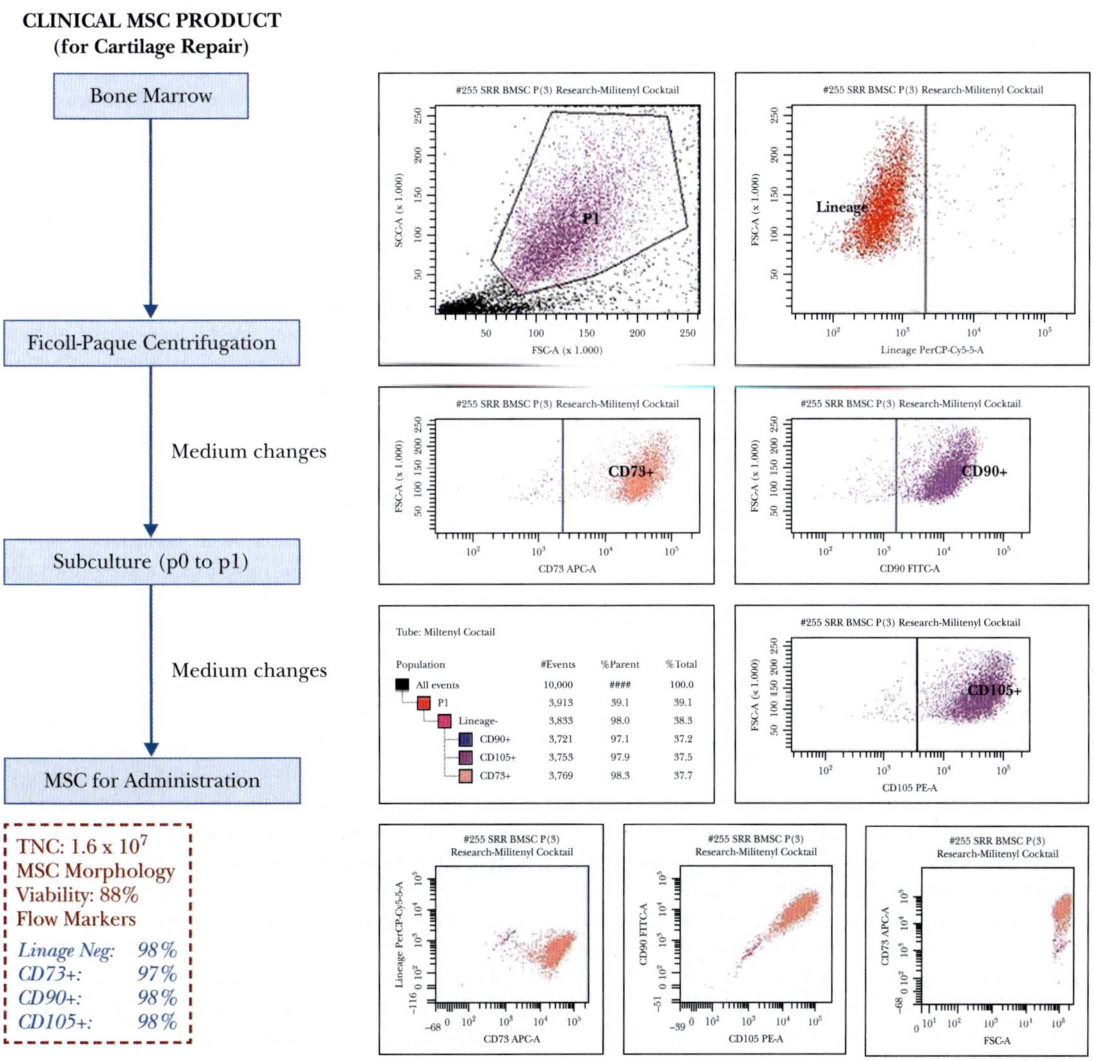

Figure 27.3. Flowchart for culture of MSCs.

ing leukocyte-rich fraction is washed and cultured for MSCs. These cells are cultured in 5 to 6 T75 cm^2 flasks with an initial culture medium consisting of Dulbecco's Modified Eagle's Medium (DMEM) containing 10% fetal bovine serum, 50 mg/mL L-ascorbic acid 2-phosphate sesquimagnesium salt hydrate (all from Invitrogen), and 1% antibiotic-antimycotic (penicillin 100 U/mL, streptomycin 0.1 mg/mL, amphotericin B 0.25 mg/mL) (Sigma) in a humidified atmosphere of 5% CO_2 at 37°C. Cells are seeded at a density of 10,000 cells/cm^2. After adherent cells are recognized, at days 5 to 7, the culture media is changed to that without antibiotics and subsequently changed every 2 to 3 days until harvest.

Sheets of cells for open surgery are formed in the presence of ascorbic acid (passage 1), whereas for injectable BMSCs, cells undergo passaging (p0 to p1) when they reach greater than 30% confluency (usually after 10 to 13 days) by treating with trypsin (Invitrogen) and washes.

Autologous serum is prepared from 70 mL of uncoagulated whole blood previously collected. The sample is centrifuged with slow acceleration; the serum is carefully aspirated and transferred to a new tube. Repeated centrifugation is performed with slow acceleration for 3 minutes at 3,000 rpm at ambient temperature.

Between 9 and 11 days, culture supernatant is sent for assays for mycoplasma and microbial contamination (aerobic and anaerobic bacteria as well as fungus).

The autologous serum is aspirated into a syringe; filtered with a sterile 0.2-mm filter and tested for sterility, anti-HIV, and hepatitis B antigen; and stored at a temperature of 20°C.

Total nucleated cell (TNC) count and viability is performed at days 9 to 12. Microscopic examination and changing of culture medium is continued regularly every 2 to 3 days till the cells are ready for harvest.

MSCs are trypsinized with collagenase and washed. A small fraction from each sample is removed to assess the cell count, viability, and flow cytometry. MSCs are ready for collection at greater than 70% confluence (estimated number of cells at time of harvest is 1.5 to 3 × 10^6/T75).

Viability is determined by fluorescent acridine orange, and propidium iodide staining and flow cytometry (MSC phenotyping kit, Miltenyi Biotec, Bergisch Gladbach, Germany) using FACSCanto II with FACSDiva software (BD, Franklin Lakes, NJ) is performed to stain for MSC markers—$CD90^+$, $CD105^+$, CD14, and CD3—to confirm that the cultured cells are MSCs.

MSC release criteria for administration include the following: no growth on mycoplasma and microbial culture, confluency greater than 70%, normal MSC morphology, and greater than 75% viable.

For direct implantation of cultured MSCs into the chondral defect, at least four sheets of cells are prepared with approximately 2 million cells/cm^2 (at least 10 to 15 million cells with 96% viability). Cell sheets are transported within the patient's serum to the operating theatre. During the arthrotomy, a periosteal patch from the proximal tibia or distal femur is harvested according to the measured size of the débrided chondral defect. The harvested periosteal patch is sutured precisely to the rim of defect, and BMSCs are implanted beneath the patch. Microsuture 7-0 and fibrin glue are used to hold the periosteum to the defect and to create a watertight seal.

For delivery of BMSCs via intra-articular injections, cultured cells are trypsinized and washed as mentioned earlier and resuspended in 0.5 to 1 mL of autologous serum in a sterile container. This, along with 2 mL of HA, is injected into the intra-articular space with a 19-gauge needle under local anesthesia.

Complications

Preliminary results from the use of MSC injections show that it is a safe procedure (in terms of serious adverse events during administration of MSC) and the rate of microbial contamination is low (1 in 218 processes during a 6-year span from 2006 to 2011).

Follow-up

Patients are reviewed on the 10th postoperative day for wound inspection and again at 3 weeks. The intra-articular injection of the cultured MSCs is given at this visit.

Patients are followed up for the first 6 months at 6 weekly intervals then at 1-year and 2-year intervals. The ICRS Cartilage Injury Evaluation Package[36] is used for patients who underwent cell-based treatment for OCD. The package included questions from the International Knee Documentation Committee (IKDC) scores, the knee scale reported by Lysholm and Gillquist,[37] and the Tegner and Lysholm Knee score.[38] MRI is performed after 1 year to look for cartilage regeneration based on the Magnetic Resonance Observation of Cartilage Repair Tissue (MOCART) scoring system.[39] MRI was performed on a 1.5T Signa HDxt MRI scanner (GE Medical Systems, Milwaukee, WI) with a dedicated extremity surface coil (HD TR knee PA). The normal knee sequences used were axial T2, coronal proton density fat saturated, coronal T1, sagittal proton density, and sagittal T2 fat saturated. The cartilage sequences used were axial spoiled gradient recalled (SPGR), sagittal SPGR, axial fast imaging employing steady-state acquisition (FIESTA), and sagittal FIESTA. Each MRI scan consists of 19 slices for the normal knee protocol and 32 slices for the cartilage sequences. All patients were positioned consistently with the joint space in the middle of the coil and the knee extended in the coil.

Rehabilitation

The goal of rehabilitation is to facilitate recovery of the patient's range of motion/mobility, walking, and cardiovascular capacity and strength; strict adherence to the protocol is encouraged to derive maximum benefits from the treatment.

The process begins on postoperative day 0 and includes passive range of motion and isometric muscle contractions. Regular continuous passive mobilization (CPM) is prescribed for 8 hours per day until 4 weeks postoperatively, starting at 30 degrees with gradual increments. This is made available during the inpatient stay and for rental when the patient is discharged. Patients unable to be reimbursed for CPM would undergo physiotherapy with 500 flexion and extension exercises per day. Patients are kept on non–weight bearing for 6 weeks, after which they are allowed active motion and partial weight bearing as comfortable, with gradual progression to full weight bearing status after 12 weeks. Thereafter, the rehabilitation protocol focuses on restoring muscular function through the use of stationary bicycles, elliptical trainers and treadmills, and closed-chain exercises.

The rehabilitation protocol is customized according to the patient's age, previous activity level, and the type of procedure performed.

Discussion

A retrospective review led by Teo et al.[33] looked at 23 patients between 12 and 21 years of age, with ICRS grade 3 or 4 OCD lesions involving the patella. These lesions were treated using cell-based therapy in conjunction with distal realignment or lateral release surgery from 2001 to 2008.

Twenty patients had ACI and three patients had cultured bone marrow stem cell implantation. The mean IKDC score, Tegner-Lysholm outcomes, and Lysholm-Gillquist scale improved from 45, 2.5, and 50, respectively, at surgery to 75, 4, and 70, respectively, at 24-month follow-up. However, not all patients returned to the activity level expected for their age. Additionally, two of the patients who had ACI were found to have asymptomatic periosteal hypertrophy noted on MRI scanning as early as 6 months follow-up. The periosteum appeared to have overgrown the defect likely as a result of cartilage hypertrophy and remodelling, and this complication has been well documented in the literature in patients treated with ACI.[40,41]

ACI have shown to be not superior to BMSCs in the treatment of cartilage defects but with increased complications such as donor site morbidity, periosteal pain, and periosteal hypertrophy.[30] In our use of BMSCs, we are moving increasingly toward an intra-articular delivery instead of direct implantation via surgery, as we found no benefits with using an open technique of delivery.[32] The usage of intra-articular injections, in addition, has the advantage of being minimally invasive and requires only a single operation. Intra-articular injections of BMSCs in HA have been compared with just HA in patients with varus knees and cartilage defects who underwent high tibial osteotomy and microfracture.[42]

Results at 2-year follow-up of 56 patients (28 cell recipient, 28 control) show that the cell-recipient group had significantly better scores (Figs. 27.4 to 27.6). The effect of treatment showed an added improvement of 7.65 (95% confidence interval [CI], 3.04 to 12.26; $P < .001$) for IKDC scores, 7.61 (95% CI, 1.44 to 13.79; $P < .016$) for Lysholm scores, and 0.64 (95% CI, 0.10 to 1.19; $P < .021$) for Tegner scores. MRI scans performed 1 year after surgical intervention showed significantly better MOCART scores for the cell-recipient group. The age-adjusted mean difference in MOCART score was 19.6 (95% CI, 10.5 to 28.6; $P < .001$).

This supports our belief that the injected MSCs have the ability to home in on the site of injury/microfracture and adhere to the site of lesion. The homing ability of MSCs have been proven by other authors.[43,44]

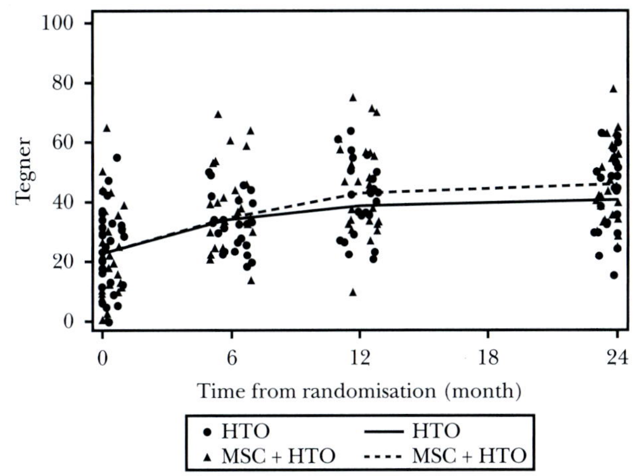

Figure 27.5. Effect of intra-articular BMSCs on Tegner scores. *HTO,* control group (high tibial osteotomy and HA); *MSC + HTO,* MSC group (high tibial osteotomy and MSC and HA). (From Wong KL, Lee KB, Tai BC, et al. Injectable cultured bone marrow-derived mesenchymal stem cells in varus knees with cartilage defects undergoing high tibial osteotomy: a prospective, randomized controlled clinical trial with 2 years' follow-up. *Arthroscopy.* 2013;29[12]:2020–2028.)

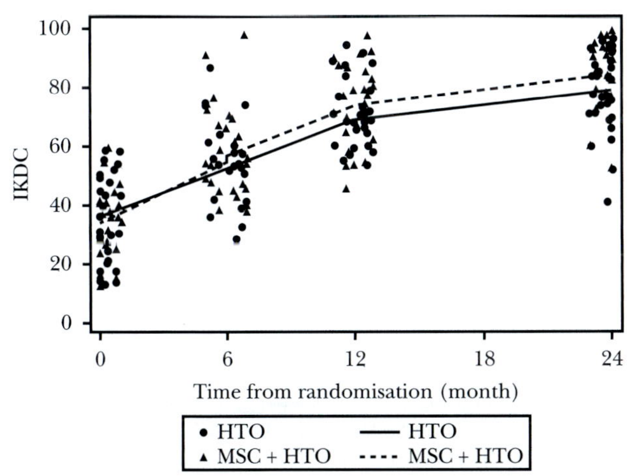

Figure 27.4. Effect of intra-articular BMSCs on IKDC scores. *HTO,* control group (high tibial osteotomy and HA); *MSC + HTO,* MSC group (high tibial osteotomy and MSC and HA). (From Wong KL, Lee KB, Tai BC, et al. Injectable cultured bone marrow-derived mesenchymal stem cells in varus knees with cartilage defects undergoing high tibial osteotomy: a prospective, randomized controlled clinical trial with 2 years' follow-up. *Arthroscopy.* 2013;29[12]:2020–2028.)

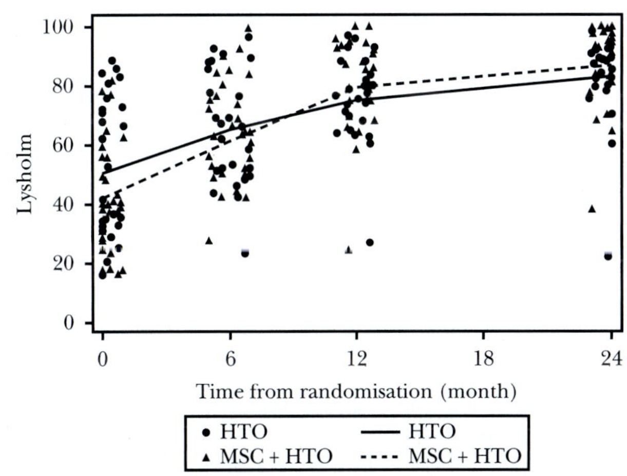

Figure 27.6. Effect of intra-articular BMSCs on Lysholm scores. *HTO,* control group (high tibial osteotomy and HA); *MSC + HTO,* MSC group (high tibial osteotomy and MSC and HA). (From Wong KL, Lee KB, Tai BC, et al. Injectable cultured bone marrow-derived mesenchymal stem cells in varus knees with cartilage defects undergoing high tibial osteotomy: a prospective, randomized controlled clinical trial with 2 years' follow-up. *Arthroscopy.* 2013;29[12]:2020–2028.)

CONCLUSION

In the setting of cartilage repair, it is feasible to translate longitudinally from laboratory studies and animal models to clinical studies and the initiation of human trials (bench to bedside). Clinical trials have shown short-term clinical and radiologic improvements after the use of intra-articular BMSCs, and the future of BMSC is promising. We await the results of large, multicenter trials to further deepen our understanding of cartilage restoration.

REFERENCES

1. Harris JD, Brophy RH, Siston RA, et al. Treatment of chondral defects in the athlete's knee. *Arthroscopy.* 2010;26(6):841–852.
2. Engström B, Forssblad M, Johansson C, et al. Does a major knee injury definitely sideline an elite soccer player? *Am J Sports Med.* 1990;18:101–105.
3. Aichroth P. Osteochondritis dissecans of the knee. A clinical survey. *J Bone Joint Surg Br.* 1971;53:440–447.
4. Outerbridge RE. The etiology of chondromalacia patellae. *J Bone Joint Surg Br.* 1961;43-B:752–757.
5. Fox A, Bedi A, Rodeo S. The basic science of articular cartilage: structure, composition, and function. *Sports Health.* 2009;1(6): 461–468.
6. Hunziker EB. Articular cartilage repair: basic science and clinical progress. A review of the current status and prospects. *Osteoarthritis Cartilage.* 2002;10:432–463.
7. Cugat R, Garcia M, Cusco X, et al. Osteochondritis dissecans: a historical review and its treatment with cannulated screws. *Arthroscopy.* 1993;9(6):675–684.
8. Dervin GF, Keene GC, Chissell HR. Biodegradable rods in adult osteochondritis dissecans of the knee. *Clin Orthop Relat Res.* 1998;(356): 213–221.
9. Hangody L, Füles P. Autologous osteochondral mosaicplasty for the treatment of full-thickness defects of weight-bearing joints: ten years of experimental and clinical experience. *J Bone Joint Surg Am.* 2003;85:25–32.
10. Gudas R, Kalesinskas RJ, Monastyreckiene E, et al. Osteochondral transplantation (mosaicplasty) in the treatment of knee joint cartilage [in Lithuanian]. *Medicina.* 2003;39(5):469–475.
11. Namdari S, Baldwin K, Anakwenze O, et al. Results and performance after microfracture in National Basketball Association athletes. *Am J Sports Med.* 2009;37:943–949.
12. Gobbi A, Nunag P, Malinowski K. Treatment of full thickness chondral lesions of the knee with microfracture in a group of athletes. *Knee Surg Sports Traumatol Arthrosc.* 2005;13:213–221.
13. Pridie K. A method of resurfacing knee joints. *J Bone Joint Surg Br.* 1959;41:618–619.
14. Steadman JR, Miller BS, Karas SG, et al. The microfracture technique in the treatment of full-thickness chondral lesions of the knee in National Football League players. *J Knee Surg.* 2003;16(2):83–86.
15. LaPrade RF, Bursch LS, Olson EJ, et al. Histologic and immunohistochemical characteristics of failed articular cartilage resurfacing procedures for osteochondritis of the knee: a case series. *Am J Sports Med.* 2008;36:360–368.
16. Mithoefer K, Williams RJ III, Warren RF, et al. The microfracture technique for the treatment of articular cartilage lesions in the knee. A prospective cohort study. *J Bone Joint Surg Am.* 2005;87:1911–1920.
17. Goyal D, Keyhani S, Lee EH, et al. Evidence-based status of microfracture technique: a systematic review of level I and II studies. *Arthroscopy.* 2013;29:1579–1588.
18. Brittberg M, Lindahl A, Nilsson A, et al. Treatment of deep cartilage defects in the knee with autologous chondrocyte transplantation. *N Engl J Med.* 1994;331:889–895.
19. Peterson L, Brittberg M, Kiviranta I, et al. Autologous chondrocyte transplantation. Biomechanics and longterm durability. *Am J Sports Med.* 2002;30:2–12.
20. Kon E, Filardo G, Berruto M, et al. Articular cartilage treatment in high-level male soccer players: a prospective comparative study of arthroscopic second generation autologous chondrocyte implantation versus microfracture. *Am J Sports Med.* 2011;39:2549–2557.
21. Bentley G, Biant LC, Carrington RW, et al. A prospective, randomised comparison of autologous chondrocyte implantation versus mosaicplasty for osteochondral defects in the knee. *J Bone Joint Surg Br.* 2003;85:223–230.
22. Johnstone B, Hering TM, Caplan AI, et al. In vitro chondrogenesis of bone marrow-derived mesenchymal progenitor cells. *Exp Cell Res.* 1998;238(1):265–272.
23. Mackay AM, Beck SC, Murphy JM, et al. Chondrogenic differentiation of cultured human mesenchymal stem cells from marrow. *Tissue Eng.* 1998;4(4):415–428.
24. Zuk PA, Zhu M, Ashjian P, et al. Human adipose tissue is a source of multipotent stem cells. *Mol Biol Cell.* 2002;13(12):4279–4295.
25. Hui JH, Li L, Teo YH, et al. Comparative study of the ability of mesenchymal stem cells derived from bone marrow, periosteum, and adipose tissue in treatment of partial growth arrest in rabbits. *Tissue Eng.* 2005;11(5–6):904–912.
26. Afizah H, Yang Z, Hui JH, et al. A comparison between the chondrogenic potential of human bone marrow stem cells (BMSCs) and adipose-derived stem cells (ADSCs) taken from the same donors. *Tissue Eng.* 2007;13(4):659–666.
27. Wakitani S, Goto T, Pineda SJ, et al. Mesenchymal cell-based repair of large, full thickness defects of articular cartilage. *J Bone Joint Surg Am.* 1994;76:579–592.
28. McIlwraith CW, Frisbie DD, Rodkey WG, et al. Evaluation of intraarticular mesenchymal stem cells to augment healing of microfractured chondral defects. *Arthroscopy.* 2011;27(11):1552–1561.
29. Wakitani S, Nawata M, Tensho K, et al. Repair of articular cartilage defects in the patello-femoral joint with autologous bone marrow mesenchymal cell transplantation: three case reports involving nine defects in five knees. *J Tissue Eng Regen Med.* 2007;1: 74–79.
30. Nejadnik H, Hui JH, Feng Choong EP, et al. Autologous bone marrow-derived mesenchymal stem cells versus autologous chondrocyte implantation: an observational cohort study. *Am J Sports Med.* 2010;38:1110–1116.
31. O'Driscoll SW. The healing and regeneration of articular cartilage. *J Bone Joint Surg Am.* 1998;80:1795–1812.
32. Lee KB, Hui JH, Song IC, et al. Injectable mesenchymal stem cell therapy for large cartilage defects. A porcine model. *Stem Cells.* 2007;25:2964–2971.
33. Teo BJ, Buhary K, Tai BC, et al. Cell-based therapy improves function in adolescents and young adults with patellar osteochondritis dissecans. *Clin Orthop Relat Res.* 2013;471(4):1152–1158.
34. Steadman JR, Rodkey WG, Rodrigo JJ. Microfracture: surgical technique and rehabilitation to treat chondral defects. *Clin Orthop Relat Res.* 2001;391(suppl): S362–S369.
35. Simmons PJ, Torok-Storb B. Identification of stromal cell precursors in human bone marrow by a novel monoclonal antibody, STRO-1. *Blood.* 1991;78:55–62.
36. International Cartilage Repair Society. The cartilage standard evaluation form/knee. *ICRS Newsletter.* 1998;1:5–7.
37. Lysholm J, Gillquist J. Evaluation of knee ligament surgery results with special emphasis on use of a scoring scale. *Am J Sports Med.* 1982;10:150–154.
38. Tegner Y, Lysholm J. Rating systems in the evaluation of knee ligament injuries. *Clin Orthop Relat Res.* 1985;(198):43–49.
39. Marlovits S, Striessnig G, Resinger CT, et al. Definition of pertinent parameters for the evaluation of articular cartilage repair tissue with high-resolution magnetic resonance imaging. *Eur J Radiol.* 2004;52:310–319.

40. Peterson L, Minas T, Brittberg M, et al. Two- to 9-year outcome after autologous chondrocyte transplantation of the knee. *Clin Orthop Relat Res.* 2000;(374):212–234.
41. Henderson IJ, Gui J, Lavigne P. Autologous chondrocyte implantation: natural history of postimplantation periosteal hypertrophy and effects of repair-site debridement on outcome. *Arthroscopy.* 2006;22:1318–1324.
42. Wong KL, Lee KB, Tai BC, et al. Injectable cultured bone marrow-derived mesenchymal stem cells in varus knees with cartilage defects undergoing high tibial osteotomy: a prospective, randomized controlled clinical trial with 2 years' follow-up. *Arthroscopy.* 2013;29(12):2020–2028.
43. Horie M, Sekiya I, Muneta T, et al. Intra-articular injected synovial stem cells differentiate into meniscal cells directly and promote meniscal regeneration without mobilization to distant organs in rat massive meniscal defect. *Stem Cells.* 2009;27(4):878–887.
44. Motoyama M, Deie M, Kanaya A, et al. In vitro cartilage formation using TGF-beta-immobilized magnetic beads and mesenchymal stem cell-magnetic field conditions. *J Biomed Mater Res A.* 2010;92(1):196–204.

SECTION

4

Discoid Meniscus

Christine M. Goodbody
R. Jay Lee
Victor M. Ho-Fung
Theodore J. Ganley

CHAPTER

28

Discoid Meniscus: Overview, Epidemiology, Classification, Assessment

INTRODUCTION AND ANATOMY

Discoid meniscus is an anatomic variant, usually affecting the lateral meniscus, in which the meniscus is abnormal in shape and/or in its attachments within the knee joint. The normal medial meniscus is a C-shaped piece of cartilage covering about 50% of the medial tibial plateau. It is fixed to the joint capsule by the meniscotibial (i.e., coronary) ligament and the meniscocapsular ligament; the latter connects to the deep medial collateral ligament.[1] The size, shape, thickness, and mobility of the lateral meniscus tend to be more variable than for its medial counterpart. In general, the lateral meniscus covers about 70% of the lateral tibial plateau and is more ring-shaped.[2] On average, it is approximately 12 mm in width and 4 to 5 mm in height. Connections to the joint capsule are less strong than for the medial meniscus. Similar to the medial meniscus, the lateral meniscus has a meniscocapsular ligament, but in this case, it attaches to the joint capsule only, with no attachment to the lateral collateral ligament. The lateral meniscus also lacks any fixation to the joint capsule in the region of the popliteal hiatus.[1] Consequently, the lateral meniscus is more mobile than the medial meniscus, translating 9 to 11 mm on the tibia during knee flexion[3] versus 2 to 5 mm. Frequent anatomic variant attachments include the ligaments of Humphry and Wrisberg (or the anterior and posterior meniscofemoral ligaments, respectively), which attach the posterior horn of the lateral meniscus to the medial femoral condyle.[2]

EPIDEMIOLOGY

Abnormal development of the meniscus, particularly the lateral meniscus, may cause it to be larger, thicker, and more hypertrophic than usual as well as more discoid in shape. A discoid meniscus also tends not to taper centrally. Its anomalous size and shape, and its subsequent decreased vascularity, cause it to be more prone to tears than a normally formed meniscus. In fact, the actual discoid shape of the meniscus is asymptomatic, and it tends to present to medical attention secondary to symptoms of a tear.

It is thought that discoid lateral meniscus affects 3% to 5% of the population, and in those affected, about 20% have bilateral involvement.[1,2] Notably, Asian and, particularly, Japanese populations are thought to have an increased prevalence of this condition, with estimates approaching 15%.[3] Discoid medial meniscus has been reported but is significantly less common. Prevalence estimates of discoid medial meniscus range from 0.06% to 0.3%, and bilateral involvement is thought to be rare.[4] Historically, the true prevalence of discoid meniscus has been difficult to estimate given that many patients with the condition are asymptomatic, and the pathology is often noted only incidentally or in the setting of a tear.[3,4] Of note, in children younger than 10 years of age, traumatic meniscal injury is rare in the absence of discoid meniscus, and this condition should always be suspected in a child presenting with symptoms of meniscus tear.[1,3] Discoid meniscus has also been referred to as *popping knee syndrome* or *snapping knee syndrome*. Presentation with a snapping knee is not typical, and this classic presentation occurs most commonly in the Wrisberg variant of the condition, which affects a minority (0% to 33%) of patients with discoid meniscus.[1,2,5–8] The classification of discoid meniscus variants and the importance of distinguishing between them will be discussed in the following text.

The pathologic nature of a discoid meniscus is evidenced by the fact that up to 70% of discoid menisci noted at arthroscopy have tears.[3,9] In patients with discoid menisci, the most common tear pattern is the horizontal cleavage tear, which lies in contrast to patients who traumatically tear normal menisci, in which case, peripheral longitudinal tears are most ubiquitous.[3] Of symptomatic tears of discoid menisci, between 58% and 98% have been reported to be of the degenerative horizontal cleavage type.[1,4,10–12] This information is significant, as tear type directly affects the treatment decision-making process. Assessment of the pathology of tears of discoid menisci has often revealed mucoid fibrinous degeneration, likely secondary to repetitive microtrauma and consequent delamination, predisposing these menisci to the cleavage tears that are seen clinically.[3] Although tears are less common in type III discoid menisci than in types I and II (classification discussed in the following text), these may be predisposed to complex degenerative tears of the posterior horn of the lateral meniscus, which is abnormally hypermobile and often enlarged compared to normal.[3]

CLASSIFICATION

Discoid meniscus has traditionally been classified into three categories: complete, incomplete, and Wrisberg ligament type (Fig. 28.1). These were described by Watanabe et al.[13] in 1967 and were based on the arthroscopic appearance of the involved portion of the meniscus. The complete and incomplete types are discoid in shape and have normal anatomic attachments to the tibia, and they vary only in the amount of the tibial plateau that they cover.[14] Those that cover the entire or most of the tibial plateau are considered complete or type I. Those that cover less than 80% of the tibial plateau are classified as incomplete or type II. Types I and II are abnormal both in shape and in width. The width of a type I or II discoid meniscus generally ranges from 8 to 10 mm, which is much larger than a normal meniscus.[3] Type III discoid lateral meniscus is also called the *Wrisberg ligament type*. Kaplan[6] initially described this type in 1957. This meniscus type may be discoid but can also be near normal in shape, with the defining characteristic being the lack of normal posterior capsular/tibial attachments. In a type III discoid meniscus, the posterior meniscotibial ligament is absent and the only posterior fixation is by the posterior meniscofemoral, or Wrisberg, ligament. The lack of attachments makes the meniscus unstable and pathologically more mobile. This hypermobility of the lateral meniscus may manifest with the classic complaint of snapping knee as the meniscus moves within the joint during knee motion.[3] Namely, in the presence of a posterior meniscofemoral ligament and absence of a posterior meniscotibial ligament, during knee extension, the lateral meniscus can be drawn into the joint toward the intercondylar notch instead of its normal anteroposterior gliding motion, and this causes symptoms of locking, popping, and snapping.[3]

More recently, Jordan et al.[15] expanded on this classification system to include both arthroscopic and clinical findings in order to more completely describe discoid meniscus type and therefore provide more insight into appropriate treatment.[1,2,14,15] This classification system stratifies discoid lateral meniscus pathology into stable and unstable categories. Stable variants have normal anterior and posterior tibial attachments, irrespective of the presence of a Wrisberg ligament, and therefore have normal mobility.[14] These types include the Watanabe type I (complete) and type II (incomplete) meniscal variants. The unstable types are defined as those without a posterior meniscotibial ligament, that is, the Watanabe type III, or Wrisberg, variant. These tend to be hypermobile given their anomalous attachments. The unstable category is then subdivided into unstable with a discoid shape and unstable with normal shape. Each of these—stable, unstable discoid, and unstable normal—are then stratified based on whether they are torn or not torn and whether they are symptomatic or asymptomatic.[2,19]

PRESENTATION AND ASSESSMENT

Evaluation of a patient with suspected discoid meniscus involves detailed history taking, clinical examination, and imaging. As previously stated, stable variants of discoid meniscus tend to present in association with a tear, whereas uninjured, stable discoid menisci are usually detected only incidentally during imaging or arthroscopy for another condition. The Wrisberg variant, on the other hand, may present as snapping knee, and symptoms are not contingent on meniscal injury. Consequently, presentation may be highly variable and dependent on meniscal type, stability, and presence or absence of a tear.[1] Of note, the classic complaint of snapping knee can occur in a formerly stable type I or II discoid meniscus if a tear occurs such that the posterior meniscotibial attachment is avulsed, causing a Wrisberg-type pathology.[4] An unstable discoid meniscus that presents with snapping is more likely to cause pain and discomfort with activity in older children (8 to 10 years of age) and is highly unlikely to cause uncomfortable symptoms or pain in younger patients (age 3 to 4 years).[3]

Symptoms that occur in the setting of a torn, stable discoid meniscus are similar to those of a tear in a normal-shaped meniscus and include pain, swelling, catching, locking, a sense of "giving out," and decreased range of motion. However, in contrast to tears of normal menisci, discoid tears differ in that they may not always present in the setting of acute trauma and may instead have a more subacute course without a known inciting event.[1,4] Snapping on terminal extension, or symptoms of a meniscal tear without known trauma, particularly in younger children, should increase suspicion for discoid meniscal pathology.

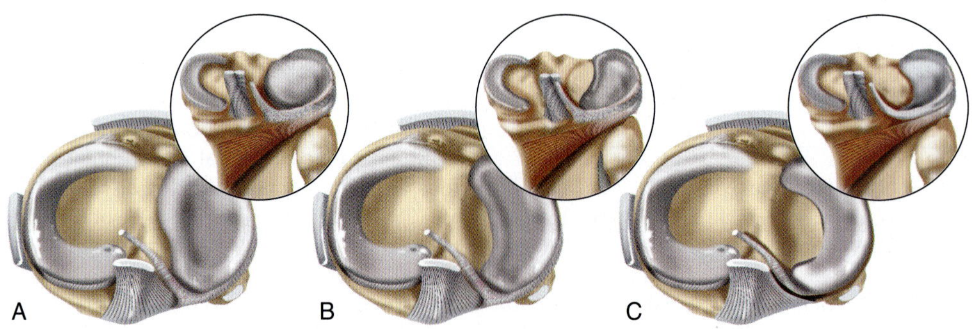

Figure 28.1. Watanabe classification of discoid meniscus: (**A**) complete, (**B**) incomplete, and (**C**) Wrisberg variant.

On examination, physical findings may include block to or pain with terminal motion, particularly extension; flexed stance during ambulation (to avoid uncomfortable snapping with extension); and a prominent bulge at the anterolateral joint line with maximal flexion.[2] Unstable discoid menisci may present earlier, as a tear is not required to elicit symptoms, and may be associated with a palpable, visible, or audible popping/snapping during extension as the meniscus reduces into its normal anatomic position.[1] Physical examination in a patient with a torn discoid meniscus will reveal similar findings to those with torn normal menisci. On top of those findings associated with discoid pathology, examination may reveal knee effusion, joint line tenderness, loss of range of motion, and positive McMurray and/or Apley maneuvers.[1] A positive McMurray is particularly rare to find in young children, and so absence of positive provocative maneuvers to detect meniscal pathology should not necessarily decrease suspicion in these patients. Imaging remains critical to the diagnosis given the variability in presentation and in examination findings. Estimates of clinical examination accuracy have ranged from 29% to 93% when compared to arthroscopic findings and are likely dependent on the experience of the practitioner.[4,16–18] Nonetheless, if discoid meniscus is suspected based on symptoms and examination, a detailed examination and possibly imaging of the contralateral, asymptomatic knee may be indicated, given the high rate of bilaterality in this condition.[3]

IMAGING

Due to the variability of clinical examination, imaging is an essential component in the diagnosis of discoid meniscus. Imaging generally begins with plain radiographs, although these are frequently normal, particularly in younger children. However, when typical findings are present, they may greatly aid in arriving at the correct diagnosis. Four views, namely, anteroposterior, lateral, sunrise, and tunnel views, are generally recommended. Findings on plain radiographs vary but may include a widened lateral joint line (secondary to widened lateral meniscus), cupping of the lateral tibial plateau, squaring or flattening of the lateral femoral condyle, calcification of the lateral meniscus, tibial eminence hypoplasia, and fibular head elevation.[1,2,4] Other musculoskeletal abnormalities that have been associated with discoid meniscus include fibular muscle defects, abnormally contoured lateral malleolus, and enlarged inferior lateral geniculate artery.[4] Specifically of concern for the pediatric sports surgeon is the association between discoid meniscus and osteochondral pathology of the lateral femoral condyle.[4] If present, these findings should increase suspicion for discoid meniscal pathology.

After plain radiographs, and particularly if initial radiographic findings are concerning for discoid meniscus, magnetic resonance (MR) imaging is indicated. Multiple findings on MR may suggest a diagnosis of discoid meniscus. Presence of any one of three criteria is consistent with a diagnosis of discoid meniscus. One criterion is continuity of anterior and posterior meniscal horns on at least three consecutive sagittal images (Fig. 28.2). Given that the normal meniscus is 12 mm in diameter and MR images are spaced by a standard 5 mm, this appearance of anteroposterior continuity should only be present on a maximum of two slices. When present on three

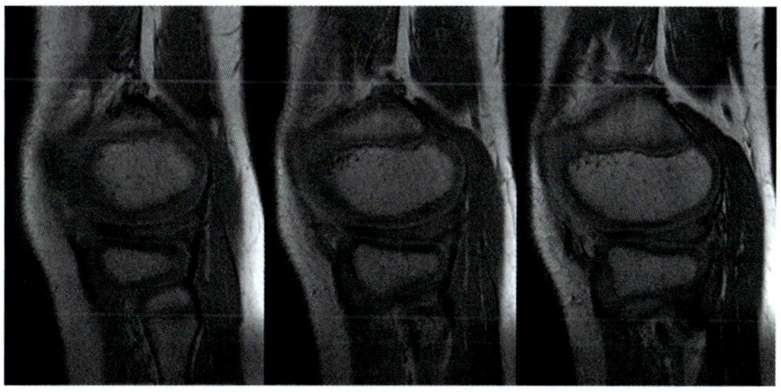

Figure 28.2. MR of a discoid lateral meniscus demonstrating anteroposterior continuity on three consecutive sagittal images.

of more, it is known as a *bow tie sign* and is indicative of discoid pathology. Another diagnostic criterion is a transverse meniscal diameter of greater than 15 mm, and the last is a transverse meniscal diameter that is greater than 20% of the total tibial width on any axial image (Fig. 28.3). The ratio of the sum of the width of both lateral meniscal horns to the maximal meniscal diameter (all on sagittal view) of greater than 75% has also been considered by some to be diagnostic.[4] Other MR evidence of discoid meniscus may include an abnormally thick, flat meniscus on any view, possibly demonstrating a thickened, extruded meniscus spanning the entire lateral tibial plateau on coronal images (Fig. 28.4) and increased thickness of the anterior horn, the posterior horn, or the entire meniscus.[2] MR imaging is also critical in evaluation of meniscal tears (Fig. 28.5), intrasubstance pathology, and presence of concomitant osteochondritis dissecans.[4]

Complete discoid menisci tend to be easier to diagnose by MR imaging than incomplete discoid menisci. It is useful to note that although MR imaging has been proven highly specific for discoid meniscus, and therefore there is a high positive predictive value for having a discoid meniscus if any of the earlier findings is present, it is not very sensitive, and so absence of these findings has low negative predictive value and does not necessarily rule out discoid pathology.[1] Moreover, due to their often near-normal morphology, Wrisberg-variant discoid menisci can be particularly difficult to detect and the previously mentioned diagnostic criteria may erroneously lead the evaluating physician to rule out discoid meniscus in these patients. Despite advancements in MR technology and expertise, accurate diagnosis of a missing posterior meniscotibial ligament may prove difficult. Subtle findings that may be present on MR in the case of Wrisberg-variant discoid meniscus are anterior subluxation of the posterior horn and increased T2 signal intensity between the lateral meniscus and the joint capsule.[3]

For any type of discoid meniscus, if clinical suspicion is high and imaging has not yielded a diagnosis, diagnostic arthroscopy may be indicated[1] (Figs. 28.6 and 28.7). This may prove beneficial in determining the presence or absence of normal meniscal attachments, in assessing meniscal stability, in visualizing the exact morphology of the meniscus, and in evaluating for meniscal tears. Limitations do exist to diagnostic arthroscopy and include difficulty accessing and visualizing the lateral joint space, particularly in the presence of a thick, wide discoid meniscus, and inability to appreciate midsubstance or undersurface tears.[2]

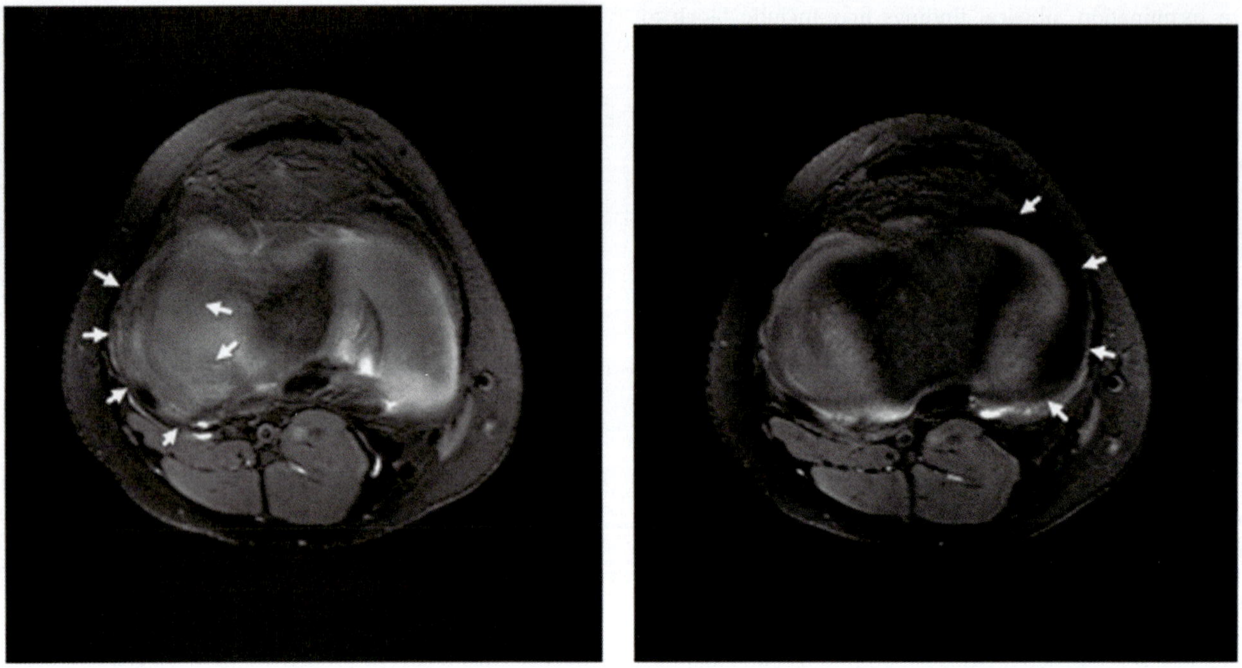

A B

Figure 28.3. **A.** Axial proton density image demonstrating a discoid lateral meniscus covering an abnormal amount of the lateral tibial plateau, with heterogeneous high signal intensity of the discoid lateral meniscus (*arrows*). **B.** Axial proton density image demonstrating normal homogenous low signal intensity of the medial meniscus (*arrows*).

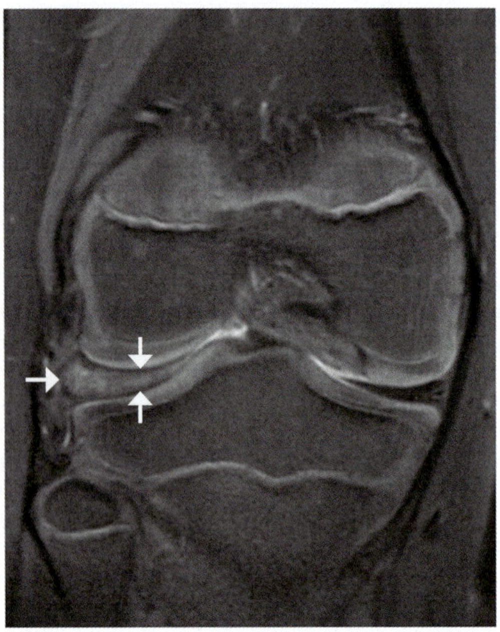

Figure 28.4. Coronal MR image demonstrating a thickened (*vertical arrows*) and extruded (*horizontal arrow*) discoid lateral meniscus.

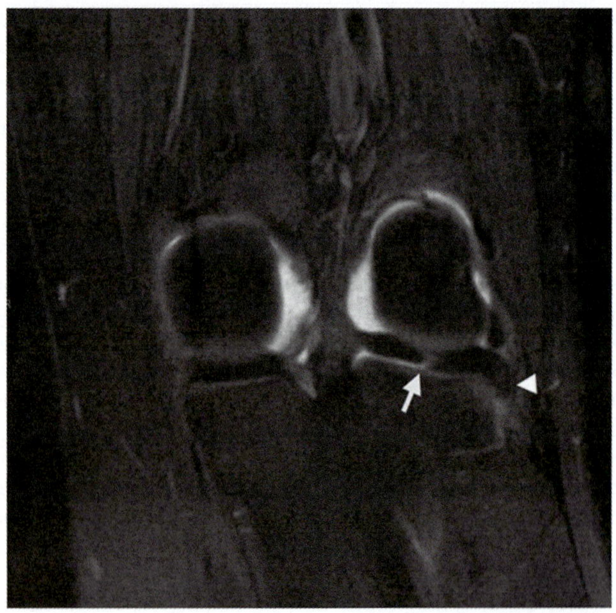

Figure 28.5. Coronal proton density image demonstrating posterior horn tear (*arrow*) and inferior displacement of peripheral portion of the lateral meniscus (*arrowhead*).

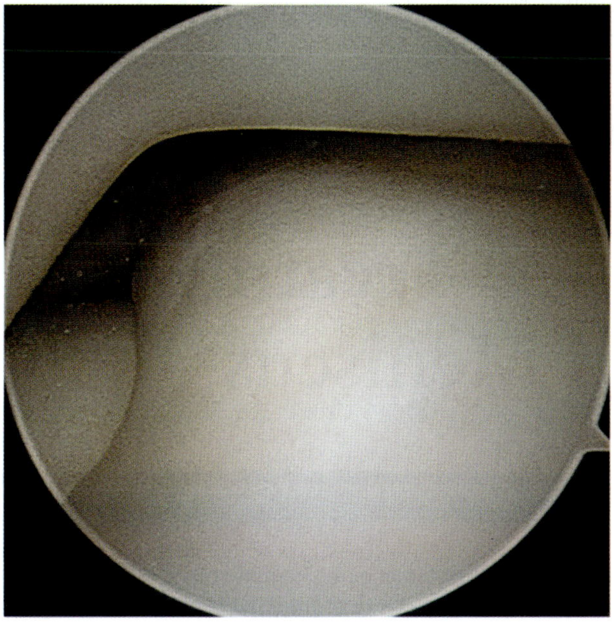

Figure 28.6. Arthroscopic view of a complete discoid meniscus in the lateral compartment of the knee. The meniscus is abnormally thickened and covers most of lateral tibial plateau, extending to the intercondylar notch. Note also the squaring of the lateral femoral condyle.

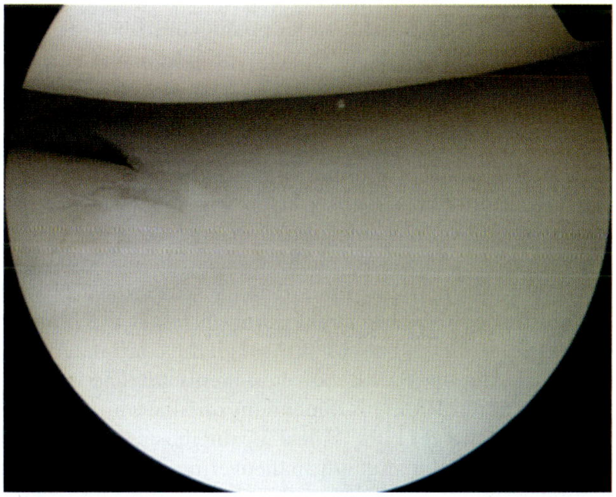

Figure 28.7. Arthroscopic view of an incomplete discoid meniscus in the lateral compartment of the knee. It covers a large amount of the lateral tibial plateau but does not extend into the intercondylar notch.

REFERENCES

1. Kocher MS, Klingele K, Rassman SO. Meniscal disorders: normal, discoid, and cysts. *Orthop Clin North Am.* 2003;34(3):329–340.
2. Jordan M. Lateral meniscal variants: evaluation and treatment. *J Am Acad Orthop Surg.* 1996;4:191–200.
3. Kramer DE, Micheli LJ. Meniscal tears and discoid meniscus in children: diagnosis and treatment. *J Am Acad Orthop Surg.* 2009;17(11):698–707.
4. Yaniv M, Blumberg N. The discoid meniscus. *J Child Orthop.* 2007;1(2):89–96.
5. Vandermeer R, Cunningham F. Arthroscopic treatment of the discoid lateral meniscus: results of long-term follow-up. *Arthroscopy.* 1989;5:101–109.
6. Kaplan EB. Discoid lateral meniscus of the knee joint. *Bull Hosp Joint Dis.* 1955;16:111–124.
7. Hayashi LK, Yamaga H, Ida K, et al. Arthroscopic meniscectomy for discoid lateral meniscus in children. *J Bone Joint Surg Am.* 1988;70:1495–500.
8. Ikeuchi H. Arthroscopic treatment of lateral discoid meniscus. Technique and long-term results. *Clin Orthop Relat Res.* 1982;(167): 19–28.
9. Klingele KE, Kocher MS, Hresko MT, et al. Discoid lateral meniscus: prevalence of peripheral rim instability. *J Pediatr Orthop.* 2004;24(1):79–82.
10. Aichroth PM, Patel DV, Marx CI. Congenital discoid lateral meniscus in children. A follow-up study and evaluation of management. *J Bone Joint Surg Br.* 1991;73:932–936.
11. Bellier G, Dupont JY, Larrain M, et al. Lateral discoid meniscus in children. *Arthroscopy.* 1989;5:52–56.
12. Pellacci F, Montanari G, Prosperi P, et al. Lateral discoid meniscus: treatment and results. *Arthroscopy.* 1992;8:526–530.
13. Watanabe M, Takada S, Ikeuchi H. *Atlas of Arthroscopy.* Tokyo, Japan: Igaku-Shoin; 1969.
14. Kelly BT, Green DW. Discoid lateral meniscus in children. *Curr Opin Pediatr.* 2002;14(1):54–61.
15. Jordan MR, Duncan JB, Bertrand SL. Discoid lateral meniscus: a review. *South Orthop J.* 1993;2(4):239–253.
16. Harvell JC Jr, Fu FH, Stanitski CL. Diagnostic arthroscopy of the knee in children and adolescents. *Orthopedics.* 1989;12:1555–1560.
17. Morrissy RT, Eubanks RG, Park JP, et al. Arthroscopy of the knee in children. *Clin Orthop Relat Res.* 1982;(162):103–107.
18. Kocher MS, DiCanzio J, Zurakowski D, et al. Diagnostic performance of clinical examination and selective magnetic resonance imaging in the evaluation of intraarticular knee disorders in children and adolescents. *Am J Sports Med.* 2001;29:292–296.
19. Good CR, Green DW, Griffith MH, et al. Arthroscopic treatment of symptomatic discoid meniscus in children: classification, technique, and results. *Arthroscopy.* 2007;23(2):157–163.

CHAPTER

29

Jacqueline Munch
Marcia Voigt
Daniel W. Green
Scott A. Rodeo

Surgical Techniques for Treatment of Symptomatic Discoid Meniscus

Discoid menisci become symptomatic due to instability and/or meniscal tearing. A discoid meniscus may have abnormal excursion with knee motion due to lack of attachments to the surrounding capsule, most commonly lack of posterior root attachment. Tibiofemoral impingement can cause the abnormally shaped meniscus to get caught, tearing the meniscal tissue. A torn discoid meniscus most often exhibits a horizontal cleavage tear.

Surgical treatment of symptomatic discoid menisci is indicated based on the type of meniscus (complete vs. incomplete) and the stability of the meniscal rim attachments (stable vs. unstable).

Table 29.1 depicts a treatment algorithm based on the morphology and stability of the meniscus.

Although early recommendations for treatment of symptomatic discoid meniscus consisted primarily of total or subtotal meniscectomy, our understanding of the role of the meniscus in load-sharing and stability of the knee has led to expanded indications for meniscal preservation and meniscocapsular repair. The lateral meniscus distributes up to 70% of the loads in the lateral compartment of the knee and plays a role in stabilizing the knee against rotational forces.[1–3]

Current strategies for the surgical treatment of symptomatic discoid menisci involve the creation of as normally shaped a meniscus as possible while stabilizing and preserving as much meniscus tissue as possible. A meniscus tear is addressed as indicated in the course of creating a more normally shaped meniscus. If the tear is in the midsubstance of a stable, completely discoid meniscus, simple saucerization is the treatment of choice. If the tear is at the periphery, repair should be undertaken. In the case of an unstable discoid meniscus that is not torn, saucerization is likely also required in order to provide adequate exposure for stabilization of the meniscus.

Saucerization involves removing the central tissue in a discoid meniscus. This is accomplished using arthroscopic biting and shaving instruments. The discoid tissue leaves less space than normal in the knee joint, causing difficulty with visualization and exposure. In addition, the patients are often young and may have very small knees compared to the average adult. In rare cases, the surgeon may even elect to use smaller arthroscopic instruments, such as the 2.7-mm arthroscope and the smaller arthroscopic biting equipment used in wrist, elbow, and ankle surgeries. However, discoid menisci consist of uniformly thick tissue rather than the central taper of a normally shaped meniscus. Although the discoid meniscus exhibits mucoid degeneration on histologic examination,[4] it often maintains the thick, rubbery texture of an intricate collagen network. This abnormal collagen content can also be visualized on magnetic resonance imaging (MRI). Thus, smaller biting instruments may be inadequate to obtain control of the entire thickness. In order to be adequately prepared in a small patient, it is recommended to have both sizes of instruments and arthroscopes available. If a central horizontal cleavage tear is present, it can serve as an entry point for instruments to access the central portion of the meniscus and begin to taper it toward the periphery. A 70-degree arthroscope may prove helpful for visualization within the confined space.

A typical set of arthroscopic biting instruments is shown in Figure 29.1. Straight and upward-going biters (Fig. 29.1A,B) are used through the ipsilateral portal to resect the posterior horn of the affected meniscus or through the contralateral portal to resect the body of the affected meniscus. The choice of straight or upward-going is dependent on anatomy and portal placement: A straight biter is ideal for the most central portion of the meniscal tissue, but any maneuvering around the femoral condyle might benefit from an upward-going biter. Right and left biters (Fig. 29.1C) are used through the ipsilateral portal to resect the body of the affected meniscus or through the contralateral portal to resect the anterior horn of the affected meniscus. For extensive resection of the anterior horn, a backbiter (Fig. 29.1D) should be available for use through the ipsilateral portal. The backbiter is not uniformly available in standard sets and must be requested specifically. Likewise, for very thick tissue, the large biter, or "fat boy" biter (Fig. 29.1E), should be requested in addition to standard instruments.

Portal placement must be carefully considered in order to reach the entirety of the discoid meniscus and achieve variable angles of approach. Initial viewing portal placement must be individualized to the patient's size and relative location of the patella with respect to the tibiofemoral joint line. The anterolateral portal must not cause injury to the meniscus or the articular surfaces of the knee with instrument passage but must

TABLE 29.1 Surgical Treatment of Discoid Menisci with Respect to Morphology and Stability

Discoid Type	*Meniscal Stability*	*Treatment*
Complete	Stable	Saucerization
Incomplete	Stable	Partial saucerization
Complete	Unstable—anterior Unstable—posterior	Saucerization plus outside-in meniscocapsular suture Saucerization plus inside-out meniscocapsular suture
Incomplete	Unstable—anterior Unstable—posterior	Partial saucerization plus outside-in meniscocapsular suture Partial saucerization plus inside-out meniscocapsular suture

be sufficiently inferior as to allow access to the posterior aspect of the joint without injury to the femoral condyle. Once the arthroscope has been inserted into the joint, the anteromedial portal can be established under direct visualization, taking care to avoid injury to the anterior horn of the medial meniscus. An approach to the lateral meniscus from the medial side of the knee must allow clearance of the tibial spines, but it should not be so high as to preclude passage under the lateral femoral condyle. Localization with a small instrument such as a spinal needle prior to establishing the skin incision is recommended. Accessory portals, including the midpatellar portal and the posterolateral accessory portal, can also aid in visualization.

The amount of resection required to prevent continued impingement of the discoid tissue is a matter of some debate. Some surgeons recommend use of the curve of the lateral condyle as a guide, but the condyle adjacent to a discoid meniscus is known to have a larger average radius of curvature compared with a knee containing a normally shaped meniscus (Fig. 29.2—plain film of a knee with a discoid lateral meniscus). Others recommend leaving 6- to 8-mm rim of tissue in order to mimic a "normal" meniscus. In the case of a saucer ized discoid meniscus (Fig. 29.3), however, this remaining rim is more of a trapezoid than the typical triangular tissue of a normal meniscus (Fig 29.4), and the implications of this increased remaining central thickness are unknown. At the minimum, the remaining meniscal tissue must have a stable rim, and dynamic assessment for impingement with range of motion can aid in intraoperative decision making.

Thermal ablation is a technique favored by some authors for contouring of meniscal tissue during adult meniscectomy. In pediatric patients, however, the proximity of the articular cartilage in the confined space of a compartment with a discoid meniscus makes the technique too high risk for tissue necrosis. If thermal instruments are used, we recommend using an outflow cannula in order to minimize the risk of elevated intra-articular temperatures.

In general, repair of a torn discoid meniscus and fixation of an unstable meniscocapsular junction should be suture-based. All-inside implants offer simplicity and speed compared to traditional inside-out or outside-in repair techniques, but they create larger defects in the meniscus with implant passage than do simple needles with suture. In pediatric patients in particular, small needles offer the advantage of multiple suture passes with minimal trauma, on both the femoral and tibial sides of the meniscus, in order to gain secure control of unstable and/or torn tissue.

Inside-out repair of the posterior horn and body of the meniscus and meniscocapsular junction requires an additional incision, generally on the posterolateral side of the knee. Vertical and horizontal mattress patterns may be used to obtain stable tissue fixation. The neurovascular structures are typically inferior to the trajectory of the needles on the lateral side of the knee, but care must be taken to avoid capture of the popliteus tendon as the sutures are passed. In the rarer circumstance of medial discoid meniscus, the saphenous nerve is at risk during inside-out repair of the posterior horn and body.

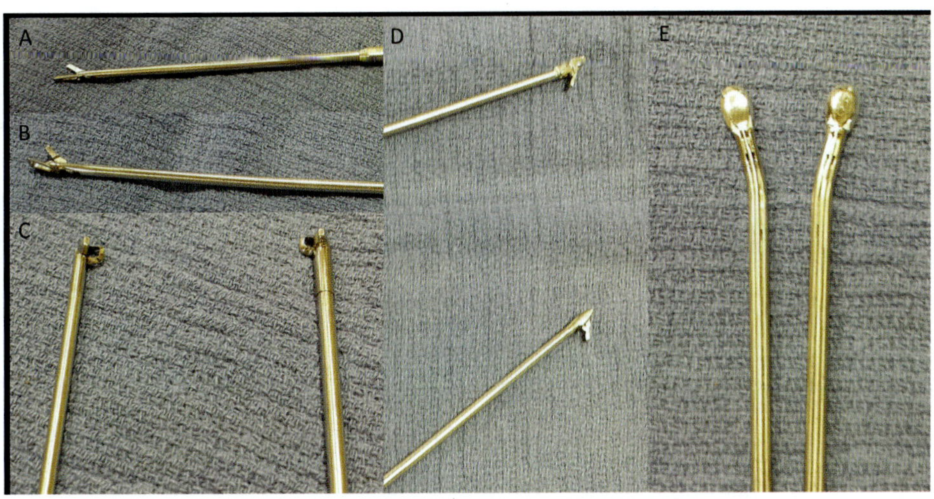

Figure 29.1. Biting instruments for resection of discoid meniscus tissue during saucerization. **A.** Straight biter. **B.** Upward-going biter. **C.** Right and left side biters. **D.** Right and left back-biters. **E.** Large, "fat boy" biters angled left and right.

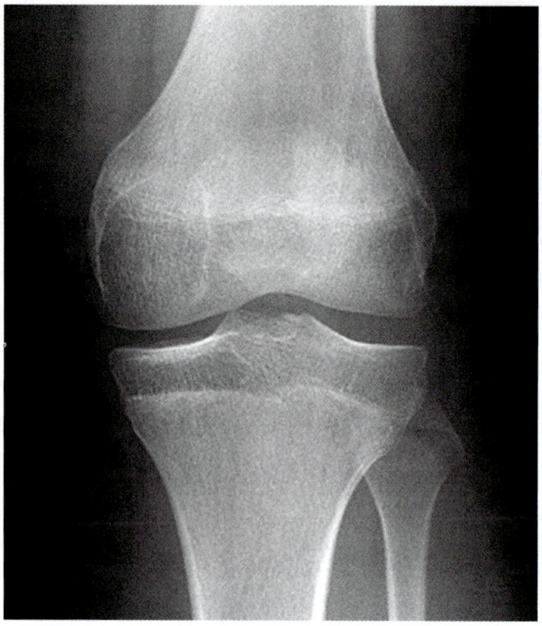

Figure 29.2. X-ray depicting typical findings in the setting of discoid lateral meniscus: increased lateral joint space and flattened femoral condyle.

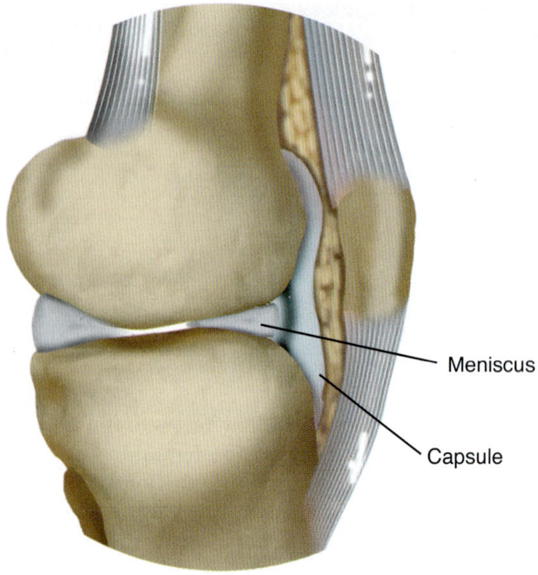

Figure 29.4. Cross-sectional shape of a normal meniscus.

Because the interior of the knee is viewed from an anterior to posterior direction through the arthroscope, instability of the anterior horn of the discoid meniscus can be subtle and may be missed unless specifically investigated during the diagnostic portion of the procedure. Specific attention must be paid to this portion of a discoid meniscus, however, because the prevalence of instability has been reported to be as high as 53%.[5] A probe or arthroscopic grasper can be used to exert pressure on the anterior horn, and instability is noted when the anterior horn of the meniscus displaces into the compartment.

When the anterior horn of the meniscus is torn, or the anterior meniscocapsular junction is unstable, outside-in repair can be used arthroscopically. Figures 29.5 to 29.7 depict a technique for outside-in anterior horn repair: Two spinal needles are inserted through the meniscus from the anterior aspect of the knee at the level of the joint line. If the anterior horn is prone to flipping posteriorly during repair, traction sutures may be placed. When the anterior horn is successfully reduced, a shuttling suture is inserted through each spinal needle and drawn out through the arthroscopic portal using a grasper. A rigid

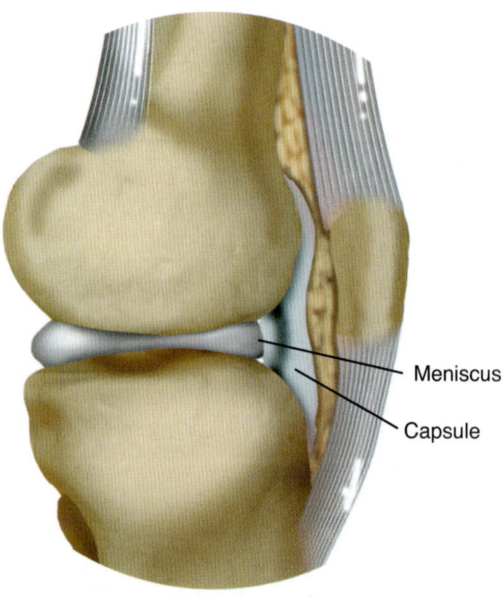

Figure 29.3. Diagram representing a complete discoid meniscus.

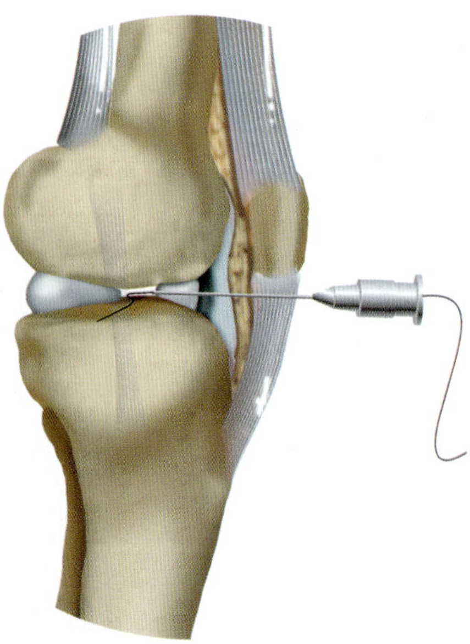

Figure 29.5. Trajectory of approach for arthroscopic outside-in repair of an anterior tear or unstable anterior horn of a discoid meniscus.

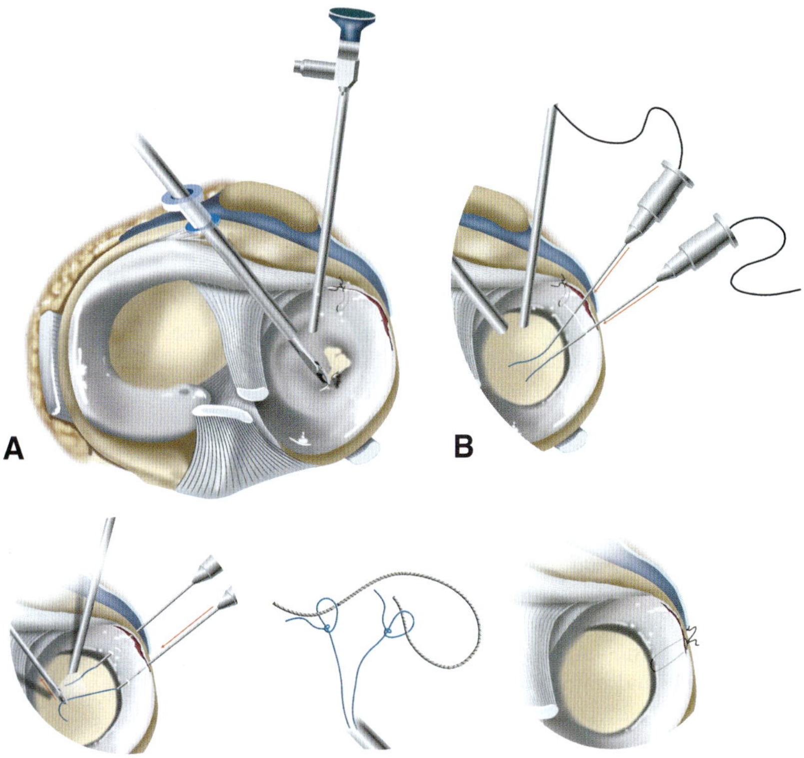

Figure 29.6. **A.** Saucerization: Biting instruments are used to create a more normally shaped meniscus prior to repair of a torn meniscus that is completely or partially discoid. **B.** Arthroscopic approach to meniscus repair: The camera views the compartment from an anterolateral portal, and a cannula is placed within the anteromedial portal. A small suture is passed through each of two spinal needles traversing the anterior horn tear. **C.** Each suture is grasped and drawn out of the joint, where **(D)** they are tied to each end of a single-braided suture. **E.** The passing sutures are drawn back across the tear as the spinal needles are removed. The ends of the braided suture are tied over the anterior joint capsule.

monofilament suture of polydioxanone (PDS) or Prolene is easiest to push into the spinal needle. Care must be taken to ensure that no tissue bridge is interposed between the shuttling suture limbs—to avoid this, a cannula may be used or the shuttling sutures must be drawn out of the portal together. One limb of a braided doubled suture is then tied to each shuttling suture. The skin bridge between the spinal needles is incised, and the two suture ends are drawn across the anterior horn as the spinal needles are removed. The two suture ends are then tied over the anterior knee capsule, creating a mattress suture across the meniscus. If a vertical mattress suture can be managed within the available space, it provides a more even approximation of the meniscus to the capsule.

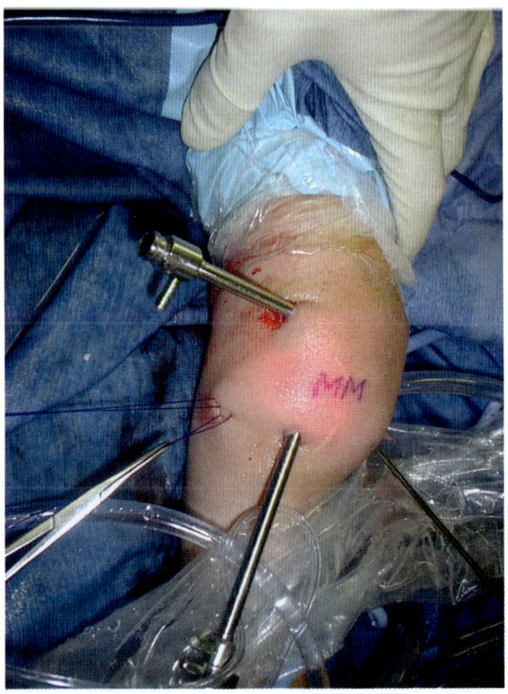

Figure 29.7. View of anterior horn meniscus repair from outside the pediatric knee.

Discoid medial menisci have been reported sporadically in the literature, and their incidence is much lower than that of discoid lateral menisci. They should be treated according to the algorithm mentioned earlier, with an understanding that discoid medial menisci are more often stable than discoid lateral menisci, given their typically more robust capsular attachments. Like their lateral counterparts, torn discoid medial menisci often exhibit horizontal cleavage tears, along with anatomic changes within the medial compartment: widening of the joint space on x-ray, cupping of the medial tibial plateau, and even confluence of the medial meniscus with the anterior cruciate ligament (ACL) anteriorly.[6–12]

AUGMENTATION OF REPAIRED DISCOID MENISCUS

Augmentation of meniscal repair and meniscocapsular suture fixation is an attractive concept in the setting of discoid meniscus. The tissue of a discoid meniscus is known to be abnormal in terms of structure and vascularity, and normal meniscal healing might not be expected after repair as a result.[4] Studies have shown improved meniscal healing in the setting of ACL reconstruction, likely due to the hemarthrosis resulting from creation of bony tunnels.[13–17] As a result, some authors have suggested augmenting an isolated meniscal repair with the components of the hemarthrosis that are thought to be responsible for the improved healing rate. Suggested surgical techniques include mechanical abrasion techniques and the use of a fibrin clot, platelet-rich fibrin matrix, growth factors, and bone marrow–derived mesenchymal cells.[18,19] These techniques aim to increase the vascular supply and healing response at the meniscus repair site.[17]

Trephination, or perforation of the meniscus to create channels between the avascular and vascularized regions of the meniscus, has been criticized as an inadequate technique for stimulating meniscal healing while maintaining positive patient outcomes. Although it does stimulate healing in the avascular portion of the meniscus, the creation of the channels disrupts the structural integrity of the meniscus. This potentially leads to a weaker meniscus and a decreased ability to distribute load across the meniscus.[17,20]

Fibrin clot placement within a meniscus repair has been proposed as one means of stimulating and facilitating meniscal healing after repair. In a dog model, Arnoczky et al.[21] found that the fibrin clot stimulated healing in the avascular zone of the meniscus. The authors suggest that the fibrin clot acts as a chemotactic and mitogenic stimulus and provides a scaffold for reparative cells. The fibrin clot is created from peripheral blood via aspiration and agitation. Its consistency allows for surgical accommodations, as it can be trimmed to size without compromising its integrity.[17] Studies have demonstrated improved rates of healing in repairs of normal (nondiscoid) torn menisci. Henning et al.[16] reported a reduction in the failure rate of isolated meniscal repairs when augmented with a fibrin clot from 41% to 8%. Van Trommel et al.[22] demonstrated that a fibrin clot may enhance meniscal healing and prevent future meniscal degeneration. Using second-look arthroscopy, the authors found healing of the peripheral menisci in all cases. In addition, all of the patients were able to return to their initial level of sporting activity after the procedure.

Platelet-rich fibrin matrix is another option for augmentation, which offers the additional benefit of growth factors that are released from the alpha and dense granules in the platelet cytoplasm.[23] The activation of the platelets leads to a cascading healing action. The release of various growth factors such as platelet-derived growth factor (PDGF), fibroblast growth factor (FGF), transforming growth factor-β (TGF-β1), insulin-like growth factor (IGF-1), hepatocyte growth factor (HGF), vascular endothelial growth factor (VEGF), epidermal growth factor (EGF), and bone morphogenic protein (BMP) help induce healing. Cytokines such as interleukin-1, tumor necrosis factor-α, and matrix metalloproteinases have been shown to inhibit meniscal healing.[20,24]

Bone marrow aspiration, microfracture, and/or stem cells may be used to augment isolated meniscal repairs to increase healing rates. The concept behind the marrow-introduction technique is to mimic the healing response that ensues after an ACL reconstruction or hemarthrosis, in which subchondral bone of the intercondylar notch is penetrated and allows for the release of marrow elements into the joint.[14,17] Mesenchymal stem cells are present in human tissue, such as bone marrow, synovium, and adipose tissues, and may differentiate into various mesenchymal lineages, including bone and cartilage.[25] Bone marrow aspirate contains multipotent cells. Aspiration from the intercondylar notch of the knee has been found to have a lower cell density than iliac crest aspirate.[21,26] In a rat model, Izuta et al.[27] found that mesenchymal stem cells can proliferate in meniscal defects and create an extracellular matrix that promotes healing in the avascular portion of the meniscus. Such cells are present up to 8 weeks after being introduced.

Pabbruwe et al.[28] developed a stem cell/collagen-scaffold implant system to promote meniscal healing. In this system, bone marrow mesenchymal stem cells are placed on a biodegradable scaffold, which is integrated into the meniscus surface. Scaffolds that have a more open and/or spongy structure adjacent to the meniscal cartilage surfaces have higher integration rates than scaffolds that are designed for osteoinduction.[28]

POSTOPERATIVE CARE

Following simple saucerization, patients are generally permitted to pursue gentle range of motion and weight bearing as tolerated. The rehabilitation of pediatric patients after meniscus repair or meniscocapsular stabilization can be more difficult: Patients are limited to toe-touch or non–weight bearing after meniscal and/or meniscocapsular repair and range of motion limitations vary depending on the location of the repair. When the posterior horn and capsule are repaired, knee flexion is generally limited to 90 degrees in order to protect the meniscal repair from loading during femoral rollback in deep flexion. Weight bearing and range of motion restrictions are maintained for 4 to 6 weeks. Pediatric patients may have increased difficulty maintaining compliance with weight bearing and range of motion restrictions, and very young children may benefit from casting in full extension for 3 weeks. Studies have demonstrated that even adult patients have difficulty maintaining weight-bearing restrictions,[29] and concerns arise for pediatric patients in particular based on activity and maturity levels.

OUTCOMES OF DISCOID MENISCUS SURGERY

The outcomes of surgical treatment of discoid menisci have been reported in several studies, with a variety of treatment approaches based on morphology and the current standard of care. In their retrospective review with an average of 54 months of follow-up, Vandermeer and Cunningham[30] noted a return to normal activities in 64% of patients with a discoid lateral meniscus. Of the 20 knees treated with arthroscopic partial meniscectomy (with a goal of 4 to 5 mm of stable rim) for symptomatic, torn discoid menisci, only 5 (25%) were rated as having an excellent result. Fair and poor results were found in 6 (30%) and 3 (15%), respectively.[30] Pellacci et al.[31] reviewed 46 patients who underwent arthroscopic, open, or "mixed" (arthroscopically assisted) meniscectomy for discoid lateral meniscus and found that 3 out of the 30 (10%) with medium-term follow-up (mean 27.7 months) noted slight pain and a click but no limitation of motion. Total meniscectomy was performed on 21 patients, and the authors noted a lower rate of excellent results after total meniscectomy compared to partial meniscectomy (83% vs. 94%). Six patients were found to have degenerative changes on x-ray, and these patients had the most variable clinical results of the group.[31]

Räber et al.[32] evaluated 17 knees in 14 patients who underwent total meniscectomy for a discoid lateral meniscus and found that 10 of the 17 knees showed clinical and radiographic evidence of osteoarthritis at a mean follow-up of 19.8 years.[32]

Atay et al.[33] reviewed 33 patients treated with meniscectomy for symptomatic discoid lateral meniscus, with an average follow-up of 5.6 years. The single patient with a completely hypermobile meniscus received a total meniscectomy, and the remainder of patients were treated with partial meniscectomy. Fair results were noted in 5 patients (15%), and no patient was found to have a poor result. The patient who underwent total meniscectomy was rated postoperatively as "good."[33]

Oğüt et al.[34] reviewed 11 patients younger than 18 years of age who underwent simple arthroscopic partial meniscectomy/saucerization for a discoid lateral meniscus. At an average of 4.5 years of follow-up, nine of the knees were rated as asymptomatic, whereas two exhibited occasional pain. No degenerative changes were found on follow-up x-rays.[34]

Adachi et al.[35] treated five patients with saucerization and suture of a peripheral tear in a discoid meniscus and performed second-look arthroscopy on three of the patients at the 3- to 4-month postoperative point. One of the three patients who underwent second-look arthroscopy demonstrated a failure to heal at the repair site. This patient also demonstrated persistent pain and clicking, whereas the other four patients in the study were rated as having an excellent result.[35]

Good et al.[5] retrospectively reviewed patients treated surgically according to their pattern of tear and meniscus stability and found that 6 of 21 patients demonstrated persistent symptoms at a mean follow-up of 29.8 months. Of note, 3 of the 4 patients younger than 4 years of age required nearly 1 year of physical therapy to regain range of motion. The fourth patient recovered by 4 months postoperatively and was the only child of the younger subset to undergo casting postoperatively.[5]

In their 2009 study of 43 knees comparing partial versus subtotal/total meniscectomy for treatment of discoid lateral meniscus, Lee et al.[36] demonstrated that arthritic changes were significant in both study cohorts. Although their clinical outcomes did not differ, the severity of the arthritic changes was higher at mid- to long-term follow-up for patients who received subtotal and total meniscectomies.[36]

Although Manzione et al.[37] showed that children aged 5.3 to 16.4 years with normal (nondiscoid) menisci often develop osteoarthritis in the lateral compartment of the knee, Washington et al.[3] demonstrated in long-term follow-up that children aged 6 to 16 years who underwent total meniscectomy for a discoid meniscus do not necessarily show degeneration over time. This discrepancy raises the possibility of plasticity of the knee in very young patients. Okazaki et al.[38] noted that patients who underwent subtotal meniscectomy for discoid lateral meniscus achieve better clinical outcomes than their counterparts with normal menisci and theorized that the discrepancy may be due to the flattening of the femoral condyle and tibial plateau in the discoid compartment.

Given the relative rarity of discoid meniscus, we are unlikely to determine clinically whether the young knee is able to adapt to dramatic changes in force distribution in settings such as total meniscectomy of a discoid meniscus. The literature is clear on the risks of subtotal and total lateral meniscectomy in older patients, however. Total or partial meniscectomy increases peak contact stresses on articular cartilage up to 700% due to a decrease in 75% of contact area within the knee joint, resulting in cartilage damage and an increased risk of osteoarthritis over time.[39–42] Thus, our current standard of care in the treatment of symptomatic discoid meniscus consists of preserving as much meniscal tissue as possible via repair of torn meniscus and stabilization of meniscocapsular attachments. In patients who underwent total or subtotal meniscectomy, concerns arise for persistent symptoms over the long term, requiring further intervention such as meniscus allograft transplant (MAT).

REFERENCES

1. McDermott ID, Amis AA. The consequences of meniscectomy. *J Bone Joint Surg.* 2006;88(12):1549–1556.
2. Walker PS, Erkman MJ. The role of the menisci in force transmission across the knee. *Clin Orthop Relat Res.* 1975;(109):184–192.
3. Washington ER III, Root L, Liener UC. Discoid lateral meniscus in children. Long-term follow-up after excision. *J Bone Joint Surg Am.* 1995;77(9):1357–1361.
4. Nathan PA, Cole SC. Discoid meniscus. A clinical and pathological study. *Clin Orthop Relat Res.* 1969;64:107–113.
5. Good CR, Green DW, Griffith MH, et al. Arthroscopic treatment of symptomatic discoid meniscus in children: classification, technique, and results. *Arthroscopy.* 2007;23(2):157–163.
6. Yaniv M, Blumberg N. The discoid meniscus. *J Child Orthop.* 2007;1(2):89–96. doi:10.1007/s11832-007-0029-1.
7. Flouzat-Lachaniette CH, Pujol N, Boisrenoult P, et al. Discoid medial meniscus: report of four cases and literature review. *Orthop Traumatol Surg Res.* 2011;97(8):826–832. doi:10.1016/j.otsr.2011.07.011.
8. Joshi D, Jain V, Goyal A, et al. Discoid medial meniscus completely coalesced with the anterior cruciate ligament. *Orthopedics.* 2013;36(11):e1461–e1463.
9. Kim SJ, Seo YJ. Bilateral discoid medial menisci: incomplete type in one knee and complete type in opposite knee. *Knee.* 2006;13:255–257. doi:10.1016/j.knee.2006.01.009.
10. Tachibana Y, Yamazaki Y, Ninomiya S. Discoid medial meniscus. *Arthroscopy.* 2003;19(7):E12–E18. doi:10.1016/S0749-8063(03)00688-1.
11. Kim SJ, Lubis AM. Medial and lateral discoid menisci: a case report. *Sports Med Arthrosc Rehabil Ther Technol.* 2010;2:21. doi:10.1186/1758-2555-2-21.
12. Auge WK II, Kaeding CC. Bilateral discoid medial menisci with extensive intrasubstance cleavage tears: MRI and arthroscopic correlation. *Arthroscopy.* 1994;10(3):313–318.
13. Cannon WD Jr, Vittori JM. The incidence of healing in arthroscopic meniscal repairs in anterior cruciate ligament-reconstructed knees versus stable knees. *Am J Sports Med.* 1992;20(2):176–181.
14. Freedman KB, Nho SJ, Cole BJ. Marrow stimulating technique to augment meniscus repair. *Arthroscopy.* 2003;19(7):794–798.
15. Gill SS, Diduch DR. Outcomes after meniscal repair using the meniscus arrow in knees undergoing concurrent anterior cruciate ligament reconstruction. *Arthroscopy.* 2002;18(6):569–577.
16. Henning CE, Lynch MA, Yearout KM, et al. Arthroscopic meniscal repair using an exogenous fibrin clot. *Clin Orthop Relat Res.* 1990;(252):64–72.
17. Swenson TM. The use of exogenous fibrin clot to supplement meniscal surgery techniques. *Orthopedics.* 2007;30(9):718–723.
18. Taylor SA, Rodeo SA. Augmentation techniques for isolated meniscal tears. *Curr Rev Musculoskelet Med.* 2013;6:95–101.
19. Tu K, Cole BJ, Freedman K. Augmentation of meniscus repair. *Op Tech Sports Med.* 2003;11(2):127–133.
20. Delos D, Rodeo SA. Enhancing meniscal repair through biology: platelet-rich plasma as an alternative strategy. *Instr Course Lect.* 2011;60:453–460.

21. Arnoczky SP, Warren RF, Spivak JM. Meniscal repair using an exogenous fibrin clot. *J Bone Joint Surg Am.* 1988;70(8):1209–1217.
22. van Trommel MF, Simonian PT, Potter HG, et al. Arthroscopic meniscal repair with fibrin clot of complete radial tears of the lateral meniscus in the avascular zone. *Arthroscopy.* 1998;14(4):360–365.
23. Lucarelli E, Beretta R, Dozza B, et al. A recently developed bifacial platelet-rich fibrin matrix. *Eur Cell Mater.* 2010;20:13–23.
24. Middleton KK, Barro V, Muller B, et al. Evaluation of the effects of platelet-rich plasma (PRP) therapy involved in the healing of sports-related soft tissue injuries. *Iowa Orthop J.* 2012;32:150–163.
25. Centeno CJ, Busse D, Kisiday J, et al. Regeneration of meniscus cartilage in a knee treated with percutaneously implanted autologous mesenchymal stem cells. *Med Hypotheses.* 2008;71(6):900–908.
26. Beitzel K, McCarthy MB, Cote MP, et al. Comparison of mesenchymal stem cells (osteoprogenitors) harvested from proximal humerus and distal femur during arthroscopic surgery. *Arthroscopy.* 2013;29(2):301–308.
27. Izuta Y, Ochi M, Adachi N, et al. Meniscal repair using bone marrow-derived mesenchymal stem cells: experimental study using green fluorescent protein transgenic rats. *Knee.* 2005;12(3):217–223.
28. Pabbruwe MB, Kafienah W, Tariton JF, et al. Repair of meniscal cartilage white zone tears using a stem cell/collagen-scaffold implant. *Biomaterials.* 2010;31(9):2583–2591.
29. Vasarhelyi A, Baumert T, Fritsch C, et al. Partial weight bearing after surgery for fractures of the lower extremity: is it achievable? *Gait Posture.* 2006;23:99–105.
30. Vandermeer RD, Cunningham FK. Arthroscopic treatment of the discoid lateral meniscus: results of long-term follow-up. *Arthroscopy.* 1989;5(2):101–109.
31. Pellacci F, Montanari G, Prosperi P, et al. Lateral discoid meniscus: treatment and results. *Arthroscopy.* 1992;8(4):526–530.
32. Räber DA, Friederich NF, Hefti F. Discoid lateral meniscus in children: long-term follow-up after total meniscectomy. *J Bone Joint Surg Am.* 1998;80(11):1579–1586.
33. Atay OA, Doral MN, Leblebicioglu G, et al. Management of discoid lateral meniscus tears: observations in 34 knees. *Arthroscopy.* 2003;19(4):346–352.
34. Oğüt T, Kesmezacar H, Akgün I, et al. Arthroscopic meniscectomy for discoid lateral meniscus in children and adolescents: 4.5 year follow-up. *J Pediatr Orthop B.* 2003;12(6):390–397.
35. Adachi N, Ochi M, Uchio Y, et al. Torn discoid lateral meniscus treated using partial central meniscectomy and suture of the peripheral tear. *Arthroscopy.* 2004;20(5):536–542.
36. Lee DH, Kim TH, Kim JM, et al. Results of subtotal/total or partial meniscectomy for discoid lateral meniscus in children. *Arthroscopy.* 2009;25(5):496–503. doi:10.1016/j.arthro.2008.10.025.
37. Manzione M, Pizzutillo PD, Peoples AB, et al. Meniscectomy in children: follow-up study. *Am J Sports Med.* 1983;11(3):111–115.
38. Okazaki K, Miura H, Matsuda S, et al. Arthroscopic resection of the discoid lateral meniscus: long-term follow-up for 16 years. *Arthroscopy.* 2006;22(9):967–971. doi:10.1016/j.arthro.2006.04.107.
39. Pengas IP, Assiotis A, Nash W, et al. Total meniscectomy in adolescents: a 40-year follow-up. *J Bone Joint Surg Br.* 2012;94(12):1649–1654. doi:10.1302/0301-620X.94B12.30562.
40. Baratz ME, Fu FH, Mengato R. Meniscal tears: the effect of meniscectomy and of repair on intraarticular contact areas preliminary report. *Am J Sports Med.* 1986;14(4):270–275.
41. Korkala O, Karaharju E, Gronblad M, et al. Articular cartilage after meniscectomy. Rabbit knees studied with the scanning electron microscope. *Acta Orthop Scand.* 1984;55(3):273–277.
42. Lanzer WL, Komenda G. Changes in articular cartilage after meniscectomy. *Clin Orthop Relat Res.* 1990;(252):41–48.

Donald E. Fowler III
Marcia Voigt
Scott A. Rodeo

CHAPTER 30

Meniscal Allograft Transplantation

INTRODUCTION

Injury and loss of the meniscus has been shown to alter load transmission in the knee by decreasing contact area and increasing contact pressure and shear stress across the articular surface. Over time, this can lead to progressive degenerative changes and osteoarthritis. Meniscal allograft transplantation (MAT) offers a biologic solution for managing patients with meniscal deficiency. The following chapter outlines meniscal function; biomechanical changes after meniscectomy; and the indications, techniques, and outcomes associated with MAT.

MENISCAL FUNCTION

Once considered a vestigial component of the knee, the meniscus is responsible for many essential functions that influence long-term knee health and stability. The knee contains medial and lateral menisci whose collagen architecture, biochemical fluid composition, and proteoglycan-collagen meshwork allow them to function in shock absorption and load transmission between the femur and tibia.[1–3] The menisci also aid in knee stability, knee joint proprioception, joint lubrication and cartilage nutrition, and prevention of osteoarthrosis.[1,3–8] As load transmitters, the menisci distribute stress across the tibiofemoral joint by increasing the contact surface area of the joint and improving the congruence of the articulating surfaces.[3] The improved tibiofemoral congruency and increased joint contact area allows the menisci to function in load sharing.[9] This aids in the knee's ability to withstand the load forces associated with walking, running, and standing while preventing damage to the articular cartilage and the subchondral bone of the femur and tibia.

The composition of the meniscus allows it to withstand high compressive forces. The meniscus is composed of 70% water, and type I collagen makes up 60% to 70% of its dry weight. Proteoglycans and water provide a swelling pressure that decreases the peak stress across the articulating surfaces of the femur and tibia. This prevents hyaline cartilage from progressive degeneration. The meniscus may also support articular cartilage nutrition by compressing synovial fluid into articular cartilage and maintaining a lubricating film over the articular surface.[7,8]

During weight bearing, the meniscus experiences tensile or "hoop" stress in the circumferential collagen fibers as it withstands radially extrusive force. The percentage of joint load that occurs across the knee depends on knee flexion angle along with femoral translation and rotation and differs between the medial and lateral menisci. The menisci transmit 50% of the joint load in the extended knee and 90% of the load in the flexed knee.[3,10] The medial meniscus transmits 40% of the joint load in its compartment, whereas the lateral meniscus transmits 70% of joint load in the lateral compartment.[3,6,11] Total or partial meniscectomy can increase the peak contact stresses on the articular cartilage between 40% and 700%.[11] These high contact stresses may result in hyaline articular cartilage degeneration with time.

The menisci also play a role in knee joint stability. The medial meniscus is a secondary stabilizer to anterior tibial translation and thus a significant restraint to anterior translation in the anterior cruciate ligament (ACL)–deficient knee.[12] In the setting of a medial meniscal–deficient knee, the forces on the ACL graft are increased.[13] Additionally, the medial meniscus plays a role in the varus–valgus stability of the knee, as biomechanical studies have shown increased varus–valgus rotation in the ACL insufficient and medial meniscal–deficient knee.[14]

The lateral meniscus plays a key role in the stability of the knee during a pivoting maneuver.[15,16] Lateral meniscal loss may contribute to instability as well as rapid progressive joint degeneration because of the convexity of the articulating surfaces in the lateral compartment. The presence of nerve endings and mechanoreceptors near the anterior and posterior horn insertions, as well as the capsular attachments of the menisci, may also contribute to joint proprioception.[8]

It is clear that the meniscus plays several important roles in knee function. The rationale behind MAT is to prevent articular cartilage degeneration and its associated clinical symptoms by restoring the important functions provided by healthy meniscal tissue.

CONSEQUENCES OF MENISCECTOMY

Clinical outcome studies, in addition to radiographic imaging and biomechanical assessments, have been consistent in identifying the consequences of meniscectomy on the knee. The protective properties and load transmission capabilities have been demonstrated in comparisons of knee health with an intact meniscus versus partial and total meniscectomy. Outcomes are dependent on the presence of articular cartilage defects or degenerative changes, the amount and location of meniscal tissue removed, ligament instability, and malalignment. Secondary factors that also play a role are patient sport and activity level, which are of increased importance and consideration in adolescent patients.

Biomechanical studies following meniscectomy have shown that meniscal loss can lead to a decrease in contact area of approximately 75% and an increase in peak contact stresses of approximately 235%.[17] Increased contact stress and decreased contact area are thought to overload the articular cartilage, resulting in damage ranging from surface fibrillation to full-thickness cartilage loss.[18,19]

Such biomechanical changes have been verified with clinical and radiographic outcome studies following meniscectomy. Fairbank[20] reported radiographic hallmarks of osteoarthritis following meniscectomy as the formation of a ridge on the margin of the condyle, joint space narrowing, and flattening of the condyle. The progression of arthritis following meniscectomy has been documented in many studies. A study following patients 21 years after meniscectomy found that the relative risk for advanced radiographic changes representing definitive osteoarthritis following meniscectomy was 14.0.[21]

The severity of each of these factors has been outlined via comparisons between operative and nonoperative knees. In an 11.5-year follow-up study of medial meniscectomy surgeries, Chatain and colleagues[22] reported that radiographic imaging revealed a 22.4% greater prevalence of joint space narrowing in the operative knee when compared to their contralateral, nonoperative knee. Similarly, in a 17-year follow-up study conducted by Johnson et al.,[23] the patients' operative knee was diagnosed with degenerative joint disease 40% of the time as compared to 6% in the nonoperative knee. In the longest follow-up study to date, Pengas et al.[24] reported that at mean follow-up of 40 years in adolescents who underwent open total meniscectomy, all patients were symptomatic; a greater than 4-fold relative risk increase for osteoarthritis existed as well as a 132-fold increase in the rate of total knee replacements.

Partial meniscectomies tend to have more positive outcomes than total meniscectomies. A direct comparison of radiographic results by McGinity and colleagues[25] found that there were radiographic changes in 60% of those who received total meniscectomies compared to 30% for those who had partial meniscectomies over the span of 5.5 years. Schimmer et al.[26] reported excellent to good results for 91.7% of patients at 4 years following partial meniscectomy and 78.1% at 12 years postoperatively. Partial meniscectomies offer a quicker return to function, faster rehabilitation, and lower morbidity rates following surgery, as the amount of meniscal tissue resected appears to be inversely related to knee function.[6] This timeline for recovery may be more appealing to patients, particularly in adolescents.

It must be noted that the long-term follow-up of partial meniscectomy is not overwhelmingly advantageous for patients with meniscal injuries; partial meniscectomies in ACL-deficient knees may result in more than twice the incidence of Fairbank's changes when compared to meniscal repairs, stable tears left untreated, and normal menisci.[27] It is important to consider the degree to which circumferential collagen fibers are disrupted and whether it affects the ability of the meniscus to functionally distribute forces across the knee. In the case of significant disruption, a partial meniscectomy may be equivalent to a total meniscectomy.[6] Damage to articular cartilage plays a key role in patient outcomes as well. Schimmer et al.[26] reported that following partial meniscectomy, 62% of patients with additional cartilage damage reported good to excellent results as compared to the 94.8% of patients with isolated meniscal tears.

As there are differences in the geometry of the articular surfaces and meniscal shapes in the medial and lateral compartments, there are also differences in the outcomes following functional meniscal loss in each compartment. The literature suggests that patients who undergo medial meniscectomy tend to achieve better outcomes than those who undergo lateral meniscectomy.[6,23] A 30-year longitudinal study by McNicholas and colleagues[28] reported good to excellent results for 80% of patients with medial meniscectomy compared to 47% of patients with lateral meniscectomy. This is primarily due to a slower progression of degenerative changes for those undergoing medial compared to lateral meniscectomy.[29] The anatomic differences between the medial and lateral compartments of the knee account for this variability: The convexity of the medial femoral condyle aligns with the concavity of the medial tibial plateau, whereas the convexity of the lateral femoral condyle is mirrored by the convexity of the lateral tibial plateau. In the case of a meniscectomy, the distribution of force within the medial and lateral compartments of the knee joint will differ, as peak stresses in the lateral compartment are significantly greater.

The cause of meniscal tears and functional meniscal deficiency may also play a role in the outcomes and possible indications for meniscal transplantation. McBride et al.[30] reported satisfactory results in 96% of patients following partial meniscectomy for nondegenerative tears versus 65% satisfactory outcomes for degenerative tears. The best results were in those patients who had mechanical symptoms. Schimmer et al.[26] reported 95% satisfaction following partial meniscectomy with no degenerative joint disease versus 62% with degenerative joint disease. Burks and colleagues[31] reported 88% satisfactory results 15 years following partial meniscectomy in ACL-intact knees versus only 48% satisfactory results in ACL-deficient knees.

There are many variables to consider when making the decision to perform a meniscectomy. Although the risk factors for degenerative change and knee instability are significant, patients may benefit from a partial or total meniscectomy based on preoperative symptoms, goals, and lifestyle. This is an especially important discussion to have with adolescent patients and their parents. Patients with functional meniscal deficiency may be candidates for MAT when certain indications are met.

BIOMECHANICAL STUDIES OF MENISCAL TRANSPLANT

The goal of MAT is to replace the biomechanical function of the meniscus. MAT provides increased joint surface area and decreased joint contact stress compared to a meniscectomy; however, it does not fully reproduce the properties of an intact meniscus. For example, Paletta et al.[32] reported that allograft replacement of the lateral meniscus decreases peak contact pressures in the knee joint by 55% to 65% when compared to the 235% to 335% increases in peak pressures after total meniscectomy. They also found that lateral meniscectomy resulted in a 45% to 50% decrease in total contact area compared to the native knee versus allograft transplantation with bone plug fixation which increased the contact area by 42% to 65% compared to the meniscectomy condition. These stress distributions with allograft transplantation only occurred with bone plug fixation of the anterior and posterior meniscal horn attachments. Paletta et al.[32] concluded that MAT can distribute joint stresses more effectively than a meniscal deficient knee but not as well as the native meniscus. Cummins and colleagues[33] found that articular cartilage showed histologic evidence of fewer degenerative changes with meniscal allografts compared to meniscectomy. Kelly et al.[34] demonstrated in a sheep model that meniscal kinematics and cartilage contact mechanics were closer to normal following MAT compared with the meniscectomized knee.

The biomechanical performance of a meniscal allograft in the human knee depends on the fixation method, material properties of the graft, and the placement and surgical technique. Alhalki et al.[35] reported that medial meniscal transplantation requires anatomic fixation of bone plugs attached to meniscal horns in order to most closely replicate normal tibiofemoral contact mechanics. Bone block meniscal transplantation is significantly stronger and stiffer than suture-only fixation. Chen and colleagues[36] reported that a joint with an intact meniscus provides the largest contact area and smallest peak contact pressure, whereas a total meniscectomy gives the smallest contact area and largest peak contact pressure. A MAT that either has a tibial bony bridge or both horns securely attached provides similar results to an intact joint. If only one horn is secured, results lie between an intact joint and meniscectomized joint. If neither horn is secured, contact mechanics are similar to a meniscectomized joint.

Although meniscal transplantations may increase the longevity of the knee joint, the long-term function of the transplant is variable. Patients who receive a transplant are typically allowed to return to daily function and low-impact sports but are advised to avoid high-impact, cutting, and pivoting activities.

INDICATIONS FOR MENISCAL TRANSPLANTATION

The clinical indications for meniscal transplantation have expanded over recent years due to more comprehensive outcome assessment in specific patient populations. Traditionally, MAT was reserved for patients younger than 50 years old with pain localized to a meniscal-deficient compartment. In order to maximize success and predictability of the procedure, the knee had to have minimal arthrosis with no chondral lesions greater than grade II, normal axial alignment, and a stable ligamentous exam. Current practice has now broadened to consider concomitant procedures such as ACL reconstruction, cartilage restoration/resurfacing, and osteotomy.

Articular Cartilage

The most common indication for MAT is pain and swelling localized to a meniscal-deficient tibiofemoral compartment. Multiple studies have shown that patients with severe joint space narrowing, condylar flattening, or other signs of advanced arthrosis have poor clinical outcomes in the setting of meniscal transplantation.[8,37,38] As a result, the majority of surgeons limit MAT to patients with early partial-thickness cartilage loss or a focal lesion amenable to resurfacing as an adjunct procedure.

In addition to depth, size and location of an articular cartilage lesion are critical features when assessing a patient for meniscal transplantation. Some lesions may not be in the weight-bearing zone, and others, if small enough, allow load transmission around the periphery of the lesion to normal hyaline cartilage. Many patients who have undergone meniscectomy develop posterior cartilage lesions that are loaded during knee flexion.[20] Appropriate preoperative evaluation includes flexion weight-bearing radiographs and magnetic resonance imaging (MRI). The meniscal transplant will be loaded in flexion similar to the native meniscus; consequently, these lesions should be small and partial thickness in those indicated for MAT. Larger lesions require careful evaluation for concomitant cartilage procedures in an effort to ensure more predictable outcomes.

Cartilage Restoration/Resurfacing

Many surgeons will now consider a combined procedure, using MAT with cartilage restoration, if there is a more significant cartilage lesion present in a meniscal-deficient compartment. In theory, the two are mutually beneficial; meniscal transplantation reduces contact stress and protects the healing articular surface, whereas the restored cartilage aids in the incorporation and survivorship of the meniscus. There is growing literature which supports improved meniscal healing and clinical outcomes in patients undergoing this combined approach.[39–41] Microfracture and autologous chondrocyte implantation (ACI) require extended time and non–weight-bearing status for potential healing and incorporation. As a result, most surgeons favor osteochondral autograft or allograft tissue, depending on the size of the lesion, for immediate restoration and protection. Further studies are required to assess the indications and long-term outcomes of these concomitant procedures.

Axial Malalignment

Varus malalignment is often seen in conjunction with medial compartment pathology, whereas valgus malalignment is associated with lateral compartment degeneration. The mechanical axis of both lower extremities should be evaluated with standing hip-to-ankle radiographs. If the deformity is severe enough, osteotomy should be considered to offload the affected compartment. Several studies have shown that MAT has higher failure rates in the setting of axial malalignment.[37,42,43] When considering concomitant osteotomy with MAT, patients should have normal condylar geometry and relatively well-preserved articular cartilage. There is still limited data outlining the true effect of osteotomy and MAT on preventing or delaying arthritis in the long term.[44]

Ligamentous Instability

The medial meniscus has long been established as an important secondary stabilizer to anterior tibial translation, particularly in an ACL-deficient knee.[12,13] More recent data suggests the lateral meniscus plays a key role in controlling the pivot shift maneuver.[16] In the long term, ACL insufficiency is commonly associated with early arthrosis due to altered loading patterns as well as previous meniscectomy. Keays et al.[45] found that meniscectomy was most predictive of tibiofemoral arthritis in a cohort of patients 6 years post ACL reconstruction. As a result, patients with an unstable knee and meniscal-deficient compartment may benefit from concomitant ACL reconstruction and MAT. Several studies have shown that meniscal transplantation may improve ACL graft survivorship and knee stability by reducing forces on the ACL graft.[38,46] Likewise, the ACL reconstruction should exert a protective effect on the incorporation and longevity of the meniscal transplant, similar to what has been documented in the setting of meniscal repair.[47] In the rarer case of both medial and lateral meniscal deficiency, MAT in both compartments may be considered to confer improved varus/valgus stability.[14] Ultimately, meniscal transplantation is not recommended unless ligamentous stability can be appropriately restored.

Early Transplantation

Meniscal transplantation is not currently indicated in patients who are truly asymptomatic; however, the goal moving forward is to identify those who are "high risk" before progressive articular cartilage degeneration can occur. The lateral meniscus bears a greater load than the medial meniscus due to the convex geometry of the lateral compartment and thus leads to more rapid degeneration in the setting of meniscal deficiency.[20] Common examples include a radial split tear that compromises the integrity of hoop-stress transmission, resection of a symptomatic discoid meniscus, or an irreparable bucket-handle tear. As a result, early MAT can be considered for the lateral compartment.

The concept of prophylactic MAT may evolve as we develop more sophisticated tools for predicting cartilage breakdown and eventual arthritis. High-resolution MRI[48,49] shows promise as an early indicator as well as synovial fluid analysis focusing on cytokine composition and matrix breakdown products.[50] Future studies incorporating these measures may help to delineate which meniscal-deficient, asymptomatic patients are at greatest risk before cartilage pathology actually develops.

CONTRAINDICATIONS

The prominent contraindications reported for meniscal transplantation consist of advanced articular cartilage degeneration including radiographic evidence of osteophyte formation, change in condylar geometry (flattening of the condyle), joint space narrowing on weight-bearing films, ligament instability, and axial malalignment. Secondary contraindications include skeletal immaturity, synovial disease, knee joint infections, inflammatory arthritis, and obesity.[51]

Advanced degenerative changes of the cartilage and presence of diffuse subchondral bone exposure have a significant effect on the success of a transplant procedure. Unfavorable results have been reported in patients with grade IV articular changes of the femoral condyle.[38,52] In addition to the size and depth of the chondral lesions, their locations play an important role in determining whether a transplant is indicated. For example, full-thickness articular cartilage lesions on the posterior portion of the femoral condyle or tibia greater than 10 to 15 mm in width or length should be noted because these areas articulate with the meniscus in flexion and may predispose to failure.[37,39,42,43]

Varus–valgus malalignment and ligament instability may cause early transplant failure. The increased pressure placed on the knee due to malalignment may result in graft degeneration and tearing. Staged or concomitant malalignment correction via osteotomy or a ligament reconstruction procedure for stability may be necessary for more favorable outcomes.[37,39,42,43]

ALLOGRAFT SIZING/PREPARATION

Accurate size matching of the allograft to the native meniscus is paramount to the success of meniscal transplantation.[8] Oversized meniscal allografts may extrude from the knee joint and lead to greater contact forces across the articular cartilage, whereas undersized allografts result in poor congruity and place higher loads on the meniscus.[53,54] Allografts are side- and compartment-specific due to distinctions in size, shape, and horn attachments. Currently, there are multiple methods and formulas used for measuring the size of the graft, with no consensus on the best approach. Most tissue banks size the graft based on bone measurements, as what remains of the involved meniscus is difficult to quantify and translate to the allograft. Anteroposterior (AP) and lateral radiographs have traditionally been used for meniscal sizing, but inconsistencies still exist between meniscal geometry and tibial plateau dimensions.[55,56] Other authors feel MRI is a more accurate imaging modality for proper size matching, yet variability persists in these results as well.[57–59] The senior author (SAR) recommends radiographs with size markers to correct for magnification along with MRI to calculate tibial plateau dimensions. Tissue banks can then provide a matching tibial or hemitibial plateau with the attached meniscus, allowing several options for incorporation. If the tissue bank provides only the meniscus alone, the surgeon must rely on the most appropriate formula for size matching that correlates with the technique of that particular bank.

Donor tissue goes through a strict screening process to ensure a disease-free allograft, with testing for HIV, hepatitis B, hepatitis C, and syphilis among others. Additionally, there are various forms of graft processing to include pulsatile washing, gamma irradiation, sterilization with ethylene oxide, and newer proprietary techniques that can further reduce the risk of disease transmission. The four types of preserved meniscal allograft tissue currently available are fresh, fresh frozen, cryopreserved, and freeze dried. Traditionally, fresh frozen allografts have been most commonly used. However, fresh tissue is now being transplanted with increasing frequency due to the potential benefit of viable cells, with minimal risk of immunogenicity as processing techniques improve. Cryopreservation has fallen out of favor because only cells in the superficial aspect of the tissue are preserved, and freeze-dried meniscal allografts are no longer implanted due to tissue shrinkage.[60,61]

SURGICAL TECHNIQUE

Our institution almost exclusively uses spinal/regional anesthesia with sedation, although general anesthesia can be used as well. The patient is laid supine and a nonsterile tourniquet is placed on the proximal thigh of the operative leg. A leg holder or post is used to control the knee during valgus stress. Standard exam under anesthesia is performed, assessing range

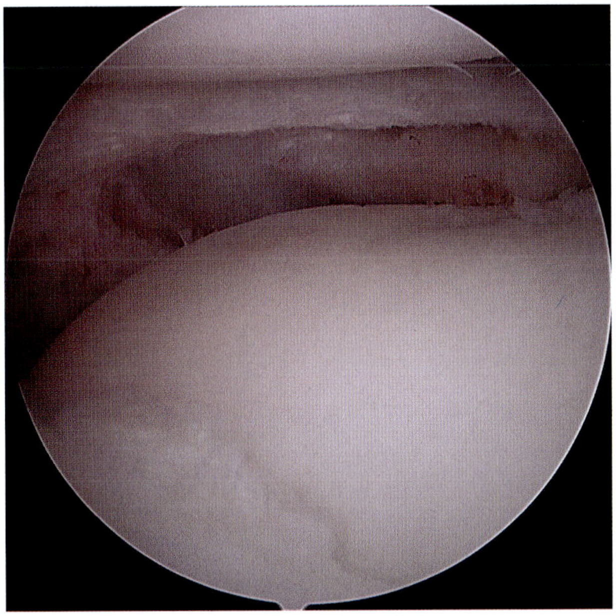

Figure 30.1. Lateral compartment with nearly complete absence of lateral meniscus.

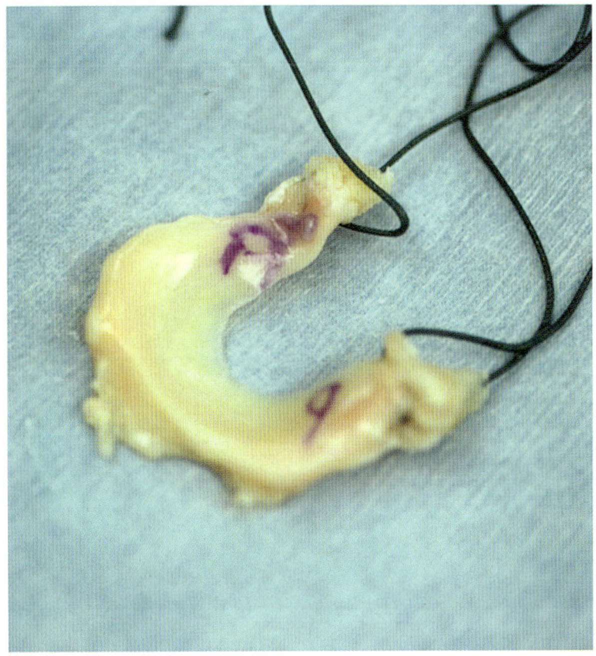

Figure 30.2. Meniscus prepared for transplantation with bone plugs attached to anterior and posterior horns.

of motion, anterior and posterior drawer, Lachman, pivot shift maneuver, varus and valgus stress at 0 and 30 degrees, and external rotation of the knee. A standard diagnostic arthroscopy is done to accurately define cartilage, meniscus, and ligament status. There is typically a small amount of remaining meniscus attached to the capsule (Fig. 30.1). Portals should be made vertically to allow for easy extension and conversion to arthrotomy. Both open and arthroscopically assisted techniques have been described for MAT with comparable results.[8,62]

Restoring the native anatomy of the anterior and posterior horn attachment sites, while providing sufficient fixation, is central to the success of meniscal transplantation. A small stump of remaining meniscal tissue can frequently be used to identify the horn insertion sites. Attachment options include suture-only fixation through transosseous tunnels, bone plugs with horn attachments, or the bone slot technique containing both the anterior and posterior horns. There is still debate in the literature regarding which should be considered the gold standard of fixation. Some authors[44,63] advocate suture-only fixation without attached bone; however, most cadaveric studies demonstrate superior results with meniscal horn bone plug fixation.[32,35,36,64] This is further supported in the clinical setting, as Rodeo[8] found an 88% success rate with bone plug fixation compared to a 47% success rate using the suture-only technique.

For a medial MAT, we recommend using 9-mm diameter bone plugs for both the anterior and posterior horns (Fig. 30.2). The tunnel for the posterior horn bone plug can be drilled using an ACL or posterior cruciate ligament (PCL) guide, whereas the anterior horn bone plug can be drilled antegrade using an enlarged arthroscopic portal (Fig. 30.3). The meniscal allograft can then be shuttled through the same small medial arthrotomy (enlarged anterior portal). In order to facilitate passage, a small amount of bone should be shaved from the medial tibial spine and medial femoral condyle. An arthroscopic probe can be used to temporarily retract the PCL so the graft can be placed posteriorly (Fig. 30.4). A long meniscal repair needle with attached suture should be passed through the posterior horn, then the posteromedial capsule, and retrieved out an accessory posteromedial incision. This suture is used to pull the graft into the joint and can be later employed for meniscal suturing. In the rare instance where the medial compartment is excessively tight and there is still difficulty with graft insertion, a partial release of the deep medial collateral ligament

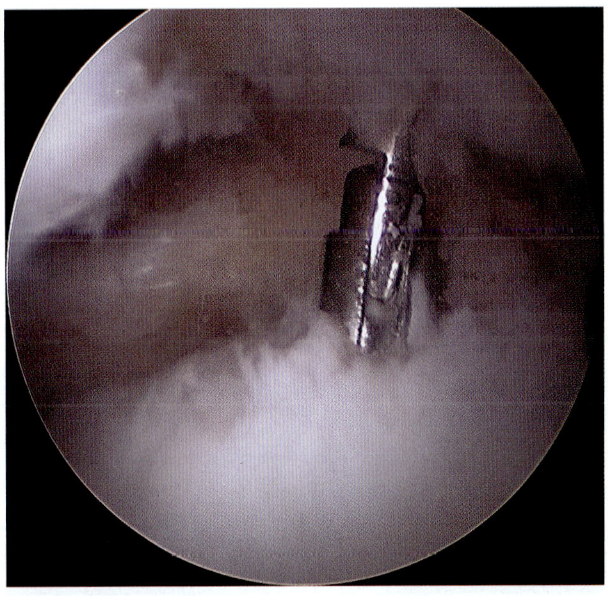

Figure 30.3. Guide pin placed for drilling of tunnel for bone plug of posterior horn of meniscus transplant.

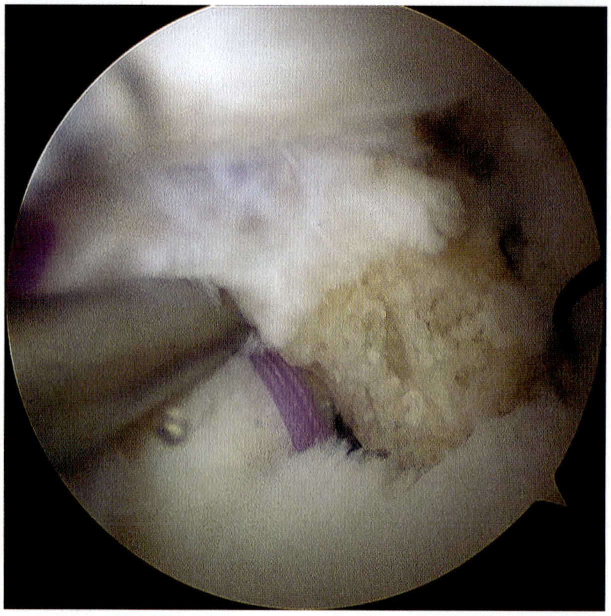

Figure 30.4. Bone plug being seated into posterior horn tunnel.

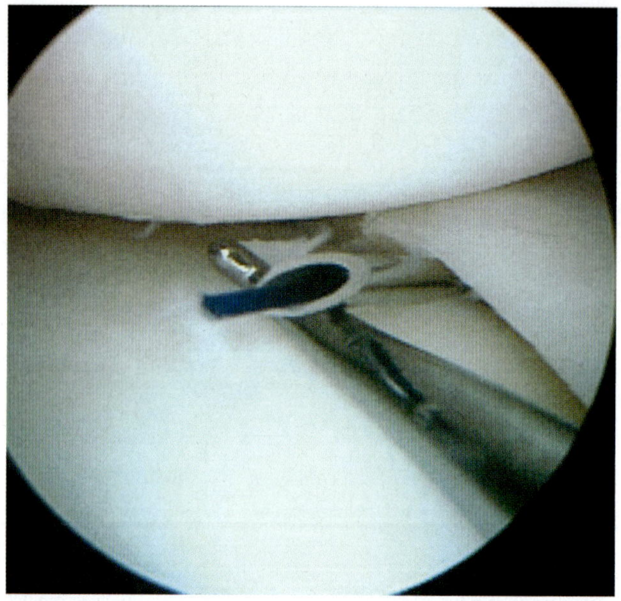

Figure 30.6. Outside-in suture passage to secure the anterior horn of the transplanted meniscus.

(MCL) can be performed. Once the bone plugs are appropriately docked in their tunnels, the sutures attached to the bone plugs are tied together over a bone bridge on the anterior tibia. Vertical mattress sutures are then used for circumferential repair of the meniscal allograft to the surrounding capsule, as this has shown superior repair strength compared to absorbable meniscal fixation devices (Fig. 30.5).[65,66] An inside-out technique with nonabsorbable suture is used for the posterior horn around to the mid-body, whereas the anterior portion can be repaired using an outside-in approach or under direct visualization using the small anterior incision (Fig. 30.6).

When performing a lateral MAT, we recommend using either individual bone plugs or the bone slot technique (Fig. 30.7). If the latter is employed, a trough in the recipient tibia is made before the graft is shuttled through a small lateral arthrotomy (Fig. 30.8). Generally, arthroscopic burrs are used to create the trough, and care must be taken to remain central while not causing damage to the ACL. Supplemental suture fixation through drill holes in the bone slot can be used to augment attachment, but typically, the graft is stable with an appropriate interference fit. The meniscus is then circumferentially repaired to the capsule as described earlier for the medial side.

Certain considerations must be taken into account when performing concomitant procedures in association with MAT. If ACL reconstruction is performed with medial meniscal transplantation, the starting point for the ACL tibial tunnel is moved medially to accommodate the central placement of the two smaller tunnels for the meniscal horn bone plugs. Proper spacing must be used to prevent tunnel confluence. For combined ACL reconstruction with lateral meniscal transplantation, the

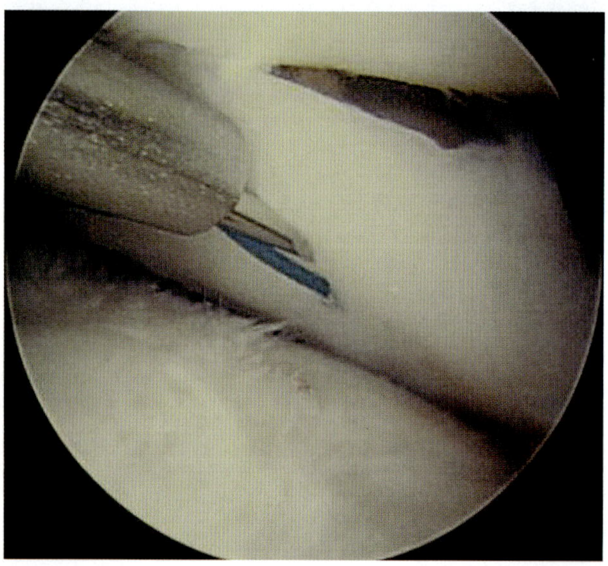

Figure 30.5. Inside-out suture placed on tibial side of meniscus alograft

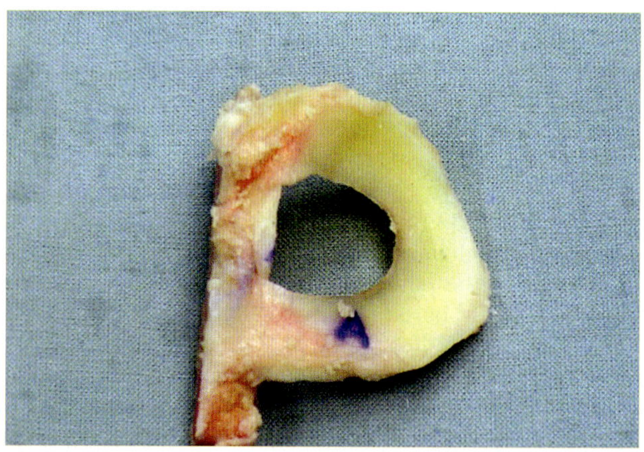

Figure 30.7. Lateral meniscus prepared with a common bone bridge connecting the anterior and posterior horns.

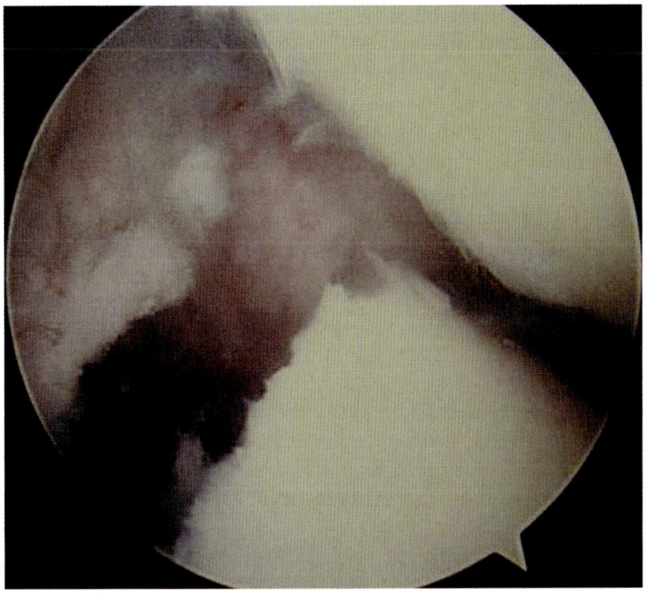

Figure 30.8. Recipient slot in tibia for lateral meniscus transplantation using bone slot technique.

bone slot is implanted first, followed by creation of the ACL tibial tunnel. There is a small chance the ACL tunnel could partially violate the bone slot; however, the overall integrity and fixation of the graft should not be compromised. If both medial and lateral MATs are performed simultaneously, a common bone bridge containing the attachments of both menisci is used for fixation. Finally, in conjunction with either cartilage resurfacing or osteotomy, meniscal transplantation is always completed first. This ensures the cartilage graft is not damaged during the passage of meniscal needles, and excessive stress is not placed on the osteotomy during knee positioning for meniscal suturing.

RESULTS OF MENISCAL TRANSPLANTATION

Recent mid- and long-term follow-up studies have produced more conclusive results for meniscal allograft procedures; however, there is still a need for additional long-term studies that limit variability in protocol and/or provide isolated MAT results. Although MAT is one of the most effective alternative treatments for meniscectomized knees and may delay articular cartilage degeneration, restore the chondroprotective function of the meniscus to some degree, and provide pain relief and functional improvement, there are several unfavorable outcomes from the procedure that may result. These include degeneration, deformation, tearing, and structural changes of the transplant during the graft remodeling process.[67] Factors that affect graft remodeling include graft type and size, degree of arthrosis, meniscocapsular healing, and extrusion.[8,67] Thorough evaluation of outcomes requires analysis of both clinical and objective parameters. Objectively, graft condition and joint preservation are evaluated using MRI or second-look arthroscopy.[8,67,68] Validated patient-reported outcome scales are used to assess subjective symptoms and overall knee function.

The method of graft preparation and storage used in MAT is a significant factor as well. The two types of graft that are currently preferred over lyophilized (freeze-dried) grafts are fresh and fresh frozen size-matched allografts.[67,69] In a clinical outcome study, Wirth et al.[61] reported that lyophilized graft recipients had comparable results to the meniscus-deficient group, whereas fresh frozen graft recipients experienced better clinical outcomes that were similar to the intact meniscus control group. On MRI and second-look arthroscopy, the lyophilized grafts showed greater shrinkage compared to fresh frozen grafts. Long-term clinical results were variable, with Lysholm scores ranging from 21 to 97 points at the 20-year postoperative milestone; however, there was clear radiographic evidence of degenerative change. Due to expanding literature corroborating this data, lyophilized grafts are not recommended due to shrinkage and significant changes in the tissue properties of the transplant.[61,67]

Cryopreserved grafts have more extensive follow-up in the literature. Van Arkel et al.[37] reported on a minimum 2-year follow-up of meniscal allografts using cryopreserved transplants with arthroscopic evaluation. Of 23 meniscal transplants, there was partial detachment in 5, and degenerative changes in 5. Cameron and Saha[42] examined clinical outcomes, reporting good to excellent results in 19 of 21 (90%) patients who had an isolated meniscal transplant. The midterm failure rate of cryopreserved grafts, defined by reoperation, has been reported to be between 30% and 35%. Failure rates associated with persistent pain and meniscal tear produced cumulative survival rates of the lateral, medial, and bilateral allografts of 76%, 50%, and 67%, respectively.[67,70] Long-term follow-up studies have evaluated clinical and objective results, producing a survival rate of 45% at 10 years.[67,70] Radiographs and MRI show joint space narrowing and meniscal shrinkage.[67] Van der Wal and colleagues[71] reported an overall failure rate of 29% at a mean follow-up of 13.8 years postoperatively in cryopreserved MATs. Although Lysholm scores decreased to as low as 61 points, the authors concluded that MAT is a good salvage option for meniscectomized knees. Proposed reasons for cryopreserved graft failure include chondrocyte apoptosis and failure of revascularization.[37,60,69]

Irradiation of the graft may be detrimental to the success of MAT due to the change in material properties of the meniscal transplant. Yahia and Zukor[72] reported that frozen irradiated allograft transplants were less viscous in rabbits when compared to allograft transplants that were nonirradiated fresh or frozen. Noyes and Barber-Westin[62] reported high failure rates of fresh frozen allografts that were irradiated with 2.5 mrad. They suggest that irradiation of the meniscus may weaken and denature the tissue, leading to poor results. Of 96 fresh frozen, irradiated transplants, MRI showed that 9 (9%) of the transplants healed, 30 (31%) partially healed, 56 (58%) failed, and 1 (2%) was unknown.

Several studies suggest improved healing rates in patients who have a meniscal transplant with attached bone plugs. Healing of the bone plugs in a bone tunnel is thought to be more secure and reproducible than that of the meniscus to bone, allowing for improved load transmission.[8,32,36] Rodeo and Johnson[73] reported on 33 meniscus transplants at 2-year follow-up evaluated with MRI and arthroscopy. Arthroscopic inspection in a subset of the patients showed normal appearance, consistency, and position in the knee joint. There was minimal articular cartilage degeneration, although some degenerative changes were commonly noted in the posterior horn on MRI. Based on objective findings, 8 of 33 transplants were rated as good; 14, moderate; 4, poor; and 7, failed. Outcome measures including the International Knee Documentation Committee (IKDC) and Lysholm scales as well as pain and function scores showed clinical improvements. Transplantation with attached bone plugs yielded significantly better results than those without bone plugs: 88% of menisci transplanted with bone plugs were rated as good or moderate in comparison to 47% transplanted with no bone plugs.

Extrusion of the transplant from the tibiofemoral compartment has also been shown on MRI. The greatest amount of extrusion was present in patients with more advanced articular degeneration.[73] Using MRI, Potter et al.[48] confirmed that extrusion is seen in patients who have flattening of the femoral condyle or advanced degenerative changes in the articular cartilage or posterior horn of the meniscus.

Cameron and Saha[42] concluded that the most frequent complication was a traumatic tear of the posterior horn of the meniscus due to unsuccessful healing and graft incorporation. Associated pathology of the knee, such as ACL deficiency, also increases the failure rate due to instability.[67] Early failure of MATs may be due to articular cartilage degeneration, malalignment, or ligamentous instability that results in abnormal loads on the knee joint. Malalignment of the joint and abnormal load bearing of the meniscus may lead to accumulation of microscopic damage prior to revascularization and cellular repopulation.[67] Cameron and Saha[42] suggest that a realignment osteotomy in combination with MAT may be beneficial in these patients, as they reported good to excellent results in 85.3% (29 of 34) of cases.

Failure rates are closely associated with the degree of arthrosis in the knee. Histologic evaluation of failed transplants show abnormal tissue remodeling, including minimal or incomplete cellular repopulation, disorganized collagen orientation, an increase in water content, and decrease in proteoglycan concentration within the meniscus.[68,74] All meniscal allograft transplants undergo remodeling at some point, but the timing and extent to which they do varies and influences survival rates.[73]

Garrett[38] suggests that less favorable outcomes in MAT are associated with grade IV articular changes. In his study, there were 2 failures out of 32 patients who had grade III chondral changes versus 6 failures out of 11 patients who had grade IV chondral changes at the time of surgery. Wirth et al.[61] similarly concluded that long-term results were negatively influenced by advanced degenerative changes in the articular cartilage.

Patient-reported outcome measures following MAT demonstrate improvements in pain, function, and swelling. Favorable results are closely associated with the degree of arthrosis at the time of transplantation: The less arthrosis present, the better the outcomes.[38,62,68,73] Improved load transmission also plays a significant role in reduced pain and increased functionality.[38,69,73,75] Most patients who are young and healthy with minimal degenerative articular changes have been able to return to light sport.[62]

A review of current literature by Lee et al.[67] shows that recent reports of clinical and objective meniscal allograft outcomes are favorable. Ha et al.[76] reported complete healing in 80% of patients who underwent a medial MAT. Kim and colleagues[77] reported satisfactory results in 69% of patients who underwent a lateral MAT. Marcacci et al.[78] found pain relief and functional improvement in 94% of patients at 40 months follow-up. They also reported improved cartilage condition on the femur and tibia at 36 months follow-up. Kim et al.[79] reported that 81.8% of patients had satisfactory results following meniscal transplantation.

COMPLICATIONS/FAILURE

Complications of MAT include infection, arthrofibrosis, neurovascular injury, deep vein thrombosis (DVT), incomplete healing of the meniscocapsular repair, meniscal retear, and allograft failure. Rates vary throughout the literature but have been reported anywhere from 0% to 45%.[80] In general, these complications correlate with those seen in meniscal repair, and as techniques evolve, these numbers should continue to decrease.[81,82]

Advanced articular cartilage degeneration appears to be the primary factor associated with meniscal transplant failure, as excessive load is transmitted through the graft. Flattening of the femoral condyle has been shown to be predictive of MAT failure.[62] Most meniscal tears and degeneration occur in the region of the posterior horn where contact pressures are highest. Several other factors likely contribute to ultimate failure. The significance of appropriate size matching has already been identified, as oversized grafts fail to normalize articular cartilage loading, and undersized grafts lead to increased loads on the meniscus. Anatomic placement of the anterior and posterior horns is vital to best restore proper contact stress and load distribution.[83,84]

The role of biologic factors is also being studied in association with meniscal transplant failure. Meniscal allografts undergo a process of host cell repopulation and graft revascularization and may be susceptible to tears during the healing process. Rodeo and colleagues[85] used immunohistochemistry and histology to examine biopsies of both intact and failed transplants and discovered microscopic evidence of a subclinical immune response. This may lead to graft shrinkage, persistent effusions, and impaired cellular repopulation and incorporation.

SUMMARY

MAT is a viable procedure when using the proper indications, particularly in the younger patient. Concomitant procedures, such as ligament reconstruction, cartilage resurfacing, and osteotomy, have expanded applications of MAT. Although native mechanics and anatomy are not entirely restored, there is clearly an improvement in pain and functional outcome. Additionally, the chondroprotective effect of MAT is encouraging, although further long-term studies are needed for validation. Patients should be educated regarding the postoperative condition of their knee joint in providing realistic expectations for return to activity. We generally advise against high load, repetitive impact sports while allowing lighter sporting activity. In the future, various biologics and scaffold implants currently in development will likely join MAT as legitimate treatment options for meniscal deficiency.

REFERENCES

1. Aagaard H, Verdonk R. Function of the normal meniscus and consequences of meniscal resection. *Scand J Med Sci Sports.* 1999;9(3): 134–140.
2. Masouros SD, McDermott ID, Amis AA, et al. Biomechanics of the meniscus-meniscal ligament construct of the knee. *Knee Surg Sports Traumatol Arthrosc.* 2008;16(12):1121–1132.
3. Walker PS, Erkman MJ. The role of the menisci in force transmission across the knee. *Clin Orthop Relat Res.* 1975;(109):184–192.
4. Kurosawa H, Fukubayashi T, Nakajima H. Load-bearing mode of the knee joint: physical behavior of the knee joint with or without menisci. *Clin Orthop Relat Res.* 1980;(149):283–290.
5. Maitra RS, Miller MD, Johnson DL. Meniscal reconstruction. Part I: indications, techniques, and graft considerations. *Am J Orthop.* 1999; 28(4):213–218.
6. McDermott ID, Amis AA. The consequences of meniscectomy. *J Bone Joint Surg Br.* 2006;88(12):1549–1556.
7. Messner K, Gao J. The menisci of the knee joint. Anatomical and functional characteristics, and a rationale for clinical treatment. *J Anat.* 1998;193(pt 2):161–178.
8. Rodeo SA. Meniscal allografts—where do we stand? *Am J Sports Med.* 2001;29(2):246–261.
9. Sekiya JK, Ellingson CI. Meniscal allograft transplantation. *J Am Acad Orthop Surg.* 2006;14(3):164–174.
10. Ahmed AM, Burke DL. In-vitro measurement of static pressure distribution in synovial joints—Part I: tibial surface of the knee. *J Biomech Eng.* 1983;105(3):216–225.
11. Seedhom BB, Hargreaves D. Transmission of load in the knee joint with special reference to the role of the menisci, part II: experimental results, discussion, and conclusions. *Eng Med Biol.* 1979;8: 220–228.
12. Levy IM, Torzilli PA, Warren RF. The effect of medial meniscectomy on anterior-posterior motion of the knee. *J Bone Joint Surg Am.* 1982;64(6):883–888.
13. Allen CR, Wong EK, Livesay GA, et al. Importance of the medial meniscus in the anterior cruciate ligament-deficient knee. *J Orthop Res.* 2000;18(1):109–115.
14. Markolf KL, Kochan A, Amstutz HC. Measurement of knee stiffness and laxity in patients with documented absence of the anterior cruciate ligament. *J Bone Joint Surg Am.* 1984;66(2):242–252.
15. Petrigliano FA, Musahl V, Suero EM, et al. Effect of meniscal loss on knee stability after single-bundle anterior cruciate ligament reconstruction. *Knee Surg Sports Traumatol Arthrosc.* 2011;19(suppl 1): S86–S93.
16. Musahl V, Citak M, O'Loughlin PF, et al. The effect of medial versus lateral meniscectomy on the stability of the anterior cruciate ligament-deficient knee. *Am J Sports Med.* 2010;38(8):1591–1597.
17. Baratz ME, Fu FH, Mengato R. Meniscal tears: the effect of meniscectomy and of repair on intraarticular contact areas and stress in the human knee. A preliminary report. *Am J Sports Med.* 1986;14(4):270–275.
18. Lanzer WL, Komenda G. Changes in articular cartilage after meniscectomy. *Clin Orthop Relat Res.* 1990;(252):41–48.
19. Korkala O, Karaharju E, Grönblad M, et al. Articular cartilage after meniscectomy. Rabbit knees studied with the scanning electron microscope. *Acta Orthop Scand.* 1984;55(3):273–277.
20. Fairbank TJ. Knee joint changes after meniscectomy. *J Bone Joint Surg Br.* 1948;30B(4):664–670.
21. Roos H, Laurén M, Adalberth T, et al. Knee osteoarthritis after meniscectomy: prevalence of radiographic changes after twenty-one years, compared with matched controls. *Arthritis Rheum.* 1998;41(4):687–693.
22. Chatain F, Robinson AH, Adeleine P, et al. The natural history of the knee following arthroscopic medial meniscectomy. *Knee Surg Sports Traumatol Arthrosc.* 2001;9(1):15–18.
23. Johnson RJ, Kettelkamp DB, Clark W, et al. Factors effecting late results after meniscectomy. *J Bone Joint Surg Am.* 1974;56(4):719–729.
24. Pengas IP, Assiotis A, Nash W, et al. Total meniscectomy in adolescents: a 40-year follow-up. *J Bone Joint Surg Br.* 2012;94(12):1649–1654.
25. McGinity JB, Geuss LF, Marvin RA. Partial or total meniscectomy: a comparative analysis. *J Bone Joint Surg Am.* 1977;59(6):763–766.
26. Schimmer RC, Brülhart KB, Duff C, et al. Arthroscopic partial meniscectomy: a 12-year follow-up and two-step evaluation of the long-term course. *Arthroscopy.* 1998;14(2):136–142.
27. Henning CE, Lynch MA. Current concepts of meniscal function and pathology. *Clin Sports Med.* 1985;4(2):259–265.
28. McNicholas MJ, Rowley DI, McGurty D, et al. Total meniscectomy in adolescence. A thirty-year follow-up. *J Bone Joint Surg Br.* 2000;82(2):217–221.
29. Yocum LA, Kerlan RK, Jobe FW, et al. Isolated lateral meniscectomy. A study of twenty-six patients with isolated tears. *J Bone Joint Surg Am.* 1979;61(3):338–342.
30. McBride GG, Constine RM, Hofmann AA, et al. Arthroscopic partial medial meniscectomy in the older patient. *J Bone Joint Surg Am.* 1984;66(4):547–551.
31. Burks RT, Metcalf MH, Metcalf RW. Fifteen-year follow-up of arthroscopic partial meniscectomy. *Arthroscopy.* 1997;13(6):673–679.
32. Paletta GA Jr, Manning T, Snell E, et al. The effect of allograft meniscal replacement on intraarticular contact area and pressures in the human knee. A biomechanical study. *Am J Sports Med.* 1997;25(5):692–698.
33. Cummins JF, Mansour JN, Howe Z, et al. Meniscal transplantation and degenerative articular change: an experimental study in the rabbit. *Arthroscopy.* 1997;13(4):485–491.
34. Kelly BT, Potter HG, Deng XH, et al. Meniscal allograft transplantation in the sheep knee: evaluation of chondroprotective effects. *Am J Sports Med.* 2006;34(9):1464–1477.
35. Alhalki MM, Howell SM, Hull ML. How three methods for fixing a medial meniscal autograft affect tibial contact mechanics. *Am J Sports Med.* 1999;27(3):320–328.
36. Chen MI, Branch TP, Hutton WC. Is it important to secure the horns during lateral meniscal transplantation? A cadaveric study. *Arthroscopy.* 1996;12(2):174–181.
37. van Arkel ER, de Boer HH. Human meniscal transplantation. Preliminary results at 2 to 5-year follow-up. *J Bone Joint Surg Br.* 1995;77(4):589–595.
38. Garrett JC. Meniscal transplantation. *Am J Knee Surg.* 1996;9(1):32–34.
39. Noyes FR, Barber-Westin SD, Rankin M. Meniscal transplantation in symptomatic patients less than fifty years old. *J Bone Joint Surg Am.* 2004;86-A(7):1392–1404.
40. Farr J, Rawal A, Marberry KM. Concomitant meniscal allograft transplantation and autologous chondrocyte implantation: minimum 2-year follow-up. *Am J Sports Med.* 2007;35(9):1459–1466.
41. Rue JP, Yanke AB, Busam ML, et al. Prospective evaluation of concurrent meniscus transplantation and articular cartilage repair: minimum 2-year follow-up. *Am J Sports Med.* 2008;36(9):1770–1778.
42. Cameron JC, Saha S. Meniscal allograft transplantation for unicompartmental arthritis of the knee. *Clin Orthop Relat Res.* 1997;(337): 164–171.
43. de Boer HH, Koudstaal J. Failed meniscus transplantation. A report of three cases. *Clin Orthop Relat Res.* 1994;(306):155–162.
44. Verdonk PC, Verstraete KL, Almqvist KF, et al. Meniscal allograft transplantation: long-term clinical results with radiological and magnetic resonance imaging correlations. *Knee Surg Sports Traumatol Arthrosc.* 2006;14(8):694–706.
45. Keays SL, Newcombe PA, Bullock-Saxton JE, et al. Factors involved in the development of osteoarthritis after anterior cruciate ligament surgery. *Am J Sports Med.* 2010;38(3):455–463.
46. Papageorgiou CD, Gil JE, Kanamori A, et al. The biomechanical interdependence between the anterior cruciate ligament replacement graft and the medial meniscus. *Am J Sports Med.* 2001;29(2):226–231.

47. Morgan CD, Wojtys EM, Casscells CD, et al. Arthroscopic meniscal repair evaluated by second-look arthroscopy. *Am J Sports Med.* 1991;19(6):632–637; discussion 637–638.
48. Potter HG, Rodeo SA, Wickiewicz TL, et al. MR imaging of meniscal allografts: correlation with clinical and arthroscopic outcomes. *Radiology.* 1996;198(2):509–514.
49. Potter HG, Chong le R. Magnetic resonance imaging assessment of chondral lesions and repair. *J Bone Joint Surg Am.* 2009;91(suppl 1): 126–131.
50. Scanzello CR, Umoh E, Pessler F, et al. Local cytokine profiles in knee osteoarthritis: elevated synovial fluid interleukin-15 differentiates early from end-stage disease. *Osteoarthritis Cartilage.* 2009;17(8):1040–1048.
51. Lee SR, Kim JG, Nam SW. The tips and pitfalls of meniscus allograft transplantation. *Knee Surg Relat Res.* 2012;24(3):137–145.
52. Garrett JC, Steensen RN. Meniscal transplantation in the human knee: a preliminary report. *Arthroscopy.* 1991;7(1):57–62.
53. Dienst M, Greis PE, Ellis BJ, et al. Effect of lateral meniscal allograft sizing on contact mechanics of the lateral tibial plateau: an experimental study in human cadaveric knee joints. *Am J Sports Med.* 2007;35(1):34–42.
54. Yoon JR, Kim TS, Wang JH, et al. Importance of independent measurement of width and length of lateral meniscus during preoperative sizing for meniscal allograft transplantation. *Am J Sports Med.* 2011;39(7):1541–1547.
55. Pollard ME, Kang Q, Berg EE. Radiographic sizing for meniscal transplantation. *Arthroscopy.* 1995;11(6):684–687.
56. Donahue TL, Hull ML, Howell SM. New algorithm for selecting meniscal allografts that best match the size and shape of the damaged meniscus. *J Orthop Res.* 2006;24(7):1535–1543.
57. Haut TL, Hull ML, Howell SM. Use of roentgenography and magnetic resonance imaging to predict meniscal geometry determined with a three-dimensional coordinate digitizing system. *J Orthop Res.* 2000;18(2):228–237.
58. Shaffer B, Kennedy S, Klimkiewicz J, et al. Preoperative sizing of meniscal allografts in meniscus transplantation. *Am J Sports Med.* 2000;28(4):524–533.
59. Prodromos CC, Joyce BT, Keller BL, et al. Magnetic resonance imaging measurement of the contralateral normal meniscus is a more accurate method of determining meniscal allograft size than radiographic measurement of the recipient tibial plateau. *Arthroscopy.* 2007;23(11):1174.e1–1179.e1.
60. Villalba R, Peña J, Navarro P, et al. Cryopreservation increases apoptosis in human menisci. *Knee Surg Sports Traumatol Arthrosc.* 2012;20(2):298–303.
61. Wirth CJ, Peters G, Milachowski KA, et al. Long-term results of meniscal allograft transplantation. *Am J Sports Med.* 2002;30(2):174–181.
62. Noyes FR, Barber-Westin SD. Prospective evaluation of allograft meniscus transplantation: a minimum 2-year follow-up. *Am J Sports Med.* 2006;34(12):2038–2039.
63. Stone KR, Walgenbach AW, Turek TJ, et al. Meniscus allograft survival in patients with moderate to severe unicompartmental arthritis: a 2- to 7-year follow-up. *Arthroscopy.* 2006;22(5):469–478.
64. McDermott ID, Lie DT, Edwards A, et al. The effects of lateral meniscal allograft transplantation techniques on tibio-femoral contact pressures. *Knee Surg Sports Traumatol Arthrosc.* 2008;16(6):553–560.
65. Albrecht-Olsen P, Lind T, Kristensen G, et al. Failure strength of a new meniscus arrow repair technique: biomechanical comparison with horizontal suture. *Arthroscopy.* 1997;13(2):183–187.
66. Dervin GF, Downing KJ, Keene GC, et al. Failure strengths of suture versus biodegradable arrow for meniscal repair: an in vitro study. *Arthroscopy.* 1997;13(3):296–300.
67. Lee BS, Kim JM, Sohn DW, et al. Review of meniscal allograft transplantation focusing on long-term results and evaluation methods. *Knee Surg Relat Res.* 2013;25(1):1–6.
68. Noyes FR, Barber-Westin SD. Meniscus transplantation: indications, techniques, clinical outcomes. *Instr Course Lect.* 2005;54:341–353.
69. Verdonk R, Volpi P, Verdonk P, et al. Indications and limits of meniscal allografts. *Injury.* 2013;44(suppl 1):S21–S27.
70. Hommen JP, Applegate GR, Del Pizzo W. Meniscus allograft transplantation: ten-year results of cryopreserved allografts. *Arthroscopy.* 2007;23(4):388–393.
71. van der Wal RJ, Thomassen BJ, van Arkel ER. Long-term clinical outcome of open meniscal allograft transplantation. *Am J Sports Med.* 2009;37(11):2134–2139.
72. Yahia L, Zukor D. Irradiated meniscal allotransplants of rabbits: study of the mechanical properties at six months postoperation. *Acta Orthop Belg.* 1994;60(2):210–215.
73. Rodeo SA WR, Johnson D. Meniscus and cartilage injury: does meniscal allograft transplantation prevent articular cartilage degeneration? In: Williams RJ, Johnson DP, eds. *Controversies in Knee Surgery.* Oxford, United Kingdom: Oxford University Press; 2004:553.
74. Jackson DW, McDevitt CA, Simon TM, et al. Meniscal transplantation using fresh and cryopreserved allografts. An experimental study in goats. *Am J Sports Med.* 1992;20(6):644–656.
75. Lubowitz JH, Verdonk PC, Reid JB III, et al. Meniscus allograft transplantation: a current concepts review. *Knee Surg Sports Traumatol Arthrosc.* 2007;15(5):476–492.
76. Ha JK, Sung JH, Shim JC, et al. Medial meniscus allograft transplantation using a modified bone plug technique: clinical, radiologic, and arthroscopic results. *Arthroscopy.* 2011;27(7):944–950.
77. Kim CW, Kim JM, Lee SH, et al. Results of isolated lateral meniscus allograft transplantation: focus on objective evaluations with magnetic resonance imaging. *Am J Sports Med.* 2011;39(9):1960–1967.
78. Marcacci M, Zaffagnini S, Marcheggiani Muccioli GM, et al. Meniscal allograft transplantation without bone plugs: a 3-year minimum follow-up study. *Am J Sports Med.* 2012;40(2):395–403.
79. Kim JM, Lee BS, Kim KH, et al. Results of meniscus allograft transplantation using bone fixation: 110 cases with objective evaluation. *Am J Sports Med.* 2012;40(5):1027–1034.
80. Hergan D, Thut D, Sherman O, et al. Meniscal allograft transplantation. *Arthroscopy.* 2011;27(1):101–112.
81. Abat F, Gelber PE, Erquicia JI, et al. Prospective comparative study between two different fixation techniques in meniscal allograft transplantation. *Knee Surg Sports Traumatol Arthrosc.* 2013;21(7): 1516–1522.
82. Lee AS, Kang RW, Kroin E, et al. Allograft meniscus transplantation. *Sports Med Arthrosc.* 2012;20(2):106–114.
83. Choi NH, Yoo SY, Victoroff BN. Position of the bony bridge of lateral meniscal transplants can affect meniscal extrusion. *Am J Sports Med.* 2011;39(9):1955–1959.
84. Lee DH, Kim JM, Lee BS, et al. Greater axial trough obliquity increases the risk of graft extrusion in lateral meniscus allograft transplantation. *Am J Sports Med.* 2012;40(7):1597–1605.
85. Rodeo SA, Seneviratne A, Suzuki K, et al. Histological analysis of human meniscal allografts. A preliminary report. *J Bone Joint Surg Am.* 2000;82-A(8):1071–1082.

SECTION

5

Pediatric and Adolescent Knee Fractures

Benedict U. Nwachukwu
Ryan C. Rauck
Shevaun M. Doyle

CHAPTER 31

Tibial Tubercle Avulsion Fractures in Children and Adolescents

INTRODUCTION

Tibial tubercle fractures are uncommon injuries that most frequently occur during maximal proximal tibial physeal growth. These fractures account for less than 1% of all physeal injuries.[1] Most studies are limited to case reports or relatively small series of patients with this fracture pattern. Despite being uncommon, tibial tubercle fractures have been associated with severe complications, including compartment syndrome, intra-articular damage, limb length discrepancy, extensive soft tissue damage, and limited knee range of motion.[2–6] This chapter provides an overview of this uncommon clinical entity, including presentation, diagnosis, and management. We also present an operative strategy for addressing these injuries.

ANATOMY AND FUNCTION

The tibial tubercle is a bony elevation on the anterior proximal tibia and is the distal attachment site for the patellar ligament. The tibial tubercle serves as the terminal attachment for the knee's extensor mechanism. The proximal part of the extensor system is the quadriceps muscle that consists of the rectus femoris, vastus medialis, vastus intermedius, and vastus lateralis. The quadriceps muscles attach distally to the superior pole of the patella through the quadriceps tendon. The patellar ligament extends from the inferior pole of the patella and attaches distally on the tibial tubercle. When the quadriceps muscles contract, the force is transmitted distally through the tibial tubercle and the knee extends.

The proximal tibia has two ossification centers. The primary ossification center is the proximal tibial physis. The secondary ossification center is the tibial tubercle apophysis. The tibial tubercle develops in four stages.[7] The first stage involves a completely cartilaginous tubercle, prior to the development of the secondary center of ossification. The second stage occurs when the apophysis develops via the secondary ossification center but is not yet connected to the proximal tibial physis. This stage occurs at approximately age 8 to 12 years in females and 9 to 14 years in males. The third stage of development, referred to as the *epiphyseal phase*, is defined as when the tibial physis and the apophysis become contiguous. This typically occurs at age 10 to 15 years for females and 11 to 17 years for males. The fourth and final stage of tibial tubercle development arises when the physis is fused completely and is no longer cartilaginous.

During the apophyseal stage of development, the patellar tendon inserts in an area that corresponds to the fibrocartilage proximal and anterior to the secondary ossification center.[8] The patellar tendon mainly attaches proximally at the level between the secondary ossification center and the proximal tibial epiphysis. As development of the tibial tubercle progresses to the epiphyseal phase, the patellar tendon inserts through fibrocartilage on to the downward-projecting tongue of the proximal tibial epiphysis. During the final stage of tibial tubercle development, the patellar tendon inserts directly into bone and fractures of the tibial tubercle rarely occur.

EPIDEMIOLOGY

Tibial tubercle fractures are rare injuries that account for less than 1% of all physeal injuries.[1] The reported incidence is relatively low and ranges from 0.4% to 2.7%.[9,10] However, given the disastrous sequelae of a missed fracture, accurate injury assessment and diagnosis is critical. These injuries occur mostly in boys while engaged in sports activities during a growth period when there is maximal epiphyseal growth.[11] The age range at the time of injury is typically between 13 and 16 years.[12] During this phase, the epiphysis is still open and the apophysis between the tibial tubercle and the rest of the tibia is a weak location for potential fracture. The predominance of males sustaining these fractures could relate to the delayed closure of their proximal tibial epiphysis and their increased participation in vigorous sporting activity.[13]

Tibial tubercle fractures can be confused with Osgood-Schlatter (OS) lesions by the inexperienced clinician. In fact, some studies have shown an association between OS lesions and subsequent tibial tubercle fractures.[11,14] Ogden et al.[4] described an OS lesion as primarily involving the anterior portion of the epiphysis or ossification center of the tuberosity, but there is no involvement of the physis. Furthermore, tibial tubercle fractures are acute disruptions, whereas OS disease tends to be chronic and symptomatic.[4]

MECHANISM OF INJURY

In 1903, Dr. Osgood[5] described that the majority of tibial tubercle fractures result from violent quadriceps contraction during exercise or activity. He also acknowledged some documented cases where the injury occurred from a fall on a hard surface with a flexed knee. In 1955, Watson-Jones[15] described the injury mechanism a result of violent knee flexion against a contracting quadriceps mechanism. Hand et al.[6] reiterated Watson-Jones' postulated mechanism. A now classic case series completed by Levi and Coleman[11] in 1976 added that tibial tubercle fractures can occur when the quadriceps contracts with a fixed foot. Each of these mechanisms can overlap with the other.

Biomechanically, avulsion of the tibial tubercle arises when the patellar tendon traction exceeds the strength of the underlying physis. This can take place during jumping or landing, times when there is sudden acceleration or deceleration of the knee extensor mechanism.[8] The phases of development are associated with specific injury patterns recognized in tibial tubercle fractures. Bolesta and Fitch[9] illustrate this in a patient who suffered an injury through the proximal tibial physis at 16 years of age, which healed with a closed reduction. Five months later, the same patient suffered a tibial tubercle avulsion through the epiphysis and diaphysis with a similar mechanism of injury as the proximal physis was closing from posterior to anterior.[9]

Some risk factors have been identified that predispose children to tibial tubercle fractures. Maffulli and Grewal[17] hypothesized that patients with this fracture may have quadriceps strength that is greater than their peers. There are also reports of pathologic fractures of the tibial tubercle in patients with underlying myelomeningocele or skeletal dysplasia.[4] Many individuals with tibial tubercle fractures have a history of OS lesions.[4,18] The association with OS lesions could indicate an underlying vulnerability of the tibial tubercle in certain patient populations. This could be the result of stronger quadriceps, inflexible knee flexors, or impaired coordination of these opposing forces about the knee.[8]

HISTORY

Typically, tibial tubercle fractures occur during violent quadriceps contraction in an athletic youth.[5] Most injuries happen during activity or vigorous play.[11] Examples include attempts to prevent oneself from falling,[5,16,19] gymnastics,[4,11,19] soccer,[13,19,20] jumping,[4,6,9,11,19,21] climbing,[11] playing football or basketball,[4,6,9,11,19–21] running,[4,13] hurdling,[13,19] skateboarding,[4] or high jumping.[6,13,19] Another possible history for injury involves falling on a flexed knee on a hard surface.[5,11,13,20]

There is acute pain after the injury, usually referred to below the patella.[5,13] Swelling also develops and is accompanied by point tenderness over the tibial tubercle. In minimally displaced fractures, there is often only a slightly diminished ability to use the leg, and the acute pain is soon replaced by a feeling of weakness with exertion. The patient usually seeks medical care as a result of the pain, weakness, and continued localized swelling or tenderness.[5] Although this condition rarely causes a complete loss in function, it is often a severe handicap in the young, active athlete.[5] In more severe fractures (*classification system for severity and fracture quality described in the following text*), patients are unable to extend the knee and are more likely to present sooner.[4]

PHYSICAL EXAMINATION

Physical examination of the knee will reveal swelling, pain, and tenderness directly over the tuberosity. Patients with less severe injury types typically can actively extend the knee but with obvious discomfort. Patients with more severe injury often are unable to extend the knee, even with gravity eliminated.[4] There may be a joint effusion and knee hemarthrosis present.[4] One may be able to palpate a movable triangular fragment of bone between the proximal tibia and distal femur. Often, the knee is held in 20 to 40 degrees of flexion secondary to hamstring spasm.[8] Patients may also present with patella alta depending on degree of involvement of the patellar tendon. It is crucial for the clinician to perform a thorough neurovascular examination and evaluate for the presence of increased compartment pressures in the leg. Injury to the nearby branches of the anterior tibial recurrent artery predisposes patients to the development of compartment syndrome.[2]

IMAGING

As with all fractures, the initial imaging study in the diagnosis of tibial tubercle avulsion fractures is plain radiography. Anteroposterior (AP) and lateral views are essential to diagnose this entity; the lateral view in particular provides best visualization of the size and displacement of any avulsed tubercle fragment. Oblique radiographs are less useful in the diagnosis of this entity (Fig. 31.1).

Tibial tubercle avulsion injuries often involve complex fracture patterns, and although standard radiographs may help in the diagnosis of injury, they are insufficient in the characterization of fracture pattern. Computed tomography (CT) is required for a precise understanding of fracture configuration (Fig. 31.2). In some cases, the fracture visualization afforded by CT allows for more accurate classification of the fracture and targeted preoperative planning as compared to what was originally provided in plain radiographs. In particular, CT allows the surgeon to gauge whether there is fracture extension into the joint (Fig. 31.3). Magnetic resonance imaging may be performed if there is a high index of suspicion for meniscal injury, ligamentous injury, or cartilage damage through the physis and epiphysis.

CLASSIFICATION

Classification of tibial tubercle avulsion fractures is based primarily on the Watson-Jones classification. Type I fractures involve a small avulsion from part of the tubercle. Type II extend through the physis without entering the joint. Type III, unlike type II, involve fracture extension into the joint. There are modifications to this original classification system. The Ogden classification was derived with types I to III modifiers to describe the injury severity for each various type of frac-

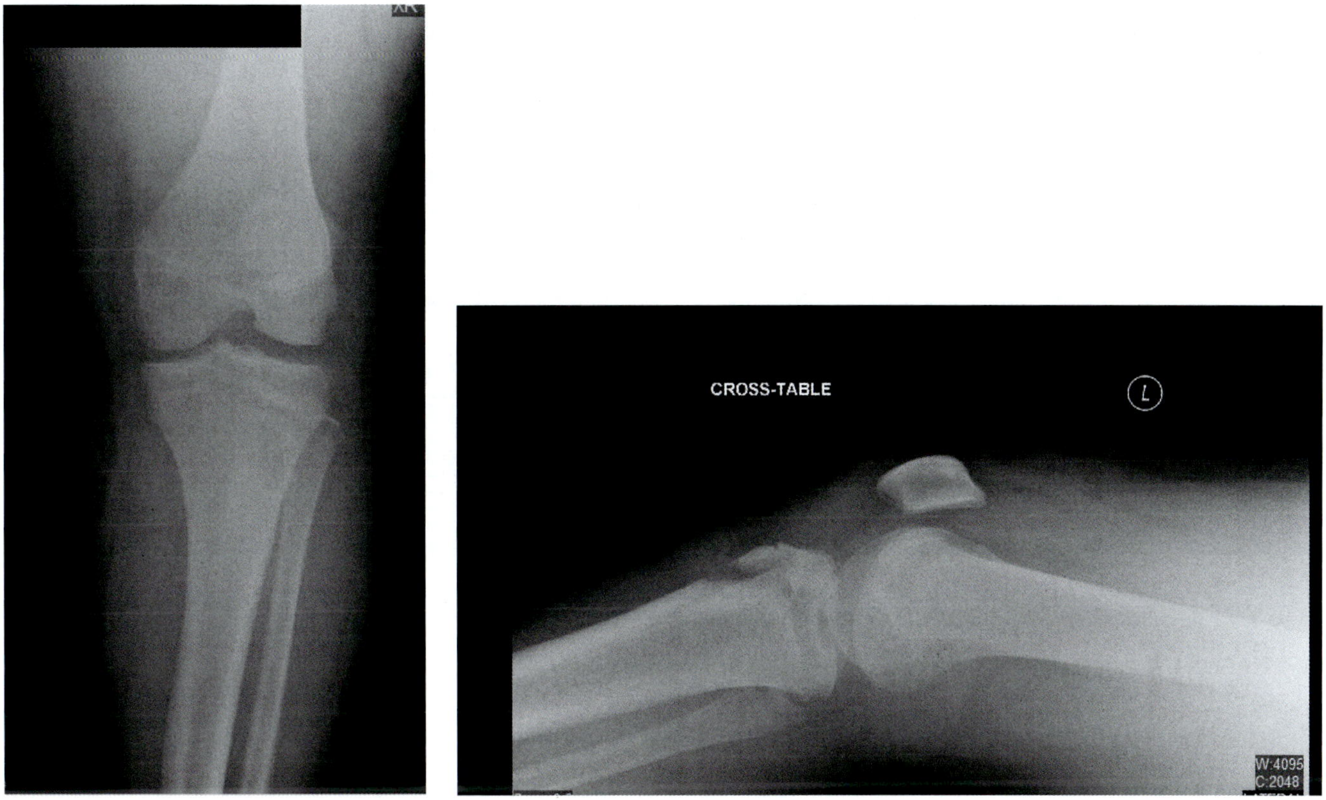

A B

Figure 31.1. **A,B.** AP and lateral radiographs of a 14-year-old male with a tibial tubercle fracture sustained while playing basketball.

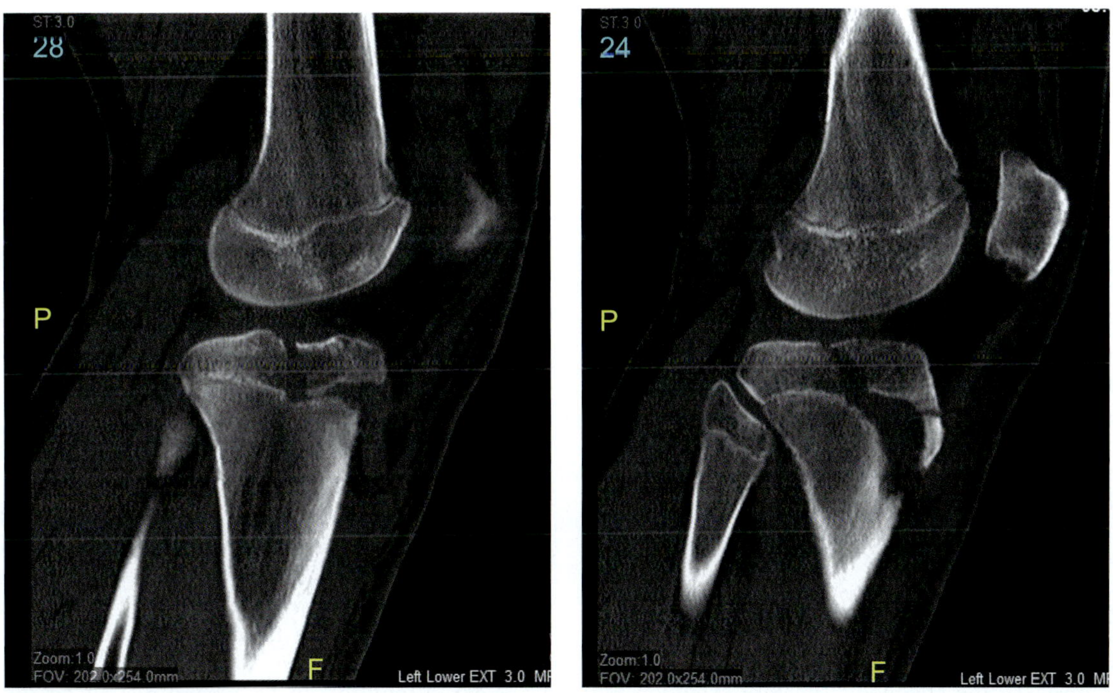

A B

Figure 31.2. **A,B.** Sagittal CT slices demonstrating the fracture pattern seen in Figure 31.1.

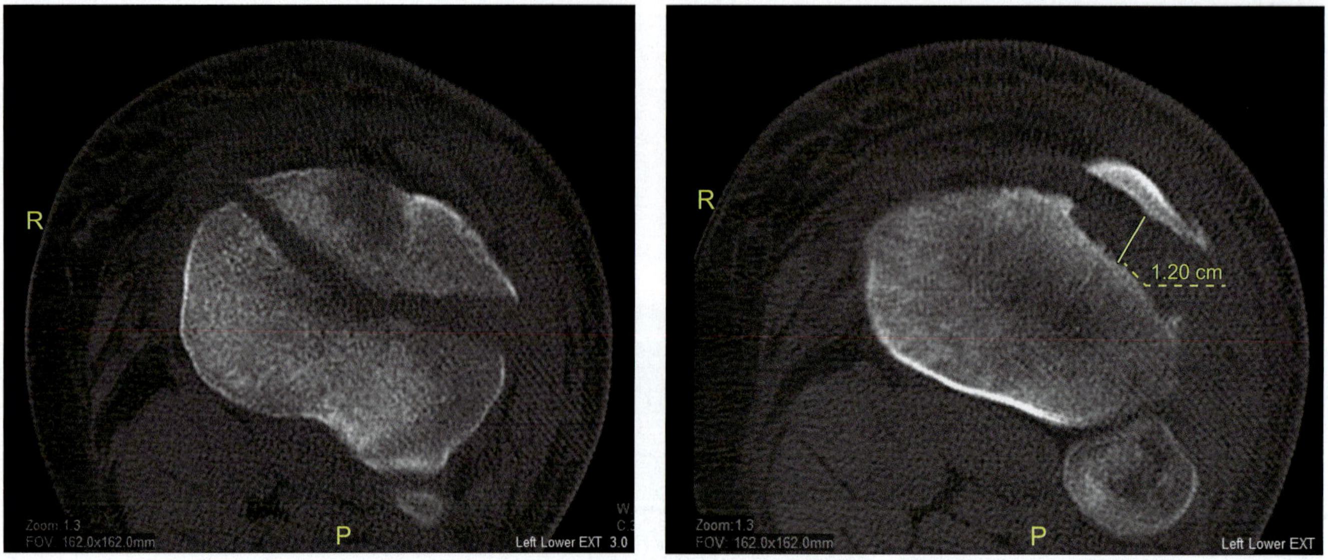

A B

Figure 31.3. **A,B.** Axial slices of the involved fracture demonstrating 1.2 cm of displacement at the widest interval.

ture.[22] Ogden added A and B subtypes in order to indicate displacement and comminution. A type C has been added and this describes associated patellar ligament avulsions.[23] Types IV and V classification also have been described.[24,25] Type IV injury involves complete tibial epiphysis involvement, whereas type V has been described as a type IIB with an associated type IV, thereby creating a "Y" fracture configuration.

MANAGEMENT

Management of tibial tubercle avulsion fractures is dictated by the fracture type and classification. Types IA and IB fractures can be treated successfully with conservative management: closed reduction and casting with the knee in extension. Type IC fractures, however, are better treated with open reduction internal fixation (ORIF) of the avulsed osseous fragment and patellar ligament.

ORIF is also performed for types IIB, IIC, IIIA, IIIB, IIIC, and any IV and V tibial tuberosity avulsion fractures. In addition to addressing the primary fracture, associated quadriceps or patellar tendon avulsions also are repaired at the time of surgery in order to maintain an intact extensor mechanism. Fixation methods typically comprise tension band wiring or cannulated screw fixation of the avulsed fragment. For fractures involving the joint, arthroscopy or submeniscal arthrotomy may be considered to address internal derangement.

OPERATIVE TECHNIQUE

We describe our preferred surgical technique to address a type III fracture involving the knee joint (fracture extension into the tibial plateau). The described technique can be modified and used for less extensive fracture types.

A midline anterior approach to the knee is performed, with an incision made from the midportion of the patella, centered over the patellar tendon, extending distally to the tibial tubercle. Then the skin and subcutaneous tissues are incised, along with the paratenon over the patellar tendon. The patellar tendon, distal portion of the patella, and the fracture site are exposed at this stage. A medial parapatellar arthrotomy is performed extending down to the fractured fragment of the proximal tibial metaphysis. Subsequently, the fracture is visualized fully, proximally to distally, and throughout the entire fracture site. At this point, a prophylactic anterior compartment release can be performed based on the clinical index of suspicion for impending compartment syndrome. In addition, a visual assessment of soft tissue injury and muscle viability are completed.

After these steps, a tourniquet will be inflated typically. Next, dissection is carried proximally to the proximal tibial plateau (lateral or medial depending on the side to which the fracture extends). A submeniscal arthrotomy is performed and two no. 2 FiberWire sutures are placed through the involved meniscus to retract the meniscus and allow for visualization of the joint surface. At this stage, it can be noted whether there is a cartilaginous defect that requires attention. Once the articular fracture site is cleaned of all hematoma and debris, the fracture can be reduced under direct visualization. Cartilaginous flaps with bony attachments should also be reduced at this point. During this critical step, the goal is primarily anatomic fracture reduction with direct apposition of the fracture at the cartilage surface. The proximal fracture fragment then may be fixed provisionally with two 1.6-mm K-wires.

Next, attention can be turned distally to the tibial tubercle fracture fixation. Any remaining alignment and reduction can be performed using a tamp and fluoroscopic

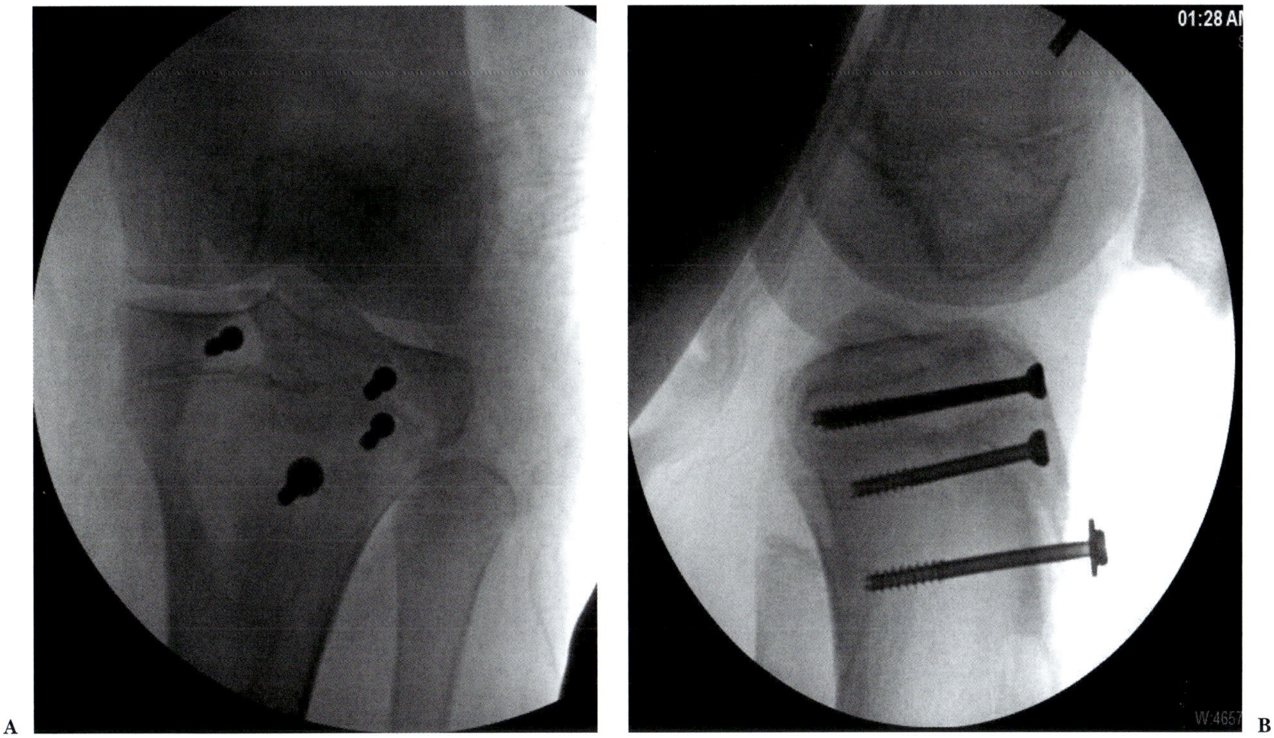

Figure 31.4. **A,B.** Intraoperative AP and lateral views of a tibial tubercle injury status post ORIF.

guidance. Once appropriate bony alignment is achieved, two 3.5-mm epiphyseal screws are placed under fluoroscopic guidance from anterior to posterior. Both screws should be placed in standard fashion: measured for depth, followed by screw placement. AP and lateral fluoroscopic views then should be used to confirm proper implant position. Next, a third screw of the same size typically is placed more distally through the center of the tibial tubercle, just below the level of the physis. In cases where the patellar tendon is avulsed distally, the distal portion can be secured with suture anchors. Typically, we use DePuy Mitek four-prong suture anchors. These are placed through drill holes in the anterior cortex and tamped into place. Then, the tendon is secured to the bone with the use of four suture strands placed in a simple fashion. At this point, final fluoroscopic views are obtained (Fig. 31.4), and the tourniquet is released in order to identify any active bleeders. The submeniscal arthrotomy is repaired with two no. 2 FiberWire sutures. The median parapatellar arthrotomy is repaired with a 0 vicryl suture. The wound is closed in layers in the usual fashion.

Postoperatively, patients are placed in a knee brace which is locked in extension. Patients are made toe-touch weight bearing and are initiated in an early physical therapy program with an emphasis of maintaining knee range of motion and performing isokinetic muscle exercises. There is no standard rehabilitation protocol; however, in most cases, the goal is a return to sports.

REFERENCES

1. Burkhart SS, Peterson H. Fractures of the proximal tibial epiphysis. *J Bone Joint Surg Am.* 1979;61(7):996–1002.
2. Pape JM, Goulet JA, Hensinger RN. Compartment syndrome complicating tibial tubercle avulsion. *Clin Orthop.* 1993;295:201–204.
3. Mosier SM, Stanitski CL. Acute tibial tubercle avulsion fractures. *J Pediatr Orthop.* 2004;24(2):181–184.
4. Ogden JA, Tross RB, Murphy MJ. Fractures of the tibial tuberosity in adolescents. *J Bone Joint Surg Am.* 1980;62(2):205–215.
5. Osgood RB. Lesions of the tibial tubercle occurring during adolescence. *Boston Med J.* 1903;148(5):114–117.
6. Hand WL, Hand CR, Dunn AW. Avulsion fractures of the tibial tubercle. *J Bone Joint Surg.* 1971;53(8):1579–1583.
7. Ehrenborg G. The Osgood-Schlatter lesion. A clinical study of 170 cases. *Acta Chir Scand.* 1962;124:89–105.
8. Beaty JH, Kasser JR. Fractures and dislocations about the knee. In: Beaty JH, Kasser JR, eds. *Rockwood and Wilkin's Fractures in Children.* 5th ed. Philadelphia, PA: Lippincott Williams & Wilkins; 2001:1019–1024.
9. Bolesta MJ, Fitch RD. Tibial tubercle avulsions. *J Pediatr Orthop.* 1986;6(2):186–192.
10. Shelton WR, Canale ST. Fractures of the tibia through the proximal tibial epiphyseal cartilage. *J Bone Joint Surg Am.* 1979;61(2):167–173.
11. Levi JH, Coleman CR. Fracture of the tibial tubercle. *Am J Sports Med.* 1976;4(6):254–263.
12. Rang M. *Children's Fracture.* Philadelphia, PA: Lippincott Williams & Wilkins; 1983.
13. Chow SP, Lam JJ, Leong JC. Fracture of the tibial tubercle in the adolescent. *J Bone Joint Surg Br.* 1990;72(2):231–234.

14. Ogden JA, Southwick WO. Osgood-Schlatter's disease and tibial tuberosity development. *Clin Orthop Relat Res.* 1976;(116):180–189.
15. Watson-Jones SR. *Fractures and Joint Surgeries.* 4th ed. Baltimore, MD: Williams & Wilkins Company; 1955.
16. Bolesta MJ, Fitch RD. Tibial tubercle avulsions. *J Pediatr Orthop.* 1986;6(2):186–192.
17. Maffulli N, Grewal R. Avulsion of the tibial tuberosity: muscles too strong for a growth plate. *Clin J Sport Med.* 1997;7(2):129–133.
18. Bang J, Broeng L. Spontaneous avulsion of the tibial tuberosity following Osgood-Schlatter disease [in Danish]. *Ugeskr Laeger.* 1995;157(21):3061–3062.
19. Pace JL, McCulloch PC, Momoh EO, et al. Operatively treated type IV tibial tubercle apophyseal fractures. *J Pediatr Orthop.* 2013;33(8):791–796.
20. Pandya NK, Edmonds EW, Roocroft JH, et al. Tibial tubercle fractures: complications, classification, and the need for intra-articular assessment. *J Pediatr Orthop.* 2012;32(8):749–759.
21. Abalo A, Akakpo-Numado K, Dossim A, et al. Avulsion fractures of the tibial tubercle. *J Orthop Surg.* 2008;16(3):308–311.
22. Ogden JA, Tross RB, Murphy MJ. Fractures of the tibial tuberosity in adolescents. *J Bone Joint Surg Am.* 1980;62(2):205–215.
23. Frankl U, Wasilewski SA, Healy WL. Avulsion fracture of the tibial tubercle with avulsion of the patellar ligament. Report of two cases. *J Bone Joint Surg Am.* 1900;72(9):1411–1413.
24. McKoy BE, Stanitski CL. Acute tibial tubercle avulsion fractures. *Orthop Clin North Am.* 2003;34(3):397–403.
25. Ryu JO, Debenham RK. An unusual avulsion fracture of the proximal tibial epiphysis. Case report and proposed addition to the Watson-Jones classification. *Clin Orthop Relat Res.* 1985;(194):181–184.

Benedict U. Nwachukwu
Daniel W. Green

CHAPTER 32

Tibial Spine Avulsion Fractures: Overview and Arthroscopic Technique for Internal Fixation with Cannulated Screws

INTRODUCTION

Children and adolescents are increasingly involved in competitive sporting activities, and as such, there continues to be a need to understand the sport-related injuries affecting the pediatric age population. Tibial spine fractures (also known as *tibial eminence fractures*) are a type of knee injury that most commonly occur in children and adolescents. Tibial spine fractures are best described as a bony avulsion of the anterior cruciate ligament (ACL) from its insertion on the intercondylar eminence of the tibia. Although these type of fractures have a low prevalence in the general population (incidence of approximately 3 per 100,000 per year[1]), they have been estimated to represent 2% to 5% of knee injuries in children and adolescents presenting with a knee effusion.[2,3] Inadequately treated tibial spine fractures can have deleterious effects on the function, quality of life, and health of the pediatric patient.

In this chapter, we provide an overview of tibial spine fractures and we present a technique for arthroscopic internal fixation using screw fixation. The method presented in this text is one method used by the senior author for the treatment of this condition.

ANATOMY

The tibial spines are bony prominences in the middle of the proximal tibia. The medial spine structure serves as the attachment site of the ACL. The broad attachment of the ACL fans out from the tibial spine and confluences with anterior horn of the medial and lateral meniscus.[4–6]

MECHANISM AND EPIDEMIOLOGY

Epidemiologic studies suggest that motor vehicle and sporting accidents (fall during skiing and fall from bike) are the most common causes of the index injury in the pediatric population.[7,8] The mechanism of injury for tibial spine avulsion fractures is thought to be similar to that for intrasubstance ACL tears where patients hyperextend the knee with a valgus or rotational force.[9,10] However, in children, tibial spine avulsion fractures occur because the tibial plateau has an incompletely ossified tibial plateau and because the ACL is stronger than its bony attachment; the bone is the point of failure when a pathophysiologic tensile load is applied. Some authors have postulated that prior to bone failure, an in situ stretch phenomenon can occur on the ACL, thereby resulting in some ligamentous laxity of the ACL even after appropriate fracture fixation.[11]

In this chapter, we discuss this unique injury for the pediatric and adolescent population; however, it should be noted that tibial spine fractures are being increasingly recognized in the adult population. One prior study proposed a higher prevalence of tibial spine fractures in the adult population than had been previously recognized.[12] There has since been continuing recognition of this fracture entity in the adult population.[13] Among adults, tibial spine fractures appear to be more common in women.[14] As such, one proposed mechanism for the occurrence of tibial spine fractures in adults is that osteopenic bone quality in adults leads to a similar injury pattern as is found in children and thus failure occurs at the bone with pathophysiologic load application on the ACL.

EVALUATION

As with any patient encounter, a thorough history and physical is a critical first step in evaluating the patient presenting with possible tibial spine fracture. Tibial spine fractures should be suspected in a skeletally immature individual presenting to clinic with painful knee hemarthrosis, decreased range of motion (ROM), and difficulty with weight bearing. History will likely be positive for a sporting or traumatic maneuver in which the leg is forcefully loaded often with a valgus stress. As with

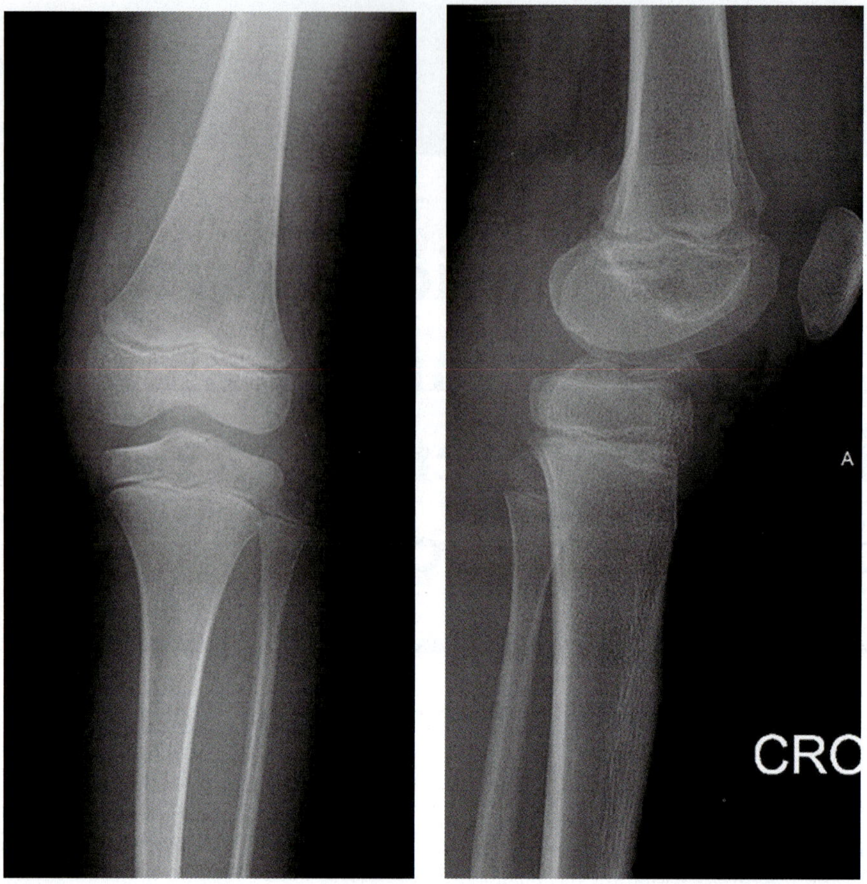

A B

Figure 32.1. **A.** AP view of a knee in an 8-year-old patient with a tibial spine fracture while skiing. **B.** Lateral view of the knee in the same patient.

ACL injuries, these patients will similarly feel a "popping" sensation; however, unlike ACL disruption, the "pop" is the breach of the tibial spine integrity and the ACL pulling the tibial spine away from the tibia. Physical examination should also include a thorough examination of the knee, being careful to detect any associated injury.

Radiographic assessment of the knee should include standard anteroposterior (AP), lateral, and tibial tunnel views of the knee (Figs. 32.1 and 32.2). Lateral views of the knee are useful in determining the degree of displacement of the fracture fragment and tibial tunnel views can assist in further defining subtle fractures in the AP plane (see Fig. 32.2). Contralateral view of the knee may be helpful as a comparison not only to define normal anatomy in this region but also to disaggregate tibial spine fractures from fractures of the inferior pole of the patellar or femoral condyle.

Some may choose to get additional diagnostic studies such as a computed tomography (CT) scan, which has been shown to have some use in better defining fracture characteristics as well as degree of comminution.[15] CT studies, however, are not part of the routine workup of tibial spine fractures at our institution. A high rate of concomitant injury with tibial spine fractures has been reported in the literature.[16,17] As such, magnetic resonance imaging (MRI) for further radiographic assessment of tibial spine injuries is recommended. MRI is useful in preoperative planning for assessing the structural integrity of the knee and ruling out interstitial injury of the ACL. Furthermore, MRI defines the fracture fragment compared to soft tissue structures (Fig. 32.3). This information is informative regarding potential obstacles to fracture reduction. One prior study reported on the MRI findings associated with tibial spine fractures.[16] Associated injuries include intrasubstance ACL and posterior cruciate ligament injuries, medial collateral ligament tears, posterior lateral corner injury, and meniscal tears—specifically meniscal entrapment within the spine fracture segment.

CLASSIFICATION

Tibial spine avulsion fractures are most commonly classified based on an algorithm devised by Meyers and McKeevers.[18] The classification scheme relies on the degree of displacement of the avulsed fragment from the fracture base. In this fracture scheme, tibial spine fractures are classified from types I to III, with type I being the least displaced and type III the most.

Type I fractures are characteristically nondisplaced fractures of the tibial spine. In type II fractures, the anterior portion of the fracture is displaced superiorly while the posterior portion remains hinged. Type III fractures are completely displaced from the fracture base and are divided into two subcategories: IIIA and IIIB. Type IIIA fractures have complete separation from the fracture base, whereas type IIIB fractures are not only

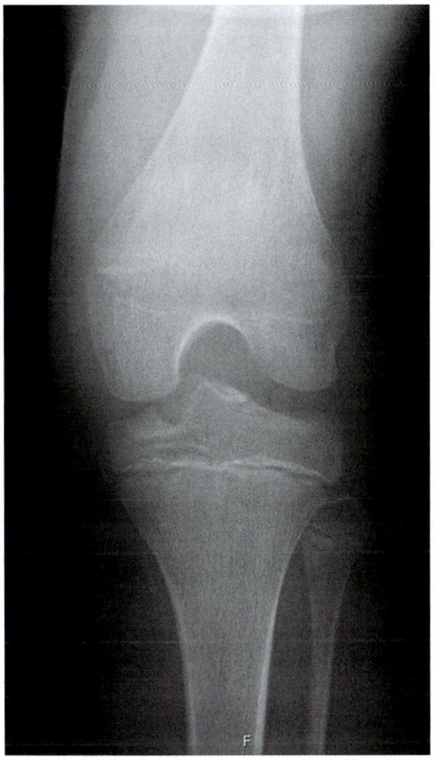

Figure 32.2. Tibial tunnel view of a tibial spine fracture may better define the fracture.

completely displaced but are also rotated cephalad. Zaricznyj[19] later added a type IV category which includes displaced fractures with comminution of the fragment.

Although not yet formally described, the authors propose that there is a fifth subset of tibial spine fractures that could be classified as type 0. In type 0, the fractures would not be seen on standard radiographs but could be detectable on MRI.

MANAGEMENT

Tibial spine fracture management is typically based on the type of underlying fracture. These fractures show significant variation in fracture characteristics and associated injury. The common goal, however, is to restore the integrity and function of the ACL as well as to restore the contour of the tibial plateau.

Management of tibial spine fractures is typically operative versus nonoperative. Type I fractures by nature of nondisplacement can be managed nonoperatively with knee immobilization. Adequate immobilization can be obtained with either a brace or a cast. Type I fractures failing nonoperative management typically have late displacement, which can occur despite adequate immobilization. For this reason, patients with type I fractures being managed nonoperatively should be closely monitored for this complication during the first 6 weeks after injury.[20] Early motion after evidence of fracture union is important to prevent knee stiffness.

Treatment of type II fractures is more controversial, and historically good results have been reported from both the operative and nonoperative management of type II fractures.[21] Similar to type I fractures, mild forms of type II fractures can be managed nonoperatively with cast or knee immobilization if there is near-anatomic reduction. Residual displacement from a malreduced tibial spine fragment leads to lack of full extension and impingement of the displaced tibial eminence in the notch. Soft tissue entrapment within the fracture is the most common etiology for an irreducible fracture. We indicate most type II fractures for arthroscopic fixation to improve reduction, take care of any meniscal entrapment, and promote early ROM.

Advances in arthroscopic techniques have expanded the surgical management of tibial spine fractures. Prior to the widespread use of knee arthroscopy, arthrotomy and open reduction internal fixation of the fracture fragment were the standards of care for types III, IV, and irreducible type II. In the modern era, surgical intervention is the standard of care for types III and IV fractures. Arthroscopy now provides the benefit of decreased morbidity, and as such, the trend is to offer arthroscopic fixation even for type II fractures. Furthermore, arthroscopy allows the surgeon to rule in/out injury to the intra-articular structures under direct visualization.

There are two primary modalities for the surgical management of tibial spine fractures: suture versus screw fixation. In this chapter, we focus on the surgical technique for screw fixation. We use a suture fixation approach for fractures consisting of a small bone fragment or with significant comminution. Both the suture and screw fixation are technically challenging.[22] Suture fixation will be further discussed in Chapter 33.

OPERATIVE TECHNIQUE

We describe here the authors' preferred surgical technique for the management of larger sized tibial spine fractures. We present a method for arthroscopic internal fixation using screw fixation (see Table 32.1 for equipment).

The patient is prepped and draped in the usual sterile fashion in the supine position. A standard anterolateral arthroscopic portal is first established. The arthroscope is introduced via the anterolateral portal and then an anteromedial portal is established under direct visualization from the anterolateral portal. A diagnostic knee arthroscopy is initially performed including the patellofemoral joint and both the medial and the lateral compartments. The presence of a chondral defect is assessed (Fig. 32.4) and the structural continuity of the ACL is determined. The ACL is inspected as is the tibial spine itself. The medial, lateral, and anterior borders of the fragment are evaluated, with particular attention to potential blocks of reduction and extension into the weight-bearing surface of the tibial plateau. Next, the menisci are inspected for involvement of the anterior meniscus in the fracture fragment (Fig. 32.5). Meniscal entrapment, although suspected on MRI, is definitively diagnosed during the diagnostic arthroscopy. One prior study by Kocher et al.[8] identified an entrapment of the anterior horn of the medial meniscus, intermeniscal ligament, or anterior horn of the lateral meniscus in 26% of type II fractures and 65% of type III fractures. In cases where there is interdigitation of the meniscus between the plateau and the fracture fragment, a probe can be used to carefully elevate the meniscus from below the tibial spine fragment. With the knee

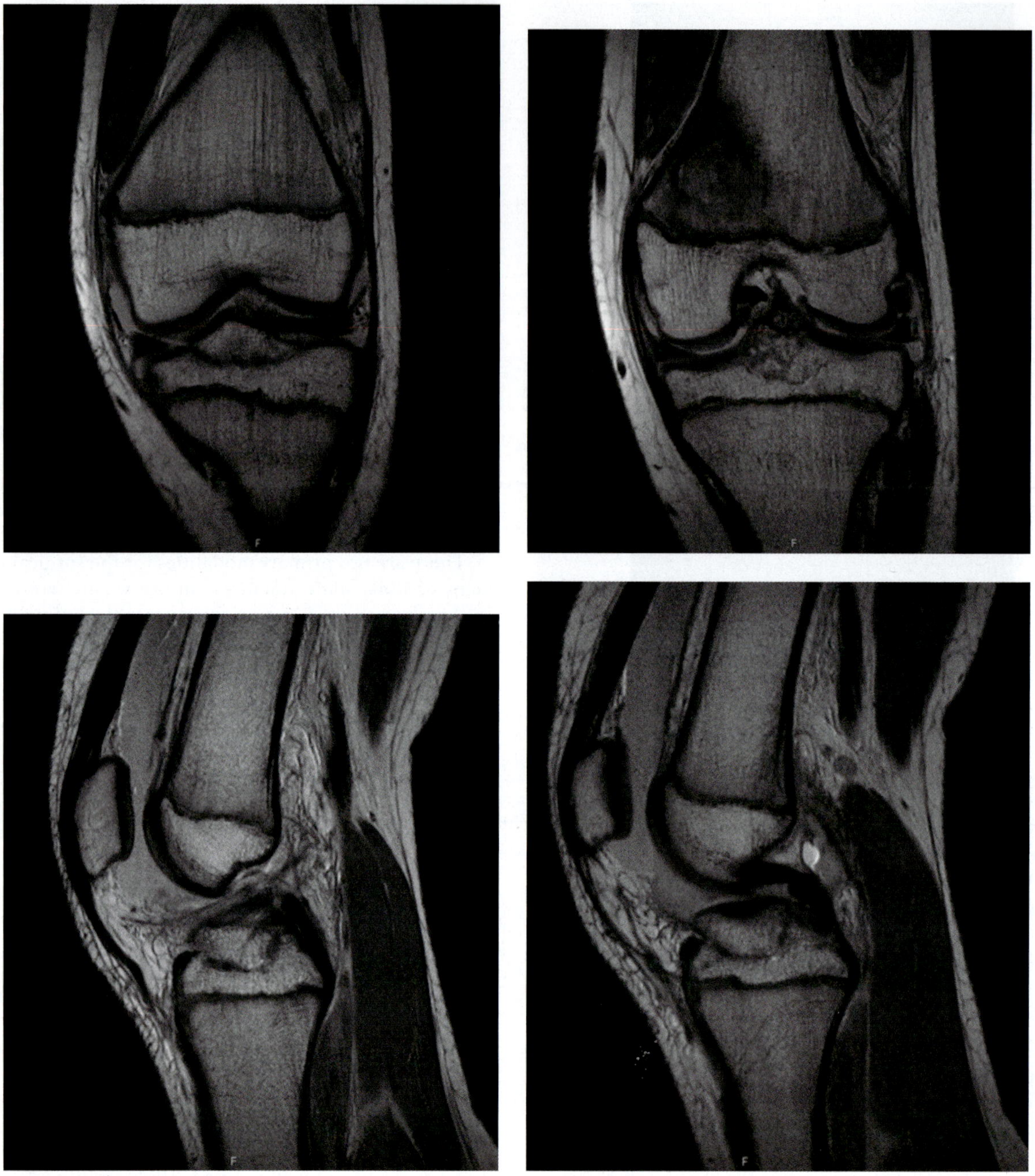

A B C D

Figure 32.3. **A–D.** AP and sagittal views of a knee with a tibial spine fracture (an incidental benign bone lesion is noted in figure **B**).

flexed, the tibial spine avulsion fragment is anatomically reduced back into its bed on the tibia. We usually use an ACL tibial guide to manipulate the fracture fragment (an angled microfracture pick or K-wire can also be used). The ACL insertion on the tibia can be used as an anatomic guide for reduction, and reduction should be confirmed by direct visualization under arthroscopy.

Next, with the knee flexed 80 to 90 degrees, a third portal (superior medial portal) is established. This portal is established just medial to the patellar tendon at the inferior pole of the patella. Using this portal, two guide wires are placed into the base of the tibial spine fragment and advanced with a K-wire driver approximately 2 cm. A mini C-arm can be used at this point to confirm reduction and pin placement on a lateral view. To avoid bending the K-wire, care must be taken not to flex or extend the knee while obtaining the lateral radiograph. Following radiographic confirmation, two 18- to 20-mm partially threaded, self-drilling, cannulated 4.0-mm screws are introduced into the fragment over the guide wires, making sure to obtain an excellent bite with each fixation. For large fracture fragments, an additional screw can be placed through a superior lateral accessory portal. Fluoroscopic images in the AP and lateral planes can then be taken after the k-wires are removed to confirm reduction of the fracture fragment and that the screws remain in

TABLE 32.1 Equipment Required for Operative Technique

Equipment
Tourniquet
Probe
Trocar
Motorized arthroscopic shaver
Kirschner wires
ACL tibial guide
Power drill
Synthes 4.0-mm cannulated, partially threaded screws
Screwdriver
Mini C-arm

ACL, anterior cruciate ligament.

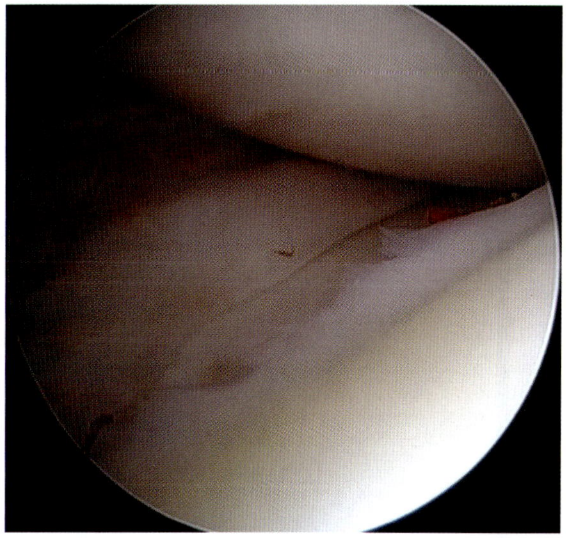

Figure 32.5. Anterior horn of the medial meniscus and the intermeniscal ligament entrapped underneath a tibial spine fracture fragment.

the epiphysis and do not violate the physis once the K-wires are removed (Fig. 32.6).

Following screw placement and fracture fixation, the knee is taken through a full ROM under direct visualization. Impingement and tracking of the screws is noted during knee ROMs. The screws should be well fixed in the tibia and safely away from the femoral condyles during knee extension.

REHABILITATION

There is no gold standard physical therapy modality for the postoperative management of tibial spine fractures. At our institution, the senior author applies a standardized protocol to all patients after fixation of their tibial spine fracture. Our program presented here is a modified ACL rehabilitation program.

Immediately postoperative, patients are placed in a knee brace, which is locked in extension, and patients are made toe-touch weight bearing (TTWB). During postoperative weeks 1 to 4, patient is maintained in TTWB status with brace locked in extension for ambulation. Crutches are used for assistance. ROM exercises are initiated immediately postoperatively with a goal of full passive knee extension. Typical exercises in our patient population include towel roll extension, quadriceps sets, and quadriceps reeducation using electrical stimulation. Active flexion and active-assisted extension is allowed during this time. During these first 4 postoperative weeks, the fixation construct is protected with continuous brace wear. Brace is worn during most hours of the day and is worn locked in extension at night for sleep. It is permissible to remove brace daily to check skin and as needed for dedicated physical therapy and ROM modalities. During weeks 4 to 6 postoperatively, the patient is then progressed to weight bearing as tolerated. Daytime brace wearing is adjusted from locked in extension to a motion range of 0 to 45 degrees. Exercises during this phase can be progressed to include straight-leg raises, hamstring/hip progressive resistance exercises, and proprioceptive tasks (once stably bearing weight), including the proprioception board and progressive gait training with crutches.

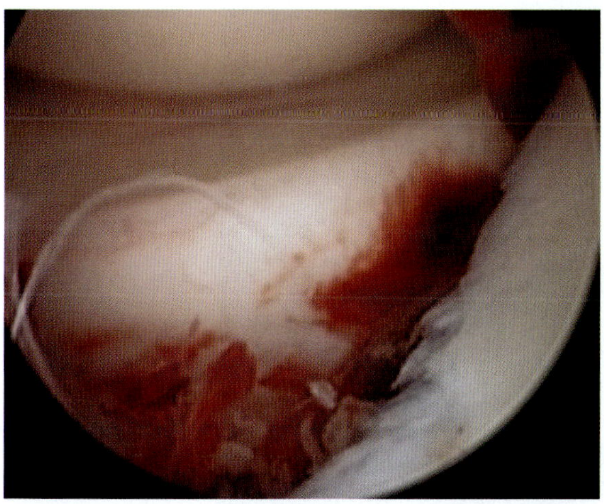

Figure 32.4. Bed of fracture fragment with cartilage defect extending into medial compartment.

During weeks 6 to 12, patient is then progressed to be fully weight bearing and is weaned off brace wear. If at the 6-week follow-up patients have knee ROM beyond 115 degrees, they can also be progressed to bicycling activities. The elite athlete with demonstrated high level of function at this phase can be progressed to more advanced activities such as retrograde treadmill ambulation and elliptical training.

At 4 months postoperatively, a forward step-down test and other functional movements are evaluated prior to advancing activities. Patients passing the step-down test demonstrate an ability to step down from a 6- to 8-in step with good eccentric control. For those passing the step-down test, a running program can be initiated. A functional brace can be used for light running or sport activities. During this final stage of rehabilitation, exercises will likely consist of plyometrics and agility-type exercises.

Most patients will be able to achieve return to sports at 4 to 6 months postoperatively. Formal radiographs can be obtained at this point or earlier to confirm healing of fixated fracture fragments (Fig. 32.7).

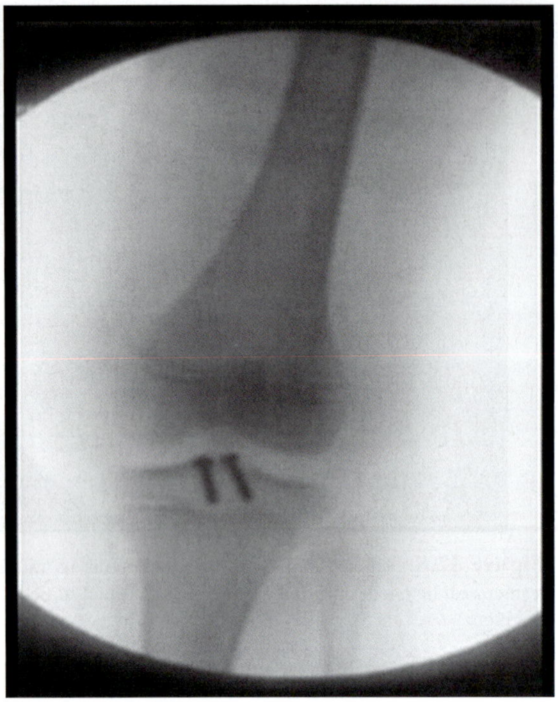

A

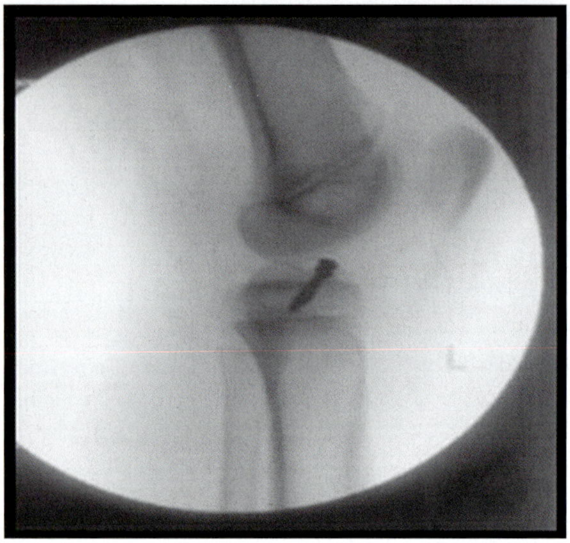

B

Figure 32.6. **A,B.** Fluoroscopic views of a tibial spine fracture status post screw fixation.

COMPLICATIONS

Fixation techniques for tibial spine fractures generally provide excellent results; however, there are some notable complications including residual laxity, loss of motion, nonunion, and growth deformity. Residual laxity after tibial spine fracture is a well-documented complication of both operative and nonoperative strategies. The incidence of laxity has been reported to be lower, however, after fracture screw fixation compared with closed reduction and immobi-

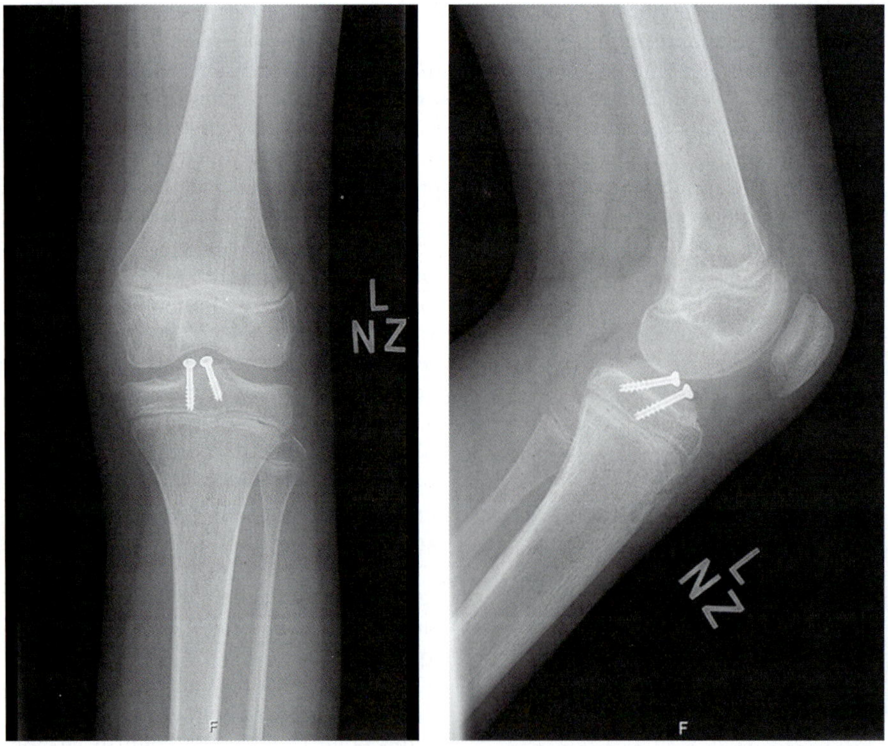

A B

Figure 32.7. **A,B.** AP and lateral radiographs of knee after screw fixation for tibial spine fracture. *(Continued)*

C

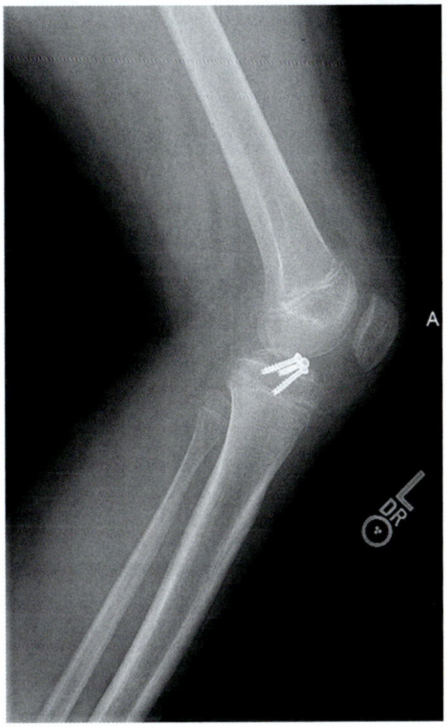

Figure 32.7. *(Continued)* **C.** Three-screw technique used for the fixation of a large tibial spine fracture.

lization.[23] Laxity is thought to be secondary to intrasubstance elongation occurring as part of the injury mechanism. Loss of motion after tibial spine fracture fixation has also been reported and is thought to be secondary to fracture malreduction versus arthrofibrosis. The causes of arthrofibrosis after pediatric knee surgery are not well understood, however, extended postoperative immobilization is likely a significant contributor.[24]

Knee stiffness (arthrofibrosis) after operative treatment of tibial spine fractures is also an increasingly recognized complication.[25] In a case series of 32 children and adolescents with arthrofibrosis after tibial spine fractures, 24 patients required reoperation to regain motion and 3 patients were unable to regain full motion at final follow-up. Intra-articular fracture hematoma and prolonged postoperative immobilization is hypothesized to be a significant risk factor in the development of arthrofibrosis. Treatment options in the event of arthrofibrosis include static/dynamic knee bracing and manipulation under anesthesia with or without lysis of adhesions. Care should be taken when performing manipulation under anesthesia to avoid chondral and physeal injury.

Growth arrest and disturbance after screw fixation of tibial spine fractures is a rare but devastating complication. Because these fractures typically occur in skeletally immature patients with an open proximal tibial physis, care should be taken to avoid violating the physis. A variety of complications have been reported after violation of the physis and these include recurvatum, distal femoral valgus deformity, and limb length discrepancy.

REFERENCES

1. Hargrove R, Parsons S, Payne R. Anterior tibial spine fracture—an easy fracture to miss. *Accid Emerg Nurs.* 2004;12(3):173–175.
2. Eiskjaer S, Larsen ST, Schmidt MB. The significance of hemarthrosis of the knee in children. *Arch Orthop Trauma Surg.* 1988;107(2):96–98.
3. Luhmann SJ. Acute traumatic knee effusions in children and adolescents. *J Pediatr Orthop.* 2003;23(2):199–202.
4. Girgis FG, Marshall JL, Monajem A. The cruciate ligaments of the knee joint. Anatomical, functional and experimental analysis. *Clin Orthop Relat Res.* 1975;(106):216–231.
5. Cabaud HE. Biomechanics of the anterior cruciate ligament. *Clin Orthop Relat Res.* 1983;(172):26–31.
6. Petersen W, Zantop T. Anatomy of the anterior cruciate ligament with regard to its two bundles. *Clin Orthop Relat Res.* 2007;454:35–47.
7. Casalonga A, Bourelle S, Chalencon F, et al. Tibial intercondylar eminence fractures in children: the long-term perspective. *Orthop Traumatol Surg Res.* 2010;96(5):525–530.
8. Kocher MS, Micheli LJ, Gerbino P, et al. Tibial eminence fractures in children: prevalence of meniscal entrapment. *Am J Sports Med.* 2003;31(3):404–407.
9. Wiley JJ, Baxter MP. Tibial spine fractures in children. *Clin Orthop Relat Res.* 1990;(255):54–60.
10. Accousti WK, Willis RB. Tibial eminence fractures. *Orthop Clin North Am.* 2003;34(3):365–375.
11. Kocher MS, Foreman ES, Micheli LJ. Laxity and functional outcome after arthroscopic reduction and internal fixation of displaced tibial spine fractures in children. *Arthroscopy.* 2003;19(10):1085–1090.
12. Kendall NS, Hsu SY, Chan KM. Fracture of the tibial spine in adults and children. A review of 31 cases. *J Bone Joint Surg Br.* 1992;74(6):848–852.
13. Aderinto J, Walmsley P, Keating JF. Fractures of the tibial spine: epidemiology and outcome. *Knee.* 2008;15(3):164–167.
14. Hunter RE, Willis JA. Arthroscopic fixation of avulsion fractures of the tibial eminence: technique and outcome. *Arthroscopy.* 2004;20(2):113–121.
15. Griffith JF, Antonio GE, Tong CW, et al. Cruciate ligament avulsion fractures. *Arthroscopy.* 2004;20(8):803–812.
16. Ishibashi Y, Tsuda E, Sasaki T, et al. Magnetic resonance imaging AIDS in detecting concomitant injuries in patients with tibial spine fractures. *Clin Orthop Relat Res.* 2005;(434):207–212.
17. Monto RR, Cameron-Donaldson ML, Close MA, et al. Magnetic resonance imaging in the evaluation of tibial eminence fractures in adults. *J Knee Surg.* 2006;19(3):187–190.
18. Meyers MH, McKeever FM. Fracture of the intercondylar eminence of the tibia. *J Bone Joint Surg Am.* 1959;41(2):209–222.
19. Zaricznyj B. Avulsion fracture of the tibial eminence: treatment by open reduction and pinning. *J Bone Joint Surg Am.* 1977;59(8):1111–1114.
20. Lafrance RM, Giordano B, Goldblatt J, et al. Pediatric tibial eminence fractures: evaluation and management. *J Am Acad Orthop Surg.* 2010;18(7):395–405
21. Anderson CN, Anderson AF. Tibial eminence fractures. *Clin Sports Med.* 2011;30(4):727–742.
22. Tsukada H, Ishibashi Y, Tsuda E, et al. A biomechanical comparison of repair techniques for anterior cruciate ligament tibial avulsion fracture under cyclic loading. *Arthroscopy.* 2005;21(10):1197–1201.
23. McLennan JG. Lessons learned after second-look arthroscopy in type III fractures of the tibial spine. *J Pediatr Orthop.* 1995;15(1):59–62.
24. Nwachukwu BU, McFeely ED, Nasreddine A, et al. Arthrofibrosis after cruciate ligament reconstruction in children and adolescents. *J Pediatr Orthop.* 2011;31(8):811–817.
25. Vander Have KL, Ganley TJ, Kocher MS, et al. Arthrofibrosis after surgical fixation of tibial eminence fractures in children and adolescents. *Am J Sports Med.* 2010;38(2):298–301.

CHAPTER

33

Itai Gans
Theodore J. Ganley

Tibial Spine/Anterior Cruciate Ligament Avulsion Fractures Overview Technique Suture

TREATMENT

It is important to review and know the Meyers and McKeever classification system for tibial spine fractures, as treatment depends on the fracture pattern observed.

Type I fractures are best managed using immobilization techniques in either a long leg cast or fracture brace. The amount of flexion recommended in the literature varies and ranges from 0 to 40 degrees.[1–7] Although few proponents argue for immobilization in hyperextension,[8] it generally is not recommended due to patient discomfort[2] and the danger of putting posterior structures such as the popliteal artery under tension, potentially causing the development of compartment syndrome.[9] The decision to evacuate the hematoma is based on physician's preference. Rapid healing occurs in skeletally immature patients; as such, most physicians treat type I fractures with 4 to 6 weeks of immobilization.[6,7,9–12] In older children, adolescents, and adults, prolonged periods of immobilization may lead to development of significant knee stiffness and muscle atrophy,[13] and the shortest period of immobilization possible that will still maintain reduction is recommended,[14–16] usually approximately 2 to 3 weeks, followed by protected range-of-motion activities. Isometric quadriceps exercises are prescribed throughout the immobilization period to minimize atrophy and the effects of disuse. Interval radiographs are obtained to ensure maintenance of fracture reduction.[17]

There are many advocates for closed reduction by knee extension under anesthesia[18–20] followed by immobilization of the knee for *type II* fractures of the tibial spine. There has been heavy debate regarding the ability of manipulation under anesthesia to cause anatomic reduction.[4,19–21] Reduction during manipulation is most likely caused by femoral notch and sulcus pressures during knee extension. Importantly, a minimal amount of fragment elevation (<4 mm) does not appreciably affect subjective knee outcomes.[10,22] Often, the inability to achieve reduction with closed manipulation is secondary to entrapment of the medial meniscus and/or intermeniscal ligament in the fracture.[23,24] If an acceptable reduction cannot be achieved or maintained by closed manipulation, operative treatment is indicated.

Surgical reduction and fixation is standard of care in types III and IV fractures, and soft tissue entrapment occurs in 65% to 100% of these fractures.[23,24] A systematic review of treatment of tibial spine fractures in pediatric patients revealed a significantly high rate of nonunion in types III and IV tibial spine fractures treated by nonoperative means.[25] As such, the authors advise operative management of all types III and IV tibial spine fractures. There are several arthroscopic techniques that have been reported, including metal screw fixation, bioabsorbable screw fixation, staple fixation, K-wire fixation, suture fixation, and suture anchor fixation. Within the orthopedic community, questions regarding the strongest method of fixation with the most stability still remain,[26] with some surgeons favoring suture fixation while others prefer screw fixation. Despite surgeon preferences, a recent systematic review of 26 articles reporting on treatment and outcomes of tibial spine fractures in pediatric patients revealed that the evidence for favoring screw or suture fixation is poor, with no appreciable benefits to one method over the other.[25]

The success of surgically treating tibial eminence fractures depends on secure fixation, early mobilization,[27] and early treatment.[8,28] Some biomechanical studies have reported that the strength of suture fixation is higher than that of screw fixation.[29,30] However, other studies have found that both suture and screw fixation had increased fracture separation during cyclic physiologic loads which could cause loss of fracture reduction.[31] More recently, reports have indicated that the use of a hybrid technique, using both suture and screw fixation, may achieve a more stable reduction, allowing early return to range of motion, thereby decreasing risk of arthrofibrosis.[32]

AUTHORS' PREFERRED TREATMENT

A diagnostic arthroscopy is performed using the usual anteromedial and anterolateral arthroscopy portals. Once the fracture is visualized, medial and lateral midpatellar portals are placed. After débridement of soft tissue beneath the fragment, the

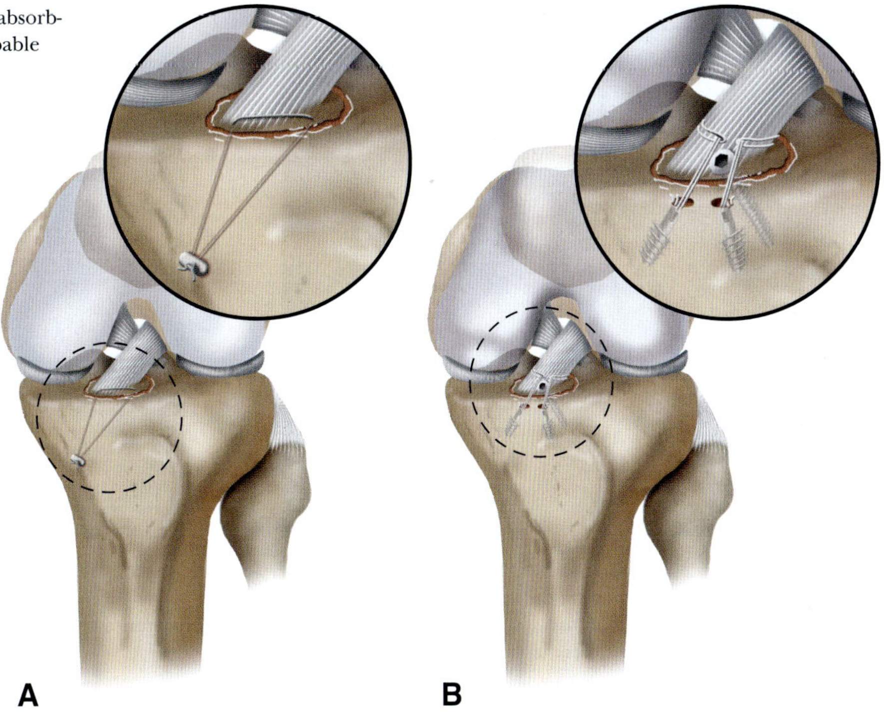

Figure 33.1. The final fixation using **(A)** bioabsorbable screw and suture fixation and **(B)** bioabsorbable screw and suture anchor fixation.

fracture is reduced and secured using a combination of two fixation techniques.

First, a bioabsorbable compression screw is used for provisional maintenance of fracture reduction (initial fixation).

Second, a high-strength suture is passed through the base of the anterior cruciate ligament (ACL) and (1) either tied over the front of the tibia through small tunnels (secondary fixation—variation A for type III tibial spine fractures) or (2) secured with shoulder anchors (secondary fixation—variation B for type IV tibial spine fractures) (Fig. 33.1).

The following technique has two variations: the first variation is best used in type III fractures using suture passed through tibial bone tunnels, and the second variation is best used in slightly comminuted type IV fractures using suture securely anchored to the anterior tibia. The initial screw fixation in both is the same.

Initial Fixation—Bioabsorbable Compression Screw

Initial fixation of the fracture fragment using a bioabsorbable screw is performed through a midpatellar portal to permit proper screw alignment and fixation.

A 0.045-in K-wire is placed through the midpatellar portal in the desired location of the compression screw to stabilize the fracture fragment. A second K-wire is placed for additional fixation that will be maintained during screw placement (Fig. 33.2).

An incision for a portal is made around the first K-wire to accommodate a small arthroscopic cannula to prevent soft tissue obstruction. After selection of a bioabsorbable compression screw of desired length, the corresponding cannulated drill, followed by the corresponding cannulated tap, is used over the top of the first K-wire to prepare the bone for screw placement (Fig. 33.3). Because the drill and tap are cannulated while the bioabsorbable compression screw is not, to proceed, the K-wire used to drill and tap must be removed while maintaining fracture reduction. This is achieved by removing the first K-wire, with the second K-wire maintaining reduction, and replacing the removed K-wire with the selected screw (Fig. 33.4). Once the screw is implanted, the second K-wire is removed and the fracture is secure and stable (Fig. 33.5), allowing for easy reinforcement of the fixation with sutures.

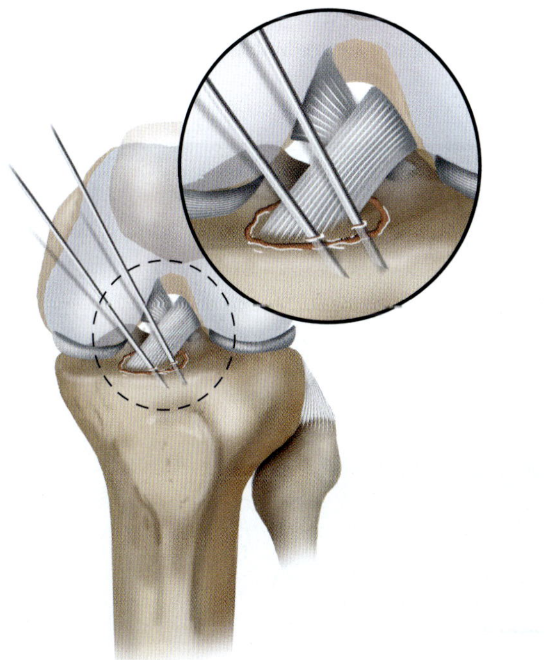

Figure 33.2. The tibial spine fracture is fixed and held in place with two K-wires to prepare for further fixation.

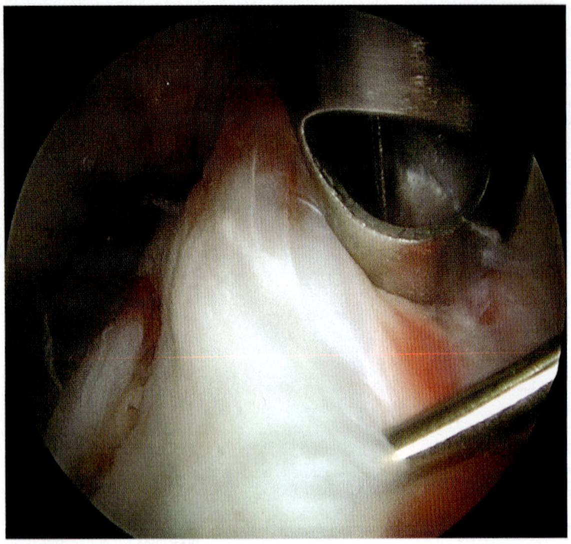

Figure 33.3. After selection of a bioabsorbable compression screw of desired length, the corresponding cannulated drill, followed by the corresponding cannulated tap, is used over the top of the first K-wire to prepare the bone for screw placement.

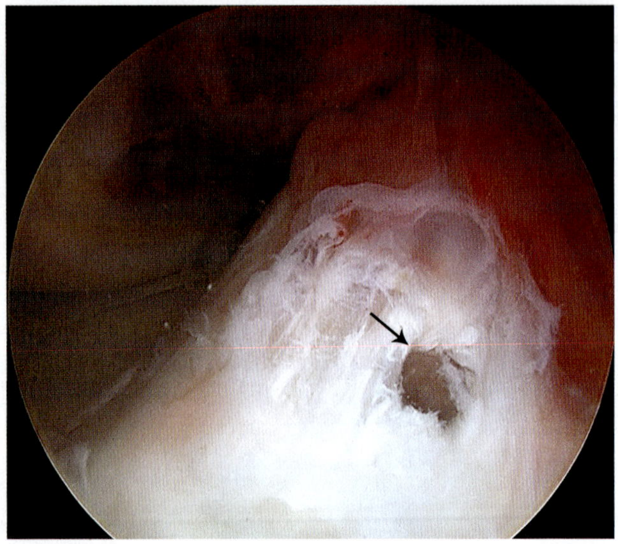

Figure 33.5. After placing the absorbable compression screw (placement indicated by the *black arrow*), the second K-wire is removed and suture or suture anchor fixation is initiated.

Secondary Fixation—High-Strength Suture (Variation A for Type III Tibial Eminence Fractures)

With the fracture fragment secured in place by the bioabsorbable compression screw, secondary fixation is made more simple. Secondary fixation is completed using ultra high-strength suture, which is passed over the fragment, down two small bone tunnels, and tied over the front of the tibia.

Two limbs of FiberWire (Arthrex, Naples, FL) are passed separately through the base of the ACL (running medial to lateral) using a suture passer (Fig. 33.6). Suture of different colors (FiberWire and TigerWire [Arthrex, Naples, FL]) can be used to help distinguish suture limbs.

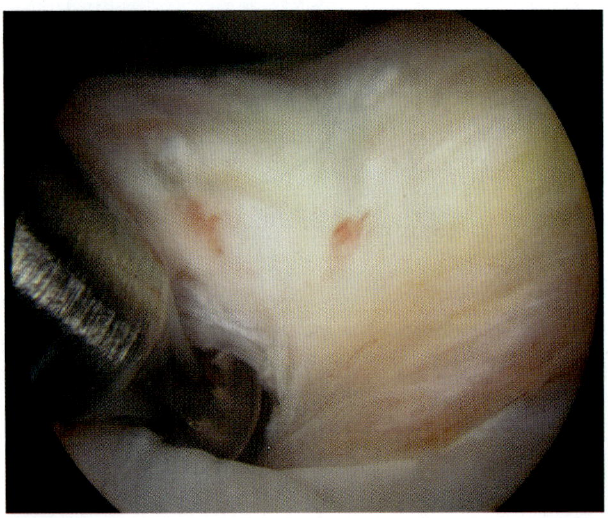

Figure 33.4. After removing one of the two K-wires, an absorbable screw is secured to provisionally hold the tibial eminence fracture in place.

An ACL tibial tunnel drill guide (Retrodrill Constant Guide [Arthrex, Naples, FL]) is then used to pass a 3-mm cannulated pin (Retrodrill Guide Pin, Cannulated [Arthrex, Naples, FL]) through the medial aspect of the fracture fragment at the base of the ACL insertion. FiberStick suture (Arthrex, Naples, FL) is passed up, through the cannula of the 3-mm pin, and retrieved through the medial portal using a grasper. The drill guide and cannulated pin allow for suture placement through the metaphyseal portion of the proximal tibia as well as the fracture fragment and the ACL. These steps are repeated to place a piece of high-strength suture, preferably of a different color than the first, through the fragment on the lateral side of the ACL. Then, both limbs of suture are pulled out through a single portal.

A loop is tied in one of the sutures (i.e., the solid suture) which is used to pull the other suture (i.e., the striped suture) down through the second bone tunnel (Fig. 33.7). The solid suture is then discarded and the striped suture is tied over the anterior bone bridge or a button (Fig. 33.8). Figure 9 is an image of the final fixation using this method with screw and suture fixation.

Secondary Fixation—High-Strength Suture (Variation B for Type IV Tibial Eminence Fractures)

In comminuted fractures of the tibial eminence, we have found that using a technique similar to basic shoulder labral repair, familiar to most arthroscopists and using the same equipment and fixation method, has been successful. After provisional fixation with a bioabsorbable compression screw, a high-strength suture fixation is achieved and secured with shoulder anchors.

As described earlier (secondary fixation for type III tibial eminence fractures), use the midpatellar portals, using a suture passer to pass two limbs of high-strength suture through the base of the ACL (see Fig. 33.6), then through the anchors, and secure the anchor(s) anterior to the tibial eminence angled slightly anterior to posterior (Fig. 33.10). Figure 33.11 is an image of the final fixation using this method with screw and anchor fixation.

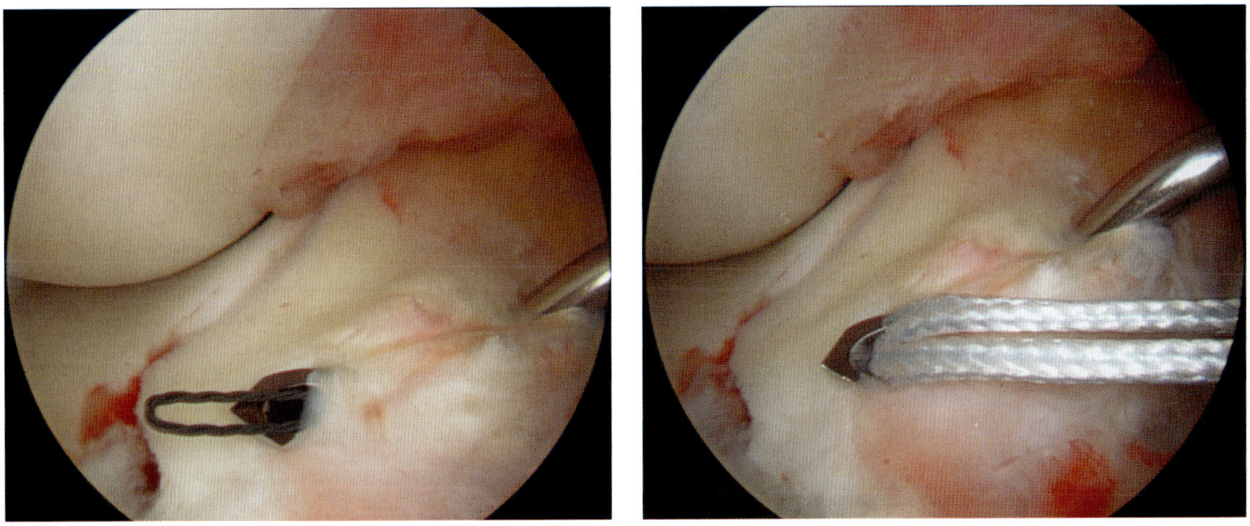

A B

Figure 33.6. Passing FiberWire through the base of the ACL using a suture passer. **A.** The suture passer is used to then feed the high-strength suture **(B)** through the base of the ACL.

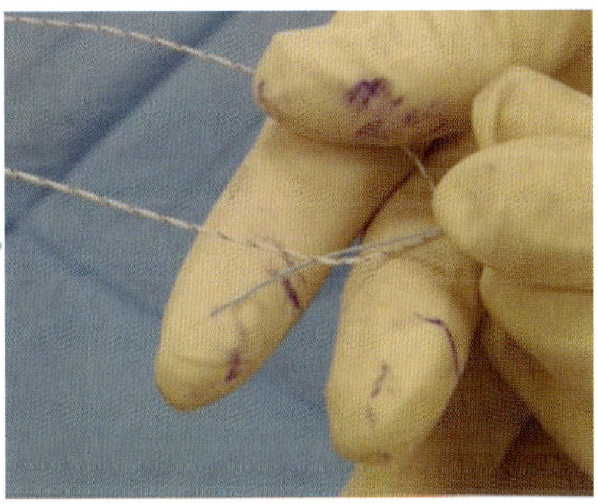

Figure 33.7. A loop is made to pull the limb of suture through the tibial bone tunnel.

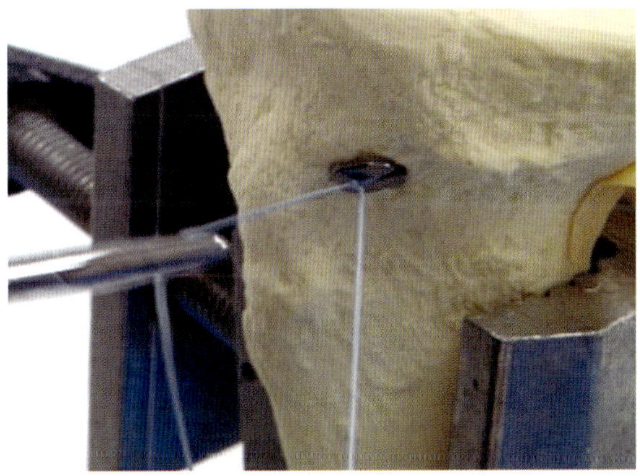

Figure 33.8. Tying the suture fixation across the tibial bone bridge. This can be done with, or without, a button as depicted.

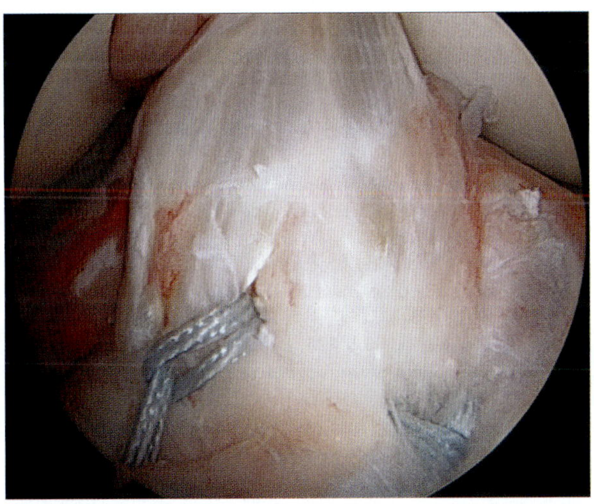

Figure 33.9. Final screw and suture fixation used to secure type III tibial eminence fractures.

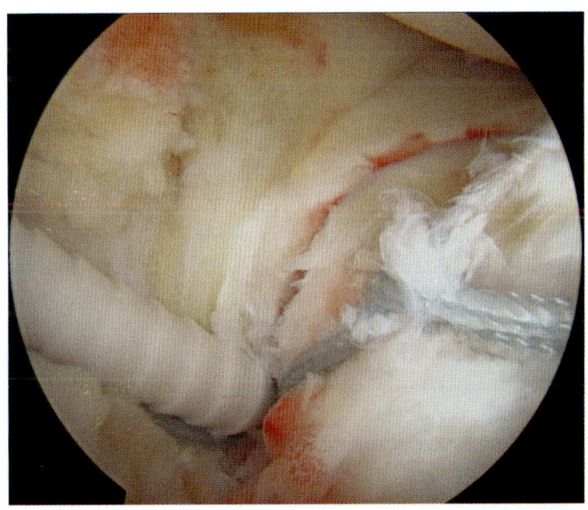

Figure 33.10. After threading the high-strength suture through anchors, the anchors are secured to the tibia, anterior to the fracture site, angled anterior to posterior.

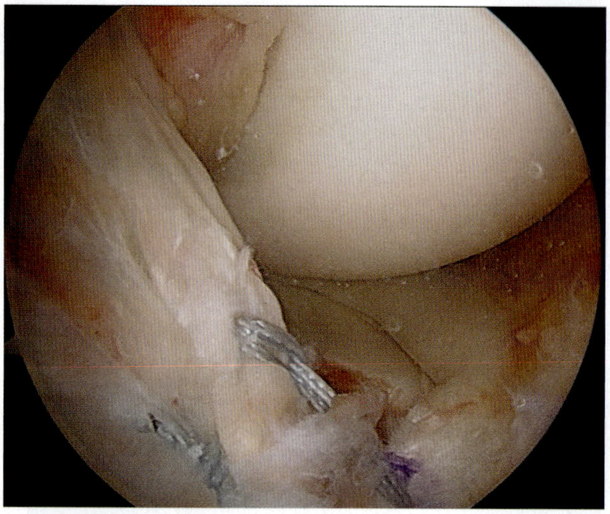

Figure 33.11. Final screw and anchor fixation used to secure type IV tibial eminence fractures.

REHABILITATION

After surgical repair, outcomes are almost uniformly excellent, with most patients returning to normal functional range of motion and activity levels within 3 to 4 months after injury when following an appropriate physical therapy and range-of-motion program. Although some stretch of the ligament occurs, most knees are stable after fixation and healing of a tibial eminence fracture.

Residual laxity is one of the most common complications and has been reported with both operative[14,33] and nonoperative[11,16,22] treatment of all fracture patterns. Laxity is increased in patients with types III and IV fractures,[25] highlighting the importance of surgical fixation, but functional outcomes remain similar in both non/minimally displaced fractures and significantly displaced fracture patterns. Anterior laxity may be due, in part, to interstitial elongation of the ACL at the time of injury[13] and/or soft tissue interposition that impedes fracture reduction.[36] Despite the presence of objective residual laxity, many researchers have found that most patients have no complaints of instability.[10,16,33,34] Residual laxity may be asymptomatic because preservation of proprioceptive feedback allows normal neuromuscular control of the knee.[6]

Another potential complication of tibial eminence fracture care is loss of range of motion. Loss of extension may arise from malunion or a mechanical block due to interposition of the intermeniscal ligament. Alternatively, arthrofibrosis alone secondary to immobilization may result in a decreased range of motion.[1] Early mobilization may help minimize the risk of arthrofibrosis.[27] Additionally, concomitant injuries of the collateral ligaments and meniscus are not uncommon in adolescents and adults. These injuries must be addressed during treatment for optimal results.

Last, given the potential severity of iatrogenic growth disturbance, physeal-sparing techniques are recommended to fix tibial spine fractures in skeletally immature patients.[35,36]

PEARLS TO AVOID PITFALLS

- To avoid misdiagnosis of fracture classification, a true lateral radiograph is necessary.
- Early treatment, secure fixation, and early mobilization can help avoid complications such as arthrofibrosis and loss of knee extension.

For those who prefer screw fixation:

- Midpatellar portals allow good visualization and easy placement of the screw perpendicular to the fracture site.
- Provisional fixation of the fracture fragment with K-wires before final fixation can help maintain reduction.
- Fixation can be aided by use of a washer when the tibial eminence fracture is thin or has slight comminution.

For those who prefer suture fixation:

- The use of cannulated ACL guides allows for easy passage of sutures from distal to proximal into the joint.
- In comminuted (type IV) fractures, use arthroscopic shoulder fixation techniques for the knee: Pass the sutures through the base of the ACL (as one would secure the capsule and labrum for a shoulder) and secure with shoulder anchors on the proximal tibia anterior to the fracture site.

REFERENCES

1. Meyers M, McKeever F. Fracture of the intercondylar eminence of the tibia. *J Bone Joint Surg Am.* 1959;41-A(2):209–220; discussion 220–222.
2. Fyfe IS, Jackson JP. Tibial intercondylar fractures in children: a review of the classification and the treatment of mal-union. *Injury.* 1981;13(2):165–169.
3. Meyers MH, McKeever FM. Fracture of the intercondylar eminence of the tibia. *J Bone Joint Surg Am.* 1970;52(8):1677–1684.
4. McLennan JG. Lessons learned after second-look arthroscopy in type III fractures of the tibial spine. *J Pediatr Orthop.* 1995;15(1): 59–62.
5. Beaty JH, Kumar A. Fractures about the knee in children. *J Bone Joint Surg Am.* 1994;76(12):1870–1880.
6. Ahmad CS, Stein BE, Jeshuran W, et al. Anterior cruciate ligament function after tibial eminence fracture in skeletally mature patients. *Am J Sports Med.* 2001;29(3):339–345.
7. Molander ML, Wallin G, Wikstad I. Fracture of the intercondylar eminence of the tibia: a review of 35 patients. *J Bone Joint Surg Br.* 1981;63-B(1):89–91.
8. Tudisco C, Giovarruscio R, Febo A, et al. Intercondylar eminence avulsion fracture in children: long-term follow-up of 14 cases at the end of skeletal growth. *J Pediatr Orthop B.* 2010;19(5):403–408.
9. Zionts LE. Fractures and dislocations about the knee. In: Green NE, Swiontkowski MF, eds. *Skeletal Trauma in Children.* Philadelphia, PA: Saunders; 2003:452–455.
10. Willis RB, Blokker C, Stoll TM, et al. Long-term follow-up of anterior tibial eminence fractures. *J Pediatr Orthop.* 1993;13(3):361–364.
11. Wilfinger C, Castellani C, Raith J, et al. Nonoperative treatment of tibial spine fractures in children-38 patients with a minimum follow-up of 1 year. *J Orthop Trauma.* 2009;23(7):519–524.
12. Kendall NS, Hsu SY, Chan KM. Fracture of the tibial spine in adults and children. A review of 31 cases. *J Bone Joint Surg Br.* 1992;74(6):848–852.
13. Geissler WB, Matthews DE. Arthroscopic suture fixation of displaced tibial eminence fractures. *Orthopedics.* 1993;16(3):331–333.

14. Kocher MS, Foreman ES, Micheli LJ. Laxity and functional outcome after arthroscopic reduction and internal fixation of displaced tibial spine fractures in children. *Arthroscopy.* 2003;19(10):1085–1090.
15. Hunter RE, Willis JA. Arthroscopic fixation of avulsion fractures of the tibial eminence: technique and outcome. *Arthroscopy.* 2004; 20(2):113–121.
16. Baxter MP, Wiley JJ. Fractures of the tibial spine in children. An evaluation of knee stability. *J Bone Joint Surg Br.* 1988;70(2): 228–230.
17. Accousti WK, Willis RB. Tibial eminence fractures. *Orthop Clin North Am.* 2003;34(3):365–375.
18. Roberts JM. Fractures of the condyles of the tibia. An anatomical and clinical end-result study of one hundred cases. *J Bone Joint Surg Am.* 1968;50(8):1505–1521.
19. Roberts JM. Operative treatment of fractures about the knee. *Orthop Clin North Am.* 1990;21(2):365–379.
20. Smillie IS. *Injuries of the Knee Joint.* 4th ed. Edinburgh, Scotland: Churchill Livingstone; 1973:155–156.
21. Lowe J, Chaimsky G, Freedman A, et al. The anatomy of tibial eminence fractures: arthroscopic observations following failed closed reduction. *J Bone Joint Surg Am.* 2002;84-A(11):1933–1938.
22. Janarv PM, Westblad P, Johansson C, et al. Long-term follow-up of anterior tibial spine fractures in children. *J Pediatr Orthop.* 1995; 15(1):63–68.
23. Senekovic V, Veselko M. Anterograde arthroscopic fixation of avulsion fractures of the tibial eminence with a cannulated screw: five-year results. *Arthroscopy.* 2003;19(1):54–61.
24. Kocher MS, Micheli LJ, Gerbino P, et al. Tibial eminence fractures in children: prevalence of meniscal entrapment. *Am J Sports Med.* 2003;31(3):404–407.
25. Gans I, Baldwin KD, Ganley TJ. Treatment and management outcomes of tibial eminence fractures in pediatric patients: a systematic review. *Am J Sports Med.* 2013;42(7):1743–1750.
26. Hapa O, Barber FA, Suner G, et al. Biomechanical comparison of tibial eminence fracture fixation with high-strength suture, EndoButton, and suture anchor. *Arthroscopy.* 2012;28(5):681–687.
27. Patel NM, Park MJ, Sampson NR, et al. Tibial eminence fractures in children: earlier posttreatment mobilization results in improved outcomes. *J Pediatr Orthop.* 2012;32(2):139–144.
28. Vander Have KL, Ganley TJ, Kocher MS, et al. Arthrofibrosis after surgical fixation of tibial eminence fractures in children and adolescents. *Am J Sports Med.* 2010;38(2):298–301.
29. Bong MR, Romero A, Kubiak E, et al. Suture versus screw fixation of displaced tibial eminence fractures: a biomechanical comparison. *Arthroscopy.* 2005;21(10):1172–1176.
30. Eggers AK, Becker C, Weimann A, et al. Biomechanical evaluation of different fixation methods for tibial eminence fractures. *Am J Sports Med.* 2007;35(3):404–410.
31. Mahar AT, Duncan D, Oka R, et al. Biomechanical comparison of four different fixation techniques for pediatric tibial eminence avulsion fractures. *J Pediatr Orthop.* 2008;28(2):159–162.
32. Gans I, Babatunde OM, Ganley TJ. Hybrid fixation of tibial eminence fractures in skeletally immature patients. *Arthroscopy Techniques.* 2013;2(3):e237–e242.
33. Perugia D, Basiglini L, Vadala A, et al. Clinical and radiological results of arthroscopically treated tibial spine fractures in childhood. *Int Orthop.* 2009;33(1):243–248.
34. Wiley JJ, Baxter MP. Tibial spine fractures in children. *Clin Orthop Relat Res.* 1990;(255):54–60.
35. Ahn JH, Lee YS, Lee DH, et al. Arthroscopic physeal sparing all inside repair of the tibial avulsion fracture in the anterior cruciate ligament: technical note. *Arch Orthop Trauma Surg.* 2008;128(11): 1309–1312.
36. Ahn JH, Yoo JC. Clinical outcome of arthroscopic reduction and suture for displaced acute and chronic tibial spine fractures. *Knee Surg Sports Traumatol Arthrosc.* 2005;13(2):116–121.

CHAPTER

34

Lauren E. Lamont
Matthew R. Garner
Roger F. Widmann

Salter-Harris Distal Femur and Proximal Tibia Fractures

INTRODUCTION

Knee injuries in adolescents commonly result in fractures of either the distal femoral or proximal tibial physis. When abnormal loads are sustained by maturing bone, the weaker physis fails more commonly than the surrounding ligaments and musculotendinous units. The Salter-Harris classification describes these patterns of injury. The severity of injury and the Salter-Harris classification often correlate with the risk of growth arrest. Resultant growth arrest may result in either leg length discrepancy or angular deformity of the knee due to the large contribution of these physes to lower limb growth.

The Salter-Harris classification ranges from types I to V (Fig. 34.1). Salter-Harris I is a transphyseal fracture involving the hypertrophic and calcified zones that tends to have a good prognosis when nondisplaced. When the transphyseal component of the fracture exits through the metaphysis, it is classified as a Salter-Harris II. The metaphyseal fragment is called the *Thurston-Holland fragment*; the periosteum is usually intact on the metaphyseal side and these fractures tend to heal well. A Salter-Harris III fracture is an intra-articular fracture as the transphyseal fracture exits the epiphysis. The reserve and proliferative zones of the physis are usually involved. These fractures usually need operative intervention to ensure an anatomic reduction of the joint surface. When the transphyseal fracture traverses the epiphysis, the physis, and exits in the metaphysis, it is a Salter-Harris IV. In these fractures, all four zones of the physis are disrupted. As with Salter-Harris III fractures, these fractures must be anatomically reduced to prevent bony bridge formation. Salter-Harris IV fractures have a worse prognosis if there is unreduced articular displacement. Last, a Salter-Harris V is a crush injury to the physis; this diagnosis is generally made retrospectively after growth arrest is seen. Here we review the physeal fractures of the distal femur and proximal tibia.

DISTAL FEMUR FRACTURES

Distal femoral physeal fractures in children may be difficult to treat and are associated with a high rate of complications including growth arrest.[1] Close follow-up is necessary to detect early angular deformity that may result from a partial growth arrest. The greater the severity of fracture and displacement across the physis, the higher the risk of growth arrest.[2] There should be a low threshold for obtaining computed tomography (CT) or magnetic resonance imaging (MRI) of the affected physis when a bony bridge is suspected in order to allow early intervention.

Anatomy

The distal femur is the most rapidly growing physis in the human body and the first epiphysis to ossify. In a full-term infant, the distal femoral ossification center is usually present at birth. The distal femur contributes approximately 70% of the growth of the femur and 40% of the overall limb.[3,4] The distal femur's average growth is 1 cm a year until closure between 14 and 16 years of age in girls and 16 to 18 years of age in boys.[5]

The majority of the distal femoral epiphysis is covered by the articular cartilage and articulates with the patella and proximal tibia. The distal femoral physis is an extra-articular structure; the capsule originates distal to the physis from the epiphysis. The undulating contour of the physis may be more resistant to shear forces; however, when shearing injury does occur, there is greater risk of growth arrest. Liu et al.[6] described the lateral and anteromedial peripheral notches located at the metaphyseal–epiphyseal junction of the distal femur. Additionally, three major undulations within the epiphysis were identified across cadaveric specimens. These ridges were identified centrally, laterally, and medially and found to decrease with age especially in the central ridge.

The stabilizing medial and lateral collateral ligaments originate from the distal femoral epiphysis. The gastrocnemius takes its origin from the posterior surface of the epiphysis. Whereas in adults the ligaments may be injured due to varus and valgus stress on the knee, in skeletally immature patients, the distal femoral physis is more commonly injured.

Multiple neurovascular structures are at risk with injury to the distal femur. Most vulnerable are the popliteal artery and peroneal and posterior tibial nerves. The popliteal artery may be injured by the metaphyseal spike of distal femoral fracture. This vulnerability is in part due to the tethering of the artery

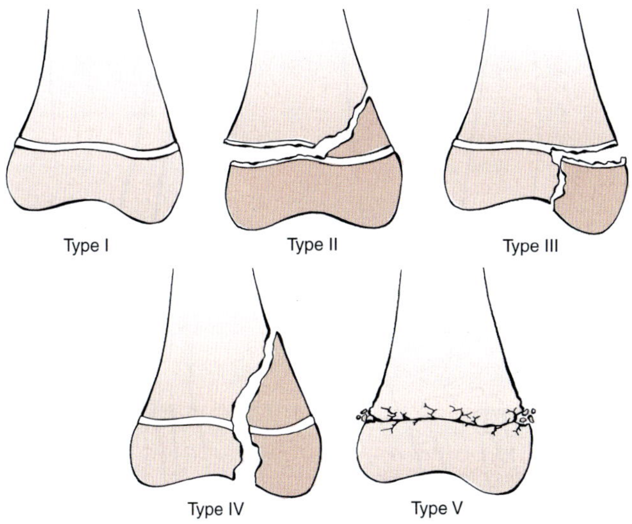

Figure 34.1. Illustration showing the Salter-Harris classification for physeal fractures.

above at the adductor hiatus and distally by the fibrous tissue over the soleus muscle. Injuries may lead to thrombosis or bleeding from intimal tears. Displaced physeal fractures also have a risk of compartment syndrome, as arterial injury is more likely to occur. In a series of distal femoral physeal fractures, compartment syndrome occurred in 1.3% of patients.[7] Injury to nervous structures may also occur with displacement. The posterior tibial and peroneal nerves form after the sciatic nerve branches in the popliteal space. Both are subject to traction injuries with displaced fractures. The incidence of peroneal nerve injuries was 7.3% in the same clinical series.[7]

Classification

The Salter Harris classification is commonly used and easily applied to these fractures. This classification can help dictate treatment as well as predict outcomes and rate of complications associated with individual fracture. The classification for distal femur fractures can be seen in Figure 34.1 and is defined as follows[8]:

A Salter-Harris I fracture is defined as a separation through the distal femoral physis with no involvement of either the metaphysis or the epiphysis. Salter-Harris II fractures are a separation through the distal femoral physis fracture exiting through the metaphysis. The resulting metaphyseal fragment is called the *Thurston-Holland fragment*. The portion of the physis that is "unprotected" by the Thurston-Holland fragment is at risk of growth arrest.

A Salter-Harris III is a physeal fracture in which the fracture line exits through the epiphysis and into the knee joint. Fractures of the medial femoral condyle that originate at the medial physis and exit into the notch have been compared to transitional fractures of the ankle given their relation to physeal closure.[9] Coronal shear fractures of the lateral condyles have also been described.[10] Salter-Harris IV injuries originate in the physis and the fracture exits through both the metaphysis (with a *Thurston-Holland fragment*) and the epiphysis. Salter-Harris V injuries are a crush injury to the physis and are unable to be definitively identified until resulting growth arrest manifests.

Epidemiology

Classification and displacement of distal femur physeal fractures has been shown to be predictive of overall outcome.[1] Overall, these fractures account for between 1.4% and 5.5% of all physeal injuries in children.[11–13] Of all fractures in children, these represent little more than 1%.[11]

Mechanism of Injury

Epidemiologic studies have shown that when physeal fractures of the distal femur occur in younger children, they are usually due to severe trauma or a high-energy injury.[13] However, Salter-Harris I and II fractures in older children and adolescents are generally related to lower energy injuries or sports-related activities.[2] For Salter-Harris I and II injuries, the knee is generally in a position of hyperextension with or without varus or valgus strain (Fig. 34.2).[5] Patients will usually present complaints of significant knee pain and have associated knee swelling.

A Salter-Harris II fracture is more likely when both compression and distraction forces occur across the knee. This simultaneously creates tension and compression sides to the fracture and metaphyseal failure occurs due to compressive shear.[14]

Salter-Harris type III fractures are relatively rare injuries compared with the more common Salter-Harris I and II. They can lead to poor outcomes but have similar mechanisms of injury. Fractures of the medial femoral condyle result from a valgus force on the knee. These fractures will demonstrate valgus laxity on presenting exam; this has been shown to resolve after fracture healing.[9] Coronal fractures involving the lateral femoral condyles result from a shear-type mechanism. The fracture types with an epiphyseal component such as a Salter-Harris III usually result in a larger effusion than types I and II injuries. Sports-related twisting or high-energy motor vehicle trauma can be the cause of a Salter-Harris IV. Similar to a Salter-Harris III, the patient will likely have a knee effusion due to the intra-articular component. The mechanism of a Salter-Harris V is unclear, but trauma causes a crush injury to the physis.

Diagnosis

For Salter-Harris I and II fractures that are nondisplaced, patients will present with localized tenderness to palpation at the level of the growth plate. An anatomic reference is that in the extended knee, the equator of the patella generally aligns with the physis unless the patient has significant patella baja or alta.[15] Given the extra-articular nature of this fracture, patients may have swelling but not a joint effusion. This contrasts with Salter-Harris III and IV fractures in which there will generally be an effusion. For all these fractures, range of motion as well as any varus or valgus stress will likely elicit pain. Pain with weight bearing will also be seen. Displaced fractures will have a more dramatic presentation with potential gross deformity of the knee in the direction of displacement.

Imaging

Careful inspection of the physis on plain radiographs is necessary in order to identify minimally displaced fractures. At presentation, Salter-Harris I radiographs may demonstrate a

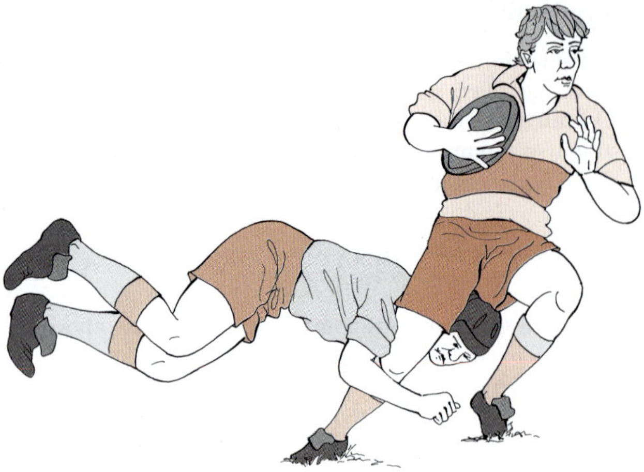

A

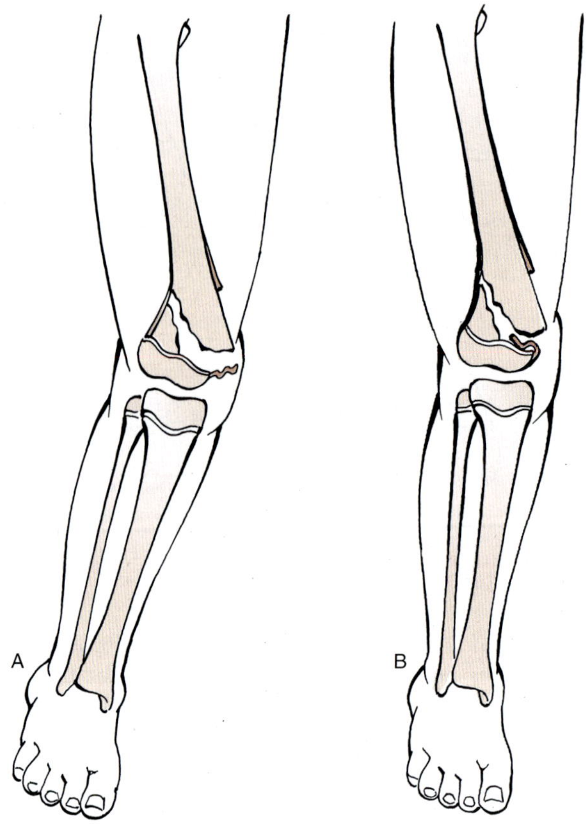

B

Figure 34.2. **A,B.** Valgus load causing injury to distal femoral physis.

widening or irregularity of the physis (Fig. 34.3). Sometimes a small fleck of bone may be evident adjacent to the physis. In nondisplaced fractures, the only sign of fracture may be periosteal reaction 2 to 3 weeks after the injury. Plain radiographs including anteroposterior, lateral, and oblique views of the knee are usually adequate for diagnosis. Although historically stress radiographs were used to document Salter-Harris I fractures, this has largely been abandoned. The impetus behind this shift in thinking is that given the nonoperative management of these injuries, the risk of stressing the physis and potentially causing additional injury to an already damaged physis is not indicated.[16] MRI has largely replaced stress radiographs and should be considered in any case of knee trauma, pain and swelling, and negative plain radiographs in order to confirm the diagnosis of a nondisplaced Salter-Harris I fracture.

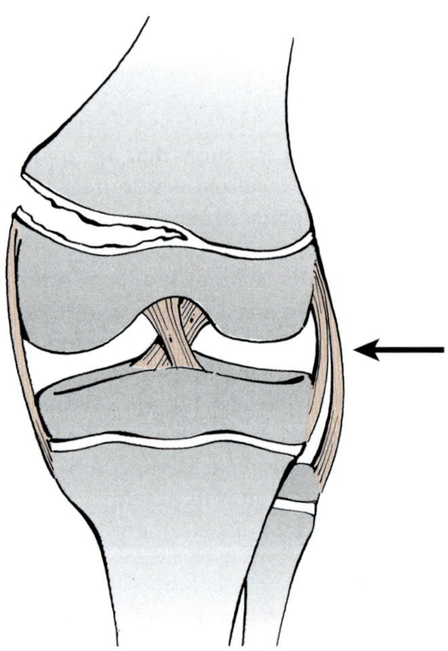

Figure 34.3. Asymmetrical physeal widening of the distal femoral physis representing a Salter-Harris I fracture.

For Salter-Harris II fractures, it is important to identify the metaphyseal component of these injuries, the size of which may influence surgical planning. MRI has been used to identify the frequency of posterior periosteal disruption in seemingly mild injuries. This posterior periosteal disruption was associated with a hyperextension mechanism of injury.[17]

Plain radiographs may not be sufficient for Salter-Harris III or IV fractures due to their intra-articular nature. The overlying patella may hide the epiphyseal component of the fracture, the displacement of which may not be adequately visualized on lateral imaging. Oblique radiographs will improve the sensitivity of assessing these fractures; however, radiographs have been shown to significantly underestimate displacement of Salter-Harris III fractures.[18,19] To most accurately determine the amount of articular step-off, a CT scan or MRI should be obtained. Advanced imaging has been shown to change surgical plan and is important given that many of these minimally displaced injuries are initially missed.[15]

Salter-Harris V fractures, as noted, are difficult to diagnose on imaging at time of initial presentation. These injuries are distinguished from their nondisplaced Salter-Harris I counterparts only in hindsight with growth arrest. It has been suggested that blurring of the bone structure around the physis may demonstrate a Salter-Harris V.[20] MRI may be helpful to identify physeal injury in the setting of negative plain films at the time of injury.

Treatment

Nondisplaced fractures should be managed with a long leg cast typically for 4 to 6 weeks. In patients with obese body habitus not amenable to long leg casting, and in very young patients, spica casting may be necessary.[15] Serial radiographs are important in order to identify displacement in a timely manner.

Displaced fractures must undergo gentle closed reduction under sedation. Reduction should be performed with longitudinal traction to minimize damage to the physis. Once anatomic reduction is achieved, it may be held with smooth crossed Kirschner wires (Fig. 34.4). Pins are typically placed in an antegrade manner from metaphysis across the physis into the epiphysis then bent to prevent pin migration. Avoiding entering through the joint also minimizes the risk of associated septic arthritis. Stability of fracture fixation should be confirmed through range of motion under fluoroscopy. Postoperatively, patients should be immobilized in a long leg cast until pin removal at 4 weeks. Two additional weeks of casting is generally prudent until allowing ambulation; however, this may vary based on age and healing potential.

Salter-Harris II treatment varies based on the size of the metaphyseal fragment. Nondisplaced fractures may be treated in a cast but must be followed closely to assess any interval displacement. Reduction should only be performed up to 7 to 10 days after injury in order to avoid risk of further traumatic injury

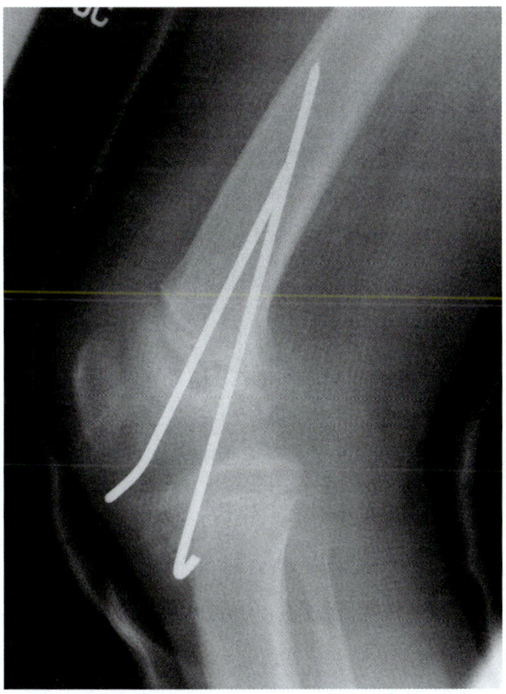

Figure 34.4. Distal femur physeal fracture with K-wire fixation.

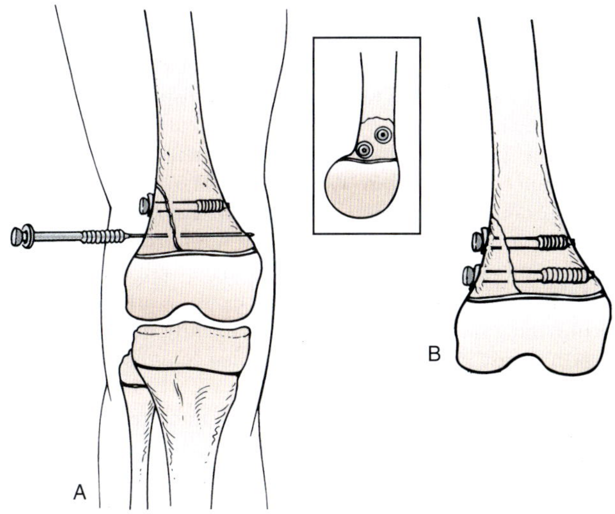

Figure 34.5. **A,B.** Fixation of a Salter-Harris II fracture with two cannulated screws across the metaphyseal fragment.

to the healing physis. Displaced Salter-Harris II fractures warrant closed or open reduction and pinning. If there is a large metaphyseal component, this may be transfixed, ideally, with two cannulated screws (Fig. 34.5). Transverse metaphyseal fixation with screws avoids crossing the physis and causing further injury to the traumatized growth plate. Postoperatively, patients should still be immobilized in a long leg cast in 20 to 30 degrees of flexion. In cases of significant soft tissue swelling and concern for a compartment syndrome or when arterial injury has occurred, apply a well-padded bivalved cast after definitive fixation.

The majority of Salter-Harris III fractures need reduction and fixation due to intra-articular nature of this fracture (see Fig. 34.1). Lippert et al.[18] asserted that if the fracture line is visible on x-ray, then it should be managed with open reduction internal fixation. This is due to the inherent instability of this fracture pattern, the intra-articular nature of the fracture, and the risk of growth arrest due to bony bridge formation without appropriate reduction and fixation. Anatomic reduction is essential, and only truly nondisplaced fractures as confirmed by axial imaging are amenable to cast immobilization.

As with Salter-Harris III fractures, Salter-Harris IV fractures should be managed with open reduction internal fixation in order to assess anatomic reduction of the epiphyseal component. When placing the transverse epiphyseal screw for fixation of the epiphyseal component, Wall and May[15] described a target triangle bordered by the growth plate, the intercondylar notch, and the trochlear groove for appropriate screw placement. It is important to avoid overpenetration of the screw tip which will cause soft tissue irritation over time.

Salter-Harris V fractures are managed nonoperatively, as the initial diagnosis is usually a nondisplaced Salter-Harris I unless abnormal physeal findings are noted and suspicion arises. The described treatment for these fractures is largely the treatment of the ultimate growth arrest as a result of the injury as opposed to the fracture itself. Skak[20] described the management of a 10-year-old female with a Salter-Harris V of the lateral distal femur that went on to growth arrest and a valgus deformity.

Outcomes

Growth disturbance is a common sequelae of distal femoral physeal fractures. Fractures that are displaced more than half of the diameter of the shaft are at greater risk for growth arrest.[21,22] In a meta-analysis of distal physeal fractures, growth disturbance was found in 36% of Salter-Harris I fractures.[23] It is important to follow the patient both radiographically and clinically to assess for growth arrest at 6 months intervals after injury. Any varus or valgus deformity may result due to medial or lateral growth arrest. On clinical exam, a knee flexion deformity may be a result of a bony deformity due to posterior growth arrest.[15] Pelvis obliquity and leg lengths on examination are also important to follow.

In a meta-analysis of distal physeal fractures, growth disturbance was found in 58% of Salter-Harris II, 49% of Salter-Harris III, and 64% of Salter-Harris IV fractures.[23] A retrospective study with 4-year follow-up of patients with Salter-Harris II injuries showed no complications for the nondisplaced injuries managed conservatively; however, there was a 70% complication rate for displaced fractures reduced under general anesthesia.[24]

Salter-Harris III and IV fractures can lead to poor outcomes; the literature has described complications including limb length discrepancy, angular deformity, knee flexion deformity, and posttraumatic arthritis. The outcomes for these intra-articular fractures are largely based on the degree of postoperative displacement, with poorer outcomes seen with greater displacement. Given the intra-articular nature of the injury, patients are at higher risk for posttraumatic osteoarthritis.

Patients who develop either limb length discrepancy or angular deformity after physeal fractures as a result of growth arrest may need secondary operative intervention. Although limb length discrepancies less than 2 cm are generally well tolerated, larger discrepancies may require contralateral epiphysiodesis or limb lengthening. Angular deformity due to partial growth arrest may be corrected by guided growth if there is sufficient growth remaining.

PROXIMAL TIBIA FRACTURES

Fractures of the proximal tibial physis are rare and mechanism of injury can vary widely. For these reasons, evaluation and treatment of these patients often requires an experienced practitioner with a high index of suspicion. Osseous injuries may involve the articular surface of the proximal tibia or may be extra-articular and involve the proximal tibial physis or metaphysis. Treatments vary based on the severity and location, and sequela may not manifest for several years after the initial injury. In this section, we specifically discuss injuries involving the proximal tibial physis.

Anatomy

The proximal tibia extends from the metaphyseal flare to the articular surface. It includes the anterior and posterior tibial spines or intercondylar eminences, which, prior to ossification, are cartilaginous structures.[25] This area also includes the tibial tubercle, which develops as an anterior extension of the proximal tibial physis in utero.[26] Pertinent anatomy and a discussion of injuries to these structures have been covered in Chapters 31 to 33 and an in-depth discussion of the anatomy of the physis will be covered in Chapter 37.

Tibial growth occurs primarily in the first 5 years of life and then slows until puberty when it accelerates again. The epiphyseal ossification center can be visualized on radiographs between the first and third months of life. Overall, this center accounts for 50% to 60% of the overall length of the tibia.[3,4] This corresponds to approximately 16 cm in females and 18 cm in males. Closure of the growth plate occurs in a posterior to anterior direction and is complete by age 13 to 15 years in girls and 15 to 18 years in boys.[27]

Anatomically, the proximal tibia is surrounded by both osseous and soft tissue structures. Laterally, the fibular head and neck abut the proximal tibial epiphysis. The fibular collateral ligament, popliteus muscle and tendon, semimembranosus, medial collateral ligament, and the structures of the pes anserinus form the surrounding soft tissue envelope without direct insertion into the epiphysis.[28,29]

Of particular importance when considering fractures of the proximal tibia is the potential for significant vascular injury as displaced injuries correlate with knee dislocation in adult. As with the distal femur, the popliteal artery courses directly behind the proximal tibial physis before branching to anterior tibial, the posterior tibial, and the peroneal artery (Fig. 34.6). Just distal to the physis, the popliteal artery is tethered as the anterior tibial artery passes through the interosseous membrane and the tibial artery passes beneath the soleus. Posterior displacement of the tibial metaphysis at this level has been implicated in injury of the popliteal artery. Although rare, this diagnosis can be devastating and leads to an increased risk of compartment syndrome, multiple surgical procedures, permanent neurologic disability, or even amputation.[30–32]

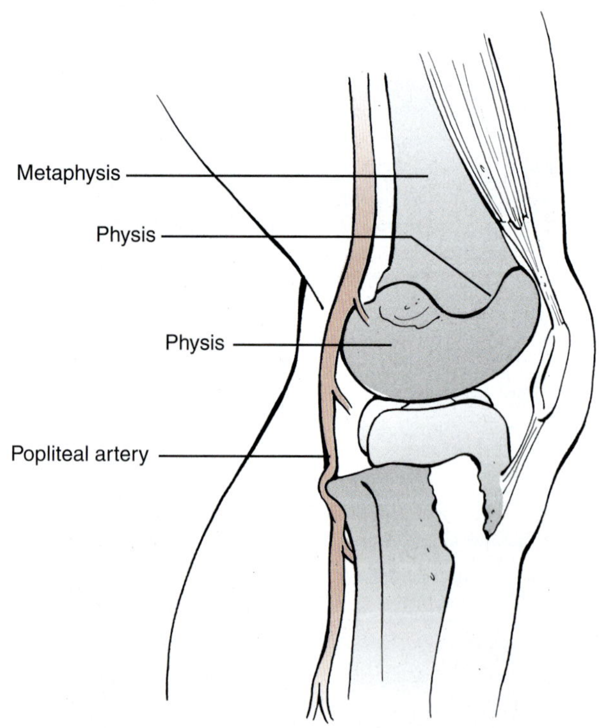

Figure 34.6. Relationship of proximal tibial physis to vascular structures.

The tibial and common peroneal nerves are also in close proximity to the tibial physis and have the potential to be damaged with fracture displacement. When evaluating patients with a suspected physeal injury of the proximal tibia, it is essential to document pedal pulses and ankle-brachial indices. Advanced arterial imaging such as magnetic resonance angiography (MRA) or a formal angiogram should be considered if there is any concern for vascular compromise. A careful sensory and motor exam as well as assessment of compartments should also be performed.

Classification

Similar to fractures of the distal femoral physis, the most common classification system used for proximal tibial growth plate fractures is the Salter-Harris Classification (see Fig. 34.1).[8] When considering fractures of the proximal tibia that include the physis, most are considered either Salter-Harris I or II injuries. Salter-Harris I fractures are a separation through the proximal tibial physis with no involvement of either the metaphysis or the epiphysis. Of the Salter-Harris I fractures, 50% are nondisplaced.[14] Salter-Harris II fractures traverse the physis and then exit obliquely through the metaphysis.[8] Salter-Harris III fractures involve the physis but exit proximally and extend into the knee joint. These fractures may produce an articular step-off, as may Salter-Harris IV fracture that extend from the joint, through the physis, and exit through the metaphysis. Salter-Harris V injuries are rare and represent a crush injury to the physis.

A triplane variant has been described in the literature and like its ankle counterpart can be attributed to the asymmetrical closure of the proximal tibial physis.[17,33–36] These are rare injuries and present as a Salter-Harris II injury on lateral films and a Salter-Harris III on anteroposterior radiographs.

Other authors have advocated a fracture classification system based on mechanism of injury and fracture displacement as a means of anticipating necessary treatment and associated complications.[2,37] Using this method, hyperextension injures result in posterior displacement of the distal fragment and therefore results in the highest risk to the posterior vascular structures. Further, varus and valgus injuries often result in an intact metaphyseal fragment and may be associated with asymmetrical growth arrest. Flexion-type injuries are typically seen in late adolescents due to the posterior to anterior ossification of the physis (Fig. 34.7).[27]

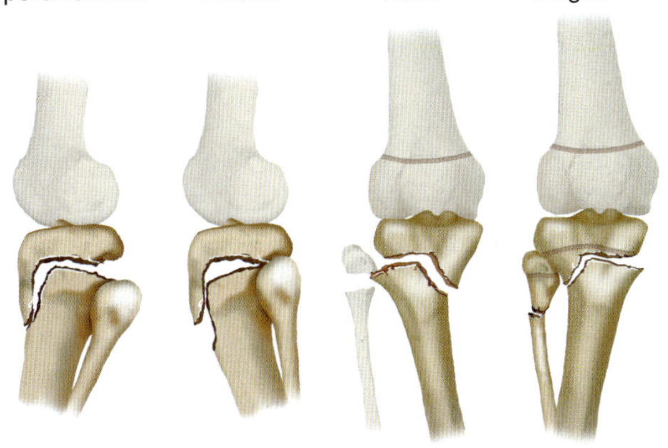

Figure 34.7. Hyperextension, flexion, varus, and valgus injuries to the proximal tibial growth plate.

Epidemiology

As mentioned previously, the incidence of proximal tibial physeal and epiphyseal fracture is low. The literature reports that these injuries represent only 1% to 3% of all physeal injuries.[11–13,29] However, despite its rarity, the injury is one that should not be missed. Patients are typically adolescents who are near maturity and who are injured during athletic events.

Mechanism of Injury

Mechanism of injury to the proximal tibial physis can often be determined based on the fracture pattern and are often the result of athletic activities or high-energy trauma such as a motor vehicle accident.[29,38] For example, a hyperextension injury typically begins at the posterior margin of the physis and typically results in a Salter-Harris I fracture with posterior displacement of the metaphyseal fragment. In an older adolescent whose growth plates have begun to close, flexion injuries also result in a Salter-Harris I fracture with propagation from the tibial tubercle, where the physis remains cartilaginous, to the posterior physis where closure has begun.[27]

Salter-Harris II to IV fractures, however, are often the result of either a varus or valgus load but may also be secondary to direct trauma. A flexion-type Salter-Harris II fracture has also been described in which there is a tibial tubercle avulsion in association with a transphyseal fracture.[27,37,39,40] These injuries tend to occur in older adolescents whose proximal tibial growth plates are near closure. Compression fractures of the growth plate, or Salter-Harris V injuries, tend to be the result of high-energy axial loading to the tibia and are uncommon.

Diagnosis

Children with fractures about the proximal tibial physis will often present to the emergency room immediately following injury with complaints of localized pain about the knee or proximal tibia. Oftentimes, these injuries occur during athletic activities and may be confused with ligamentous injury. Clinicians should have a low threshold to obtain radiographs to rule out osseous injuries in these instances and to obtain an MRI if radiographs are nonrevealing and suspicion remains high. A careful history should be taken to determine the position of the limb at the time of injury, as this may provide important insight regarding the final diagnosis.

Typically, at the time of initial presentation, patients are unable to weight bear and may require assistive devices such as crutches. Soft tissue swelling is common and a knee effusion may be present. Focal tenderness at the level of the physis may be present, but it is not uncommon to have diffuse tenderness about the proximal tibia and knee. Deformity at the physis may be easily visualized, particularly in high-energy injuries with significant displacement, but the fracture may also be partially or completely reduced prior to presentation. For this reason, it is often difficult to determine the overall zone of injury. Pulses and compartments should be palpated and an ankle-brachial index should be obtained to assess for injury to the popliteal artery. A careful neurologic exam should also be performed.

Imaging

Standard anteroposterior and lateral radiographs typically provide adequate information to make a diagnosis and form a plan of care. As with all physeal injuries, attention should be paid to subtle characteristics of the radiographs such as asymmetrical widening of the physis or significant local soft tissue swelling. Care should be taken to ensure there is no intra-articular involvement, as this may prompt axial imaging to assess for articular incongruity. As with distal femur fractures, stress radiographs are no longer recommended, as they may cause additional injury to the physis.[16] When plain radiographs are negative and significant injury is suspected, an MRI should be obtained.

If there is any concern for vascular injury, a CT or MRA is indicated to assess the patency of the popliteal artery and its major branches. It should also be noted that nondisplaced Salter-Harris I fractures and compression injuries (Salter-Harris V Fractures) to the physis are often not detectable on initial injury radiographs. In such instances, follow-up radiographs may show periosteal reaction indicating that an injury occurred; however, physeal damage may not be identified until growth arrest and deformity occurs (Fig. 34.8). MRI may

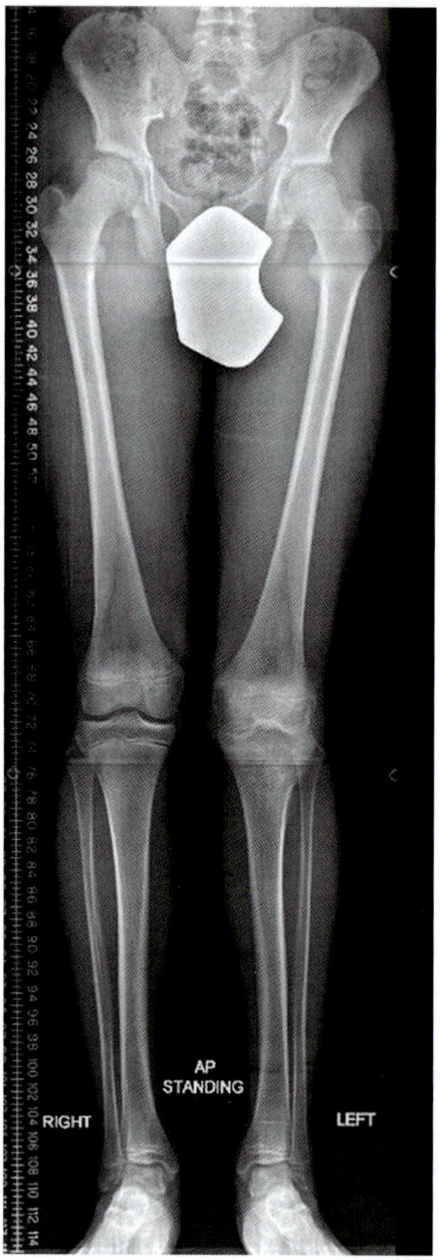

A

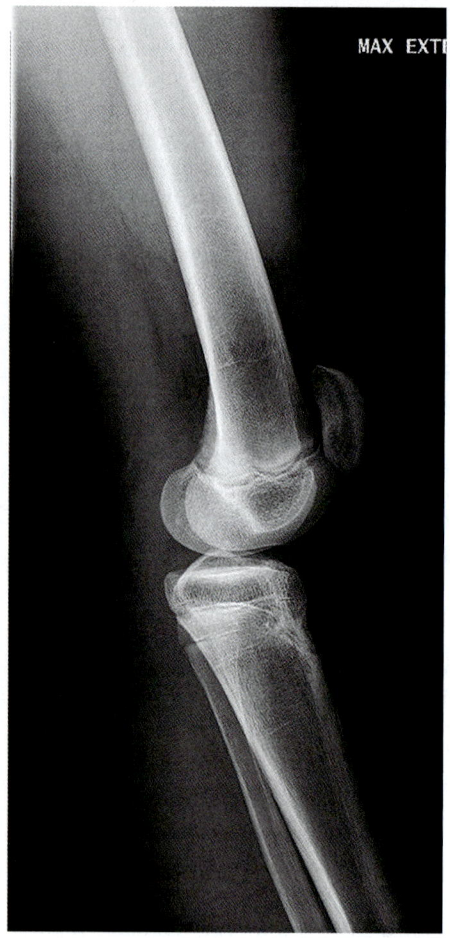

B

Figure 34.8. A,B. Salter-Harris V proximal tibia fracture resulting in recurvatum and deformity.

provide evidence of a physeal injury that cannot be seen on plain radiographs.

Treatment

As with any fracture, the goals for treatment are to obtain and maintain anatomic alignment. It is also critical to try to prevent further damage to the physis. Stable and nondisplaced injuries can typically be treated with a long leg cylinder cast for a period of 4 to 6 weeks. New radiographs should be taken 1 week after injury to ensure that no displacement has occurred and again at 3 to 4 weeks to ensure evidence of healing. Intra-articular injuries may require closer follow-up in the early postinjury period to ensure that articular incongruity and/or displacement does not develop.

Displaced Salter-Harris I and II fractures can occasionally be treated with closed reduction and casting; however, these patients need to be monitored very closely for evidence of displacement. Most authors advocate closed or open reduction and surgical fixation of displaced fractures to limit the likelihood of loss of reduction.[2,19,37] During the reduction maneuver, an image intensifier should be used and traction should be performed to minimize further damage to the physis. Based on the direction of displacement, gentle varus, valgus, flexion, or extension is typically required. If gentle closed reduction cannot be obtained with 1 or 2 attempts under sedation or general anesthesia, an open reduction should be performed.

In contrast to Salter-Harris I and II fractures, displaced Salter-Harris III fractures require open reduction to restore joint congruity. Internal fixation should be based on the fracture pattern, but care should be taken to avoid further damage to the physis. Fixation may be performed with either pins or screws, with pins being more commonly used in younger patients and screws in older patients.

After reduction is obtained, smooth, crossed transphyseal pins can be used to stabilize the fracture and to limit further insult to the physis. For some Salter-Harris II fractures with a large metaphyseal fragment, cannulated screw fixation across the metaphysis may also be warranted. Postoperatively, a well-padded long leg cylinder cast can be applied in 20 to 30 degrees of knee flexion. For flexion injuries, extension of the knee may provide additional stability but should be used with caution as the cast will have a tendency to slip distally. In cases with significant hyperextension and risk of vascular injury, fixation with pins of these fractures is indicated to stabilize and avoid necessitating a constrictive molded cast. A gentle varus or valgus mold may also be applied to the cast in cases of varus or valgus injuries. If there is concern for soft tissue swelling, the cast may be bivalved or a posterior splint may be used instead. These patients should be monitored in an inpatient setting for 24 to 48 hours with frequent compartment and neurovascular assessments. Pins should be removed in the office at the 3- to 4-week postoperative visit. Immobilization can be discontinued after 6 weeks followed by progressive weight bearing.

Salter-Harris V fractures of the proximal tibial physis are, by definition, nondisplaced and stable. These injuries are typically only diagnosed after 2 to 3 weeks when periosteal reaction is seen at the level of the physis. Occasionally, in younger patients, diagnosis is delayed until growth arrest is noted. Treatment of Salter-Harris V fractures requires a high index of suspicion and typically requires 4 to 6 weeks of immobilization in a long leg cylinder cast at 20 to 30 degrees of knee flexion, followed by progressive weight bearing and return to activity.

Outcomes

Closed injuries to the proximal tibial physis typically occur in older children and adolescents, and the proximal tibia contributes less to the overall growth of the lower extremity when compared to the distal femur.[29] These attributes limit the opportunity for issues with physeal growth arrest and angular deformities. Patients who tend to have poor outcomes include those who are younger, those who have neurovascular injury secondary to fracture displacement, and those to suffer high-energy injuries such as lawn mower accidents. Patients with low-energy or minimally displaced fractures can also have poor outcomes due to developing recurvatum deformity.[2,19,29,32]

Similar to fractures of the distal femoral physis, angular deformity and limb length discrepancy may result from an injury to the proximal tibial growth plate. Although it is not possible to determine the extent of deformity to expect at the time of injury, parents should be counseled that operative treatment may be required in the future. Such interventions may include ipsilateral hemiepiphysiodesis, contralateral epiphysiodesis, guided growth, corrective osteotomy, or limb lengthening procedures.

PROXIMAL TIBIA METAPHYSEAL FRACTURE (COZEN FRACTURE)

Although not involving the proximal tibial physis and not common injuries in children, fractures of the proximal tibia metaphysis deserve mention. These injuries are typically a minimally displaced, valgus greenstick fracture occurring in children ages 2 to 5 years and caused by low-energy trauma.[2,19] The fracture line typically extends two-thirds of the way across the metaphysis and appears innocuous. Initial treatment includes reduction of the fracture and application of a long leg cast with the knee in full extension and a varus mold. An image intensifier can be helpful, and if a reduction cannot be obtained by closed means, there may be interposition of periosteum or pes anserinus.[2,41]

Patients with this injury need to be followed well beyond evidence of fracture healing, as the most common complication is progressive valgus deformity over the first 24 months.[42,43] For this reason, it is essential to counsel families on the importance of follow-up. The cause of the valgus deformity is unknown, but it is thought to arise from localized hyperemia and relative overgrowth of the proximal tibial growth plate.[43] Osteotomy is rarely required, as the deformity tends to spontaneously correct over several years and osteotomy has resulted in recurrent deformity.[44–49] Guided growth has been used more recently in the setting of persistent valgus deformity (Fig. 34.9).

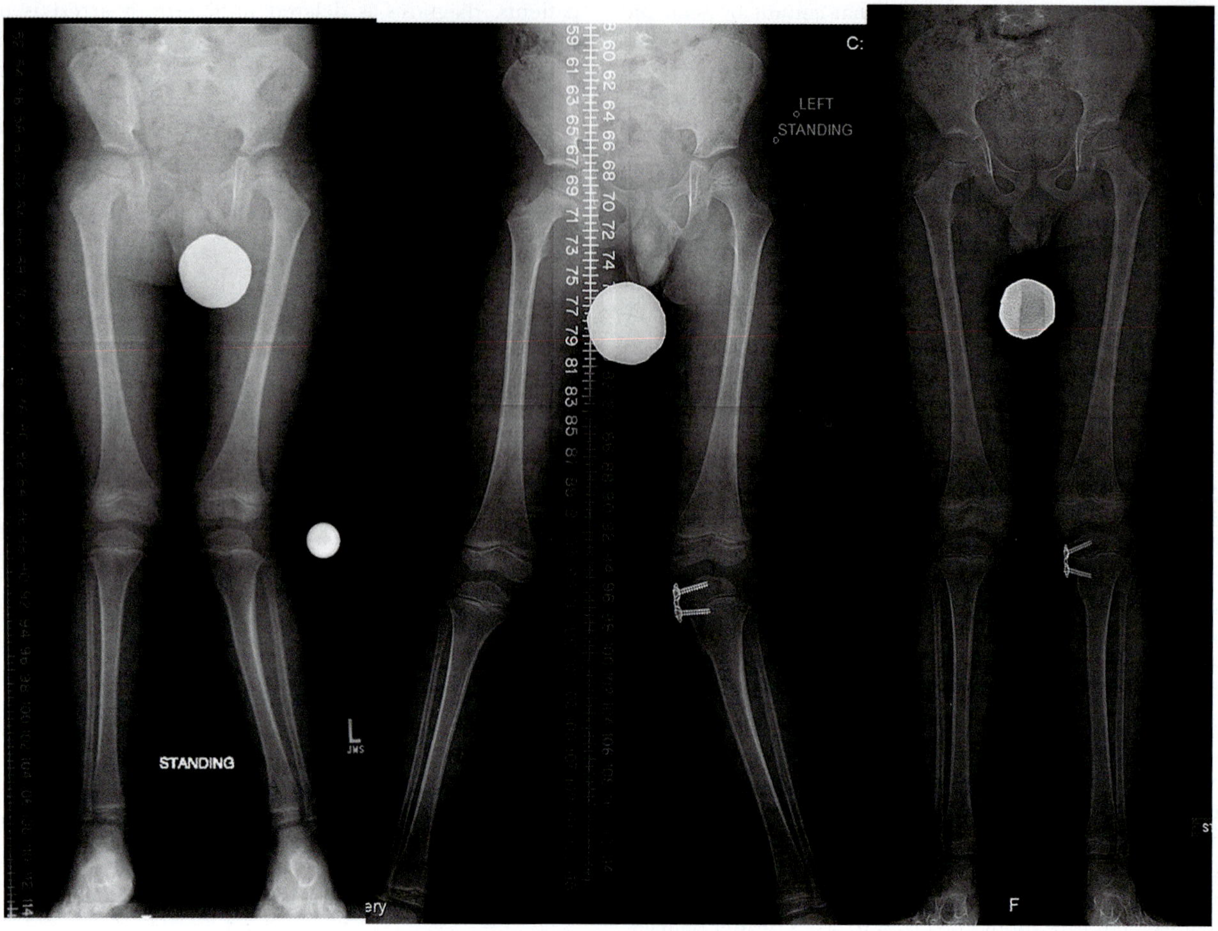

Figure 34.9. Radiographs of a patient with a proximal tibial Cozen fracture, subsequent valgus deformity, and correction of deformity with guided growth.

REFERENCES

1. Arkader A, Warner WC Jr, Horn BD, et al. Predicting the outcome of physeal fractures of the distal femur. *J Pediatr Orthop.* 2007;27(6):703–708.
2. Zionts L. Fractures and dislocations about the knee. In: Green N, Swiontkowski M, eds. *Skeletal Trauma in Children.* 4th ed. Philadelphia, PA: Saunders; 2009:425–469.
3. Anderson M, Green WT, Messner MB. The classic. Growth and predictions of growth in the lower extremities by Margaret Anderson, M.S., William T. Green, M.D. and Marie Blail Messner, A.B. from the Journal of Bone and Joint Surgery, 45A:1, 1963. *Clin Orthop Relat Res.* 1978;(136):7–21.
4. Pritchett JW. Longitudinal growth and growth-plate activity in the lower extremity. *Clin Orthop Relat Res.* 1992;(275):274–279.
5. Beaty JH, Kumar A. Fractures about the knee in children. *J Bone Joint Surg Am.* 1994;76(12):1870–1880.
6. Liu RW, Armstrong DG, Levine AD, et al. An anatomic study of the distal femoral epiphysis. *J Pediatr Orthop.* 2013;33(7):743–749.
7. Eid AM, Hafez MA. Traumatic injuries of the distal femoral physis. Retrospective study on 151 cases. *Injury.* 2002;33(3):251–255.
8. Salter R, Harris R. Injuries involving the epiphyseal plate. *J Bone Joint Surg Am.* 1963;45:587–622.
9. McKissick RC, Gilley JS, DeLee JC. Salter-Harris type III fractures of the medial distal femoral physis—a fracture pattern related to the closure of the growth plate: report of 3 cases and discussion of pathogenesis. *Am J Sports Med.* 2008;36(3):572–576.
10. Sabharwal S, Henry P, Behrens F. Two cases of missed Salter-Harris III coronal plane fracture of the lateral femoral condyle. *Am J Orthop (Belle Mead NJ).* 2008;37(2):100–103.
11. Mann DC, Rajmaira S. Distribution of physeal and nonphyseal fractures in 2,650 long-bone fractures in children aged 0–16 years. *J Pediatr Orthop.* 1990;10(6):713–716.
12. Peterson CA, Peterson HA. Analysis of the incidence of injuries to the epiphyseal growth plate. *J Trauma.* 1972;12(4):275–281.
13. Peterson HA, Madhok R, Benson JT, et al. Physeal fractures: part 1. Epidemiology in Olmsted County, Minnesota, 1979–1988. *J Pediatr Orthop.* 1994;14(4):423–430.
14. Skaggs D. Rockwood and wilkins' fractures in children. In: Beaty JH, Kasser JR, eds. *Rockwood & Wilkin's Fracture in Children.* 7th ed. Philadelphia, PA: Lippincott Williams & Wilkins; 2010:1076.
15. Wall EJ, May MM. Growth plate fractures of the distal femur. *J Pediatr Orthop.* 2012;32(suppl 1):S40–S46.
16. Stanitski CL. Stress view radiographs of the skeletally immature knee: a different view. *J Pediatr Orthop.* 2004;24(3):342.
17. Kanellopoulos AD, Yiannakopoulos CK, Badras LS. Triplane fracture of the proximal tibia. *Am J Orthop (Belle Mead NJ).* 2003;32(9):452–454.
18. Lippert WC, Owens RF, Wall EJ. Salter-Harris type III fractures of the distal femur: plain radiographs can be deceptive. *J Pediatr Orthop.* 2010;30(6):598–605.
19. Zionts LE. Fractures around the knee in children. *J Am Acad Orthop Surg.* 2002;10(5):345–355.

20. Skak SV. A case of partial physeal closure following compression injury. *Arch Orthop Trauma Surg.* 1989;108(3):185–188.
21. Lombardo SJ, Harvey JP Jr. Fractures of the distal femoral epiphyses. Factors influencing prognosis: a review of thirty-four cases. *J Bone Joint Surg Am.* 1977;59(6):742–751.
22. Thomson JD, Stricker SJ, Williams MM. Fractures of the distal femoral epiphyseal plate. *J Pediatr Orthop.* 1995;15(4):474–478.
23. Basener CJ, Mehlman CT, DiPasquale TG. Growth disturbance after distal femoral growth plate fractures in children: a meta-analysis. *J Orthop Trauma.* 2009;23(9):663–667.
24. Ilharreborde B, Raquillet C, Morel E, et al. Long-term prognosis of Salter-Harris type 2 injuries of the distal femoral physis. *J Pediatr Orthop B.* 2006;15(6):433–438.
25. Meyers MH, McKeever FM. Fracture of the intercondylar eminence of the tibia. *J Bone Joint Surg Am.* 1959;41-A(2):209–220; discussion 220–222.
26. Ogden JA. Radiology of postnatal skeletal development. X. Patella and tibial tuberosity. *Skeletal Radiol.* 1984;11(4):246–257.
27. Blanks RH, Lester DK, Shaw BA. Flexion-type Salter II fracture of the proximal tibia. Proposed mechanism of injury and two case studies. *Clin Orthop Relat Res.* 1994;(301):256–259.
28. Aitken AP. Fractures of the proximal tibial epiphysial cartilage. *Clin Orthop Relat Res.* 1965;41:92–97.
29. Burkhart SS, Peterson HA. Fractures of the proximal tibial epiphysis. *J Bone Joint Surg Am.* 1979;61(7):996–1002.
30. Chan YC, Ting AC, Qing KX, et al. Delayed presentation of popliteal pseudo-aneurysm following soccer football injury. *Ann Vasc Surg.* 2010;24(4):553.e13–553.e16.
31. Mommsen P, Zeckey C, Hildebrand F, et al. Traumatic extremity arterial injury in children: epidemiology, diagnostics, treatment and prognostic value of Mangled Extremity Severity Score. *J Orthop Surg Res.* 2010;5:25.
32. Reid JJ, Kremen TJ Jr, Oppenheim WL. Death after closed adolescent knee injury and popliteal artery occlusion: a case report and clinical review. *Sports Health.* 2013;5(6):558–561.
33. Conroy J, Cohen A, Smith RM, et al. Triplane fracture of the proximal tibia. *Injury.* 2000;31(7):546–548.
34. Hermus JP, Driessen MJ, Mulder H, et al. The triplane variant of the tibial apophyseal fracture: a case report and a review of the literature. *J Pediatr Orthop B.* 2003;12(6):406–408.
35. Patari SK, Lee FY, Behrens FF. Coronal split fracture of the proximal tibia epiphysis through a partially closed physis: a new fracture pattern. *J Pediatr Orthop.* 2001;21(4):451–455.
36. Sinigaglia R, Gigante C, Basso G, et al. Triplane fracture of the proximal tibial epiphysis. *Chir Narzadow Ruchu Ortop Pol.* 2007;72(2):149–151.
37. Mubarak SJ, Kim JR, Edmonds EW, et al. Classification of proximal tibial fractures in children. *J Child Orthop.* 2009;3(3):191–197.
38. Shelton WR, Canale ST. Fractures of the tibia through the proximal tibial epiphyseal cartilage. *J Bone Joint Surg Am.* 1979;61(2): 167–173.
39. Donahue JP, Brennan JF, Barron OA. Combined physeal/apophyseal fracture of the proximal tibia with anterior angulation from an indirect force: report of 2 cases. *Am J Orthop (Belle Mead NJ).* 2003;32(12):604–607.
40. Potenza V, Caterini R, Maglione P, et al. Simultaneous bilateral flexion-type Salter-Harris II fractures of the proximal tibia: a case report and review of the literature. *Open Orthop J.* 2011;5:315–318.
41. Weber BG. Fibrous interposition causing valgus deformity after fracture of the upper tibial metaphysis in children. *J Bone Joint Surg Br.* 1977;59(3):290–292.
42. Jackson DW, Cozen L. Genu valgum as a complication of proximal tibial metaphyseal fractures in children. *J Bone Joint Surg Am.* 1971;53(8):1571–1578.
43. Ogden JA, Ogden DA, Pugh L, et al. Tibia valga after proximal metaphyseal fractures in childhood: a normal biologic response. *J Pediatr Orthop.* 1995;15(4):489–494.
44. Balthazar DA, Pappas AM. Acquired valgus deformity of the tibia in children. *J Pediatr Orthop.* 1984;4(5):538–541.
45. Dal Monte A, Manes E, Cammarota V. Post-traumatic genu valgum in children. *Ital J Orthop Traumatol.* 1983;9(1):5–11.
46. McCarthy JJ, Kim DH, Eilert RE. Posttraumatic genu valgum: operative versus nonoperative treatment. *J Pediatr Orthop.* 1998;18(4):518–521.
47. Skak SV. Valgus deformity following proximal tibial metaphyseal fracture in children. *Acta Orthop Scand.* 1982;53(1):141–147.
48. Tuten HR, Keeler KA, Gabos PG, et al. Posttraumatic tibia valga in children. A long-term follow-up note. *J Bone Joint Surg Am.* 1999;81(6):799–810.
49. Zionts LE, MacEwen GD. Spontaneous improvement of post-traumatic tibia valga. *J Bone Joint Surg Am.* 1986;68(5):680–687.

CHAPTER

35

Sarah Hobart
Benton E. Heyworth

Patellar Sleeve Fractures

INTRODUCTION

Patella fractures are relatively rare in the skeletally immature, comprising only 1% to 6% of all patella fractures in all ages.[1,2] However, due to the developmental anatomy of the growing knee, over 50% of this small proportion are patellar sleeve fractures.[2,3] In most patellar sleeve fractures, a sudden eccentric force leads to avulsion of the inferior pole of the patella, along with a patellar chondral fragment of varying size attached to the distal fracture fragment. This articular cartilage represents the deep or posterior segment of the sleeve, whereas the patellar periosteum comprises the superficial or anterior segment of the sleeve (Fig. 35.1). For caregivers of young athletes, familiarity with the anatomic subtleties of this fracture and the age group typically affected is critical, as these fractures are frequently misdiagnosed and can be difficult to identify on radiographs.

ANATOMY AND FUNCTION

The patella, which begins to ossify between ages 3 and 6 years, is uniquely flexible in younger children.[4] Anywhere between one and six ossicles will form and merge into a single unit through intramembranous ossification, which then spreads peripherally. Until ossification is complete, the periphery of the ossifying patella may normally appear irregular on radiographs and should not be mistaken for patellar pathology. Bipartite or multipartite patella, representing incomplete coalition of ossicles, are reported in between 2% and 15% of adolescents and are important as part of any differential diagnosis that includes patella fracture in this age group.[5,6] However, the most common location of an accessory ossicle is the superolateral pole compared with patellar sleeve fractures, which more commonly occur in the distal half of the patella.

The vascular supply of the patella comes predominantly from the paired superior and inferior geniculate arteries. They converge, predominantly anteriorly, to form an anastomotic circle surrounding the patella. Additional branches enter from below the distal pole posterior to the patellar tendon.[7] Vascularity is important to take into account when considering fixation, as the blood supply of the patella arises from the anterior surface and distal pole.

EPIDEMIOLOGY/MECHANISM OF INJURY/ETIOLOGY/PATHOMECHANICS

As the skeletally immature patella is more cartilaginous than in adults, it is more accommodating to three-point bending.[8] A forceful quadriceps contraction with the knee in flexion creates a fulcrum effect. In skeletally immature patients, the collagen of the tendon blends directly with the cartilage, as opposed to adults in whom Sharpey's fibers form a robust connection between the tendon and its bony attachment site. With the eccentric force of the quadriceps, the weakest part of the construct, the connection between the cartilage and bone, is the most vulnerable site of fracture with excessive forces.[9]

Sleeve fractures of the patella are the most common type of patella fracture in preadolescents and adolescents. They usually do not occur before the age of 8 years or after skeletal maturity, with an average age of 12.7 years and a 3:1 male predominance.[2] Inferior avulsions are most common, but superior avulsions have also been reported and are more likely to be nondisplaced.[10]

EVALUATION

In the patient's described injury history, there is usually an identifiable traumatic event, with the patient reporting a jump, landing from a jump, or a sudden fall. If there is no specific event, and the patient simply began to have pain after an athletic event or after a period of significant activity, other diagnoses such as a symptomatic bipartite patella or Sinding-Larsen-Johansson syndrome—a traction apophysitis specific to the inferior pole of the patella[9]—should be considered more strongly. Questions regarding symptomatology in the preceding weeks to months, even if mild, may be helpful in identifying an acute exacerbation of more chronic pathology rather than a fracture. A direct blow to the patella is a possible mechanism of injury for a patellar sleeve fracture, but less likely. Difficulty with weight bearing is common, and patients will often be unable to bring the knee into full extension. Rapid swelling and bruising are also commonly reported.

On physical examination, prepatellar swelling and ecchymosis, as well as a tense effusion, are frequently seen. Aspiration can alleviate some symptoms and confirm hemarthrosis but is seldom performed today, compared with traditional practices.

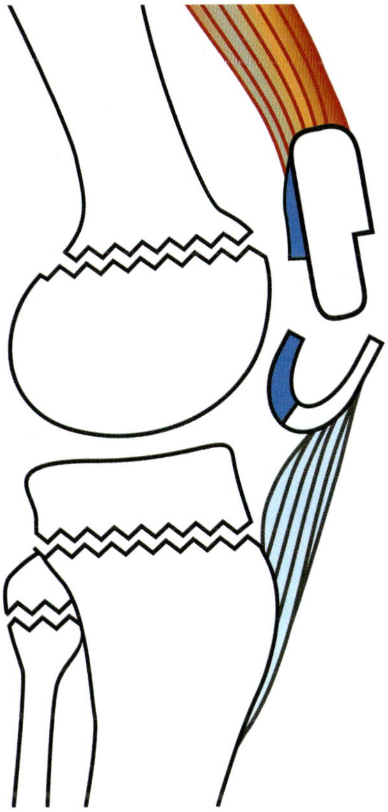

Figure 35.1. Schematic representation of sleeve fracture demonstrating both an articular cartilage (*dark blue*) component of the sleeve and, more superficially, a patellar preossification chondral and periosteal (*white*) component of sleeve, confluent with the patellar tendon. (Figure courtesy of Nathaniel Wittstruck.)

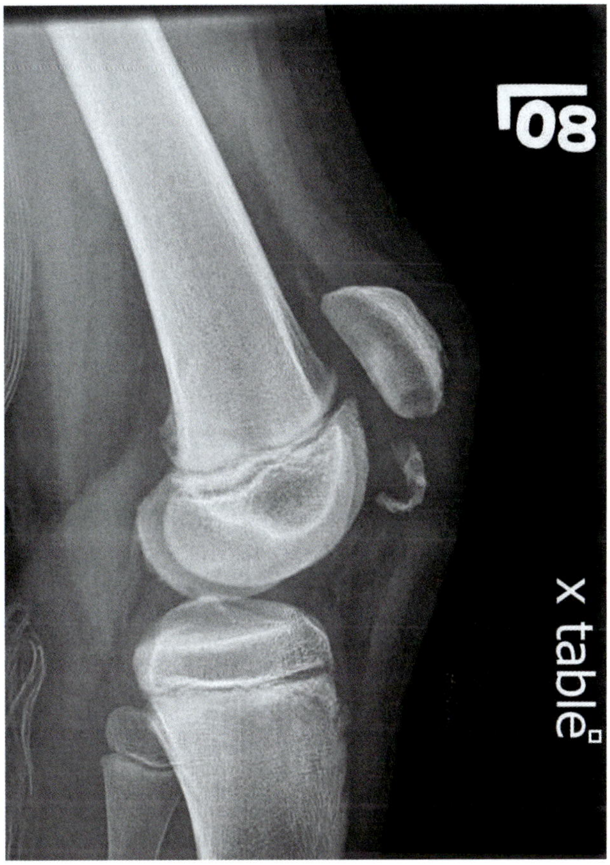

Figure 35.2. A 12-year-old male twisted his knee playing football and felt a pop. Distal fragment, although seen clearly on this lateral view, is not always so apparent.

Lack of full extension and inability to complete a straight-leg raise is common. However, if the retinaculum is intact, there may not necessarily be an extension lag. Patients may also internally rotate the leg and use the fascia lata to complete a straight-leg raise.[9] Commonly, a defect inferior to a high-riding patella, or patella alta, can be palpated.

Meticulous evaluation of imaging is paramount in the diagnosis, as patellar sleeve fractures are frequently missed or underappreciated. Two orthogonal view radiographs are usually sufficient, although oblique views may more conclusively delineate the pathoanatomy. A bony fragment distal to the inferior pole of the patella ranging in size from a small fleck of bone (within a larger unossified fragment of patellar cartilage) to a larger sleeve of ossified distal pole (Fig. 35.2) is usually best seen on the lateral view. Amount of displacement is important, as it determines treatment selection. The most important aspect of radiographic interpretation, however, is that a small osseous opacity almost always represents a much larger fractured osteochondral fragment.[11,12] Contralateral films may therefore be helpful, as a small, nondisplaced, or minimally displaced well-corticated ossicle may more likely represent Sinding-Larsen-Johansson syndrome or a bipartite patella, as opposed to a true sleeve fracture.[13] Because of the importance of understanding the precise pathoanatomy of such injuries, we consider magnetic resonance imaging (MRI) to be invaluable in determining the extent of injury in equivocal cases or those unclear from plain radiographs alone, as well as assessing the size of fragment and for preoperative planning, when applicable.[11] MRI will demonstrate the cartilage contiguous with the small osseous component (Fig. 35.3) and generally elucidate the injury pattern more precisely.

TREATMENT

Indications/Contraindications

Many patellar sleeve fractures are nondisplaced and can be treated with a cylindrical long leg cast in extension or, depending on the age, reliability, and comfort level of the patient and family, with a knee immobilizer or hinged knee brace locked in extension. Weight bearing may be progressed as symptoms permit, but the knee should remain immobilized in extension when ambulating to prevent fracture displacement. The degree to which range of motion exercises are begun when not ambulating is quite variable between surgeons and, at times, is individualized for a given patient or fracture.

Indications for operative treatment include fracture displacement greater than 2 mm, an extensor lag, or articular incongruity. For borderline fractures that appear minimally or mildly displaced, pain may preclude a young patient from performing a straight-leg raise, so temporary bracing or casting may be performed, with repeat clinical checks confirming

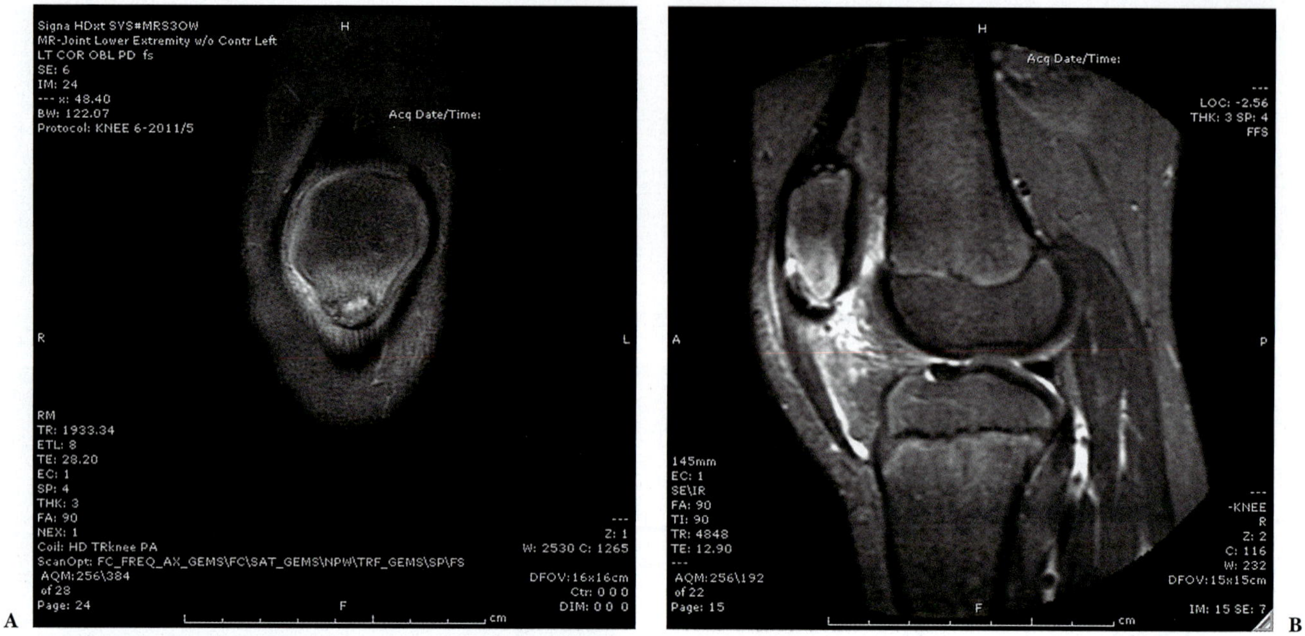

Figure 35.3. **A.** Coronal T2 weighted image demonstrating minimally displaced sleeve fracture in an 11-year-old male. **B.** Sagittal T2 weighed image of same patient, with minimally disrupted anterior periosteal extension of patellar tendon.

an intact extensor mechanism at later visits. In such cases, prognostic discussions with families should be tempered and logistical planning arranged to allow for possible surgical fixation if follow-up visits suggest a persistent extensor lag.

If the distal osseous fragment is large enough, displaced fractures can often be addressed similarly to adult patella fractures, with either a tension band construct or screw fixation. The AO tension band technique involves two fixed longitudinal wires with a wire loop over the anterior patella in a figure-of-eight fashion. John et al.[14] found that the horizontal figure-of-eight orientation had the best mechanical strength when compared with the vertical figure-of-eight.[14] Some surgeons have come to favor high-strength braided suture in place of metal wire for figure-of-eight material.

If the osteochondral avulsion is smaller, as it often is in avulsion fractures, nonabsorbable sutures can be used to attach both the fragment and the patellar tendon to the inferior pole of the remaining patella with the use of suture anchors or with suture advanced through longitudinally drilled holes or cannulated screws.[15,16]

AUTHORS' PREFERRED TECHNIQUE

Generally, larger fractures are adequately fixed with either figure-of-eight tension band K-wire constructs or screws. Cannulated, partially threaded 3.5- or 4.0-mm screws provide fixation with compression and also allow for a no. 2 or no. 5 high-strength braided suture to be fed through the screw cannulation to serve as an adjunctive tension band construct. This technique decreases the need for short-term removal of prominent hardware, which can slow the return of flexion during rehab, even when bent K-wires are cut several millimeters from the superior or inferior patellar surface. Usually, the K-wires, which are usually 0.045 or 0.062 in, are bent anteriorly at the proximal patellar exit point, with the bent tips then rotated posteriorly and tamped distally into small longitudinal rents in line with the fibers of the distal quadriceps tendon insertion. The distal tips are then cut near-flush with the level of the inferior pole of the patella, taking care to maintain the position of the suture weaved around the tips of the K-wire.

However, for the more common sleeve fractures that involve more chondral tissue than bony tissue, we have had success using biocomposite suture anchors loaded with no. 2 high-strength braided sutures. With newer generations of bioabsorbable anchors, this construct provides reliable fixation and stability without having to drill large holes through the full extent of the patella or disrupt or irritate the quadriceps insertional complex, thereby also facilitating effective early rehabilitation. Regardless of the repair technique pursued, it is important to also repair any retinaculum and periosteal tears, when possible.

REHABILITATION

Internal fixation generally allows slightly earlier knee range of motion in an advanced rehabilitation protocol than with fractures treated nonoperatively, although given the involved age group, 2 to 4 weeks of knee immobilization may be reasonable. Postoperatively, weight bearing is allowed within the first 2 weeks with either a cylindrical cast or a hinged knee brace locked in extension. Although the brace is locked in extension when weight bearing throughout the first 6 weeks, our preference is to use a brace to allow initiation of range of motion from 0 to 30 degrees in the first 2 weeks, progressed to 0 to 60 degrees for postoperative weeks 2 to 4, and 0 to 90 degrees from weeks 4 to 6.

PEARLS/PITFALLS

Patellar sleeve fractures are often misdiagnosed initially, and this delay can lead to complications such as nonunion, malunion, quadriceps atrophy and contracture, extensor lag, loss of knee flexion, and ischemia.[17–19] An extensor lag in the appropriate age group, approximately ages 8 to 13 years, should heighten suspicion for this injury. With doubts in diagnosis, there should be a low threshold for obtaining an MRI.

Operative complications include stiffness, loss of knee flexion, heterotopic bone formation, ischemic changes, patellar chondrosis, and painful hardware, especially if metal wires are used in a tension band construct over the anterior patella.[3,17,20] Although adolescents are generally quicker to regain range of motion compared to their adult counterparts, an overtensioned construct with suture extending distally into the patellar tendon may prevent full flexion as undertensioning may prevent full extension. An improperly balanced construct can also lead to ossification in the stretched patellar tendon.[9] Careful tensioning is not only important for maintenance of motion but also critical in avoiding ischemic changes, as it is easy to damage the delicate nutrient vessels entering the anterior surface and distal pole.[17,20] Lastly, anatomic alignment both of the articular cartilage and tendon insertion is important in maintaining the mechanics and preventing chondrosis. Although articular incongruity leads to uneven load sharing and eventual degenerative arthrosis, it may be unclear if this is from the initial injury or from inadequate alignment.[21–23] In addition, it is important to reattach the distal fragment anatomically so as not to alter the extensor mechanism kinematics. Although long-term follow-up on sleeve fractures is limited, it remains essential to optimize a near-anatomic reduction and tension correctly.

REFERENCES

1. Maguire JK, Canale ST. Fractures of the patella in children and adolescents. *J Pediatr Orthop.* 1993;13(55):567–571.
2. Ray JM, Hendrix J. Incidence, mechanism of injury, and treatment of fractures of the patella in children. *J Trauma.* 1992; 32:464–467.
3. Dai LY, Zhang WM. Fracture of the patella in children. *Knee Surg Sports Traumatol Arthrosc.* 1999;7:243–245.
4. Ogden JA. Radiology of postnatal skeletal development. X. Patella and tibial tuberosity. *Skeletal Radiol.* 1984;11:246–257.
5. Ogden JA, McCarthy SM, Jokl P. The painful bipartite patella. *J Pediatr Orthop.* 1982;2:263–269.
6. Zumstein M, Sukthankar A, Exner GU. Tripartite patella: late appearance of a third ossification center in childhood. *J Pediatr Orthop B.* 2006;15:75–76.
7. Scapinelli R. Blood supply of the human patella. Its relation to ischaemic necrosis after fracture. *J Bone Joint Surg Br.* 1967;49(3): 563–570.
8. Beaty JH, Kasser JR. *Rockwood and Wilkins' Fractures in Children.* 7th ed. Philadelphia, PA: Lippincott Williams & Wilkins; 2009.
9. Hunt DM, Somashekar N. A review of sleeve fractures of the patella in children. *The Knee.* 2005;12:3–7.
10. Grogan DP, Carey TP, Leffers D, et al. Avulsion fractures of the patella. *J Pediatr Orthop.* 1990;10(6):721–730.
11. Bates DG, Hresko MT, Jaramillo D. Patellar sleeve fracture: demonstration with MR imaging. *Radiology.* 1994;193:825–827.
12. King SJ. Magnetic resonance imaging of knee injuries in children. *Eur Radiol.* 1997;7:1245–1251.
13. Dupuis CS, Westra SJ, Makris J, et al. Injuries and conditions of the extensor mechanism of the pediatric knee. *Radiographics.* 2009;29(3):877–886.
14. John J, Wagner WW, Kuiper JH. Tension-band wiring of transverse fractures of patella. The effect of site of wire twists and orientation of stainless steel wire loop: a biomechanical investigation. *Int Orthop.* 2007;31:703–707.
15. Weber MJ, Janecki CJ, McLeod P, et al. Efficacy of various forms of fixation of transverse fractures of the patella. *J Bone Joint Surg Am.* 1980;62(2):215–220.
16. Carpenter JE, Kasman R, Matthews LS. Fractures of the patella. *J Bone Joint Surg Am.* 1993;75A:1550–1561.
17. Gao GX, Mahadev A, Lee EH. Sleeve fracture of the patella in children. *J Orthop Surg.* 2008;16:43–46.
18. Houghton GR, Ackroyd CE. Sleeve fractures of the patella in children: a report of three cases. *J Bone Joint Surg Br.* 1979;61-B(2):165–168.
19. Wu CD, Huang SC, Liu TK. Sleeve fracture of the patella in children. A report of five cases. *Am J Sports Med.* 1991;19(5):525–528.
20. Jacquemier M, Chrestian P, Guys JM, et al. Fracture-avulsions of the patella in children. Apropos of 3 cases [in French]. *Chir Pediatri.* 1983;24:201–204.
21. Boström A. Fracture of the patella: a study of 422 patellar fractures. *Acta Orthop Scand Suppl.* 1972;143:1–80.
22. Saltzman CL, Goulet JA, McClellan RT, et al. Results of treatment of displaced patellar fractures by partial patellectomy. *J Bone Joint Surg Am.* 1990;72(9):1279–1285.
23. Melvin J, Mehta S. Patellar fractures in adults. *J Am Acad Orthop Surg.* 2011;19(4):198–207.

SECTION

6

Physis

Shari T. Jawetz
Parina H. Shah
Hollis G. Potter

CHAPTER 36

Diagnostic Imaging of the Physis

Physeal injuries are common in the pediatric population and injury can impart significant morbidity, with the potential for long-lasting complications. Trauma is the most frequent etiology of physeal damage, with approximately 18% to 30% of pediatric fractures involving the physis.[1–3] Injury to the physis is more common during times of rapid growth in both males and females.[4] Traumatic physeal fractures are rare in children younger than 5 years of age, and the peak incidences are at ages 11 to 12 years in girls and 13 to 14 years in boys.[5] Although less common, nontraumatic causes of physeal injury include infection, ischemia, neoplasm, radiation,[6] metabolic derangement, thermal injury, sensory neuropathy, and iatrogenic injury.[7]

Physeal growth arrest occurs in 5% to 10% of all physeal fractures.[4] Factors that may influence the risk of postinjury growth disturbance include the age of the child, the degree of skeletal maturity, amount of growth remaining, and degree and area of physeal involvement.[4] Postinjury growth disturbances more commonly occur at the distal ends of the long bones compared with the proximal ends,[3] and growth arrest more commonly occurs from physeal injuries to the lower rather than upper extremities.[8]

Up to 50% of distal femoral physeal fractures result in growth arrest.[9] Growth of the proximal tibia and distal femur contribute to 55% to 70% of the growth of the lower extremity; thus, premature physeal closure about the knee joint can result in substantial limb length discrepancies.[10]

Physeal injuries may result in pathologic bars or bridges across the physis. The complications of physeal bars include limb length discrepancy, angular growth deformity, and altered joint biomechanics.[6] The younger the child is at the time of physeal injury, the greater the risk of subsequent complications.[7] The risk of physeal bar formation is also increased when a fracture is malreduced or when a fracture line extends through the osseous portions of the epiphysis.[4]

Ogden[6] defined three types of physeal bridging in the setting of partial physeal arrest: peripheral (type 1), linear (type 2), and central (type 3). Peripheral bridges can vary in size, but when they include the peripheral zone of Ranvier, which is involved in physeal widening, severe angular deformities may occur over short periods of time. Linear bridges extend linearly across the physis and may also result in angular deformities. Central bridges form across the central portion of the physis, with uninjured growth plate completely surrounding the bridge; central bridges tend to result in longitudinal growth disturbance.

Physeal bridges tend to occur at the sites of physeal undulations, such that they are most common centrally in the distal femur and peripherally in the proximal tibia. The relative location of the physeal damage will impact the types of future growth disturbances. Premature eccentric physeal closure causes angular growth deformity, whereas early central physeal closure may lead to an overall limb length discrepancy without angular abnormality.[10]

Smaller physeal bridges may be of little to no clinical significance because they can be transient. Animal models have shown that physeal bars involving less than 7% of the cross-sectional area may be transient.[11] Growth of adjacent normal areas of the physis will cause traction on and ultimately fracture a small bridge, allowing for restoration of normal growth.[12] Growth disturbance has been shown to occur in animal models once damage has occurred to more than 7% of the cross-sectional area of the physis.[11]

Physeal bars involving less than 25% of the cross-sectional area of the physis may be amenable to surgical resection with subsequent interposition of an inert material such as fat. Those patients with damage to less than 10% of the growth plate tend to have the best outcomes. Better outcome following physeal bar resection is also associated with younger age at the time of surgery, single site of bar formation, and a centrally located defect.[5] Therefore, for preoperative planning, knowledge of a physeal bridge's precise location and size is necessary.[13]

Knowledge of the normal patterns of physeal closure is vital in order to avoid incorrectly diagnosing a physeal bar in a patient who is actually maturing normally. Physiologic epiphysiodesis about the distal femur occurs in a predictable pattern, with the central physis maturing initially and subsequent physeal closure continuing in a centripetal fashion.[14] Within the proximal tibia, the posterior aspect of the physis closes initially, with subsequent progression anteriorly[4] (Fig. 36.1).

In 1963, Salter and Harris[15] initially categorized fractures involving the physis (Fig. 36.2). This remains the most commonly used classification system guiding treatment of physeal injuries.[15] Types I and II fractures are extra-articular, whereas types III to V fractures are intra-articular. Types III to V fractures may result in both joint incongruity and physeal damage.

Type I fractures are confined to the physis without extension into either the epiphysis or the metaphysis.

Type II fractures (Fig. 36.3) extend along the physis and exit through a portion of the metaphysis, often yielding a triangular-shaped metaphyseal fragment, sometimes referred to as *a Thurston Holland fragment*.

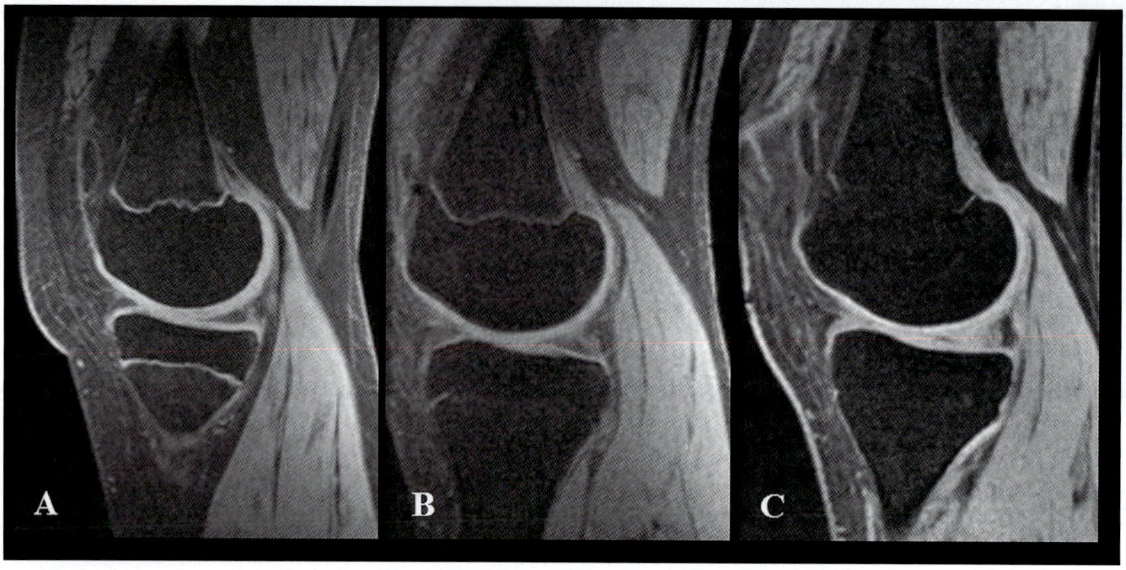

Figure 36.1. Sagittal 3-D images in a child at three time points (**[A]** age 12 years, **[B]** age 14 years, and **[C]** age 15 years) demonstrate closure of the femoral and tibial physes progressing centripetally in the distal femur and from posterior to anterior in the proximal tibia.

Type III fractures (Fig. 36.4) extend from the articular surface, through the epiphysis to the physis, through which the fracture exits.

Type IV fractures arise from the articular surface, extend through the epiphysis and physis, and exit through the metaphysis. Anatomic reduction of the physis is necessary to reduce the risk of bony bar formation.

Type V fractures are compression or crush injuries to the physis.

The Salter-Harris types III to V fractures are associated with the greatest risk of future growth disturbances.[16]

Of traumatic fractures involving the physis, the Salter-Harris type II fractures are the most common (60.9%) followed by type I (28.6%), type III (6.7%), and type IV (3.7%) fractures. No type V injuries were identified in the cohort studied by Kawamoto et al.[2]

Harris growth arrest lines, related to variations in the rate of bone growth, typically parallel the physis and can indicate physeal damage. These growth arrest lines may be seen on radiographs, computed tomography (CT), and magnetic resonance imaging (MRI) examinations. A decreased distance between the growth arrest line and the physis on the side of injury indicates a

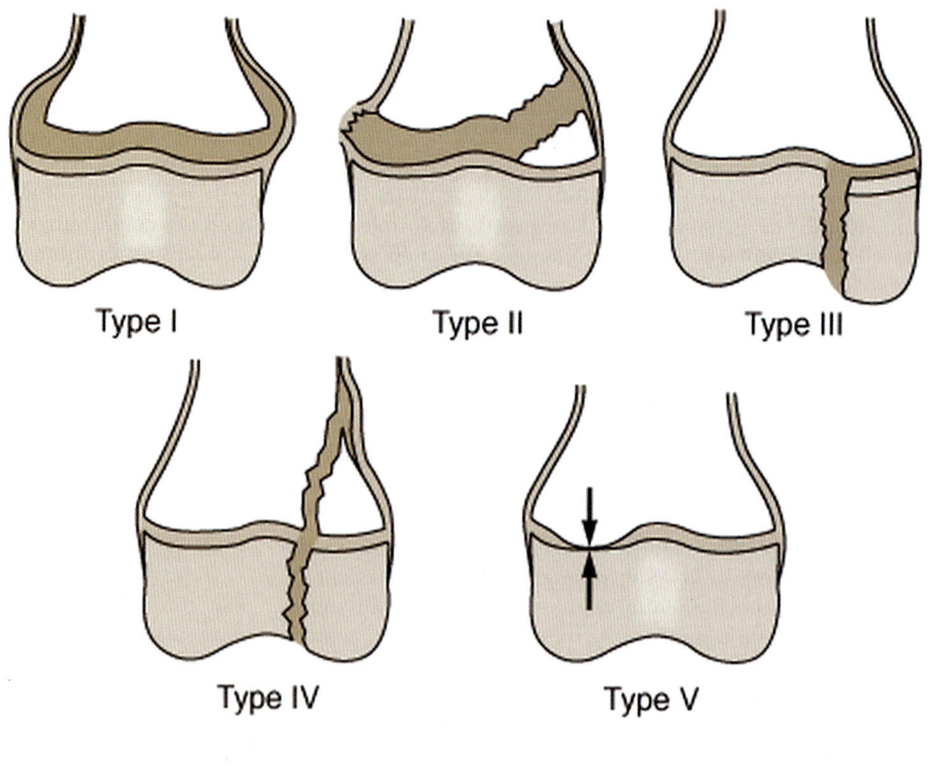

Figure 36.2. Artistic rendering of the types I to V Salter-Harris fractures. (Reprinted with permission from Mulholland MW, Lillemoe KD, Doherty GM, et al, eds. *Greenfield's Surgery: Scientific Principles and Practice.* 4th ed. Philadelphia, PA: Lippincott Williams & Wilkins; 2006.)

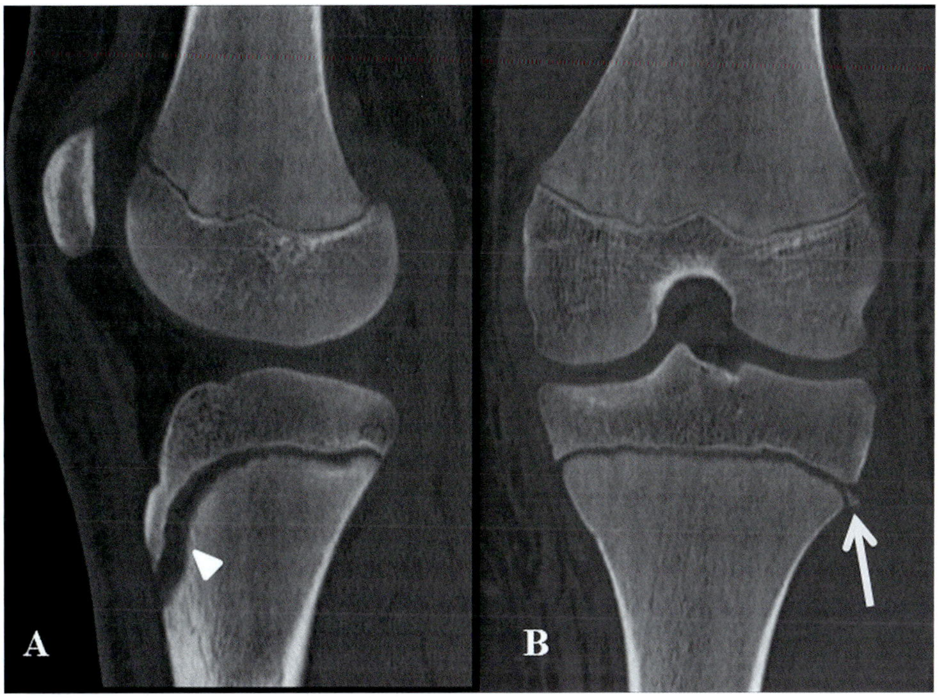

Figure 36.3. A 13-year-old male with Salter-Harris type II fracture. The sagittal CT image **(A)** demonstrates widening of the proximal tibial physis anteriorly (*arrowhead*). Coronal CT image **(B)** demonstrates a tiny fracture through the metaphysis with a Thurston Holland fragment (*arrow*).

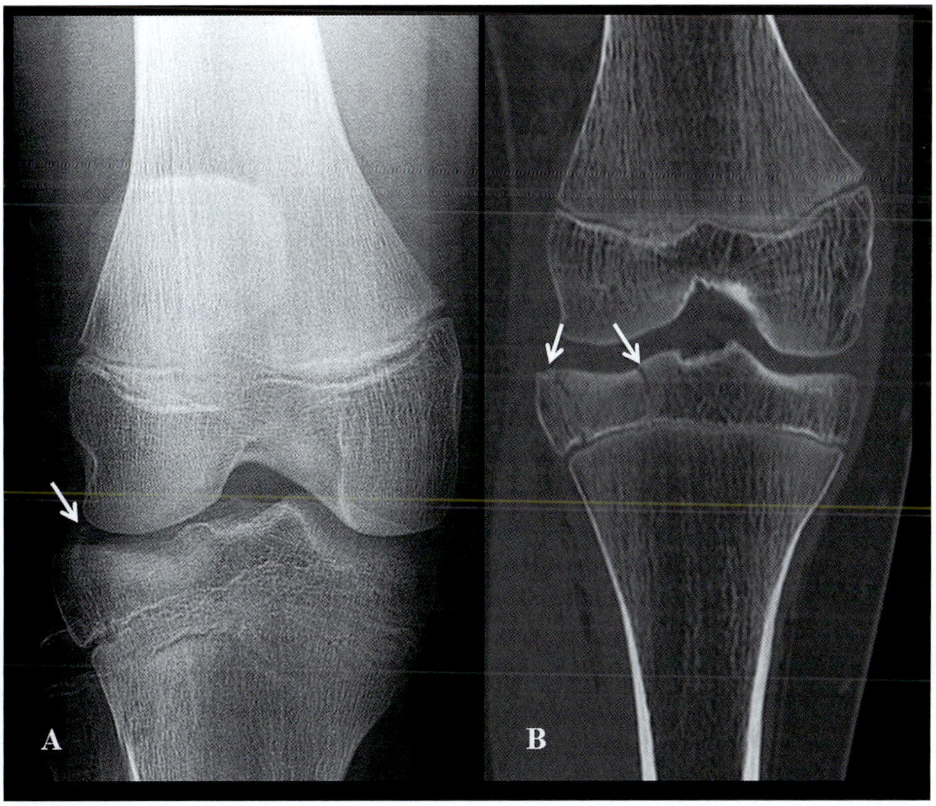

Figure 36.4. A 17-year-old male (bone age 15 years) with Salter-Harris type III fracture. Anteroposterior (AP) radiograph **(A)** demonstrates vertically oriented lucency through the lateral margin of the epiphysis extending to the physis (*arrow*). Coronal CT **(B)** image demonstrates additional vertical fracture line extending through the tibial epiphysis to the physis, and there is a subtle step-off of the articular surface (*arrows*).

deceleration of growth of the injured extremity. In contrast, complete absence of a growth arrest line in an injured extremity indicates complete cessation of growth. Growth arrest lines that are oblique rather than parallel to the physis suggest a tethering effect secondary to partial growth arrest. Other secondary signs of a partial growth arrest include progressive malalignment.[5]

RADIOGRAPHY

Radiographs are the first-line imaging approach,[7] particularly in the setting of trauma, due to their cost-effectiveness and ease of accessibility.[17] However, radiographs do not allow for direct evaluation of the cartilage, as noncalcified cartilage is lucent on radiographs and thus secondary signs of physeal injury must be relied upon to make a diagnosis.[18] Secondary findings of physeal injury on radiographs include epiphyseal displacement; physeal widening; and indistinctness of the normal, sharply defined sclerotic margins on the opposing sides of the epiphysis and metaphysis.[12]

On radiographs, signs of a type I fracture include widening, haziness, sclerosis, or irregularity of the physis. These findings can be subtle, and radiographs of the contralateral, symptom-free side may be helpful for comparison. For the types II through IV fractures, the fracture lucency may be seen in the metaphysis and/or epiphysis, but the precise degree of involvement of the physis can often not be determined. Of note, the type V injuries are often radiographically occult at initial assessment, leading to a delay in diagnosis if radiographs are the only means of imaging used to evaluate the injured patient.

Stress radiographs may be useful in evaluating posttraumatic joint stability, but they are often not possible in the acute trauma setting because of pain inhibition. In addition, there is a risk that the applied stress could cause inadvertent injury to the physis, such that a subtle Salter-Harris type I fracture might be converted into a displaced Salter-Harris type III fracture.[19]

Radiographs are indicated for evaluation of fractures, but the use of radiography in isolation has significant limitations. Evaluation of the physis can be difficult when the x-ray beam is not parallel to the physis.[20,21] The irregular three-dimensional (3-D) nature of the physis, which includes anatomic undulations and ridges, limits the use of the two-dimensional imaging used in radiographs. Subtle nondisplaced fractures may be occult on radiographs (Fig. 36.5).[12]

Only osseous bars are potentially visible on radiographs; fibrous tissue is radiolucent and a fibrous physeal bridge could not be appreciated. Even in the setting of an osseous bridge across the physis, radiographs cannot provide 3-D information regarding the size and location of the bridge (Fig. 36.6).

The widespread availability of radiography is useful in the regular follow-up of fractures to assess for fracture healing and to evaluate for potential growth disturbances and development of malalignment. Following physeal injury, the frequency at which follow-up radiographs should be obtained will vary based on the assessment of risk for subsequent growth disturbance. For example, with higher risk physeal injuries, it is reasonable to obtain radiographs every 3 months until normal growth rate can be documented, which may take up to 2 years[5] or even until skeletal maturity.[6] Without close radiologic follow-up, an angular deformity might not be identified until it is already apparent clinically[6] at which time it may be more difficult to surgically correct.

COMPUTED TOMOGRAPHY

Cross-sectional imaging modalities such as CT can demonstrate the extent of physeal involvement in more detail than radiographs. CT can demonstrate subtle alterations in fracture

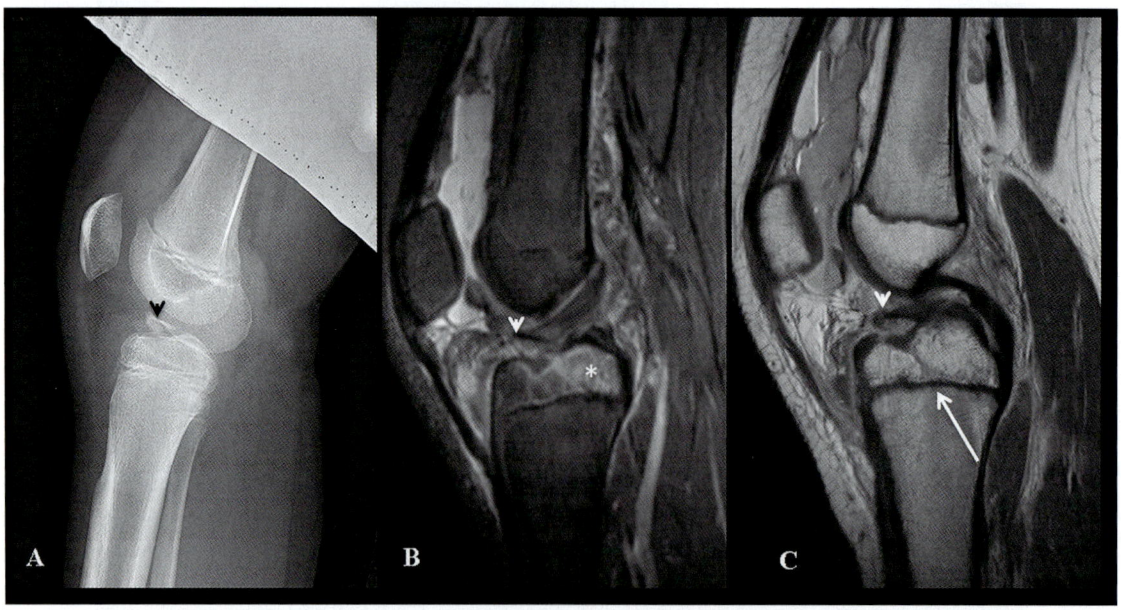

Figure 36.5. A 10-year-old female with tibial eminence avulsion seen on lateral radiograph **(A)** (*black arrowhead*). Sagittal inversion recovery **(B)** and fast spin echo **(C)** MR images demonstrate an obliquely oriented Salter-Harris type III fracture line extending from the articular surface through the epiphysis to the physis (*arrow*) with surrounding bone marrow edema pattern (*asterisk*), in addition to the tibial eminence avulsion (*white arrowheads*).

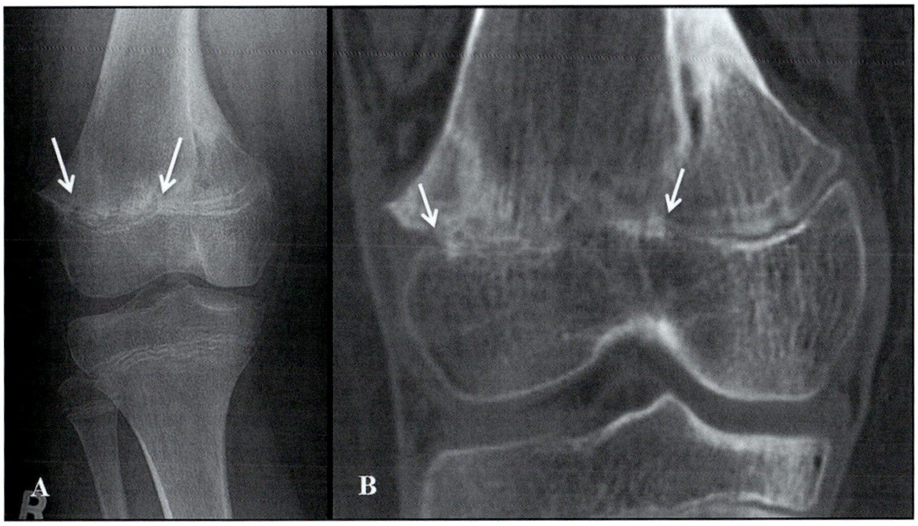

Figure 36.6. AP radiograph **(A)** and coronal CT image **(B)** of a 10-year-old male 5 months following a distal femoral fracture during a bicycle accident with an osseous bar (*arrows*) across the lateral margin of the distal femoral physis, leading to varus angulation at the knee.

alignment, which is particularly useful in Salter-Harris types III and IV fractures, which involve the epiphysis.[12] Additionally, CT can provide further detail about a bony physeal bar. However, as with radiographs, cartilage remains radiolucent on CT, and direct visualization of a physeal injury remains limited. CT is more expensive than radiography[22] and also employs ionizing radiation for image acquisition, but CT imparts higher doses of radiation to patients than radiographs do.[23] Radiation dose is of vital importance, particularly in pediatric patients whose organs are more radiosensitive and whose longer life expectancy affords a lengthier period of time during which they can potentially develop a radiation-induced cancer.[24] Radiation shielding should be always used, especially when imaging pediatric patients, with shields placed above and below the patient. Newer dual-energy CT scanners offer superior bone detail with marked reduction in dose. Table 36.1 shows suggested parameters used for scanning the knee with physeal injury on both 16- and 64-slice CT scanners.

TABLE 36.1 Computed Tomography Acquisition Parameters for Imaging the Pediatric Knee Using Both 64-Slice and 16-Slice Scanners

Scanner	*64-Slice*	*16-Slice*
Scan type	Helical	Helical
Thickness (mm)	.8	.8
Increment (mm)	.4	.4
Voltage (kV)	80	90
mAs/slice	50	100
Resolution	High	High
Pitch	.391	.438
Rotation time (s)	.5	.5
Collimation	64 × .0625	16 × .75

With acquisition of thin slices yielding isotropic data sets, the CT data can be post-processed to generate both multiplanar reconstructed images and 3-D reformations (see Fig. 36.6).[25] Thus, unlike radiography, CT can provide complex anatomic information about an osseous physeal bar.

CT is unable to provide as much direct information about physeal anatomy and pathology compared with MRI, but it remains an important imaging modality in the settings of Salter-Harris types III and IV fractures where detection and treatment of subtle joint incongruities is vital (see Figs. 36.4 and 36.5). CT is also indicated in the relatively small subset of patients in whom MRI is contraindicated.

MAGNETIC RESONANCE IMAGING

In 1990, Jaramillo et al.[18] first used MRI to evaluate physeal injuries in an animal model. Since then, MRI has proven to be clinically useful in demonstrating osseous and fibrous physeal bridges, epiphyseal and metaphyseal avascular necrosis, and growth arrest.[12] An MRI of the knee obtained soon after injury can provide meaningful information about the relative location, morphology, and type of fracture[26] or physeal injury as well as the precise size of the physeal damage.[27]

MRI is of particular value, as it offers high spatial resolution, superior soft tissue contrast, and multiplanar imaging capabilities without using ionizing radiation.[19] Although MRI is more expensive and the acquisition and postprocessing is more time-intensive than that for radiography and CT, MRI can provide direct visualization of the physeal cartilage.[20]

MRI of pediatric patients should be performed on a clinical 1.5 or 3.0 T magnet using a surface coil. Table 36.2 shows a suggested protocol for obtaining a knee MRI in pediatric patients.

The 3-D frequency-selected fat-suppressed spoiled gradient recalled (SPGR) T1 weighted images are the most useful in evaluating hyaline cartilage of the growth plate.[28] The 3-D nature of the SPGR sequence affords the opportunity to reformat the images into additional planes following image acquisition; as such, it is only necessary to acquire the 3-D SPGR images in a single plane, thereby diminishing the time of image acquisition. In evaluating the knee, the 3-D SPGR data is generally acquired

TABLE 36.2 **Magnetic Resonance Imaging Acquisition Parameters for Imaging the Pediatric Knee with Physeal Injury**

Parameters	*Sagittal PD*	*Axial PD*	*Coronal PD*	*Sagittal IR*	*3-D SPGR*
Repetition time (TR) (ms)	4,000–5,000	5,000–6,000	4,500–5,500	4,000–4,500	12–17
Echo time (TE) (ms)	20–25	20–25	20–25	15–20	1.4–1.6
Slice thickness (SL) (mm)	3–3.5	3–3.5	2.5–3.0	3.0–3.5	1.5
Bandwidth (BW) (kHz)	±20–40	±20–40	±20–40	±20–40	±20–40
Acquisition matrix	512 × 384	512 × 256	512 × 256	256 × 192	256 × 256
Field of view (FOV) (cm)	16–20	14–18	14–18	16–20	15–20
Number of excitations (NEX)	2	2	2	2	2

3-D SPGR, three-dimensional frequency-selected fat-suppressed spoiled gradient recalled.

in a plane orthogonal to the physis (either the sagittal or coronal plane), but acquisition in any plane is possible.

On gradient echo images, mineralization of the bony trabeculae results in diffuse low signal intensity in the osseous structures, whereas hyaline cartilage is higher in signal intensity.[29] The differential signal intensities yield superior contrast resolution between the physeal cartilage and the adjacent epiphyseal and metaphyseal bone. In a normal physis, the growth plate appears as a uniform high signal intensity line extending across the width of the bone. Physeal disruption will be manifest as an area of abnormal low signal intensity within the high signal intensity physis (Fig. 36.7).[10]

The 3-D SPGR can also show other features indicative of prior physeal damage including foci of metaphyseal intrusion where the physeal cartilage extends beyond the growth plate into the metaphysis (Fig. 36.8).[30] Over time, metaphyseal intrusions may become fixed within the metaphyseal bone, giving rise to discrete islands of physeal cartilage within the metaphysis.[7] Metaphyseal intrusions and metaphyseal islands of physeal cartilage are both associated with prior physeal injury, but there is no association between the prevalence of metaphyseal intrusions and the cause of physeal injury.[10]

In cases of a Salter-Harris type I fracture, MRI can demonstrate subtle physeal widening. A fluid-sensitive sequence, such as an inversion recovery (IR) or frequency-selective fat saturated T2 sequence, may demonstrate edema (high signal) along the physis, which is an additional sign of injury. In the acute to subacute Salter-Harris types II to IV injuries, in addition to the edema seen about the physis, bone marrow edema pattern will also be evident in the epiphysis and/or metaphysis depending on the fracture type. The actual fracture line can sometimes be more apparent on MRI than other imaging modalities (Figs. 36.5 and 36.9).

Although the 3-D SPGR sequence provides direct visualization of the physeal cartilage, it does have limitations. As shown in Figure 36.10, 3-D SPGR MRI offers little to no contrast between the physeal and articular cartilage. As a result, the edges

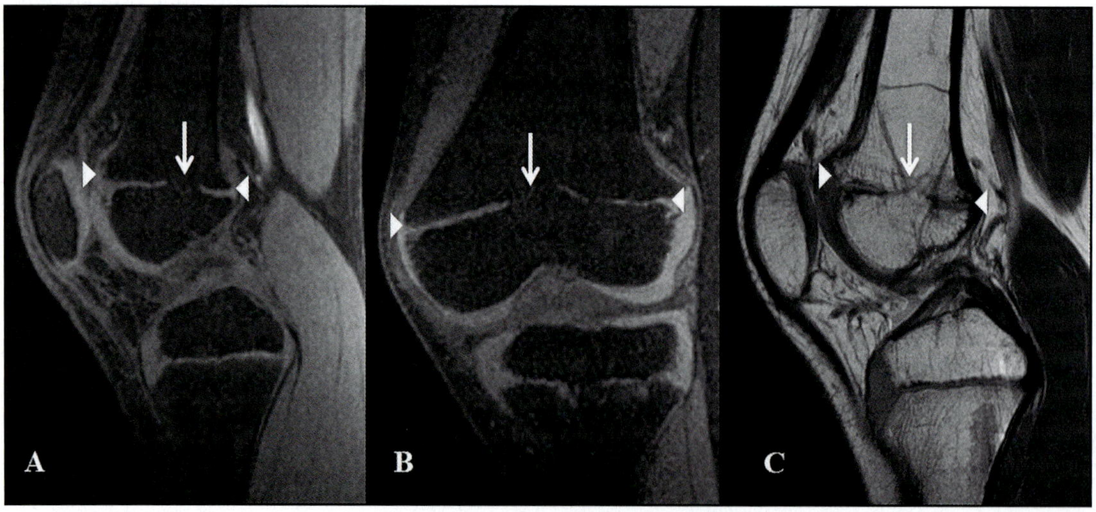

Figure 36.7. An 8-year-old male 13 months following a distal femoral fracture with an osseous bar across the central aspect of the distal femoral physis. Sagittal **(A)** and coronal **(B)** 3-D SPGR images demonstrate the bar (*white arrows*) as abnormal low signal intensity crossing the central physis (*white arrowheads*). Sagittal fast spin echo image **(C)** demonstrates that signal within the bar (*white arrow*) is isointense to the adjacent bone, indicating that it is osseous in nature.

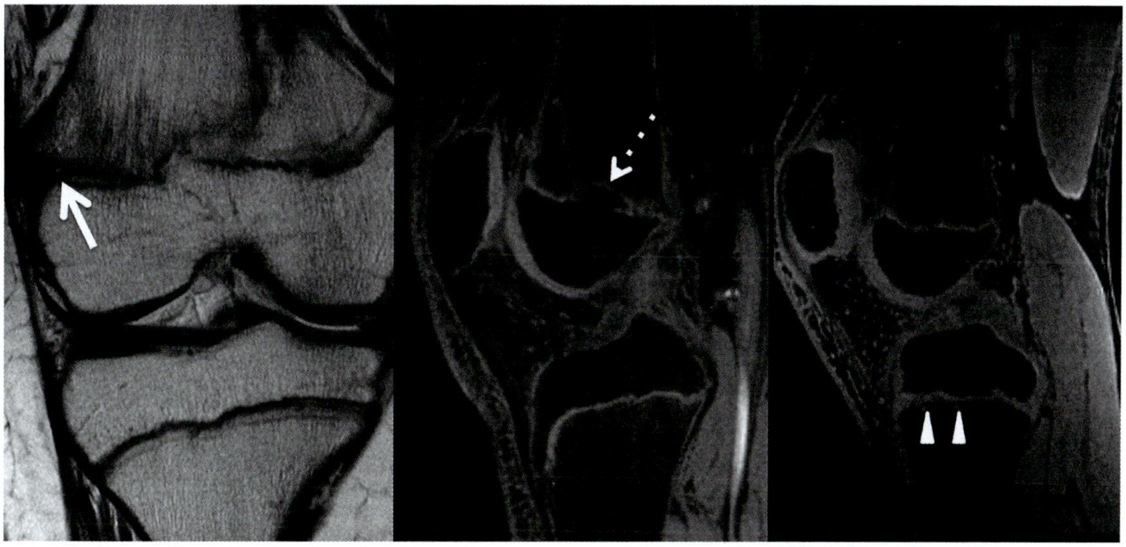

Figure 36.8. Coronal PD **(A)** and sagittal **(B)** 3-D SPGR images from the patient shown in Figure 36.7 demonstrate physeal irregularity (*solid white arrow*) and a metaphyseal island of physeal cartilage (*hatched white arrow*). Sagittal 3-D SPGR **(C)** from a different 11-year-old male demonstrates metaphyseal intrusions of physeal cartilage into the proximal tibial metaphysis (*arrowheads*).

of the physis may be difficult to distinguish from the articular surfaces at the peripheral margins.[7,20] This minor limitation can be overcome by using images in multiple planes, either using prospectively acquired or subsequently reconstructed images.

Artifact due to metal susceptibility on gradient echo images may limit the use of the SPGR sequence in the postoperative setting. Different metal compounds generate variable degrees of susceptibility. Even in the absence of metallic fixation, imperceptible tiny foci of metallic debris shed from surgical instruments can generate susceptibility that may obscure the physis. The history of prior surgery, however, is not a contraindication for use of the 3-D SPGR sequence. Postoperative MRI can offer meaningful information about iatrogenic injury. At our institution, MRI is frequently obtained following anterior cruciate or medial patellofemoral ligament reconstruction to evaluate for postoperative physeal damage (Fig. 36.11).

A baseline MRI examination of the physis may serve as a reference point from which to compare follow-up studies. The mean time to detection of a bar is 1 year (median, 10.8 months), but bars have been identified as early as 2 months post injury.[10] Typically, an MRI obtained in the acute setting following an injury will not show evidence of a physeal bar, but it can provide useful information about the pattern and extent of physeal injury as well as any other concomitant injuries about the knee joint.

Information from the proton density (PD) fast spin echo sequences in planes orthogonal to the physis can help in characterizing the nature of a physeal bar. Fibrous tissue is low

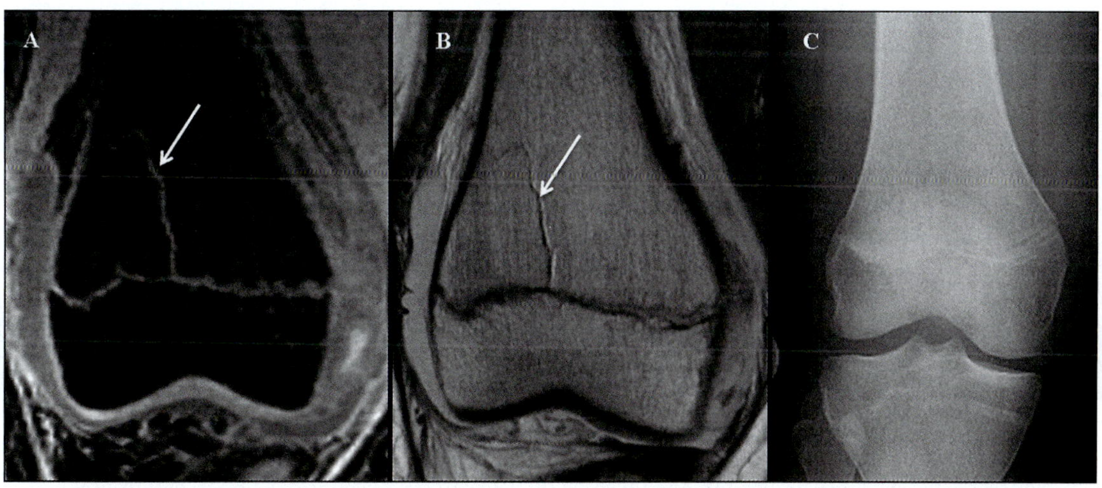

Figure 36.9. A 15-year-old female injured playing soccer. MRI was obtained to evaluate the anterior cruciate and medial collateral ligaments. Coronal 3-D SPGR **(A)** and PD **(B)** images demonstrate a Salter-Harris type II fracture (*white arrows*). A high-grade medial collateral ligament injury is not shown. Even in retrospect, the fracture is occult on the AP radiograph **(C)**.

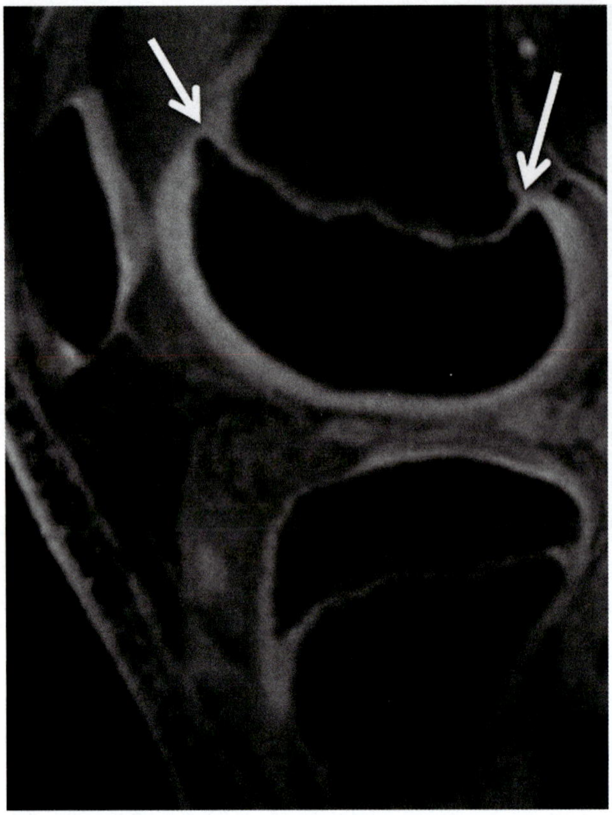

Figure 36.10. Sagittal 3-D SPGR MR image demonstrates isointensity of the physeal and articular cartilage. Anteriorly and posteriorly (*arrows*), the physeal cartilage and articular cartilage are indistinguishable.

in signal intensity, whereas osseous tissue will be high signal intensity due to the presence of fatty marrow (see Fig. 36.7). On T1 weighted images, larger osseous bridges (involving >25% of physeal cross-sectional area) appear isointense or slightly hyperintense to the metaphyseal marrow, but smaller bridges may demonstrate more variable signal intensity.[10]

PD sequences also complement the 3-D SPGR images. For example, linear low signal intensity adjacent to the growth plate can indicate sclerosis. Harris growth lines are not visible on the SPGR but are apparent on the PD images.

The 3-D SPGR data sets may be analyzed both qualitatively and quantitatively. Scrolling through the 3-D SPGR images, it is possible to qualitatively detect an area of physeal closure, either physiologic or posttraumatic. The relative location of the physeal defect can also be determined. A rough percentage of involvement can be estimated by visual analysis of the size of the defect relative to the physis.

Software included with many of the modern picture archiving and communications systems (PACS) can be used to create a maximum intensity projection (MIP) image from the MRI data to generate a physeal map.[10] Commercially available software also enables users to manually segment the physis and to subsequently calculate the physeal surface area.[13,31] Semiautomated physeal segmentation has been described using customized software.[27,30] Following segmentation, postprocessing enables calculation of the physeal damage and/or bar as both an absolute surface area and as a percent of the total physeal surface area. The physeal bar surface area calculated from the MRI data correlates with the histologic size of the defect, and such validation of software is essential for accurate, reproducible assessment of the magnitude of physeal interruption.[27] Physeal segmentation also allows for creation of 3-D models, which provide more than

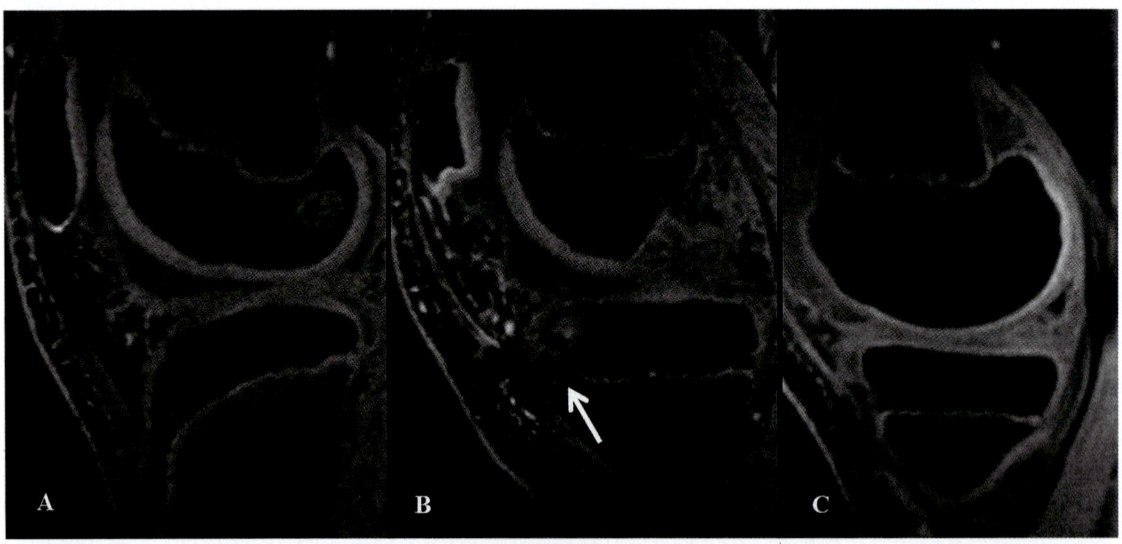

Figure 36.11. Sagittal 3-D SPGR MR images **(A and B)** from a 13-year-old female 3 months status post all epiphyseal anterior cruciate ligament reconstruction demonstrates no injury to the distal femoral physis adjacent to the epiphyseal fixation **(A)**. *Arrow* in image **(B)** demonstrates a small area of physeal disturbance anteriorly in the proximal tibia. Sagittal 3-D SPGR MR image **(C)** from a 13-year-old female 3 months status post medial patellofemoral ligament reconstruction demonstrates a normal distal femoral physis adjacent to the epiphyseal fixation.

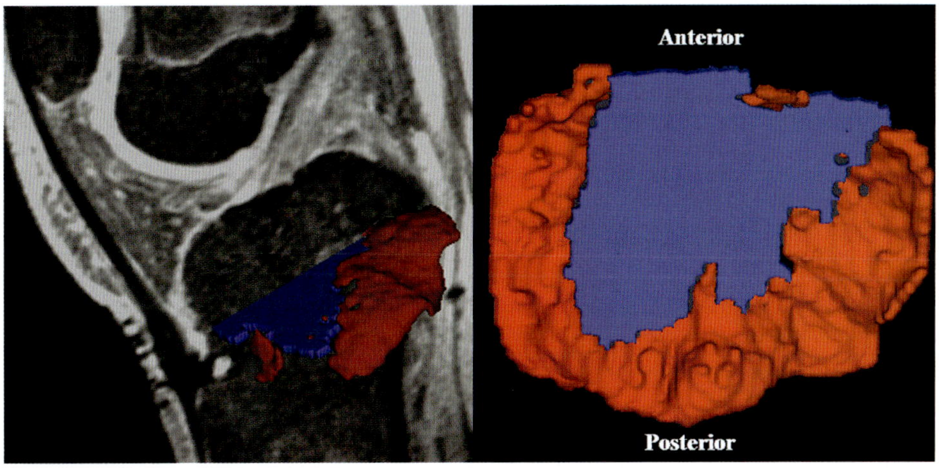

Figure 36.12. Sagittal 3-D SPGR image from a 16-year-old female with superimposed 3-D physeal model of the physeal bar where the *red* indicates the normal physis and the *blue* represents the bar. On this image, the 3-D model has been "extracted" from the planar image. The physis and bar area were calculated from the 3-D model. Physis area: 2,545.2 mm^2; bar area: 1,112.9 mm^2; percent bar: 43.7%.

just aesthetically pleasing pictures; the size, location, and geometry of the region of physeal damage and/or bar are easier to appreciate on 3-D models (Fig. 36.12).[30] These data are essential guides to operative planning and may be used to predict potential limb length discrepancy.

Ligamentous injuries occur in half of patients with epiphyseal injuries.[12] In particular, distal femoral injuries have a high incidence of associated ligamentous injuries.[10] Nonphyseal structures are best evaluated on high-resolution fast spin echo images.[19] Our recommended imaging protocol (see Table 36.2) includes the 3-D SPGR, a sagittal IR sequence, as well as three-planes (sagittal, axial, and coronal) of proton density. Injuries to articular cartilage and periarticular ligamentous, muscular, and tendinous structures as well as nearby neural and vascular structures will be most apparent on the PD and IR sequences.

Imaging plays a vitally important role in the management of pediatric patients with physeal injuries. The risk of future growth disturbance can be more comprehensively assessed with knowledge of the location and extent of physeal damage and injury to the extraphyseal structures. Imaging information helps orthopedic surgeons to assess the risk of future growth disturbance and appropriately counsel a patient and his or her parents regarding the risk of future complications. Information provided by radiologic studies can lead to significant alterations in patient care, including earlier intervention which can lead to a reduction in overall patient morbidity.

REFERENCES

1. Mizuta T, Benson WM, Foster BK, et al. Statistical analysis of the incidence of physeal injuries. *J Pediatr Orthop.* 1987;75:518–523.
2. Kawamoto K, Kim WC, Tsuchida Y, et al. Incidence of physeal injuries in Japanese children. *J Pediatr Orthop B.* 2006;15(2):126–130.
3. Mann DC, Rajmaira S. Distribution of physeal and nonphyseal fractures in 2,650 long-bone fractures in children aged 0-16 years. *J Pediatr Orthop.* 1990;10(6):713–716.
4. Dodwell ER, Kelley SP. Physeal fractures: basic science, assessment and acute management. *Orthop Trauma.* 2011;25(5):377–391.
5. Escott BG, Kelley SP. Management of traumatic physeal growth arrest. *Orthop Trauma.* 2012;26(3):200–211.
6. Ogden JA. The evaluation and treatment of partial physeal arrest. *J Bone Joint Surg Am.* 1987;69(8):1297–1302.
7. Craig JG, Cramer KE, Cody DD, et al. Premature partial closure and other deformities of the growth plate: MR imaging and three-dimensional modeling. *Radiology.* 1999;210(3):835–843.
8. Peterson HA, Madhok R, Benson JT, et al. Physeal fractures: part 1. Epidemiology in Olmsted County, Minnesota, 1979-1988. *J Pediatr Orthop.* 1994;14(4):423–430.
9. Basener CJ, Mehlman CT, DiPasquale TG. Growth disturbance after distal femoral growth plate fractures in children: a meta-analysis. *J Orthop Trauma.* 2009;23(9):663–667.
10. Ecklund K, Jaramillo D. Patterns of premature physeal arrest: MR imaging of 111 children. *AJR Am J Roentgenol.* 2002;178(4):967–972.
11. Makela EA, Vainionpaa S, Vihtonen K, et al. The effect of trauma to the lower femoral epiphyseal plate. An experimental study in rabbits. *J Bone Joint Surg Br.* 1988;70(2):187–191.
12. Rogers LF, Poznanski AK. Imaging of epiphyseal injuries. *Radiology.* 1994;191(2):297–308.
13. Craig JG, Cody DD, Van Holsbeeck M. The distal femoral and proximal tibial growth plates: MR imaging, three-dimensional modeling and estimation of area and volume. *Skeletal Radiol.* 2004;33(6):337–344.
14. Harcke HT, Synder M, Caro PA, et al. Growth plate of the normal knee: evaluation with MR imaging. *Radiology.* 1992;183(1):119–123.
15. Salter RB, Harris WR. Injuries involving the epiphyseal plate. *J Bone Joint Surg.* 1963;45(3):587–621.
16. Ogden JA. Injury to the growth mechanisms of the immature skeleton. *Skeletal Radiol.* 1981;6(4):237–253.
17. Sanchez TR, Jadhav SP, Swischuk LE. MR imaging of pediatric trauma. *Magn Reson Imaging Clin N Am.* 2009;17(3):439–450, v.
18. Jaramillo D, Shapiro F, Hoffer FA, et al. Posttraumatic growth-plate abnormalities: MR imaging of bony-bridge formation in rabbits. *Radiology.* 1990;175(3):767–773.
19. Potter HG. Imaging of the multiple-ligament-injured knee. *Clin Sports Med.* 2000;19(3):425–441.
20. Sailhan F, Chotel F, Guibal AL, et al. Three-dimensional MR imaging in the assessment of physeal growth arrest. *Eur Radiol.* 2004;14(9):1600–1608.
21. Shi DP, Zhu SC, Li Y, et al. Epiphyseal and physeal injury: comparison of conventional radiography and magnetic resonance imaging. *Clin Imaging.* 2009;33(5):379–383.

22. Murray K, Nixon GW. Epiphyseal growth plate: evaluation with modified coronal CT. *Radiology*. 1988;166(1, pt 1):263–265.
23. Vallier HA, Ahmadinia K, Forde FA, et al. Trends in musculoskeletal imaging for trauma patients: how has our practice changed over time? *J Orthop Trauma*. 2014;28(10):e236–e241.
24. Costello JE, Cecava ND, Tucker JE, et al. CT radiation dose: current controversies and dose reduction strategies. *AJR Am J Roentgenol*. 2013;201(6):1283–1290.
25. Rogalla P, Kloeters C, Hein PA. CT technology overview: 64-slice and beyond. *Radiol Clin North Am*. 2009;47(1):1–11.
26. Futami T, Foster BK, Morris LL, et al. Magnetic resonance imaging of growth plate injuries: the efficacy and indications for surgical procedures. *Arch Orthop Trauma Surg*. 2000;120(7–8):390–396.
27. Koff MF, Chong le R, Virtue P, et al. Correlation of magnetic resonance imaging and histologic examination of physeal bars in a rabbit model. *J Pediatr Orthop*. 2010;30(8):928–935.
28. Disler DG. Fat-suppressed three-dimensional spoiled gradient-recalled MR imaging: assessment of articular and physeal hyaline cartilage. *AJR Am J Roentgenol*. 1997;169(4):1117–1123.
29. Jaimes C, Chauvin NA, Delgado J, et al. MR imaging of normal epiphyseal development and common epiphyseal disorders. *Radiographics*. 2014;34(2):449–471.
30. Lurie B, Koff MF, Shah P, et al. Three-dimensional magnetic resonance imaging of physeal injury: reliability and clinical utility. *J Pediatr Orthop*. 2013;34(3):239–245.
31. Borsa JJ, Peterson HA, Ehman RL. MR imaging of physeal bars. *Radiology*. 1996;199(3):683–687.

Hannah-Noemi Ladenhauf
Gerd Seitlinger

CHAPTER 37

Growth Plate Anatomy

THE DEVELOPMENT OF BONE

During fetal development, three distinct ways of differentiation of the skeleton have been described. Somites, bilaterally paired blocks of mesoderm that form along the anterior-posterior axis, give rise to the axial skeleton. The lateral mesodermal plate generates the limb skeleton, and the cranial neural crest develops the branchial arch, craniofacial bone, and cartilage.

The formation of new bone tissue by osteoblasts is termed *ossification* or *osteogenesis*. In the process of generating new, healthy bone, there are two major pathways: *intramembranous ossification* and *endochondral ossification*. Both involve the transformation of a preexisting mesenchymal tissue into bone tissue. Intramembranous ossification occurs when flat bone needs to be built. It is an essential process during the formation of rudimentary bones of the skull.

The first step during intramembranous ossification is the formation of bone spicules, which will subsequently fuse with each other. Therefore, a small group of mesenchymal precursor cells proliferate and form a dense cluster of cells, a nodule. The cells within the nodule replicate and develop into an osteoprogenitor cell.[1] During further development, the osteoprogenitor cell changes in morphology and displays the morphologic characteristics of an osteoblast. Osteoblasts can then create an extracellular matrix containing type 1 collagen fibrils, termed *osteoid*, an immature bone, which increases the size of the bone spicules. As the spicules continue to grow, they fuse and form trabeculae. Some of the osteoblasts become incorporated within the osteoid and develop into osteocytes, which can later mineralize the immature bone tissue. As growth continues, the trabeculae become interconnected and so-called woven bone is formed. This initial trabecular network is also termed *primary spongiosa*. The periosteum is formed around the trabeculae by differentiating mesenchymal cells. Osteogenic cells that originate from the periosteum increase appositional growth and a bone collar is formed. The bone collar is then mineralized and lamellar bone is formed. Unlike endochondral ossification, intramembranous ossification does not require the preexistence of cartilage.

Endochondral ossification is the second process by which new bone tissue can be created. This pathway requires the formation of a cartilaginous template, which can then be converted into bone. This process occurs during embryonic long bone formation and longitudinal physeal growth. Endochondral ossification does not only occur at the growth plates but also at many other sites. Epiphyses and their equivalents including carpals, tarsals, sesamoids, and apophyses all develop solely by endochondral growth.[2]

The pathway of endochondral growth can be divided into several stages. First, mesenchymal cells differentiate into chondrocytes, which grow cartilage. The chondrocytes will then proliferate rapidly to form the model for the bone. The cartilage will grow in length by successive cell division of chondrocytes, accompanied by continuous secretion of extracellular matrix. This process is termed *interstitial growth*. In contrast, appositional growth happens when the cartilage model also grows in thickness through addition of more extracellular matrix on the peripheral cartilage. In a later stage, the chondrocytes will terminate their division process and increase dramatically in volume, becoming hypertrophic. This alters the matrix and thus enables it to become mineralized by calcium carbonate and to be invaded by blood vessels. The hypertrophic chondrocytes will later go into apoptosis,[3] leaving this space to become bone marrow. So-called stacked cells which earlier surrounded the cartilage model now give rise to the lineage of osteogenic cells that will later differentiate into osteoblasts, beginning to form bone matrix on the partially degraded structure of the cartilage model.[4] This pathway is responsible for the construction of new healthy bone on the basis of a cartilage model.

Endochondral growth and ossification are affected by various factors, such as biologic parameters, intrinsic genetic predisposition, and systemic chemical agents. In addition, epigenetic mechanical factors have been found to be interacting factors. In areas of intermittent high shear stress, growth may be accelerated, whereas in areas of intermittent high hydrostatic pressure, it may be decelerated, and these latter areas may remain cartilaginous. The articular cartilage or growth plates are examples of this. Today, models are available that allow for calculation of a specific growth rate for each region of cartilage as well as estimation of overall longitudinal growth, taking biologic and mechanobiologic influences into account.[5]

In the long bones of the skeleton, endochondral ossification spreads outward in both directions from the center of the bone. As the ossification process nears the edges of the cartilage model, chondrocytes proliferate and become hypertrophic, pushing out the cartilaginous end of the bone, forming an area that is termed *epiphyseal growth plate*, resulting in two centers of endochondral ossification. The primary center lies in the diaphysis, where chondrocytes replicate and form trabeculae, which are successively replaced by mineralized bone. The perichondrium layer surrounding the former cartilage forms the periosteum, leaving a small foramen for the nutrient artery in the diaphysis. The secondary center of ossification appears at the epiphysis, the region yet to be converted into mineralized bone. Growth plates were found to consist of three layers of chondrocytes during their process of maturation. This area has also been termed the *zone of maturation* and consists of a region of chondrocyte proliferation, a region of mature chondrocytes, and a region of hypertrophic chondrocytes.[6] Apart from the distal femur and the proximal tibia, these secondary ossification centers appear around or after birth.[7] With the secured blood supply via epiphyseal arteries, osteogenic cells will later invade the epiphysis and deposit osteoblasts and osteoclasts that will build bone. The process of endochondral ossification occurs in both directions, initiated from the center of long bones. The only exceptions to this are digits and ribs. In case of the formation of ribs and digits, ossification is not directly correlated with the invasion of blood vessels. For example, in ribs, new bone is separated from the perichondrium by a layer of mineralized cartilage; therefore, it cannot be classified as intramembranous ossification. Moreover, there is no preexistence of cartilage as seen in a process of endochondral ossification arising from an epiphyseal growth plate,[8] even though text books still describe two to four centers of ossification in the development of ribs.[9] The exact pathway remains unknown.

In the phalanges, the process of ossification is known to take a different course, too. Here, two centers of ossification are described. The primary center of ossification is placed in the diaphysis of the phalanx and ossification begins in the prenatal period. However, only one physis can be seen, located at the base of the phalanges. At the approximate age of 14 to 18 years, all of the epiphyses unite and form the digits.

BONE HEALING

Bone has the capability to repair itself following a fracture. During this process, both pathways to create new bone—intramembranous and endochondral ossification—are applied. However, both require the presence of mesenchymal cells that migrate to the wound site and differentiate into chondrocytes and osteoblasts in response to increased levels of growth factors and cytokines.[10] In nonrigid fractures, that is, fractures that retain a certain amount of movement (for instance those immobilized with a cast), the process of endochondral formation of bone will be triggered.

Immediately after the fracture occurs, the physiologic process of wound healing begins and a hematoma is formed. Within the inflammatory phase, the cell debris undergoes phagocytosis and is removed. Blood factors are released and cause the migration and proliferation of fibroblasts, which build granulation tissue.[11] This process is termed the *reactive phase* in the course of fracture healing. Several days after the fracture, a reparative phase is initiated. Periosteal cells proximal to the fracture gap replicate together with the fibroblasts and differentiate into chondroblasts, which form a hyaline cartilage template. The periosteal cells distal to the fracture gap differentiate into osteoblasts that form woven bone until the hyaline cartilage and the woven bone interconnect and form a heterogeneous mass. This mass is called *soft callus.*

During the next phase of fracture healing, the bone is remodeled using the pathway of endochondral ossification. The callus is invaded by microvessels and osteoblasts, which form new lamellar bone within the earlier mineralized matrix of hyaline cartilage and woven bone.[12] This new "hard callus" consists of trabecular bone, already restoring most of the bone's original strength. In a final phase, this trabecular bone is resorbed by osteoclasts, leaving space for osteoblasts to deposit compact bone within the resorption pit. In time, the callus is remodeled into a state resembling the bone's original shape and strength. This repair process is fundamentally affected by mechanical loading forces and by the geometric configuration of the fracture fragments, and its finalization may take up to 3 to 5 years.[11,13]

In comparison, highly stabilized (i.e., rigid) fractures (e.g., those treated with open reduction and stabilization with a metal plate or screws) heal by intramembranous ossification. Here, mesenchymal cells present at the site of injury differentiate directly into osteoblasts to form an osteoid that is later transformed into new bone. The exact pathway of how cells can interpret and respond to changes in the local mechanical environment still remains unclear.[14]

FORMATION OF A LONG BONE

As pointed out earlier, the long bones of the skeleton are formed on the basis of a cartilaginous model that is created during fetal development. Under the influence of vascular invasion, mesenchymal cells differentiate into osteoclasts and osteoblasts, which in the process of endochondral ossification form an osteoid matrix, from which trabecular bone and, later, mineralized bone is formed. These first centers of ossification appear in the diaphysis of long bones (Fig. 37.1). A perichondral layer of osteogenic cells encircles the cartilaginous model to ensure endochondral growth. Vascular supply is secured through nutrient arteries that invade the long bone via the nutrient foramen, a small opening in the diaphysis, allowing for the migration of osteogenic cells to the primary ossification center. By appositional growth of osteoblasts, longitudinal growth is achieved.

At specific times in the development of each long bone, two secondary centers of ossification appear—the growth plates on either end of the long bone. The growth plate, also known as *epiphyseal plate,* is an area where formation of new bone is possible. It is located at each end of long bones. Secondary ossification centers mostly occur after birth, with the exception of the growth plate of the distal femur and the proximal tibia, which develop during the perinatal period. From these centers of ossification, the end of each long bone is enlarged by centrifugal growth and allows the process of ossification to spread rapidly from the ossification centers. However, the rate of appositional growth from the secondary center is much slower than that of the primary growth plate. This development of new bone continues until closure of the growth plate at skeletal maturity.

ANATOMY OF THE GROWTH PLATE

As it is well known, a long bone is divided into its proximal epiphysis, proximal metaphysis, diaphysis (shaft), distal metaphysis, and an epiphysis at the distal end. The growth plate

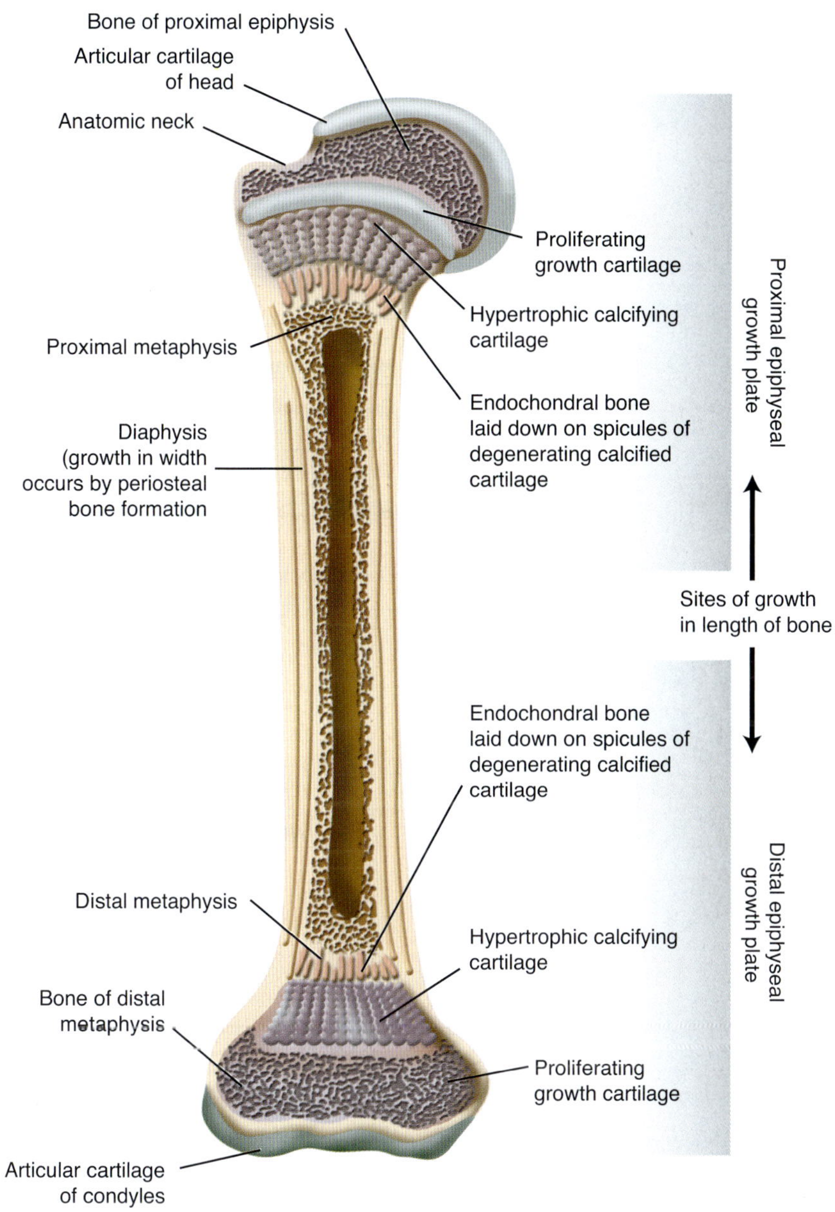

Figure 37.1. Formation of a long bone: The first centers for ossification appear in the diaphysis of long bones. By appositional growth of osteoblasts, longitudinal growth is achieved.

is found in the area of the metaphysis and holds the area of endochondral ossification. As we go from the epiphysis to the diaphysis, there first is an area of articular cartilage forming a cap onto the epiphysis (Fig. 37.2). Especially in long bones such as the femur, where the proximal epiphysis is part of the hip joint, this articular surface is essential for allowing movement in the joint. Therefore, the articular cartilage in this area will be required to transmit weight and will function as a so-called pressure epiphysis. Underneath the articular cartilage, the secondary ossification center of the epiphysis is located. It is supplied by the epiphyseal artery, which enables continuous immigration of osteogenic cells.

The growth plate can be anatomically divided into three types of tissue components: a cartilaginous component (epiphyseal plate), an ossific component (metaphysis), and a fibrous component surrounding the periphery of the plate. The cartilaginous part, which is composed of four different histologic zones, holds the essential stages during which new bone is created. This area is encircled by a fibrous component made up of the groove of Ranvier and the perichondral ring of LaCroix. Adjacent to the cartilage, we find a bony metaphysis.

During childhood, the growth plate consists of connecting cartilage, enabling the long bone to grow in length and girth. At adulthood, the components terminate growth and the growth plate completely ossifies into solid bone.

The Cartilaginous Component

The cartilaginous component of the growth plate is divided histologically into four zones, described as the resting zone, the proliferative zone, the hypertrophic zone, and the zone of provisional calcification (Fig. 37.3).

Located immediately below the secondary center of ossification, there is a zone of undifferentiated or resting cartilage cells, named the *reserve zone.* This zone contains irregularly scattered cartilage cells with a high lipid content, suggesting

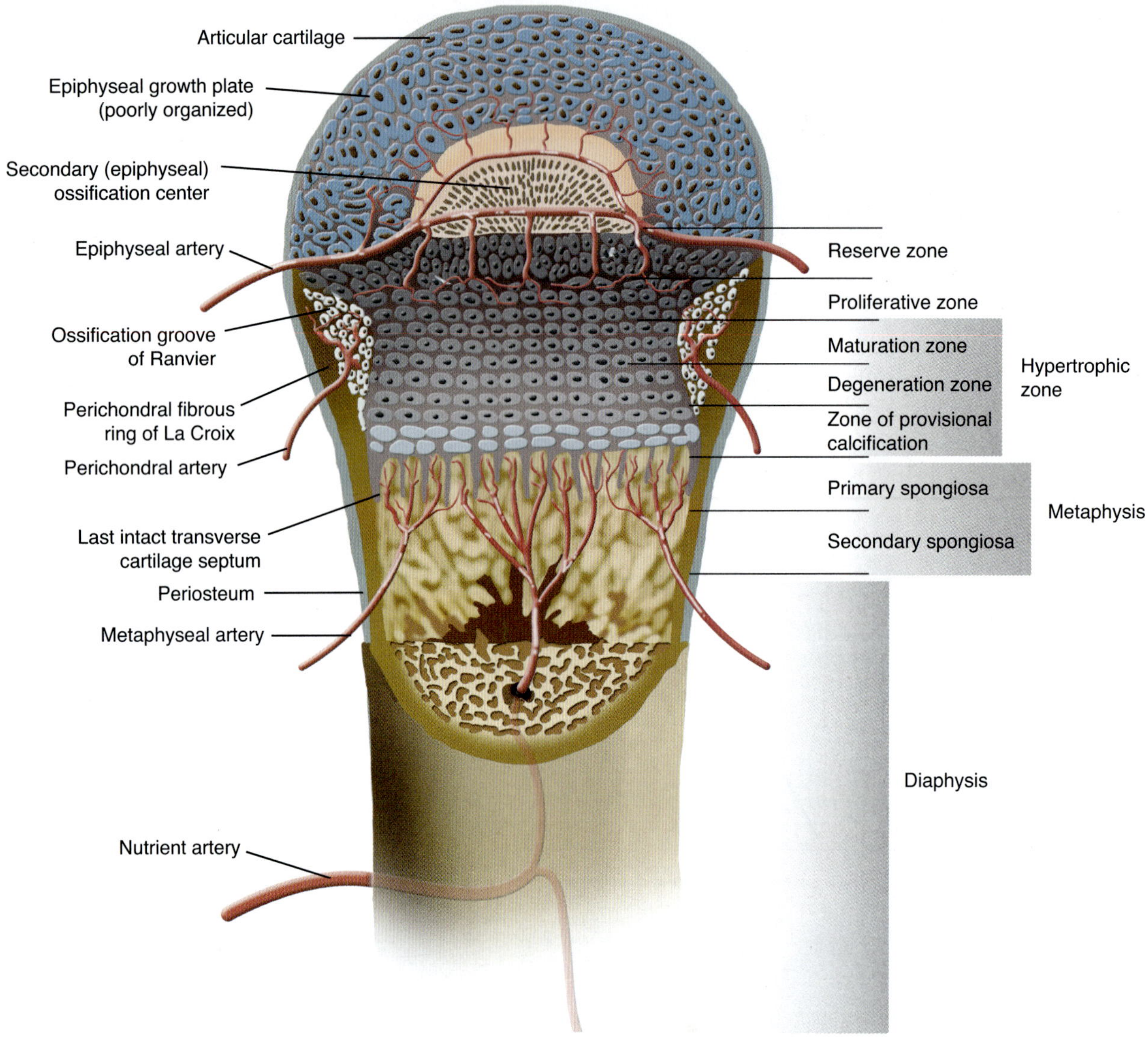

Figure 37.2. Morphologic structure and blood supply of the growth plate.

a nutrient storage potential. These cells act as precursor cells for the developing cartilage cells in the next zone. Injury to this zone is deleterious because it often results in a partial or complete arrest of growth. Adjacent to the reserve zone, there is the *zone of proliferating cartilage.* This zone comprises about half of the overall height of the physis. Although chondrocytes still appear rather flat in this area, they already start to proliferate. At the base of these columns, mitotic activity is found. Cells rapidly divide and become organized into columns, laying down a cartilage extracellular matrix that will later serve as a scaffold for future osteoblasts, which in the future allow the process of ossification. The entire growth in length of the long bone occurs at this location. In the *zone of maturation* or *hypertrophic zone,* which follows, cells are still organized in columns, but they enlarge to 5 to 10 times the size of the proliferating zone.

In this layer, there is no active growth and the chondrocytes begin to terminally differentiate, resulting in cell death, triggering blood vessel invasion and bone formation.

As the chondrocytes become hypertrophic, the extracellular matrix, consisting of collagens and proteoglycans, is diminished. This explains why the hypertrophic zone is the weakest: It lacks both collagen and calcified tissue. Therefore, most physeal separations and fractures occur through this layer because it is less resistant to stress than the other parts of the growth plate.

As endochondral ossification depends on the invasion of blood vessels and matrix remodeling, blood vessels enter the partially dismantled scaffold in the *zone of provisional calcification.* This process allows osteogenic progenitor cells to invade and deposit trabecular bone. The remodeling process causes variations in calcium and phosphate levels in the matrix at the junction of cartilage and bone. The variations in ion concentrations, matrix degradation and mineralization, and influx of new cell types all regulate the equilibrium of cartilage degradation to bone formation.

The Fibrous Structure

Surrounding the periphery of the growth plate lays a wedge-shaped groove of cells, called the *groove of Ranvier,*[15] and a ring of fibrous tissue, the perichondral ring of LaCroix.[16]

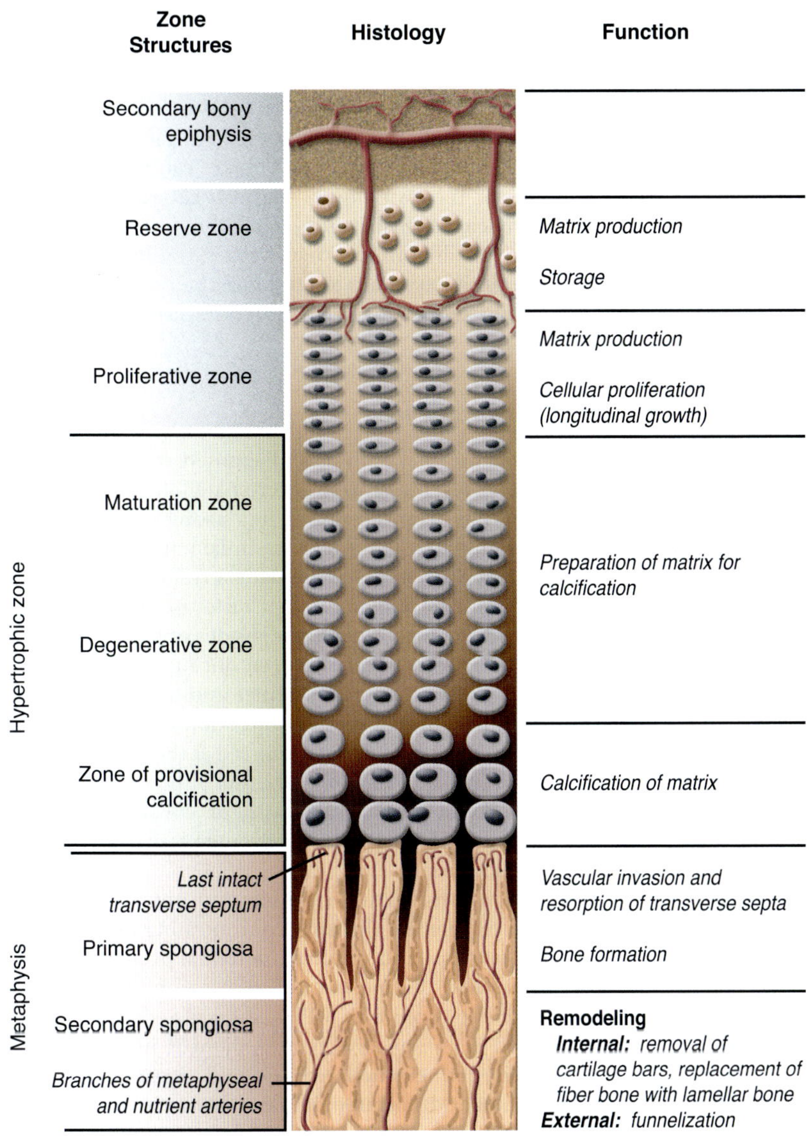

Figure 37.3. Growth plate anatomy: The cartilaginous component of the growth plate is divided histologically into four zones, described as the resting zone, the proliferative zone, the hypertrophic zone, and the zone of provisional calcification.

The groove of Ranvier contains cells, which are active in division and contribute in the increase of the width of the growth plate. The structure of the perichondral ring of LaCroix is a fibrous collagenous network that is continuous with the fibrous portion of the groove of Ranvier and the periosteum of the metaphysis. Its function is to mechanically support and stabilize the bone–cartilage junction of the growth plate.[17–20]

The Metaphysis

The metaphysis holds the function of removal of the cartilaginous matrix and its replacement with bone. Its beginning is in the last intact transverse septum of each cartilaginous cell column. Lysosomal enzymes remove the last transverse septum and allow for endothelial and perivascular cells to invade. Between capillaries and osteoblasts that line the calcified bars, osteoprogenitor cells start the process of ossification. This area of only little or no bone formation is termed the *primary spongiosa*.[21] Using the cartilaginous scaffold, osteoblasts progressively form bone, creating the secondary spongiosa. The initial fiber bone is soon replaced by lamellar bone by the process of synchronized osteoclastic bone resorption and osteoblastic bone formation.

Vascular Supply of the Growth Plate

The growth plate and the epiphyseal region are supplied by three vascular systems: the epiphyseal, metaphyseal, and perichondral blood supply.[1] The epiphyseal artery mostly secures vascular supply of the epiphysis. It divides into small branches forming a network of vessels, which enter the epiphysis from different sides. Each small branch spreads out in a tree-like fashion and supplies 4 to 10 cell columns. Therefore, the proliferative zone is well perfused to allow for cell proliferation and division.[22]

In the past, an existence of transphyseal vessels was uncertain and subject to intense controversy. However, recent studies using modern imaging techniques have revealed blood vessels that cross the growth plate.[23]

The metaphysis is richly supplied with arterial blood from the nutrient artery as well as from the metaphyseal arteries arising from the ascending cervical arteries. About 80% of the metaphyseal vessels derive from the nutrient artery, which divides into several branches that supply the central region of the metaphysis.

The perichondral vessels supply the fibrous peripheral structures of the growth plate, such as the groove of Ranvier and the perichondral ring of LaCroix. Branches surround the growth plate and send anastomoses to both the epiphyseal and the metaphyseal arteries.[24,25]

THE INFLUENCE OF RECONSTRUCTIVE SURGERY AROUND THE KNEE ON THE DISTAL FEMORAL GROWTH PLATE

Participation of children and adolescents in sports is on the rise, with young athletes training year-round and specializing at earlier ages, predisposing them to sports-related injuries. Once thought to be rare, injuries of the anterior cruciate ligament (ACL) and medial patellofemoral ligament (MPFL) are seen with a greater frequency in the pediatric population. Numerous preventive training programs have been developed but are yet to be established among the society.[26] Even though ACL injuries are among the most extensively researched orthopedic injuries and treatment options have evolved, there are still many controversies surrounding the appropriate treatment of these injuries in children and adolescents.

Anterior Cruciate Ligament Injury

Today, there seems to be a consensus among pediatric orthopedic surgeons that reconstructive surgery after a complete tear of the ACL or the MPFL yields a favorable outcome for pediatric and adolescent patients.[27–34] Although conservative management is an appealing option given the increased potential of regeneration in children, clinical results after nonoperative treatment have not been satisfactory.[35–38] In cases of partial tears of the ACL, nonreconstructive management may be successful in younger children and adolescents.[30,34]

However, reconstructive surgery allows for early mobilization and participation in sports and may prevent further meniscal injury and articular cartilage damage, which can result in early-onset osteoarthritis.[27,39–44] Especially in cases where bone bruising is detected on magnetic resonance imaging (MRI) studies, the incidence of intra-articular injuries such as meniscal tears seem to be increased.[45–47] Bisson et al.[45] stated that 90% of all subjects were found to have bone bruising on MRI after injury of the ACL. In their cohort, moderate and severe bone bruising seen on MRI was associated with an increased arthroscopic finding of medial meniscal tears.[45] Yoon et al.[47] found that medial meniscal injury was detected in 66% of cases with medial and lateral bone contusion.

In a meta-analysis from 2013, Ramski et al.[32] were able to show that benefits in multiple outcomes favor early surgical stabilization over nonoperative treatment. They found that children and adolescents suffering from an ACL injury who underwent nonoperative or delayed treatment were likely to experience more instability and pathologic laxity.

Furthermore, many were more frequently unable to return to their previous activity levels when compared to patients treated with surgical reconstruction of their ACL.[32] Many authors published similar results and concluded that up to 50% of children treated nonoperatively for a complete ACL tear did not return to athletic activity.[48]

There has been ongoing discussion and research regarding the optimal technique to reconstruct the ACL in children and adolescents. Generally, modern techniques can be categorized in extraphyseal reconstruction, transphyseal reconstruction, and all-epiphyseal reconstruction. Each one is directed toward restoring the stability of the knee, with extraphyseal and all-epiphyseal techniques trying to minimize the risk of iatrogenic physeal injury (see Section 1 on Anterior Cruciate Ligament Injury).

Patellar Dislocation

Patellar dislocation is commonly diagnosed in children and adolescents and often results in severe patellofemoral instability. The MPFL has been recognized as a strong stabilizer of the patella, providing 50% to 60% of the innate medial passive resistance. Lateral dislocation of the patella results in disruption of this ligament. The initial event of dislocation is frequently traumatic in origin, with recurrent episodes of patellar dislocation after a low-energy trauma or even during forceful flexion of the knee. In a previous study, Kepler and colleagues[49] were able to detect that in 44 children and adolescents with acute primary MPFL disruption, injury occurred at the patella in 61% of cases, at the femur in 12% of cases, and at both sites in 12%. Ligamentous laxity, skeletal dysplasia, or collagen disorders such as Marfan or Ehlers-Danlos syndrome predispose patients to patellar dislocation.

Even though conservative treatment with short immobilization followed by physical therapy (concentrating on the evaluation of gait patterns and restoring potential preexisting muscle imbalances and the mechanical axis) can be successful in cases of traumatic rupture of MPFL, surgical reconstruction is recommended if conservative management is ineffective and recurrent episodes of patellar dislocation occur. In cases of atraumatic patellar dislocation, initial conservative treatment is often ineffective and high rates of redislocation—up to 80%—have been reported.[50,51]

However, surgical treatment in skeletally immature patients is still a subject of discussion. More than 100 different surgical techniques exist to stabilize the patella and address various contributing anatomic factors that may promote recurrent dislocation of the patella, such as the patellofemoral osseous geometry, overall limb alignment, and physeal anatomy.

Many authors advocate surgical reconstruction of the MPFL, allowing skeletally immature patients to quickly return to their full level of activity.[52–55] Recent studies have shown that short-term results seem to favor reconstruction over repair of the MPFL in children and adolescents.[56,57] Therefore, several physeal-sparing operative techniques have been presented and discussed in the literature.[58–64] In order to achieve satisfactory long-term results, it is essential to restore biomechanical kinematics of the knee through an anatomic reconstruction of the MPFL.

When planning an MPFL reconstruction in a child with open physis, the anatomic relationship of the MPFL insertion around the distal femoral physis needs to be considered. The MPFL insertion on the medial condyle of the femur has been described to be distal to the adductor tendon insertion and proximal to the femoral insertion of the medial collateral

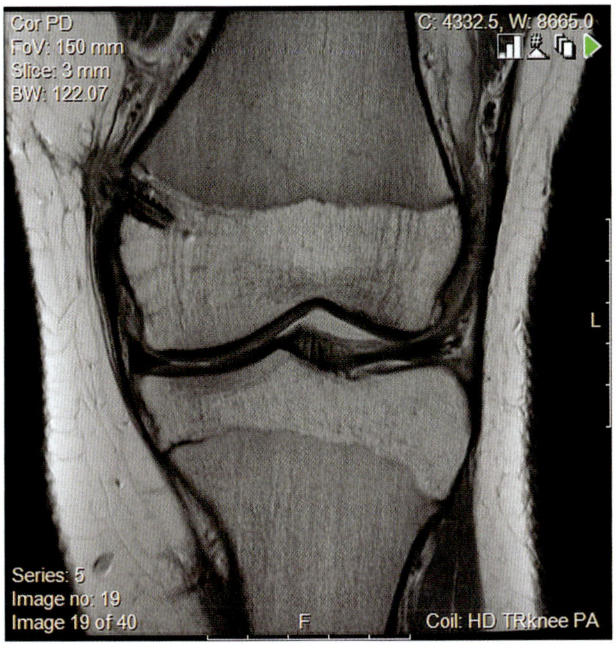

Figure 37.4. Anatomic reconstruction of the MPFL in a skeletally immature patient using a hamstring graft: femoral insertion of the reconstructed MPFL just distal to the femoral growth plate.

ligament, with close proximity to the medial aspect of the distal femoral growth plate.[55,63,65] Kepler and colleagues[49] as well as Balcarek[66] and Nelitz and colleagues[67] have further investigated the origin of the MPFL and found the zone of insertion to be just distal to the distal femoral physis. This knowledge is essential in order to avoid injury of the growth plate and to allow for an anatomically correct reconstruction (Fig. 37.4). Bone fixation proximal to the distal femoral physis may result in proximal migration of the femoral insertion of the MPFL, causing for loss of graft tension, graft isometry, and loss of motion in the knee (see Section 2 on Patellofemoral Instability).

Surgical Tendon Reconstruction and the Growth Plate

It is unclear whether the benefits of a surgical reconstruction of the ACL and MPFL in a skeletally immature patient outweigh the risk of potential injury of the distal femoral growth plate and the proximal tibial growth plate. Concern of damage to the growth plate, subsequent growth arrest, angular deformity, and limb length discrepancy after ACL or MPFL reconstruction have been discussed frequently in the literature and promoted surgeons to defer surgical management until skeletal maturity.[31,36,38,48] To circumvent physeal injury, many physeal-sparing techniques have been developed and promoted.[58–64,68–77] However, it is not clear which technique of ACL or MPFL reconstruction provides the least risk while best restoring the anatomic function of the injured ligament in the growing child.

The growth plate in children is a dynamic structure that is subject to physiologic and, in some cases, pathologic changes. Recently, ongoing research has attempted to enhance understanding of the anatomy and to identify specific landmarks around the knee in order to prevent damage to the growth plate. Harcke et al.[78] identified four stages of physeal development, analyzing 60 MRI studies obtained in male and female subjects aged 1 to 20 years. They found stage 1 to be characterized by a solely spherical ossification center, which seemed to enlarge and replace the cartilage during stage 2. As the ossification center grew in size, the growth plate gradually flattened and developed a contour that paralleled the metaphyseal contour during stage 3. Stage 4 was marked by the complete closure of the growth plate, during which the epiphysis is gradually replaced by bone. In a recent anatomic study of the distal femoral epiphysis by Liu et al.,[79] the investigators were able to characterize the shape of the growth plate, dividing its contour into three major undulations: the central ridge, lateral ridge, and medial peak. Although some previous descriptions suggested the growth plate to be a flat structure, they were able to show its undulating character in 26 specimens. Their results showed that although the growth plate is more linear in younger children, deepening of the metaphyseal–epiphyseal junctional notches increased with age.[79] This knowledge is essential when placing screws in close proximity to the distal femoral growth plate because the insertion point may falsely appear to be proximal of the physis due to the nonlinear structure of the distal femoral growth plate (Fig. 37.5). Sasaki et al.[80] found that in the proximal tibia, the central portion of the growth plate closed earlier than the peripheral portion. This suggests that use of a tibial tunnel for ACL reconstruction in skeletally immature patients does not elicit future growth disturbances.[80] Behr et al.[81] attempted to define the anatomic relationship of the femoral origin of the ACL to the distal femoral physis in the fetal knee throughout skeletal development of the knee. They found that all investigated fetal specimens clearly showed the fetal ACL originating from the posterior epiphysis of the lateral condyle. The origin site was immediately distal to the posterior aspect of the distal femoral physis. Magnetic resonance images correlated closely with the gross anatomic and histologic observations. The average distance of the ACL origin site was

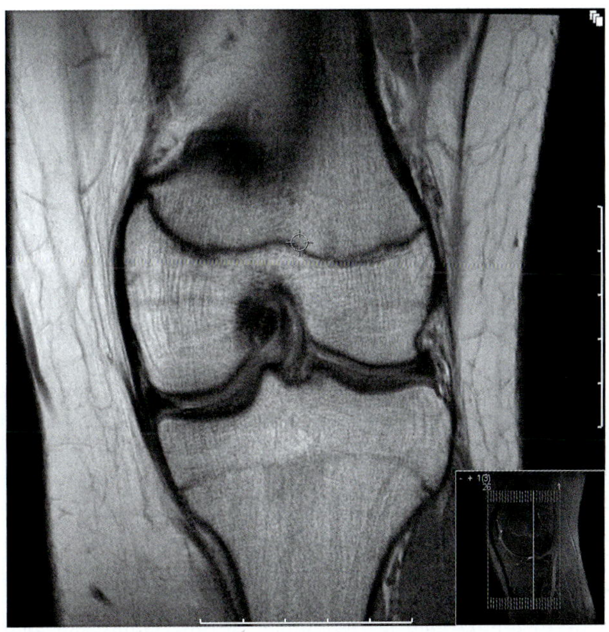

Figure 37.5. MRI of the distal femoral growth plate in a 14-year-old female demonstrating the undulating character of the growth plate.

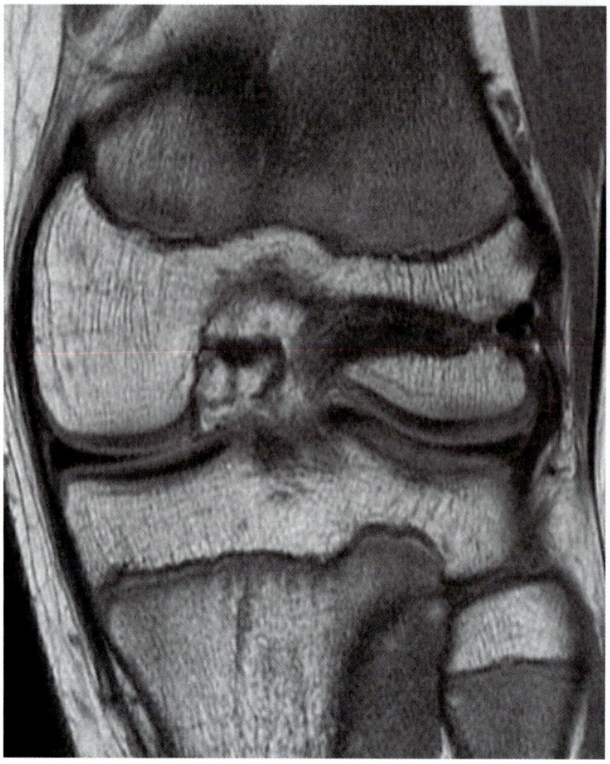

Figure 37.6. Anatomic reconstruction of the ACL in a skeletally immature patient: an all-epiphyseal technique using a hamstring graft. No injury to the distal femoral growth plate.

2.66 mm distal to the femoral physis. These results suggest that with a less than 3-mm margin for error between the physis and the attachment site of the ACL, fixation of the graft at the anatomically correct site is technically challenging due to the high risk of iatrogenic injury of the growth plate (Fig. 37.6).

Chudik et al.[82] investigated the influence of three different femoral techniques for graft placement on ACL reconstruction using a skeletally immature canine model. Their group performed unilateral ACL reconstructions using a central transphyseal tibial tunnel and one of three different femoral fixation techniques. All tunnels were created with a 4.0-mm cannulated drill. They found that in the groups where an "over-the-top" fixation or a transphyseal drill tunnel was used, the ACL graft did not attach to the lateral femoral condyle. Grafts migrated and moved away from the knee with longitudinal growth. In the group where an epiphyseal drill tunnel was used, attachment of the graft at the original site was maintained. However, although valgus deformity of the distal femur was significantly greater in the transphyseal and over-the-top groups than in the epiphyseal group, the epiphyseal and transphyseal groups exhibited increased rates of external rotation of the distal femur. Postoperative findings of chondral injuries were increased in the epiphyseal group. They concluded that although an epiphyseal technique may reduce the risk of angular deformity and allow for better femoral graft positioning, the epiphyseal technique might have an increased risk for rotational deformity, physeal injury, and articular surface injury.[82]

Even though iatrogenic injury to the epiphyseal plate should be avoided, some animal model studies using rabbits suggest that it might be possible to violate a small part of the distal femoral or proximal tibial growth plate without causing harm and promote premature physeal closure. Guzzanti et al.[83] performed intra-articular ACL reconstructions with semitendinosus tendons placed in 2-mm diameter tunnels in skeletally immature rabbits. This technique caused damage of 3% of the cross-sectional area of the proximal femoral growth plate and 4% of the proximal tibial growth plate. No alteration of growth or axial deviation of the femur resulted. However, there were two cases of valgus deformity of the tibia, and one tibia was shortened.[83] Mäkelä et al.[84] published a study including 44 rabbits that were operated on when 5 weeks old. In one group, a 2-mm hole was drilled across the intercondylar portion of the right femur in the central portion of the growth plate up to the diaphysis, whereas in the other group, a similar hole of 3.2 mm was drilled. During analysis, it was found that the 2-mm drill hole did not cause any significant shortening of the femur, whereas the 3.2-mm drill hole lead to formation of an osseous bridge, resulting in permanent growth disturbance and shortening of the femur.[84]

These results promote careful evaluation of the percentage of tissue damage to the growth plate when performing intra-articular reconstruction techniques around the knee in skeletally immature patients but also suggest that limited injury of the growth plate does not necessarily cause permanent damage and growth arrest. However, even though animal models may provide insight and direction as reconstructive procedures around the knee are developed and adapted, one has to consider that animal models have anatomic and physiologic differences that may limit direct comparison to humans.[82] Especially in adolescents reaching skeletal maturity, the incidence of growth disturbances after ACL reconstruction seems to be high. Yoo et al.[85] reported on five patients where a focal bone bridge was found on MRI after transphyseal reconstruction of the ACL. However, there was no case of clinically significant limb shortening or angular deformity.[85] It has been shown in experimental studies by Seil et al.[86] and Guzzanti et al.[83] that small focal bone bridges occur on the border of transphyseal tunnels, even if the defect of the tunnel is covered by the ACL graft. On the one hand, these small zones of fusion probably break and resolve through high expansion forces during constant growth of the physis. On the other hand, these forces decrease in patients close to skeletal maturity, as growth is drawing to an end. As a result, bone bridges cannot be overcome and may result in growth disturbances.[87]

Whenever surgical intervention in close proximity to the growth plate is indicated, one should be mindful of a number of factors that could potentially influence further growth.

REFERENCES

1. Brighton CT. Structure and function of the growth plate. *Clin Orthop Relat Res.* 1978;(136):22–32.
2. Oestreich AE. Enchondral growth: physes and acrophyses. In: Oestreich AE, ed. *Growth of the Pediatric Skeleton: A Primer for Radiologists.* New York, NY: Springer Publishing; 2008:7–11.
3. Hatori M, Klatte KJ, Teixeira CC, et al. End labeling studies of fragmented DNA in the avian growth plate: evidence of apoptosis in terminally differentiated chondrocytes. *J Bone Miner Res.* 1995;10: 1960–1968.
4. Bruder SP, Caplan AI. Cellular and molecular events during embryonic bone development. *Connect Tissue Res.* 1989;20:65–71.

5. Stevens SS, Beaupre GS, Carter DR. Computer model of endochondral growth and ossification in long bones: biological and mechanobiological influences. *J Orthop Res.* 1999;17:646–653.
6. Chen Q, Johnson DM, Haudenschild DR, et al. Progression and recapitulation of the chondrocyte differentiation program: cartilage matrix protein is a marker for cartilage maturation. *Dev Biol.* 1995;172:293–306.
7. Gray H. Osteology: the skeleton. In: Pick TP, Howden R, eds. *Anatomy, Descriptive and Surgical.* New York, NY: Gramercy Rooks; 1977:33–215.
8. Kampen WU, Claassen H, Kirsch T. Mineralization and osteogenesis in the human first rib cartilage. *Ann Anat.* 1995;177:171–177.
9. Gray H. Osteology: the ribs. In: Gray H, Lewis WH, eds. *Anatomy of the Human Body.* Philadelphia, PA: Lea & Febiger; 1918.
10. Caplan AI, Bruder SP. Cell and molecular engineering of bone regeneration. In: Lanza R, Langer R, Chick W, eds. *Textbook of Tissue Engineering.* Georgetown, TX: R. G. Landes; 1997:603–618.
11. Ham AW, Harris WR. Repair and transplantation of bone. In: Bourne GH, ed. *The Biochemistry and Physiology of Bone.* New York, NY: Academic Press; 1972:337–399.
12. Ford JL, Robinson DE, Scammell BE. Endochondral ossification in fracture callus during long bone repair: the localisation of "cavity-lining cells" within the cartilage. *J Orthop Res.* 2004;22:368–375.
13. Lacroix D, Prendergast PJ. A mechano-regulation model for tissue differentiation during fracture healing: analysis of gap size and loading. *J Biomech.* 2002;35:1163–1171.
14. Thompson Z, Miclau T, Hu D, et al. A model for intramembranous ossification during fracture healing. *J Orthop Res.* 2002;20:1091–1098.
15. Sapolsky AI, Howell DS, Woessner JF Jr. Neutral proteases and cathepsin D in human articular cartilage. *J Clin Invest.* 1974;53:1044–1053.
16. LaCroix P. *The Organization of Bone.* New York, NY: McGraw-Hill; 1951.
17. Chung SM, Batterman SC, Brighton CT. Shear strength of the human femoral capital epiphyseal plate. *J Bone Joint Surg Am.* 1976;58:94–103.
18. Ranvier L. Quelques fait relatifs au developpement du tissu osseux. *C R Acad Sci.* 1973;77:1105.
19. Rigal EM. The use of tritiated thymidine in studies of chondrogenesis. In: LaCroix P, Bud AM, eds. *Radioisotopes and Bone.* Oxford, United Kingdom: Blackwell Scientific Publications; 1962:197.
20. Shapiro F, Holtrop ME, Glimcher MJ. Organization and cellular biology of the perichondrial ossification groove of Ranvier: a morphological study in rabbits. *J Bone Joint Surg Am.* 1977;59:703–723.
21. Brighton CT. *Clinical Problems in Epiphyseal Plate Growth and Development. American Academy of Orthopaedic Surgeons Instructional Course Lectures.* Vol 23. St. Louis, MO: Mosby; 1974:105–122.
22. Tonna EA. The cellular complement of the skeletal system studied autoradiographically with tritiated thymidine (H3TDR) during growth and aging. *J Biophys Biochem Cytol.* 1961;9:813–824.
23. Wirth T, Syed Ali MM, Rauer C, et al. The blood supply of the growth plate and the epiphysis: a comparative scanning electron microscopy and histological experimental study in growing sheep. *Calcif Tissue Int.* 2002;70:312–319.
24. Haraldsson S. The vascular pattern of a growing and fullgrown human epiphysis. *Acta Anat (Basel).* 1962;48:156–167.
25. Trueta J, Buhr AJ. The vascular contribution to osteogenesis. V. The vasculature supplying the epiphyseal cartilage in rachitic rats. *J Bone Joint Surg Br.* 1963;45:572–581.
26. Ladenhauf HN, Graziano J, Marx RG. Anterior cruciate ligament prevention strategies: are they effective in young athletes—current concepts and review of literature. *Curr Opin Pediatr.* 2013;25:64–71.
27. Aichroth PM, Patel DV, Zorrilla P. The natural history and treatment of rupture of the anterior cruciate ligament in children and adolescents. A prospective review. *J Bone Joint Surg Br.* 2002;84:38–41.
28. Henry J, Chotel F, Chouteau J, et al. Rupture of the anterior cruciate ligament in children: early reconstruction with open physes or delayed reconstruction to skeletal maturity? *Knee Surg Sports Traumatol Arthrosc.* 2009;17:748–755.
29. Hinterwimmer S, Engelschalk M, Sauerland S, et al. Operative or conservative treatment of anterior cruciate ligament rupture: a systematic review of the literature [in German]. *Unfallchirurg.* 2003;106:374–379.
30. Kocher MS, Micheli LJ, Zurakowski D, et al. Partial tears of the anterior cruciate ligament in children and adolescents. *Am J Sports Med.* 2002;30:697–703.
31. McCarroll JR, Shelbourne KD, Patel DV. Anterior cruciate ligament injuries in young athletes. Recommendations for treatment and rehabilitation. *Sports Med.* 1995;20:117–127.
32. Ramski DE, Kanj WW, Franklin CC, et al. Anterior cruciate ligament tears in children and adolescents: a meta-analysis of nonoperative versus operative treatment. *Am J Sports Med.* 2014;42:2769–2776.
33. Al-Hadithy N, Dodds AL, Akhtar KS, et al. Current concepts of the management of anterior cruciate ligament injuries in children. *Bone Joint J.* 2013;95-B:1562–1569.
34. Pressman AE, Letts RM, Jarvis JG. Anterior cruciate ligament tears in children: an analysis of operative versus nonoperative treatment. *J Pediatr Orthop.* 1997;17:505–511.
35. Janarv PM, Nystrom A, Werner S, et al. Anterior cruciate ligament injuries in skeletally immature patients. *J Pediatr Orthop.* 1996;16:673–677.
36. Kannus P, Jarvinen M. Knee ligament injuries in adolescents. Eight year follow-up of conservative management. *J Bone Joint Surg Br.* 1988;70:772–776.
37. Pattee GA, Fox JM, Del Pizzo W, et al. Four to ten year followup of unreconstructed anterior cruciate ligament tears. *Am J Sports Med.* 1989;17:430–435.
38. Shelbourne KD, Patel DV, McCarroll JR. Management of anterior cruciate ligament injuries in skeletally immature adolescents. *Knee Surg Sports Traumatol Arthrosc.* 1996;4:68–74.
39. Gelber AC, Hochberg MC, Mead LA, et al. Joint injury in young adults and risk for subsequent knee and hip osteoarthritis. *Ann Intern Med.* 2000;133:321–328.
40. Graf BK, Lange RH, Fujisaki CK, et al. Anterior cruciate ligament tears in skeletally immature patients: meniscal pathology at presentation and after attempted conservative treatment. *Arthroscopy.* 1992;8:229–233.
41. Lawrence JT, Argawal N, Ganley TJ. Degeneration of the knee joint in skeletally immature patients with a diagnosis of an anterior cruciate ligament tear: is there harm in delay of treatment? *Am J Sports Med.* 2011;39:2582–2587.
42. Millett PJ, Willis AA, Warren RF. Associated injuries in pediatric and adolescent anterior cruciate ligament tears: does a delay in treatment increase the risk of meniscal tear? *Arthroscopy.* 2002;18:955–959.
43. Roos EM. Joint injury causes knee osteoarthritis in young adults. *Curr Opin Rheumatol.* 2005;17:195–200.
44. von Porat A, Roos EM, Roos H. High prevalence of osteoarthritis 14 years after an anterior cruciate ligament tear in male soccer players: a study of radiographic and patient relevant outcomes. *Ann Rheum Dis.* 2004;63:269–273.
45. Bisson LJ, Wickiewicz T, Levinson M, et al. ACL reconstruction in children with open physes. *Orthopedics.* 1998;21:659–663.
46. Terzidis IP, Christodoulou AG, Ploumis AL, et al. The appearance of kissing contusion in the acutely injured knee in the athletes. *Br J Sports Med.* 2004;38:592–596.
47. Yoon KH, Yoo JH, Kim KI. Bone contusion and associated meniscal and medial collateral ligament injury in patients with anterior cruciate ligament rupture. *J Bone Joint Surg Am.* 2011;93:1510–1518.
48. McCarroll JR, Rettig AC, Shelbourne KD. Anterior cruciate ligament injuries in the young athlete with open physes. *Am J Sports Med.* 1988;16:44–47.

49. Kepler CK, Bogner EA, Hammoud S, et al. Zone of injury of the medial patellofemoral ligament after acute patellar dislocation in children and adolescents. *Am J Sports Med.* 2011;39:1444–1449.
50. Colvin AC, West RV. Patellar instability. *J Bone Joint Surg Am.* 2008;90:2751–2762.
51. Hensler D, Sillanpaa PJ, Schoettle PB. Medial patellofemoral ligament: anatomy, injury and treatment in the adolescent knee. *Curr Opin Pediatr.* 2014;26:70–78.
52. Bitar AC, Demange MK, D'Elia CO, et al. Traumatic patellar dislocation: nonoperative treatment compared with MPFL reconstruction using patellar tendon. *Am J Sports Med.* 2012;40:114–122.
53. Camp CL, Krych AJ, Dahm DL, et al. Medial patellofemoral ligament repair for recurrent patellar dislocation. *Am J Sports Med.* 2010;38:2248–2254.
54. Nelitz M, Dreyhaupt J, Reichel H, et al. Anatomic reconstruction of the medial patellofemoral ligament in children and adolescents with open growth plates: surgical technique and clinical outcome. *Am J Sports Med.* 2013;41:58–63.
55. Schoettle PB, Fucentese SF, Romero J. Clinical and radiological outcome of medial patellofemoral ligament reconstruction with a semitendinosus autograft for patella instability. *Knee Surg Sports Traumatol Arthrosc.* 2005;13:516–521.
56. Luhmann SJ, O'Donnell JC, Fuhrhop S. Outcomes after patellar realignment surgery for recurrent patellar instability dislocations: a minimum 3-year follow-up study of children and adolescents. *J Pediatr Orthop.* 2011;31:65–71.
57. Sillanpaa PJ, Maenpaa HM. First-time patellar dislocation: surgery or conservative treatment? *Sports Med Arthrosc.* 2012;20:128–135.
58. Brown GD, Ahmad CS. Combined medial patellofemoral ligament and medial patellotibial ligament reconstruction in skeletally immature patients. *J Knee Surg.* 2008;21:328–332.
59. Deie M, Ochi M, Sumen Y, et al. Reconstruction of the medial patellofemoral ligament for the treatment of habitual or recurrent dislocation of the patella in children. *J Bone Joint Surg Br.* 2003;85:887–890.
60. Giordano M, Falciglia F, Aulisa AG, et al. Patellar dislocation in skeletally immature patients: semitendinosous and gracilis augmentation for combined medial patellofemoral and medial patellotibial ligament reconstruction. *Knee Surg Sports Traumatol Arthrosc.* 2012;20:1594–1598.
61. Kumahashi N, Kuwata S, Tadenuma T, et al. A "sandwich" method of reconstruction of the medial patellofemoral ligament using a titanium interference screw for patellar instability in skeletally immature patients. *Arch Orthop Trauma Surg.* 2012;132:1077–1083.
62. Ladenhauf HN, Berkes MB, Green DW. Medial patellofemoral ligament reconstruction using hamstring autograft in children and adolescents. *Arthrosc Tech.* 2013;2:e151–e154.
63. Nelitz M, Reichel H, Dornacher D, et al. Anatomical reconstruction of the medial patellofemoral ligament in children with open growth-plates. *Arch Orthop Trauma Surg.* 2012;132:1647–1651.
64. Yercan HS, Erkan S, Okcu G, et al. A novel technique for reconstruction of the medial patellofemoral ligament in skeletally immature patients. *Arch Orthop Trauma Surg.* 2011;131:1059–1065.
65. LaPrade RF, Engebretsen AH, Ly TV, et al. The anatomy of the medial part of the knee. *J Bone Joint Surg Am.* 2007;89:2000–2010.
66. Balcarek P, Ammon J, Frosch S, et al. Magnetic resonance imaging characteristics of the medial patellofemoral ligament lesion in acute lateral patellar dislocations considering trochlear dysplasia, patella alta, and tibial tuberosity-trochlear groove distance. *Arthroscopy.* 2010;26:926–935.
67. Nelitz M, Dornacher D, Dreyhaupt J, et al. The relation of the distal femoral physis and the medial patellofemoral ligament. *Knee Surg Sports Traumatol Arthrosc.* 2011;19:2067–2071.
68. Akinleye SD, Sewick A, Wells L. All-epiphyseal ACL reconstruction: a three-year follow-up. *Int J Sports Phys Ther.* 2013;8:300–310.
69. Anderson AF. Transepiphyseal replacement of the anterior cruciate ligament using quadruple hamstring grafts in skeletally immature patients. *J Bone Joint Surg Am.* 2004;86-A(suppl 1):201–209.
70. Bonnard C, Fournier J, Babusiaux D, et al. Physeal-sparing reconstruction of anterior cruciate ligament tears in children: results of 57 cases using patellar tendon. *J Bone Joint Surg Br.* 2011;93:542–547.
71. Guzzanti V, Falciglia F, Stanitski CL. Physeal-sparing intraarticular anterior cruciate ligament reconstruction in preadolescents. *Am J Sports Med.* 2003;31:949–953.
72. Kocher MS, Garg S, Micheli LJ. Physeal sparing reconstruction of the anterior cruciate ligament in skeletally immature prepubescent children and adolescents. Surgical technique. *J Bone Joint Surg Am.* 2006;88(suppl 1, pt 2):283–293.
73. Lubowitz JH, Ahmad CS, Anderson K. All-inside anterior cruciate ligament graft-link technique: second-generation, no-incision anterior cruciate ligament reconstruction. *Arthroscopy.* 2011;27:717–727.
74. Lykissas MG, Nathan ST, Wall EJ. All-epiphyseal anterior cruciate ligament reconstruction in skeletally immature patients: a surgical technique using a split tibial tunnel. *Arthrosc Tech.* 2012;1:e133–e139.
75. McCarthy MM, Graziano J, Green DW, et al. All-epiphyseal, all-inside anterior cruciate ligament reconstruction technique for skeletally immature patients. *Arthrosc Tech.* 2012;1:e231–e239.
76. Nakhostine M, Bollen SR, Cross MJ. Reconstruction of mid-substance anterior cruciate rupture in adolescents with open physes. *J Pediatr Orthop.* 1995;15:286–287.
77. Parker AW, Drez DJ, Cooper JL. Anterior cruciate ligament injuries in patients with open physes. *Am J Sports Med.* 1994;22:44–47.
78. Harcke HT, Synder M, Caro PA, et al. Growth plate of the normal knee: evaluation with MR imaging. *Radiology.* 1992;183:119–123.
79. Liu RW, Armstrong DG, Levine AD, et al. An anatomic study of the distal femoral epiphysis. *J Pediatr Orthop.* 2013;33:743–749.
80. Sasaki T, Ishibashi Y, Okamura Y, et al. MRI evaluation of growth plate closure rate and pattern in the normal knee joint. *J Knee Surg.* 2002;15:72–76.
81. Behr CT, Potter HG, Paletta GAJ. The relationship of the femoral origin of the anterior cruciate ligament and the distal femoral physeal plate in the skeletally immature knee. An anatomic study. *Am J Sports Med.* 2001;29:781–787.
82. Chudik S, Beasley L, Potter H, et al. The influence of femoral technique for graft placement on anterior cruciate ligament reconstruction using a skeletally immature canine model with a rapidly growing physis. *Arthroscopy.* 2007;23:1309–1319.e1.
83. Guzzanti V, Falciglia F, Gigante A, et al. The effect of intra-articular ACL reconstruction on the growth plates of rabbits. *J Bone Joint Surg Br.* 1994;76:960–963.
84. Mäkelä EA, Vainionpaa S, Vihtonen K, et al. The effect of trauma to the lower femoral epiphyseal plate. An experimental study in rabbits. *J Bone Joint Surg Br.* 1988;70:187–191.
85. Yoo WJ, Kocher MS, Micheli LJ. Growth plate disturbance after transphyseal reconstruction of the anterior cruciate ligament in skeletally immature adolescent patients: an MR imaging study. *J Pediatr Orthop.* 2011;31:691–696.
86. Seil R, Pape D, Kohn D. The risk of growth changes during transphyseal drilling in sheep with open physes. *Arthroscopy.* 2008;24:824–833.
87. Chotel F, Seil R. Growth disturbances after transphyseal ACL reconstruction in skeletally immature patients: who is more at risk? Young child or adolescent? *J Pediatr Orthop.* 2013;33:585–586.

CHAPTER

38

James F. Mooney III

Assessment of Growth Remaining in the Skeletally Immature Patient

INTRODUCTION

Assessment of growth remaining in the long bones of children and adolescents is of great importance in understanding the longitudinal and angular growth of the extremity. As the femur is the longest bone in the axial skeleton, normal or aberrant growth of the femur, particularly involving the distal femoral growth plate adjacent to the knee, greatly affects the overall length and/or angular alignment of the limb.

THE GROWTH PLATES (PHYSES) ABOUT THE KNEE

The growth plates about the knee remain open, and provide longitudinal growth, until the late teenage years. The distal femoral growth plate closes completely at an average age of 18 to 19 years in males and 17 years in females, although there is often little significant growth from this physis after 14 years of age in females and 16 years in males. The proximal tibial physis closes similarly in males at 18 to 19 years and 16 to 17 years of age in females. Typically, the proximal tibial physis closes prior to the distal femoral in most patients. Each of these is susceptible to accidental and iatrogenic injury during a very physically active part of life. Trauma (accidental or iatrogenic), infection, or vascular insufficiency are some of the primary causes of damage to the physis and thereby may cause significant limb length discrepancy and/or angular deformity that may require further surgical intervention or reconstruction (Fig. 38.1).

The growth plate of the distal femur provides more to the longitudinal growth of the lower limb than any other growth plate, and the physis of the proximal tibia is the next most important. The specifics of the histology and microscopic anatomy of the physis, both similarities and differences, are beyond the scope of this chapter. However, the orthopedic surgeon involved in the care of skeletally immature patients with knee injuries, and particularly those performing surgery about the knee, should be well aware of some basic facts regarding the anatomy of, development of, and risk of injury to these growth areas.

Distal femoral physeal injuries comprise approximately 2% of all physeal fractures.[1–3] The most common complication of distal femoral physeal fracture is growth disturbance with resultant angular growth abnormality or leg length discrepancy.[2,4–6] The distal femoral physis possesses less stability against traumatic displacement and injury than the physis of the proximal tibia, which has a rate of traumatic injury approximately half that of the distal femur.[2,7] The shape of the proximal tibial physis, with the anterior and distal projection of the tibial tubercle as well as the spanning collateral ligaments, and the buttress provided by the proximal fibula are thought to be protective against potentially injuring forces.[2,7]

Angular deformity or shortening have been reported in 39% to 50% of all patients sustaining a distal femoral physeal fracture.[2,8–10] Patients from ages 2 to 12 years appear to be at highest risk of these complications.[2] The specific mechanism of injury, the type of fracture by Salter classification, as well as the amount of potential growth remaining each play a role in this risk. In addition, there is a change in the anatomy of the distal femoral physis with increasing patient age that may contribute to this increasing rate. The gross anatomy of the distal femoral physis has been shown to be essentially "flat" up until approximately 2 years of age. After that time, the growth plate develops a more undulating course that puts more of the germinal zone of the physis at risk of injury, even in the face of a seemingly radiographically benign fracture pattern.

REVIEW OF ASSESSMENT OF SKELETAL GROWTH—DETERMINATION OF SKELETAL AGE

Management of orthopedic conditions in the face of a constantly changing skeleton is one of the fundamental issues facing the pediatric orthopedic surgeon as well as any physician involved with the care of musculoskeletal problems in children. As such, it is important to be familiar with the methods of assessing current and potential amounts of growth, as well as general development, in children. Many of these require the use of the skeletal (bone) age of the patient rather than the

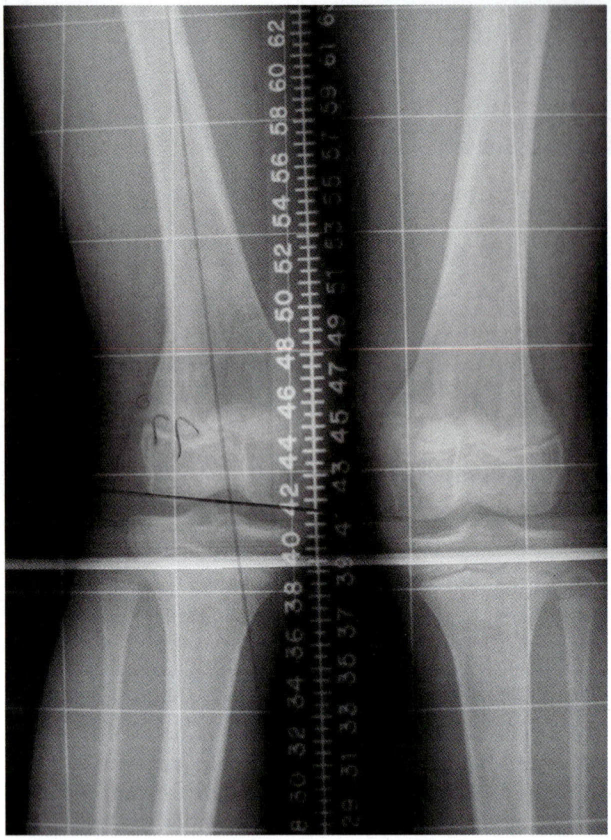

Figure 38.1. AP radiograph of valgus deformity after distal femoral physeal injury.

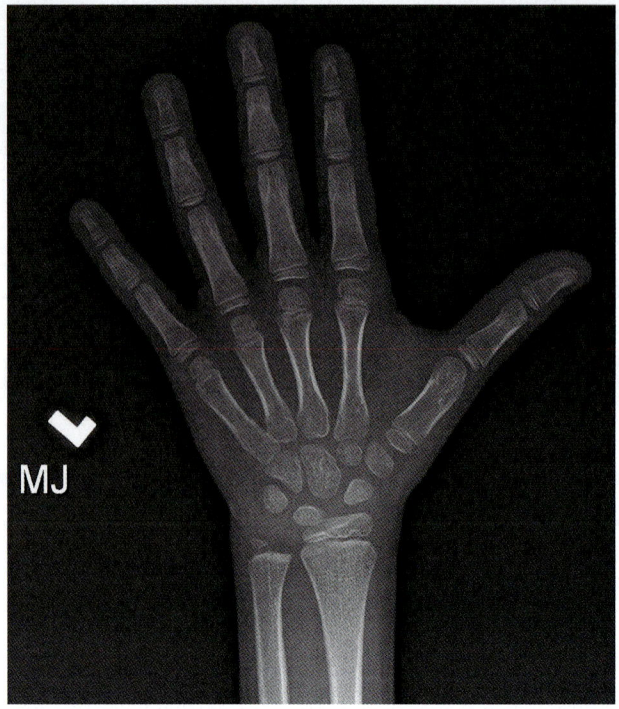

Figure 38.2. AP left hand and wrist radiograph for bone age demonstrating a bone age of 6 years and 10 months in a female.

chronologic age. There are multiple methods available to generate this value.[11]

GREULICH AND PYLE ATLAS

The Greulich and Pyle[12] *Atlas of Skeletal Development* was published originally in 1950 and was based on Todd's works that were published in 1937. Todd obtained multiple extremity images of 1,000 patients at 3-month intervals during the first year of life, every 6 months from 1 to 5 years of age, and then annually until skeletal maturity. Greulich and Pyle used these radiographs in their atlas to generate a standard for skeletal development of children based on radiographic changes that occur over time in the bones of the hand and wrist, as seen on a left hand and wrist anteroposterior (AP) radiographs (Fig. 38.2). A set of radiographs is provided for males and females due to the differences in skeletal development based on gender. The standard film that most closely resembles that of the patient in question is reported as the skeletal, or bone, age. Concerns exist regarding the validity of assumptions based on radiographic images obtained from patients with health and diet significantly different than found in modern pediatric patients. However, it is difficult to imagine a similar longitudinal radiographic study being generated at this time. Overall, the Greulich and Pyle atlas method is used most commonly at this time to determine skeletal age in pediatric orthopedic surgery.

TANNER AND WHITEHOUSE METHOD

This method is similar to the Greulich and Pyle technique in that the bone age determination is generated through examination of left hand and wrist AP radiographs of the patient in question.[11] Specific bones are considered as "regions of interest." These areas are then divided into epiphysis, metaphysis, and diaphysis. A numerical score is generated for each area, and then an overall maturity score and bone age are determined. There is some evidence that the Tanner and Whitehouse method may be more accurate and reproducible than the Greulich and Pyle technique.[13] However, the relative complexity and time-consuming nature of the Tanner-Whitehouse method compared to the Greulich and Pyle atlas limits its use by orthopedic surgeons in clinical practice.

THE SHORTHAND BONE AGE ASSESSMENT

This method was developed over a number of years of clinical practice at the Hospital for Special Surgery (HSS) in New York and reported in the literature in 2013 by Heyworth et al.[14] The shorthand bone age (SBA) assessment was derived from the Greulich and Pyle method in an attempt to simplify the determination of bone age and skeletal maturity for male patients between the ages of 12.5 and 16 years and for females between 10 and 16 years. Clinicians at HSS noted that certain specific radiographic findings on the bone age images appeared to correlate highly with specific ages within this patient population.

Briefly, the SBA uses a single radiographic finding, rather than multiple findings on the hand/wrist bone age image,

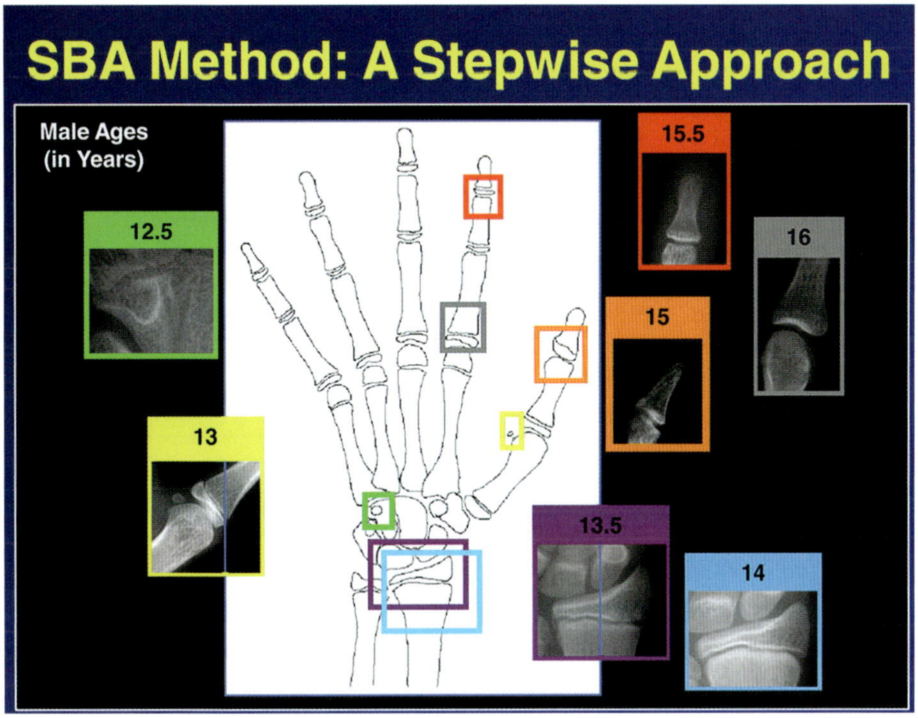

Figure 38.3. Pictorial representation of the SBA assessment for male patients. (From Heyworth BE, Osei DA, Fabricant PD, et al. The shorthand bone age assessment: a simpler alternative to current methods. *J Pediatr Orthop.* 2013;33[5]: 569–574.)

that appear to correlate with skeletal age in patients around the time of puberty. This single radiographic finding correlated with bone age can then be separated by gender in a table or single sheet format (Figs. 38.3 and 38.4), which is easier to access and use than the Greulich and Pyle atlas.

Heyworth, et al.[14] compared the SBA method with the use of the Greulich and Pyle atlas. They found substantial agreement between the two techniques with excellent intra- and interobserver reliability. As such, they felt that the SBA was a simple, valuable, and effective alternative to the use of the Greulich and Pyle method.

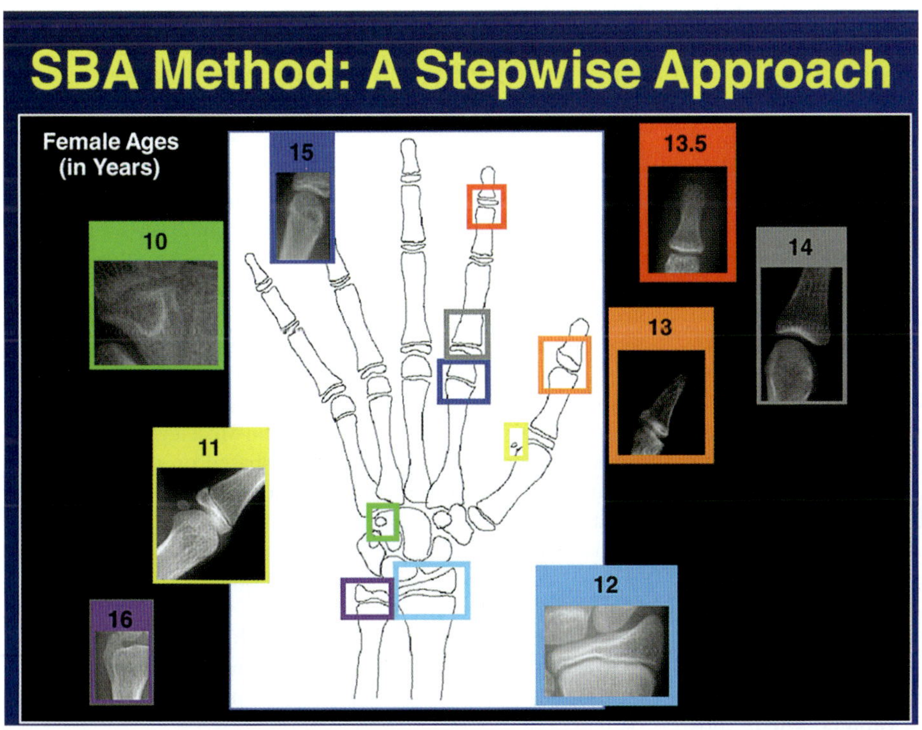

Figure 38.4. Pictorial representation of the SBA for female patients. (From Heyworth BE, Osei DA, Fabricant PD, et al. The shorthand bone age assessment: a simpler alternative to current methods. *J Pediatr Orthop.* 2013;33[5]: 569–574.)

DETERMINATION OF LEG LENGTH AND POTENTIAL LEG LENGTH DISCREPANCY

Multiple methods exist to assist in prediction of leg length and possible leg length discrepancy. Each has its own value, and it is important to have some idea of the use of each technique. As the vast majority of the longitudinal growth of the lower limb occurs through the distal femoral and proximal tibial growth plates about the knee, these are the areas involved in the determination of limb length and potential limb length discrepancy. As such, manipulation of these growth plates through timed epiphyseal arrest is one of the primary interventions to address existing and predicted discrepancies.

ARITHMETIC METHOD

Menelaus[15] described a simple method that allows determination of growth remaining in the growth plates about the knee. It is based on a number of assumptions that hold true in most cases. These include the following:

1. Boys continue to have skeletal growth up to age 16 years and girls up to age 14 years.
2. The distal femoral growth plate provides ⅜ in (9 mm) per year of growth and the proximal tibial growth plate ¼ in (6 mm) per year.

By using this method, it is possible to generate reasonably accurate determinations of growth potential without specialized graphs and with simple calculations. However, it is limited by assumptions regarding chronologic and skeletal age and fails to take into account the fact that the growth rate of the physis is not constant. Overall, this method is useful in providing a reasonable estimate, but other methods are more accurate.

THE ANDERSON-GREEN (GROWTH REMAINING) METHOD

Anderson, Green, and Messner[16] published longitudinal growth data on 100 children in 1963. They gathered data on the subjects once per year over the 8 years prior to cessation of growth. This data included orthoroentgenograms for bone length and left hand and wrist films for bone age, which was then determined using the Greulich and Pyle atlas. This information was used to generate a series of charts that depicted rates of growth of overall stature as well as growth of the femur and tibia in these patients. The data was further analyzed to generate graphs that provided growth remaining of the individual physes about the knee when reported against skeletal or bone age. These graphs are depicted in Figure 38.5.

The Anderson-Green graphs provided estimations of predicted growth remaining in male and female patients. In addition, the mean growth remaining, as well as growth remaining 1 and 2 standard deviations above and below the mean, were provided for both the proximal tibial and distal femoral physes. These graphs may be used to assess, and estimate, the growth remaining of the lower limb based on the contributions of the two primary growth centers. The graphs can be used as part of the determination of any projected leg length discrepancy as well as to assist in the timing of surgical intervention.

It is important to realize that variations do exist and that this data was generated on a group of patients from a single geographic area over a half century ago. As such, this information cannot be considered an exact and absolute prediction in this day and age. However, this level of broad demographic and radiographic data is the gold standard to date, and it is doubtful that similar evaluations and data can ever be compiled again.

THE STRAIGHT-LINE GRAPH METHOD (MOSELEY)

The straight-line method was described by Moseley[17] in 1977 as a technique to calculate the ultimate leg length discrepancy in a specific patient as well as to predict the best possible timing for an epiphysiodesis of the distal femoral and/or proximal tibial physes. Moseley's graphs were constructed through mathematical manipulation of the Anderson-Green data so as to generate straight lines representing limb length. In addition to describing the method, Moseley reviewed patients who had reached skeletal maturity after an epiphysiodesis for leg length discrepancy based on use of this graphing method. He found a mean error of 0.6 cm when he used his method versus 0.9 cm with the Anderson-Green method.[17]

There are potential problems with this technique. Moseley assumed a linear rate of growth inhibition of the limb, which has been shown by Shapiro and others to be incorrect in some patients. In addition, the technique is cumbersome, requiring manual plotting of multiple data points on specialized graph paper. Computer programs exist to limit inconvenience and to improve efficiency, thereby minimizing some negative aspects.

THE PALEY MULTIPLIER METHOD

Paley et al.[18] described what they have termed the *multiplier method* in 2000. Since then, they have provided further published reports of the clinical use of this method.[19] They extracted data from multiple limb length databases to generate a novel factor, or multiplier, for each limb. This allows prediction of eventual limb length and possible discrepancy. There are different tables of multipliers for males and females. Unlike most other methods, use of this technique does not require acquisition of bone age data (hand/wrist radiographs) and relies on the patient's chronologic age, further simplifying patient evaluation. In addition, unlike the Moseley technique, the multiplier method allows prediction based on data at a single point in time rather than requiring a minimum of two or three separate data points to generate a line on the graph. Overall, this is a simple method to use and has been documented to be as accurate as any of the other techniques.[19] Of note, a smartphone application exists for use of the multiplier method for determination of overall predicted limb length discrepancy as well as timing of epiphysiodesis and hemiepiphysiodesis for treatment of limb length discrepancy or angular deformity in patients with skeletal growth remaining.

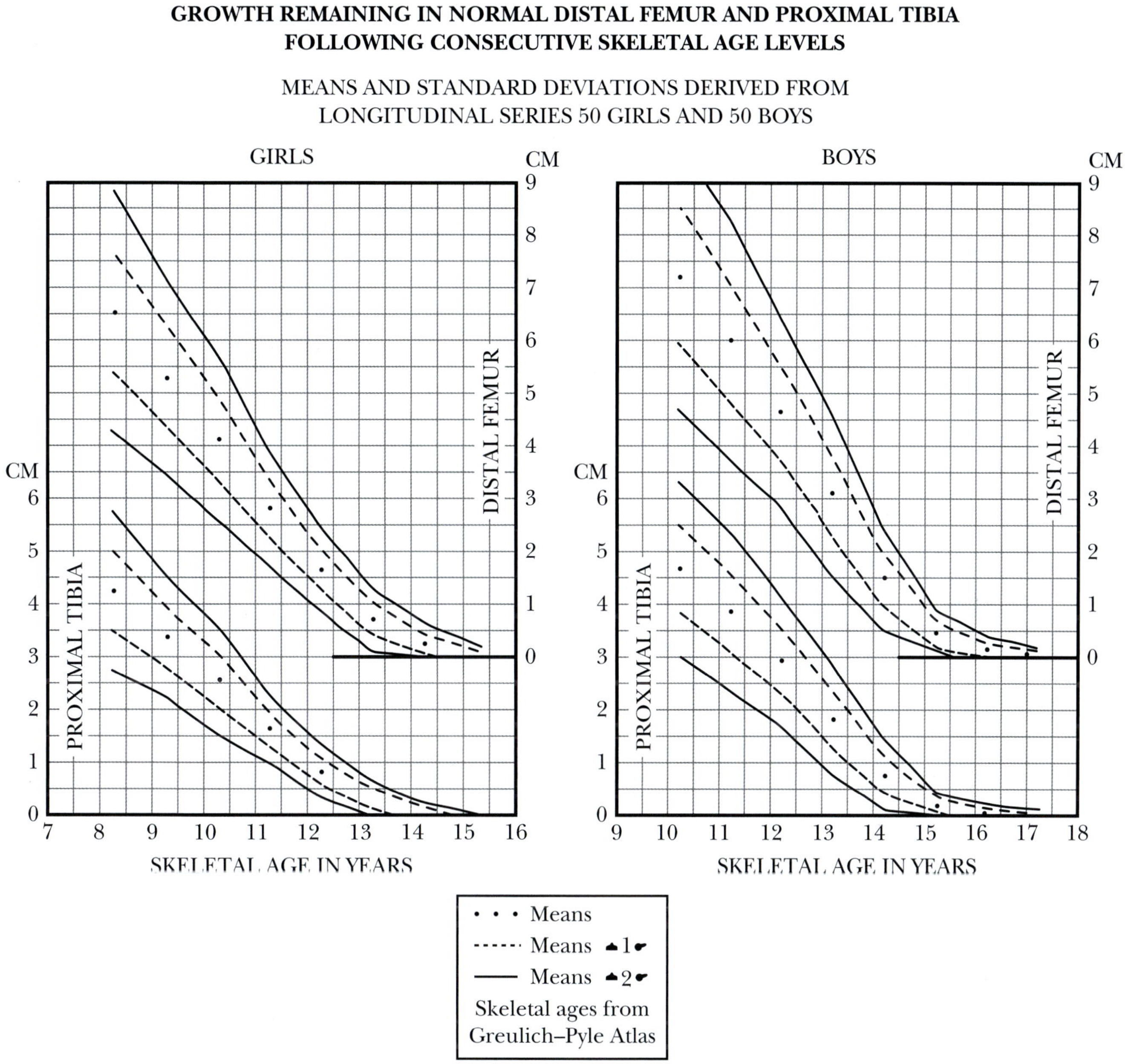

Figure 38.5. Male and female graphs of distal femoral and proximal tibial growth remaining charts as published by Anderson, Green, and Messner. (From Anderson M, Green WT, Messner MB. Growth and predictions of growth in the lower extremities. *J Bone Joint Surg Am.* 1963;45-A:1–14.)

CLINICAL APPLICATION OF INFORMATION

Injury to the growth plates about the knee may occur secondary to trauma, may be iatrogenic, or may be the result of vascular or infectious causes. The most common and problematic complication of such injuries is growth disturbance with resulting angular deformity or leg length discrepancy. It is essential that physicians involved in the care of skeletally immature patients with knee injuries and knee pathology understand the methods of assessing skeletal growth and maturation, determination of growth remaining from specific growth areas, and the effects of injury to the growth plate itself. Without this information, or without facility in using this information, the treating surgeon will be unable to formulate a plan to manage potential problems and will be unable to provide optimal patient care.

REPRESENTATIVE CASE

A 12-year-old male sustained a closed Salter-Harris II fracture of the distal femur and underwent successful closed reduction and screw fixation. The postoperative course was uneventful, and the screws were removed at 8 months post injury due to prominence. He was then lost to follow-up for approximately 18 months. He

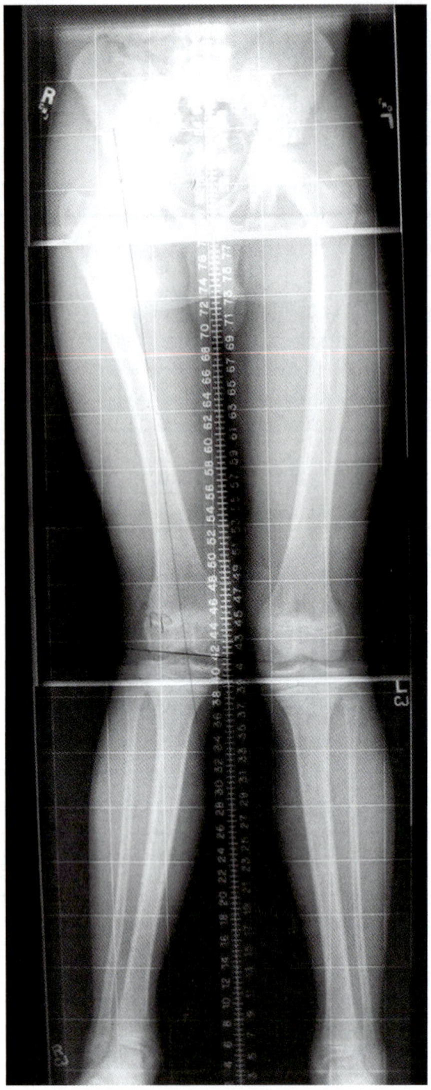

Figure 38.6. Standing bone length AP radiograph demonstrating valgus deformity and limb length discrepancy after distal femoral physeal injury.

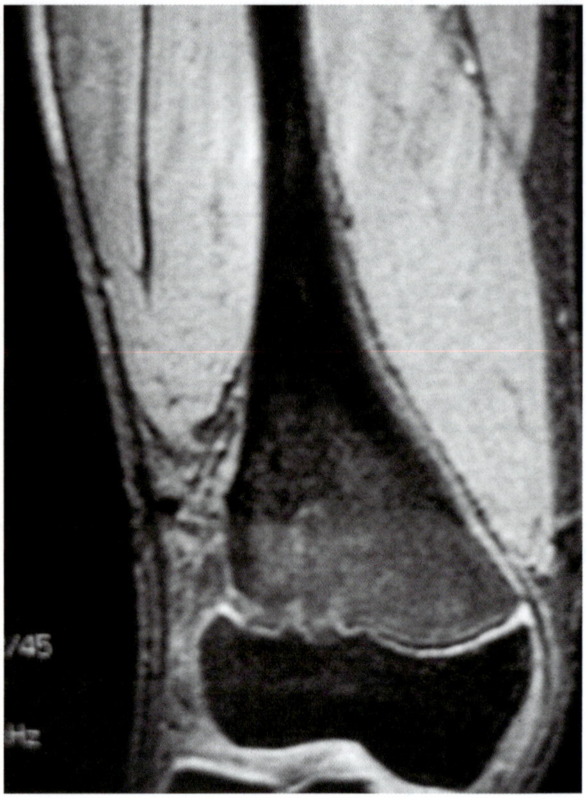

Figures 38.7. MRI illustrating lateral physeal injury and growth disturbance with bony bridging across the physis.

presented back with complaints of progressive deformity at the knee on the side of the previous injury (Fig. 38.6).

Standing radiographs demonstrated the significant valgus deformity of the femur and a moderate limb length discrepancy. Subsequent MRI showed growth disturbance of the lateral femoral physis (Fig. 38.7). His bone age was 13 years at that time, and by the arithmetic method, he had approximately 2.7 cm of femoral growth remaining, whereas the Anderson-Green charts showed that he had approximately 3.5 cm remaining. After discussion with his family, plans were made to address the deformity of the right femur as well as the current and potential future leg length discrepancy. The family chose to accept some mild decrease in overall height so as to limit the number of surgical interventions that would be necessary.

He underwent completion of the epiphysiodesis of the right distal femoral physis with staples and acute correction of the valgus deformity of the femur with a monolateral external fixator (Fig. 38.8). After a brief period of quiescence, the femur was gradually lengthened with the fixator to equalize the leg lengths

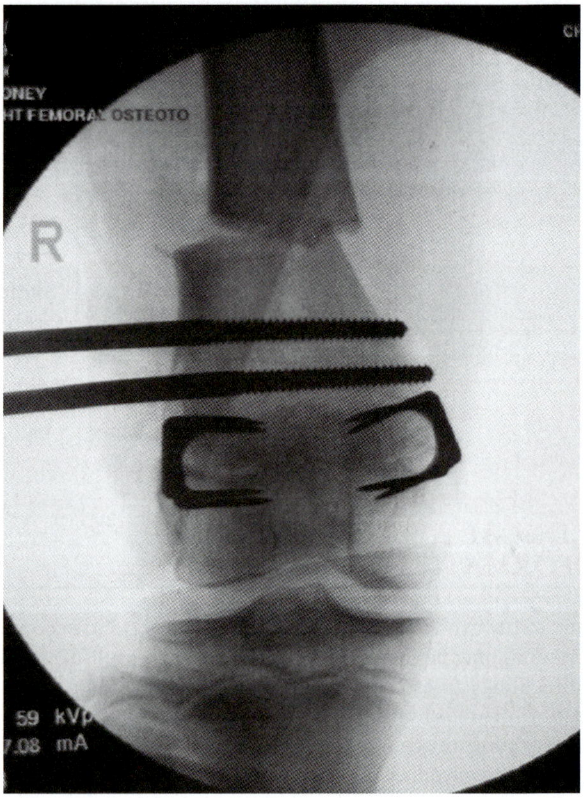

Figure 38.8. Intraoperative AP image demonstrating acute correction of the distal femoral deformity and completion of epiphysiodesis with staples.

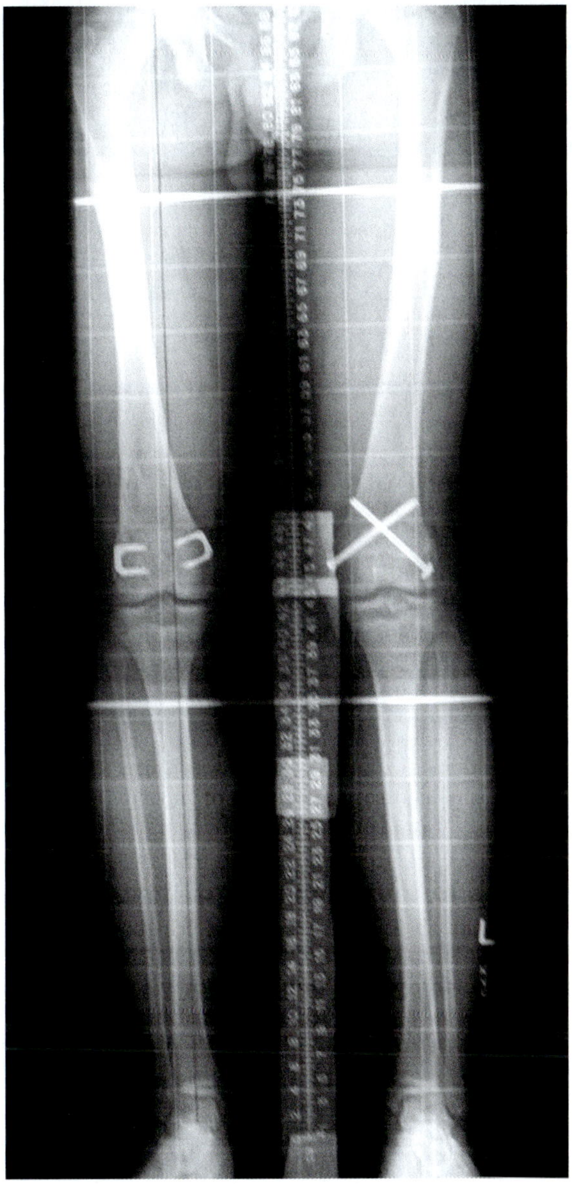

Figure 38.9. Final standing AP image demonstrating correction of the limb length discrepancy and angular deformity.

to an acceptable level and to take into account any growth of the left limb that occurred during the surgery and lengthening process. When the leg length discrepancy was corrected, he then underwent an epiphysiodesis of the contralateral distal femur using a percutaneous screw technique, which allowed maintenance of full weight-bearing status on the left side. Final standing films after formation of sufficient regenerate bone at the site of lengthening and final follow-up demonstrated restoration of an essentially normal mechanical axis on the right side as well as minimal residual limb length discrepancy (Fig. 38.9).

CONCLUSION

The growth plates about the knee provide the greatest input to overall length of the limb in the developing child and adolescent. Injuries to these areas, from whatever cause, can be devastating and extremely problematic. It is essential that the practicing orthopedic surgeon be aware of the nature of these injuries and their effects on limb development. In addition, it is imperative that those treating children for knee injuries, either with or without surgery, are aware of the methods used to determine growth of the limb and to aid in prediction of overall limb lengths.

REFERENCES

1. Mann DC, Rajmaira S. Distribution of physeal and nonphyseal fractures in 2,650 long-bone fractures in children aged 0-16 years. *J Pediatr Orthop.* 1990;10(6):713–716.
2. Price CT, Herrara-Soto J. Extra-articular injuries of the knee. In: Beaty JH, Kasser JR, eds. *Rockwood and Wilkins' Fractures in Children.* 7th ed. Philadelphia, PA: Lippincott Williams & Wilkins; 2010: 842–893.
3. Peterson HA, Madhok R, Benson JT, et al. Physeal fractures: part 1. Epidemiology in Olmsted County, Minnesota, 1979-1988. *J Pediatr Orthop.* 1994;14(4):423–430.
4. Arkader A, Warner WC Jr, Horn BD, et al. Predicting the outcome of physeal fractures of the distal femur. *J Pediatr Orthop.* 2007;27: 703–708.
5. Eid AM, Hafez MA. Traumatic injuries of the distal femoral physis. A retrospective study on 151 cases. *Injury.* 2002;33:251–255.
6. Graham JM, Gross RH. Distal femoral physeal problem fractures. *Clin Orthop Relat Res.* 1990;(255):51–53.
7. Burkhart SS, Peterson HA. Fractures of the proximal tibial epiphysis. *J Bone Joint Surg Am.* 1979;61(7):996–1002
8. Ogden JA. Distal femoral epiphyseal injuries. In: Ogden JA, ed. *Skeletal Injury in the Child.* New York, NY: Springer Publishing; 2000:896–912.
9. Riseborough EJ, Barrett IR, Shapiro F. Growth disturbances following distal femoral physeal fracture-separations. *J Bone Joint Surg Am.* 1983;65(7):885–893.
10. Thomson JD, Stricker SJ, Williams MM. Fractures of the distal femoral epiphyseal plate. *J Pediatr Orthop.* 1995;15(4):474–478.
11. Spampinato C. Skeletal bone age assessment. http://homepages.inf.ed.ac.uk/rbf/CVonline/LOCAL_COPIES/SPAMPINATO/SKELETALBONEAGEASSESSMENT.pdf. Accessed January 30, 2014
12. Greulich WW, Pyle SI. *Radiographic Atlas of Skeletal Development of the Hand and Wrist.* 2nd ed. Palo Alto, CA: Stanford University Press; 1959.
13. Bull RK, Edwards PD, Kemp PM, et al. Bone age assessment: a large scale comparison of the Greulich and Pyle and Tanner and Whitehouse (TW2) methods. *Arch Dis Child.* 1999;81:172–173.
14. Heyworth BE, Osei DA, Fabricant PD, et al. The shorthand bone age assessment: a simpler alternative to current methods. *J Pediatr Orthop.* 2013;33(5):569–574.
15. Menelaus MB. Correction of limb length discrepancy by epiphyseal arrest. *J Bone Joint Surg Br.* 1966;48B(2):336–339.
16. Anderson M, Green WT, Messner MB. Growth and predictions of growth in the lower extremities. *J Bone Joint Surg Am.* 1963; 45-A:1–14.
17. Moseley CF. A straight-line graph for leg length discrepancy. *J Bone Joint Surg Am.* 1977;59(2):174–179
18. Paley D, Bhave A, Herzenberg JE, et al. Multiplier method for predicting limb-length discrepancy. *J Bone Joint Surg Am.* 2000;82: 1432–1446.
19. Aguilar JA, Paley D, Paley J, et al. Clinical validation of the multiplier method for predicting limb length at maturity. *J Pediatr Orthop.* 2005;25(2):186–191.

CHAPTER

39

Lauren E. LaMont
Emily R. Dodwell

Surgical Treatment of Growth Arrest

OVERVIEW

Growth arrest typically occurs due to some traumatic insult to the physis. Multiple etiologies may cause this insult that leads to injury to germinal cells and, ultimately, some degree of bony bridge formation. The cartilaginous component of the physis consists of resting, germinal, and proliferating cells (Fig. 39.1). Physeal separations due to trauma typically occur in the weakest layer of the physis, the hypertrophying layer.[1] In some injuries, they can also occur within the germinal layer or at the junction between cartilage and bone.[2] The majority of growth arrests occur at the periphery of the physis.

Most growth arrests are seen in the adolescent population; they most commonly occur after trauma. Mizuta et al.[3] collected over 2,000 bony injuries in children with open physes and found 18% of fractures had physeal involvement. In this series, growth arrest occurred just over 1% of the time and the proximal tibia was the most common site.[3] The occurrence of growth arrest in adolescence does not necessarily correlate with time of injury. Bony bridges may form within 1 to 2 months after injury. However, it may take months to years before deformity or shortening due to growth arrest manifest clinically. Although there is risk stratification based on type and degree of physeal injury, it is not possible to predict which children will go on to have growth arrest. For this reason, children with a confirmed or suspected growth plate injury require surveillance for growth arrest. Early identification of a bony bridge may allow more directed and less extensive treatment. Growth arrest tends to occur more commonly in boys than in girls.[4] Growth arrests are seen more commonly in the distal femur, proximal tibia, distal tibia, and distal radius.

Etiology

All five types of Salter-Harris fractures (Fig. 39.2) have been associated with growth arrest and development of physeal bar. Bony physeal bridges typically occur when injury to the physis results in contact between epiphyseal and metaphyseal bone. This bony contact can occur as result of displacement of fracture (Fig. 39.3) or destruction of physis from injury. Growth arrest is seen more commonly in the lower than upper extremity, although this is thought to relate to mechanism and energy of injury. Growth arrest is most common in distal femoral physeal fractures and may cause significant deformity due to the large contribution of distal femoral growth to overall limb length. High rates of shortening and angular deformity have been seen with both Salter-Harris types II and IV distal femur fractures.[5] If Salter-Harris type IV fractures are not properly reduced, then the child is at particularly high risk for physeal arrest due to the risk of metaphyseal–epiphyseal contact. Epidemiologic studies have found that Salter-Harris type III fractures tend to occur near the end of growth so they do not often produce clinically significant deformity or shortening.[6]

Trauma alone is not the sole cause of growth arrest in a physis nor does it have to be acute. Repetitive loading and stress-related injuries have been suggested to be causes of growth arrest.[7] Bony bridges may also be caused by infections, tumors, disuse, irradiation (Fig. 39.4), thermal injuries, laser beam, metabolic disorders, vascular insufficiency, or hematologic disorders.[8,9] A growth arrest may also be caused iatrogenically by violating the physis with either pins or screws. Smooth pins are thought to have minimal impact on the physis, although in an animal model, they have been associated with a small percentage of growth arrests.[10] Growth arrest has been documented following anterior cruciate ligament (ACL) reconstruction in children and adolescents with transphyseal tunnel placement.[11] Any type of threaded wire or screw can cause disruption of the physis and higher risk of growth arrest. Screws across the physis are sufficiently effective at growth arrest that they are commonly used when epiphysiodesis (growth plate closure) is clinically warranted.

Pathoanatomy

The various etiologies of growth arrest result in varying patterns which help guide the surgical approach to correction. Both the size as well as the location of a growth arrest influence the deformity that develops. In patients who have a complete growth arrest, the affected limb will be shortened but is less likely to develop angular deformity. Partial growth arrests will commonly lead to angular deformity of the limb, the degree of which is determined by remaining growth of the physis.

Classification

Growth arrest is classified into three separate patterns. A type I arrest is a peripheral growth arrest and a resulting peripheral bony bar. In patients with type II arrest, there is central physeal tethering due to a central arrest. In these patients, the peripheral physis continues to develop normally and the perichondrial ring is intact. Type III growth arrest is a combination of the first two; these patients demonstrate a linear bar involving the peripheral

Figure 39.1. Layers of the physis. From Flynn J, Skaggs D, Waters P. *Rockwood and Wilkins Fractures in Children.* 8th ed. Philadelphia, PA: Wolters Kluwer; 2014, with permission.

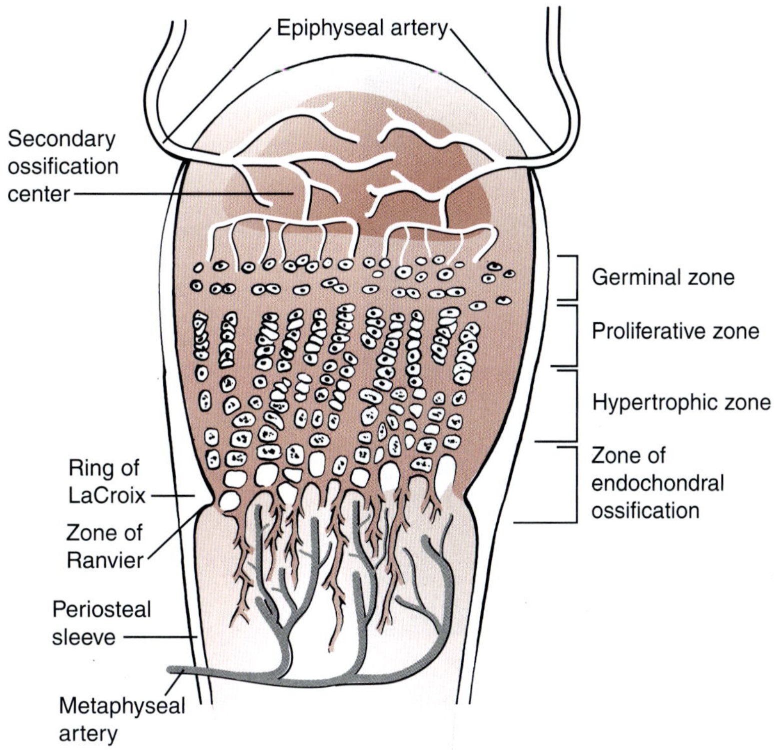

and central portions of the physeal plate (Fig. 39.5). Linear bar formation is more commonly seen after a Salter-Harris type III or IV fracture.[12] These were similarly described by Peterson[8] as peripheral bridge, elongated bridge, and central bridge formation.

Histopathology

Once insult has occurred to cells of physis, the resulting bony bridge consists of dense, sclerotic bone. Normal and abnormal physeal cartilage can be distinguished visually at time of surgery if physeal bar excision is indicated. The normal physis is opaque white with a bluish hue. In contrast, the injured physis has a more grayish, translucent color.[13]

Imaging

Radiographs are first obtained in order to evaluate planes of deformity. In patients with growth arrest over time, a physeal bar will be visible. Additionally, Harris growth arrest lines may be noted on the diaphyseal side of the physis and may be the first sign of bony bridge formation.[14] These lines indicate slowing growth of the physis that may be due to either a localized or a systemic process. When the insult is uniform, the arrest lines are parallel to the physis. When there is a partial growth arrest,

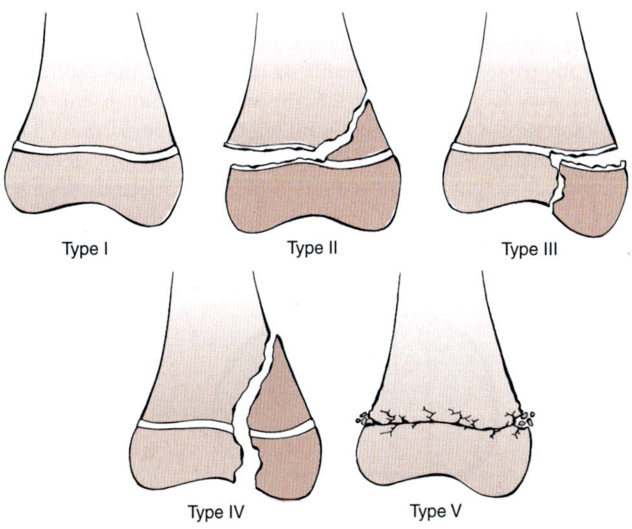

Figure 39.2. Salter-Harris Categorization of growth plate fractures. (From Flynn J, Skaggs D, Waters P. *Rockwood and Wilkins Fractures in Children.* 8th ed. Philadelphia, PA: Wolters Kluwer; 2014, with permission.)

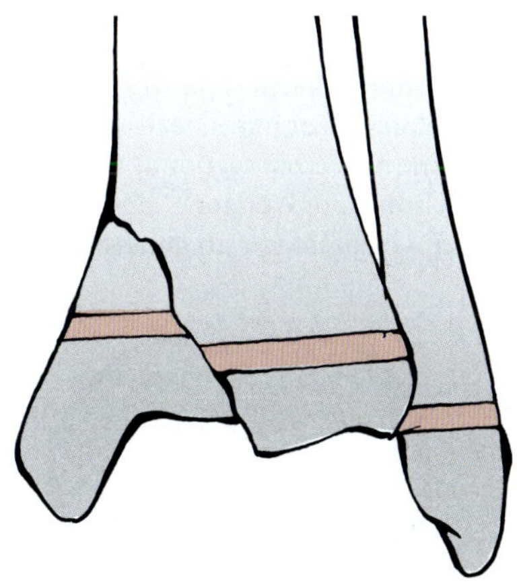

Figure 39.3. Malalignment of the growth plate fracture allows epiphyseal bone to contact metaphyseal bone. (From Flynn J, Skaggs D, Waters P. *Rockwood and Wilkins Fractures in Children.* 8th ed. Philadelphia, PA: Wolters Kluwer; 2014, with permission.)

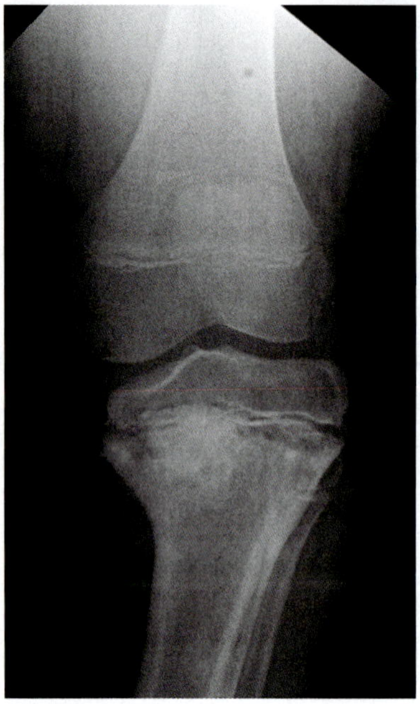

Figure 39.4. Proximal tibial physeal growth disturbance with angular deformity after irradiation for Ewing sarcoma. (From Flynn J, Skaggs D, Waters P. *Rockwood and Wilkins Fractures in Children*. 8th ed. Philadelphia, PA: Wolters Kluwer; 2014, with permission.)

these lines will be oblique or asymmetrical in nature (Fig. 39.6). When adequate time has passed since injury, often, a distinct bridge of bone or blurred or narrowed physis will be evident. When a physeal bar from a growth arrest is noted, more advanced imaging is indicated to determine size and location in every plane (Fig. 39.7).

Bone age radiographs of the left hand may also be indicated to predict remaining growth. When attempting to correct limb length discrepancy, exact leg lengths should be determined. Computed tomography (CT) scanogram is an accurate method to determine differences in leg lengths, especially in the setting of joint contractures which may be inaccurate on standing radiographs.[4] If an angular deformity is present, assessing length on both anteroposterior (AP) and lateral views of standing radiographs or low-dose biplanar radiograph (EOS) may be useful.

In order to determine the precise size and location of the bony bridge, multiplanar imaging is necessary. CT imaging can be used to determine the cross-sectional area involved by the physeal arrest. Carlson and Wenger[15] described a technique on graph paper from axial images to generate a cross-sectional map from biplane polytomography. Although CT imaging is a short exam, it does involve radiation to the child, an issue of increasing concern to parents and the general population.

Magnetic resonance imaging (MRI) provides another option for the evaluation of physeal bridges. Ecklund and Jaramillo[16] described use of fat-suppressed three-dimensional (3-D) spoiled gradient recalled echo imaging to assess growth disturbance. MRI has the benefit of no radiation exposure to the child compared with CT. The drawback to MRI is the longer length of the scan, which younger children may not be able to tolerate. Sedation may be required to obtain quality images. Findings on MRI include bridge size and location, signal intensity, growth recovery lines, avascular necrosis, and metaphyseal cartilage tongues.

Surgical Interventions

Surgical treatment is based on location, size, type of growth arrest, remaining growth, and anticipated deformity.[12] Patient goals and activity level must also be factored into management. Treatment is necessary in patients who have or are developing significant deformity with remaining growth.[17] Remaining growth for a child and ultimate limb length discrepancy can be measured in a number of ways. Commonly used techniques include the arithmetic method, the growth remaining method, the Moseley straight-line graph method, and the Paley multiplier method.[18–21] Surgical treatment for growth arrest can consist of one or a combination of corrective osteotomy, completion epiphysiodesis, contralateral epiphysiodesis, limb lengthening, deformity correction with frame, or excision of the physeal bridge.

Complete Growth Arrest

In a complete physeal arrest, the most common deformity to address is limb length inequality. Decision making for approach is largely based on remaining growth. If a patient is nearing end of growth, then a complete arrest in the lower extremity may be managed nonoperatively and followed clinically. Leg length discrepancies less than 2.5 cm have been shown to have little functional deficit, although it is unclear how those deficits affect patients into adulthood. Differences of this scale are generally treated with a shoe lift or not at all. If the estimated discrepancy is greater than 2.5 cm and less than 5 cm, then epiphysiodesis of the contralateral leg may be performed. This must be made with the understanding that this will decrease the overall height of the patient. When limb length discrepancy will be greater than 5 cm, then lengthening procedures are typically indicated.

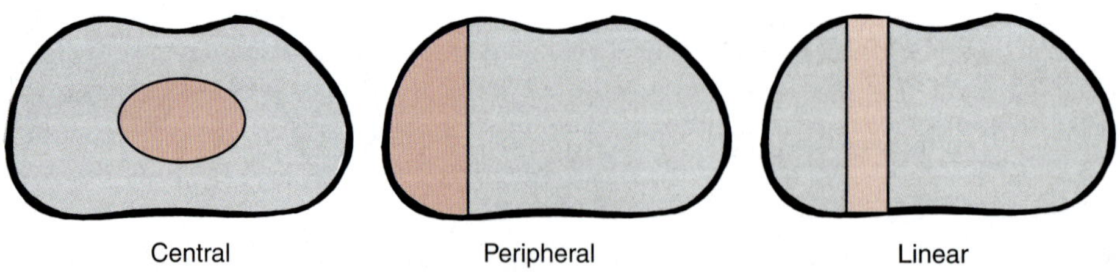

Figure 39.5. Anatomic classification of physeal arrests. Central arrests are surrounded by a perimeter of normal physis. Peripheral arrests are located at the perimeter of the physis. Linear arrests are "through-and-through" lesions with normal physis on either side of the arrest area. (From Flynn J, Skaggs D, Waters P. *Rockwood and Wilkins Fractures in Children*. 8th ed. Philadelphia, PA: Wolters Kluwer; 2014, with permission.)

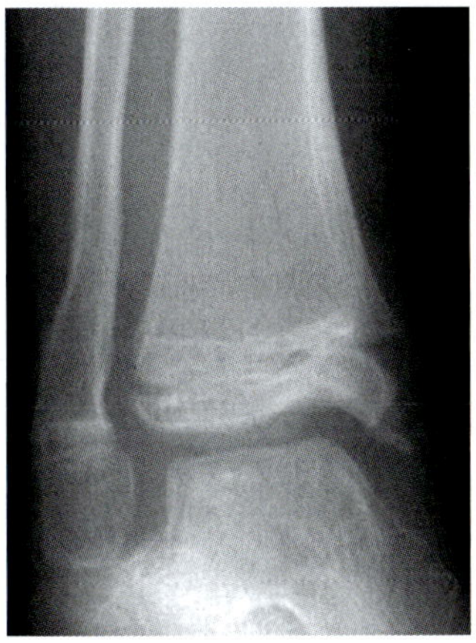

Figure 39.6. Anteroposterior x-ray of the distal tibia after Salter-Harris type IV fracture demonstrates a Harris growth arrest line tapering to the medial distal tibial physis, where a partial physeal arrest has formed. (From Flynn J, Skaggs D, Waters P. *Rockwood and Wilkins Fractures in Children.* 8th ed. Philadelphia, PA: Wolters Kluwer; 2014, with permission.)

Limb length differences have different parameters for the upper extremity and are based on the long bone affected. The humerus can tolerate a significant amount of shortening without any functional or noticeable cosmetic defect. The forearm, however, does not tolerate shortening well if only one of the bones is affected. Shortening of either the radius or ulna in relation to the other can lead to problems with wrist or elbow stability.[4] In Cannata's[22] series of 157 distal radius and ulna fractures, patients with less than 1 cm of length discrepancy were asymptomatic. Therefore, with significant remaining growth, shortening or lengthening of each respective bone may be indicated.

Partial Growth Arrest

For a partial growth arrest, if there is little remaining growth, one option is to surgically complete the arrest of the entire physis. Depending on the rate of growth of that physis and its contribution to overall limb length, this may be an acceptable option that avoids angular deformity of the limb. The location of the arrest will affect the resulting deformity. Peripheral bars such as a medially located bar will cause a genu varum deformity. A central arrest may lead to limb shortening and deformity of the metaphysis.[4]

If a growth arrest and physeal bar is small enough, it may be possible for a bar to fail with growth. Cases of spontaneous correction of partial physeal arrest have been described. Gkiokas and Brilakis[23] described a case of a 3.5-year-old female who formed a bony bridge at the distal tibial physis after a Salter-Harris type IV fracture. After refusing intervention, the bridge resolved after 6 months and all deformity and shortening had been corrected.

Historically, physeal distraction had been used to disrupt physeal bars near the end of growth for small growth arrests. In this technique, tension through the bony bridge causes failure of bridge and continued growth, although it has largely been abandoned due to high complication rates.[24]

Bar Resection

To determine if a bar is amenable to resection, first the size and exact location of the bridge should be determined on advanced imaging. The bridge should then be mapped in relation to anatomic landmarks easily identified intraoperatively if resection is planned (Fig. 39.8). For physeal arrests that involve less than half of the physis, resection of the bar may be an alternative to epiphysiodesis. This is generally performed in patients who have significant amount of growth remaining, usually stated as at least 2 cm or 2 years of residual growth.

Resection of the bar is more successful in smaller arrests, and better outcomes have been seen in patients with less than 25% of the physis affected or in patients with less than 20 degrees of angulation.[12,25] Exceptions to this may be in the very young children with a bony bridge. As there is significant growth remaining, an attempt may be made to resect a bar greater than 50%. Failure of such an operation at a young age still leaves the patients with multiple surgical options for correction of deformity and possibly obviates the need for them. The best outcomes for resection are seen with smaller bridges, identified soon after initial injury.

Peripheral growth arrests are more amenable to resection given that the bony bridge can be approached directly.

A, B

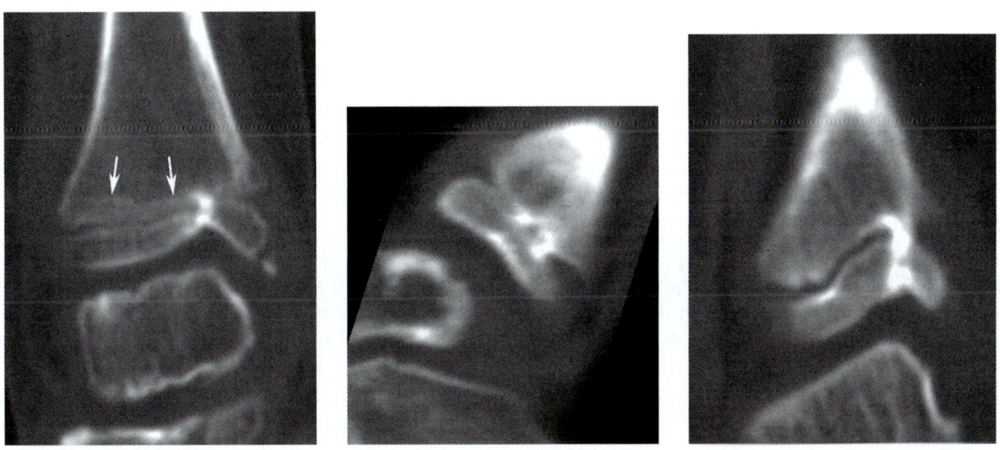

C

Figure 39.7. Harris growth arrest line as noted on CT. CT scans with coronal **(A,C)** and sagittal **(B)** reconstructions corrected for bone distortion provide excellent images of the location and size of arrest with arrows localizing growth arrest. (From Flynn J, Skaggs D, Waters P. *Rockwood and Wilkins Fractures in Children.* 8th ed. Philadelphia, PA: Wolters Kluwer; 2014, with permission.)

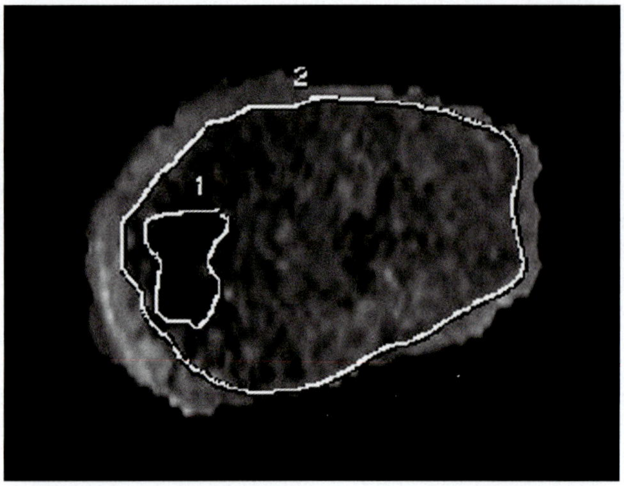

Figure 39.8. Reconstructed magnetic resonance images allow estimation of the percentage of surface area of the physis affected by a growth arrest. This workstation reconstruction delineates the perimeter of normal physis (*border 2*) and that of the physeal arrest (*border 1*). Surface area affected can be calculated from these reconstructions. (From Flynn J, Skaggs D, Waters P. *Rockwood and Wilkins Fractures in Children.* 8th ed. Philadelphia, PA: Wolters Kluwer; 2014, with permission.)

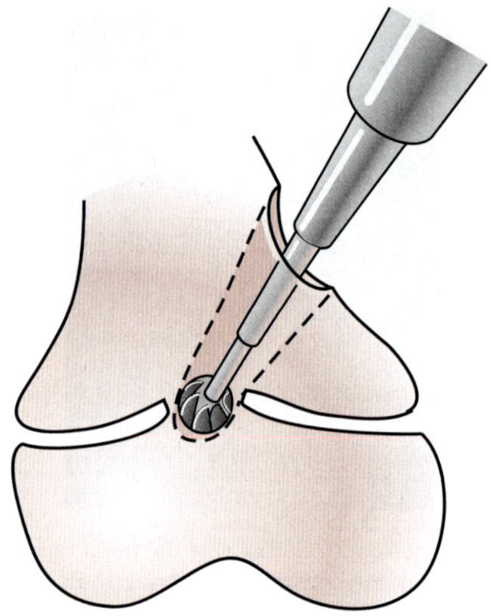

Figure 39.9. Central arrests are approached through a metaphyseal "window" or the medullary canal after metaphyseal osteotomy. (From Flynn J, Skaggs D, Waters P. *Rockwood and Wilkins Fractures in Children.* 8th ed. Philadelphia, PA: Wolters Kluwer; 2014, with permission.)

Generally, posterior peripheral bridges are more difficult to address in the lower limb given location of neurovascular structures. The bony bridge is localized on imaging, then periosteum and associated bridge are resected until normal cartilaginous physis is visualized. Due to the sclerotic nature of bridges, removal is often performed with a high-speed burr; during removal, it is crucial to irrigate and prevent thermal necrosis of surrounding bone. When removing the bridge, resection should be carried a few millimeters into healthy bone of the epiphysis and metaphysis to prevent contact and reformation.[17]

To resect a central arrest, access must avoid the healthy peripheral physis; this can be performed in several ways: A metaphyseal window may be created or a wedge removed to access the central bar (Fig. 39.9). Care must be taken to preserve the peripheral normal physis and perichondral ring of Ranvier. Intervening cancellous bone is removed with a curette in the path to the central bony bridge to adequately visualize. Once location is confirmed on imaging, the sclerotic bridge may be burred from inside out. Jackson[26] has described a window technique in which a predrilled and tapped metaphyseal wedge is removed then fixated back to bone once resection complete. Stricker[27] has described the use of the arthroscope to improve visualization. Once resection is complete, it is important to place metallic marker in the epiphysis and metaphysis to accurately determine future growth. This can also be used to help determine the amount of overgrowth of the remaining healthy physis. Markers used in the past for this purpose have been portions of K-wires, although titanium or tantalum markers may be beneficial if future MRI is anticipated.

Once resected, interposition material is inserted at the bony bridge site to prevent recurrence. Multiple interposition materials have been proposed; these include fat, polymethylmethacrylate (PMMA), bone wax, cartilage, muscle, silicone, and biologics. The most commonly used interposition grafts remain fat and PMMA, as they are readily available. Fat is easily accessible from the buttock region and is globular in nature. Drawbacks of fat interposition are that fat is typically not secure and may be displaced from the insertion site. It may be resorbed. Fat is not structural and thus a stress riser may remain at larger resection sites until healing and may therefore necessitate postoperative immobilization. PMMA has the advantage of being radiolucent, structural, and may be applied in a liquid or semisolid states, allowing molding into a cavity.

Epiphysiodesis

For partial growth arrests in which the overall limb length discrepancy will be less than 2 cm, some authors have recommended contralateral epiphysiodesis and completion epiphysiodesis of injured physis.[28] In physes with little residual growth, bilateral epiphysiodesis may be the best option to prevent both angular deformity and limb length discrepancy. This, however, must be clearly discussed with the patient and parents, as there are often gender-specific concerns about growth. An epiphysiodesis to complete a partial growth arrest can generally be considered when the remaining growth of the limb will result in a length discrepancy less than 2 cm.

When epiphysiodesis has been selected for treatment of an angular or longitudinal limb length discrepancy, then a technique must be selected. Epiphysiodesis can be performed in an open or percutaneous fashion. Methods for inciting growth arrest include placement of a bony bridge with the Phemister technique or ablation with a drill or curette, radioablation, or fixation across physis. The procedure should be performed on a radiolucent table, as fluoroscopy is necessary to localize the physis. If the lower extremity is the operative site, the extremity should be bumped and positioned to allow isolated views of the involved growth plate. Incisions should be planned to allow adequate access to the entirety of the physis. Some have recommended ablation only at the periphery of the physis, whereas others prefer central physis ablation.

When ablating a physis, a drill, burr, or curette may be used to mechanically disrupt the physis. First the physis is localized on x-ray (Fig. 39.10), then a small 5-mm incision is centered

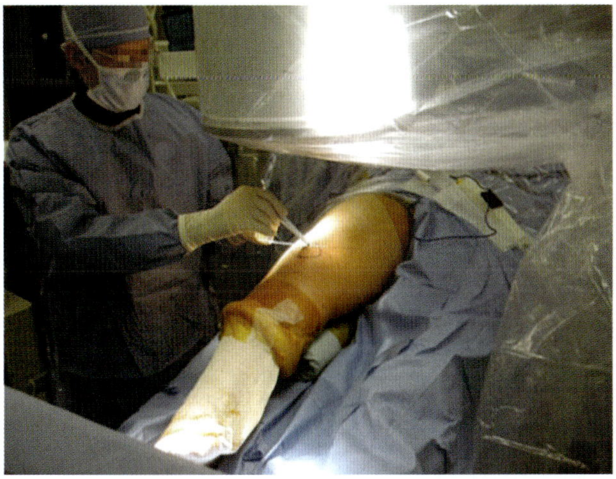

Figure 39.10. Localization of physis on imaging prior to epiphysiodesis.

over the physis, with consideration of surrounding neurovascular structures. A drill is then directed across the physis. Generally, this is repeated for both the medial and lateral aspects of the physis, although in some cases, both the medial and lateral physis can be ablated from a single approach. In the forearm and lower leg, both bones must be treated to prevent angular deformity.

Once drill holes have been created across medial and lateral physis, a curette can then be inserted through the drill holes to mechanically disrupt and remove physeal cells in each direction. Fluoroscopic images can be used to confirm the extent of physeal disruption (Fig. 39.11). Alternatively, radiopaque dye can be injected through the drill holes to show the extent of epiphysiodesis (Fig. 39.12).

Although the cortex is minimally breached by drill holes with this technique, supportive bracing of the lower extremity is frequently used for a week or two. For epiphysiodesis of the proximal tibia or distal femur, a knee immobilizer is advised in which patients may weight bear as pain allows.[29] Patients should be followed clinically and radiographically every 6 months until skeletal maturity. Physeal closure may occur as early as 1 month following drill or curette ablation.[30]

Alternatively, hardware fixation across the physis can be used to arrest growth. Typically this is permanent. Fixation options include screws, staples, or small plates across the physis. For a complete epiphysiodesis, fully threaded cannulated screws are often used. After localizing under fluoroscopy, guide wires are placed obliquely from the metaphysis into epiphysis across physis. Placement of the guide wire must avoid penetration of subchondral bone and the joint. Once guide wires are in appropriate alignment, the appropriate-sized drill is passed just beyond the physis, and fully threaded screws are placed (Fig. 39.13).

Complications of epiphysiodesis by either technique can include a failure of growth arrest, miscalculation of remaining growth leading to residual leg length discrepancy, infection, as well as wound or neurovascular complications and fracture.

Eight-plate epiphysiodesis and medial and lateral staples have been used for epiphysiodesis. Stewart et al.[31] compared dual 8-plate technique with ablation epiphysiodesis and found the improvement in leg length discrepancy to be significantly better in the ablation group compared with the 8-plate group. Staple epiphysiodesis has been associated with mechanical axis deviation when used to treat limb length discrepancy. Gorman et al.[32] followed alignment after staple epiphysiodesis of proximal tibia and distal femur and found over 50% of the patients had clinically significant deviation. Multiple options for epiphysiodesis exist; screw and ablative techniques have had the most reproducible results in the literature to date.

Distraction Osteogenesis

An alternate approach to limb length discrepancy in the setting of growth arrest is distraction osteogenesis either through monoplanar or circular/multiplanar (Ilizarov/Taylor Spatial Frame) external fixation or the newer intramedullary growing nail techniques. A large part of lengthening procedures is preoperative planning to determine the lengthening goal; optimal level for corticotomy; and, for external fixation, the arch,

A

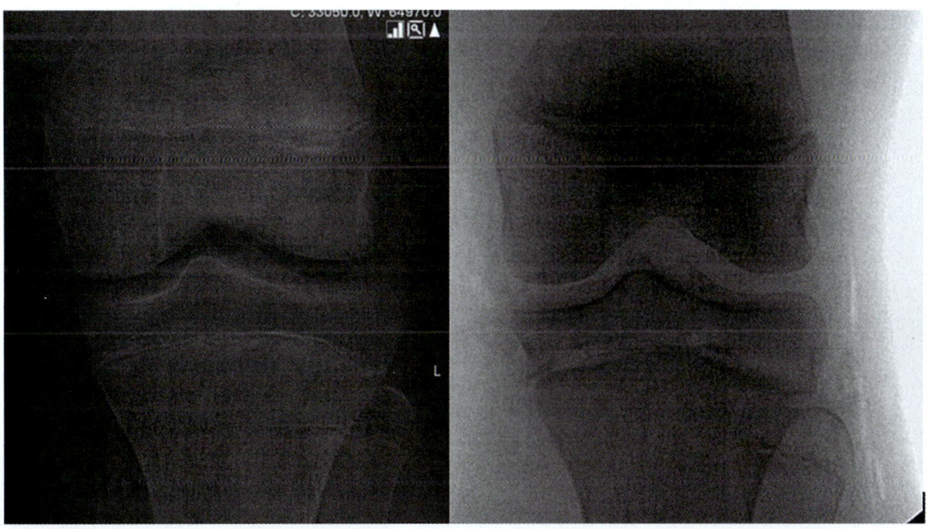

B

Figure 39.11. **A.** The proximal tibial physis preoperatively prior to mechanical disruption of the physis. **B.** The proximal tibial physis post drill and curette epiphysiodesis, showing removal of the physis.

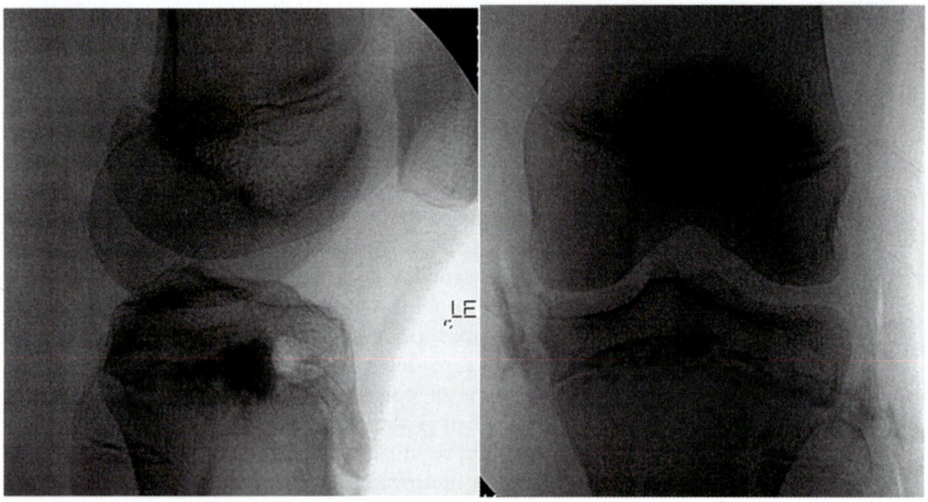

Figure 39.12. Fluoroscopic images with Omnipaque dye injected into the site of mechanical disruption, confirming disruption of the central physis.

ring, wire, and pin fixation appropriate for anatomy. A monoplanar fixation device is applied using fluoroscopic guidance; based on preoperative planning and anatomy, appropriately sized half-pins are inserted. Lower infection rates and loosening have been seen with hydroxyapatite-coated half-pins, which are inserted bicortically perpendicular to the bone segment.[33] Once pins are inserted, the frame is assembled to confirm the alignment that should be restored after the corticotomy; the assembled frame is then removed.

Corticotomy is performed by localizing the level of osteotomy with fluoroscopy then making a small incision to accommodate 5-mm osteotomes. Under imaging, multiple drill holes are made in the same plan, generally from anterior to posterior. Once adequate cortical perforation has occurred, then osteotomes are advanced in the same plane. When the osteotome reaches the far cortex, then it is rotated with a wrench to generate a controlled fracture.

Following corticotomy, the fragment is rotated to confirm completion of the corticotomy on fluoroscopy then rotated back to the previous position. The rods of the monoplanar fixation can then be reconnected in the reduced position for future lengthening. When a circular frame is used, the procedure

A

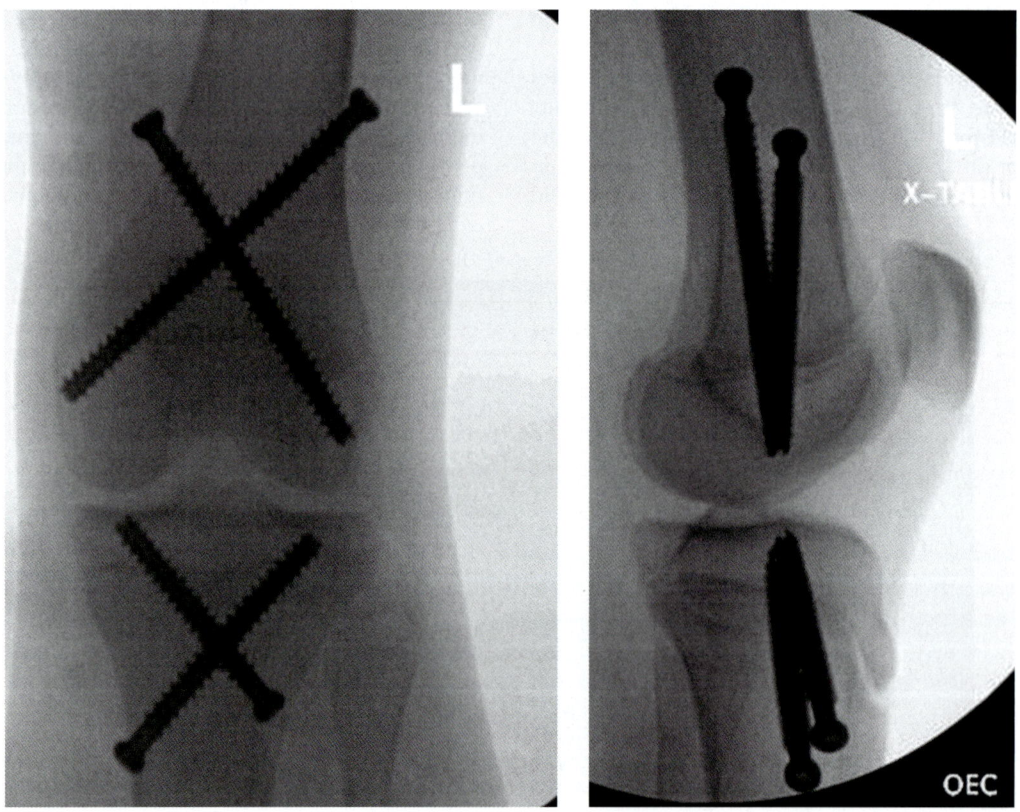

B

Figure 39.13. **A,B.** Transphyseal screw epiphysiodesis of the distal femur and proximal tibia.

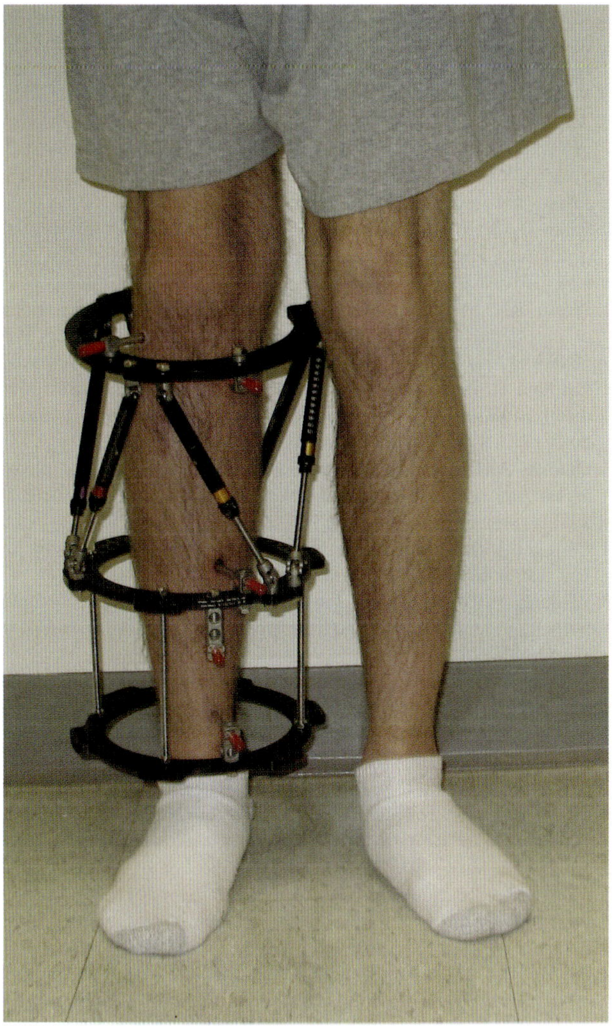

Figure 39.14. Circular frame, Taylor Spatial Frame, used for correction of leg length discrepancy.

differs in that a combination of wires and half-pins are used for fixation (Fig. 39.14). Circumferential anatomy must be considered when using a circular frame, as fixation will pass through soft tissue on either side. Similarly, the frame is preassembled, then rods disconnected at time of corticotomy. Taylor Spatial Frames are in many ways simpler than the traditional Ilizarov technique. The deformity, frame, and mounting parameters are entered in a software program. From this information, a lengthening/deformity correction program is generated for the patient over a given time period. In both the Taylor Spatial Frame and Ilizarov techniques, the child or family assists in the lengthening of the limb by turning struts on the frame multiple times per day. Generally, lengthening will be applied at 1 mm/day. The time required for lengthening depends on the child's age, quality of bone production, and the desired length to be acquired. A consolidation phase is required for the bone to regenerate, ossify, and mature. This phase may take 2 to 3 months or more. In children, frames are typically removed under sedation or general anesthetic. Although the circular frame technique has been largely described in the lower extremity, it can also be used for deformity correction and lengthening in the upper extremity.[34]

In children with minimal growth remaining, a rigid intramedullary growing nail may be considered for lengthening of the femur and tibia (e.g., Precice nail).

Correction Angular Deformity

When there is significant remaining growth in the setting of partial growth arrest, the affected limb will go on to develop angular deformity as the healthy physis continues to grow. This will lead to overall limb as well as joint malalignment. Correction of angular deformity should be addressed prior to causing additional structural changes that may predispose a joint to early degeneration or result in changes in biomechanics of adjacent joints.

When patients have an angular deformity and the bony bridge is amenable to resection, these can be addressed concurrently. The bony bridge can be resected with the previously described techniques and an osteotomy can be performed to correct the angular deformity. Although some spontaneous correction has been reported, it is difficult to predict, and spontaneous resolution of angular deformity should not be relied on for significant deformities.[25] If a patient has a deformity requiring over 20 degrees of correction, it is unlikely to correct spontaneously and corrective osteotomy is recommended.[8,13] Scheffer et al.[35] performed opening wedge osteotomies with insertion of tricortical graft for correction of 25 degrees or less. For deformity about the knee and ankle, osteotomy has been recommended for deformities over 10 degrees.[25] Remaining growth plays a role as well in surgical decision making.

The approach to angular deformity correction can either be gradual or acute and can be combined with lengthening. Noonan et al.[28] has described acute correction of deformity followed by appropriate lengthening. Patients were lengthened an average of 4.1 cm and underwent an average of 19 degrees of correction of the femur or tibia.[28] These patients were mostly adolescents, and deformities were corrected through opening wedge osteotomies. Concomitantly, a monolateral external fixation device was applied and lengthening initiated approximately 16 days after surgery. An acute correction carries the risk of a traction injury to nerve tensioned by realignment which can result in neurapraxia; however, this was not seen in this series.

Similarly, Horn et al.[36] performed combined angular correction and limb lengthening with completion epiphysiodesis of the injured physis for adolescent patients with partial growth arrest. In this series, patients had between 12 to 24 degrees of deformity and 15 to 60 mm of shortening in the lower limb.[36] Correction was achieved using either Ilizarov or Taylor Spatial Frames.

Shin et al.[37] compared two approaches to correcting angular deformity during growth; asymmetrical physeal suppression was achieved through either hemiepiphyseal stapling or percutaneous transphyseal screw placement. Both of these methods were found to be equally effective in the correction of angular deformity.

Multiple approaches to angular deformity and limb length discrepancy exist for partial and complete growth arrests. Decision making regarding algorithm is unique to each patient and deformity. Location and size of growth arrest and remaining skeletal growth must all be weighed in order to optimize treatment for the patient.

Future Directions

Another direction of research has targeted the underlying injury to the physis in attempt to restore the healing potential of the physis and lead to future growth. Although various strategies have been implemented to repair defects in the physis, biologic agents are a potential option for repair or regeneration. Mesenchymal stem cells have been one direction of this research in the animal model in attempt to create physeal regeneration.[38]

To date, there have been various animal studies; however, results are still mixed. Studies have investigated the use of biologic scaffolds to promote growth; these include chitin, collagen, and Gelfoam. Another avenue of investigation to induce repair has been use of growth factors such as transforming growth factor-β (TGF-β), insulin-like growth factor (IGF-1), bone morphogenetic proteins (BMPs), and fibroblast growth factor (FGF-2).[3] Future research may focus on the use of growth factors to incite repair with stem cell therapy for regeneration. Modulation of genes may also allow for sustainable delivery of growth factors to injury sites.[39]

REFERENCES

1. Salter RB. Injuries of the epiphyseal plate. *Instr Course Lect.* 1992; 41:351–359.
2. Ogden JA, Ganey T, Light TR, et al. The pathology of acute chondro-osseous injury in the child. *Yale J Biol Med.* 1993;66(3):219–233.
3. Mizuta T, Benson WM, Foster BK, et al. Statistical analysis of the incidence of physeal injuries. *J Pediatr Orthop.* 1987;7(5):518–523.
4. Ramachandran M, Skaggs DL. Physeal injuries. In: Green NE, Swiontkowski MF, eds. *Skeletal Trauma in Children.* 4th ed. Philadelphia, PA: Elsevier; 2008:19–37.
5. Eid AM, Hafez MA. Traumatic injuries of the distal femoral physis. Retrospective study on 151 cases. *Injury.* 2002;33(3):251–255.
6. Peterson HA, Madhok R, Benson JT, et al. Physeal fractures: part 1. Epidemiology in Olmsted County, Minnesota, 1979–1988. *J Pediatr Orthop.* 1994;14(4):423–430.
7. Caine D, Howe W, Ross W, et al. Does repetitive physical loading inhibit radial growth in female gymnasts? *Clin J Sport Med.* 1997;7(4):302–308.
8. Peterson HA. Partial growth plate arrest and its treatment. *J Pediatr Orthop.* 1984;4(2):246–258.
9. Peterson HA, Wood MB. Physeal arrest due to laser beam damage in a growing child. *J Pediatr Orthop.* 2001;21(3):335–337.
10. Dahl WJ, Silva S, Vanderhave KL. Distal femoral physeal fixation: are smooth pins really safe? *J Pediatr Orthop.* 2014;34:134–138.
11. Shifflett G, Green D, Berner N, et al. Growth arrest following ACL reconstruction with hamstring autograft in skeletally immature patients: a review of four cases. Poster presented at: European Pediatric Orthopaedic Society 33rd Annual Meeting; April 2–5, 2014; Bruges, Belgium.
12. Price CT, Flynn JM. Injury to the physis. In: Morrissy RT, Weinstein SL, eds. *Lovell and Winter's Pediatric Orthopaedics.* 6th ed. Philadelphia, PA: Lippincott Williams & Wilkins; 2006:1433–1436.
13. Ogden JA. The evaluation and treatment of partial physeal arrest. *J Bone Joint Surg Am.* 1987;69(8):1297–1302.
14. Kasser JR. Physeal bar resections after growth arrest about the knee. *Clin Orthop Relat Res.* 1990;(255):68–74.
15. Carlson WO, Wenger DR. A mapping method to prepare for surgical excision of a partial physeal arrest. *J Pediatr Orthop.* 1984;4(2): 232–238.
16. Ecklund K, Jaramillo D. Patterns of premature physeal arrest: MR imaging of 111 children. *AJR Am J Roentgenol.* 2002;178(4):967–972.
17. Khoshhal KI, Kiefer GN. Physeal bridge resection. *J Am Acad Orthop Surg.* 2005;13(1):47–58.
18. Anderson M, Green WT, Messner MB. Growth and predictions of growth in the lower extremities. *J Bone Joint Surg Am.* 1963;45-A:1–14.
19. Moseley CF. A straight-line graph for leg-length discrepancies. *J Bone Joint Surg Am.* 1977;59(2):174–179.
20. Paley D, Bhave A, Herzenberg JE, et al. Multiplier method for predicting limb-length discrepancy. *J Bone Joint Surg Am.* 2000; 82-A(10):1432–1446.
21. Westh RN, Menelaus MB. A simple calculation for the timing of epiphysial arrest: a further report. *J Bone Joint Surg Br.* 1981; 63-B(1):117–119.
22. Cannata G, De Maio F, Mancini F, et al. Physeal fractures of the distal radius and ulna: long-term prognosis. *J Orthop Trauma.* 2003;17(3):172–179; discussion 179–180.
23. Gkiokas A, Brilakis E. Spontaneous correction of partial physeal arrest: report of a case and review of the literature. *J Pediatr Orthop B.* 2012;21(4):369–372.
24. Canadell J, de Pablos J. Correction of angular deformities by physeal distraction. *Clin Orthop Relat Res.* 1992;(283):98–105.
25. Williamson RV, Staheli LT. Partial physeal growth arrest: treatment by bridge resection and fat interposition. *J Pediatr Orthop.* 1990; 10(6):769–776.
26. Jackson AM. Excision of the central physeal bar: a modification of Langenskiöld's procedure. *J Bone Joint Surg Br.* 1993;75(4):664–665.
27. Stricker S. Arthroscopic visualization during excision of a central physeal bar. *J Pediatr Orthop.* 1992;12(4):544–546.
28. Noonan KJ, Price CT, Sproul JT, et al. Acute correction and distraction osteogenesis for the malaligned and shortened lower extremity. *J Pediatr Orthop.* 1998;18(2):178–186.
29. Ghanem I, Karam JA, Widmann RF. Surgical epiphysiodesis indications and techniques: update. *Curr Opin Pediatr.* 2011;23(1):53–59.
30. Ogilvie JW, King K. Epiphysiodesis: two-year clinical results using a new technique. *J Pediatr Orthop.* 1990;10(6):809–811.
31. Stewart D, Cheema A, Szalay EA. Dual 8-plate technique is not as effective as ablation for epiphysiodesis about the knee. *J Pediatr Orthop.* 2013;33(8):843–846.
32. Gorman TM, Vanderwerff R, Pond M, et al. Mechanical axis following staple epiphysiodesis for limb-length inequality. *J Bone Joint Surg Am.* 2009;91(10):2430–2439.
33. Caja VL, Piza G, Navarro A. Hydroxyapatite coating of external fixation pins to decrease axial deformity during tibial lengthening for short stature. *J Bone Joint Surg Am.* 2003;85-A(8):1527–1531.
34. Gundes H, Buluc L, Sahin M, et al. Deformity correction by Ilizarov distraction osteogenesis after distal radius physeal arrest. *Acta Orthop Traumatol Turc.* 2011;45(6):406–411.
35. Scheffer MM, Peterson HA. Opening-wedge osteotomy for angular deformities of long bones in children. *J Bone Joint Surg Am.* 1994;76(3):325–334.
36. Horn J, Kristiansen LP, Steen H. Deformity correction during growth after partial physeal arrest. *Acta Orthop Belg.* 2009;75(2): 219–224.
37. Shin SJ, Cho TJ, Park MS, et al. Angular deformity correction by asymmetrical physeal suppression in growing children: stapling versus percutaneous transphyseal screw. *J Pediatr Orthop.* 2010;30(6):588–593.
38. Shukrimi AB, Afizah MH, Schmitt JF, et al. Mesenchymal stem cell therapy for injured growth plate. *Front Biosci (Schol Ed).* 2013;5: 774–785.
39. Sanghani A, Chimutengwende-Gordon M, Adesida A, et al. Applications of stem cell therapy for physeal injuries. *Curr Stem Cell Res Ther.* 2013;8(6):451–455.

Jonathan D. Haskel
Yong-Woon Shin
Daniel W. Green

CHAPTER 40

Applications of Implant-Mediated Guided Growth in Pediatric Knee Surgery

PRINCIPLES

Lower extremity angular alignment changes predictably under physiologic conditions during early human development. At birth, infants present with varus alignment and eventually progress to valgus alignment starting around 24 to 48 months of age. Typically, femorotibial angle stabilizes at 8 years of age.[1] Progression and increased severity of either varus or valgus angular alignment in childhood can be pathologic, resulting in abnormal gait mechanics and unfavorable functional consequences.

Varus and valgus deformities can result in altered mechanical load, and failure to treat may result in degenerative changes such as osteoarthritis.[2] Therapeutic strategies aimed at treating angular deformities have evolved over time, with an array of treatment options currently available such as corrective osteotomy, stapling, and percutaneous transphyseal screws. More recently, development of implant-mediated guided growth (IMGG) has spurred innovations in this technique, which is becoming an increasingly popular component of the treatment strategy for correcting lower limb angular deformities. In addition, other knee pathologies may also benefit from this treatment, such as recurrent patella dislocation, osteochondral injury, and meniscal insufficiency.

The gold standard for the treatment of severe angular deformities of the lower limb is corrective osteotomy; however, it is an invasive procedure characterized by substantial morbidity and a long recovery period. As such, the less invasive treatment option of IMGG (also referred to as *mechanical hemiepiphysiodesis*) may be preferred.

Unlike osteotomy, mechanical hemiepiphysiodesis allows for slow correction of angular deformities. Its use has become widespread in skeletally immature patients because subsequent bone growth after implant removal is relatively unhindered and the postoperative restrictions are much less severe. Blount and Clarke[3] first described the use of staples for hemiepiphysiodesis. Epiphyseal staples act to correct angular deformities by impeding growth via compressive forces on one side of the growth plate, while allowing unhindered growth on the opposite side. The primary drawbacks to staples include physeal damage, premature closure of the growth plates, and hardware issues such as staple breakage and staple migration.

In 2007, Dr. Peter Stevens[4] advanced the concept of IMGG further with his invention of the "8-plate," a two-holed plate secured by two 4.5-mm screws. This dynamic construct allows the screws to pivot up to 45 degrees to accommodate physis growth[5] and acts as a tension band whose fulcrum rests outside the physis. Staples, however, apply rigid compressive forces within the physis, which may lead to difficult removal and perhaps growth arrest.[4] This distinction has popularized the use of the 8-plate, and multiple short-term studies indicate that the 8 plate is as effective as staple hemiepiphysiodesis for the treatment of angular deformities in children.[5–8]

Recently, Gottliebsen et al.[9] conducted the first randomized clinical trial that compared the use of epiphyseal staples to the use of the 8-plate for the treatment of idiopathic genu valgum. Twenty children participated in the study, with 10 randomized to each treatment group. All 20 children achieved complete angular correction, and no statistically significant differences were found between the two groups in terms of time to correct the deformity or postoperative visual analog scale (VAS) pain scores. The main conclusion of this study was that, in agreement with previous research,[5–8] there is little evidence to suggest the superiority of the 8-plate over stapling in terms of time to correct the deformity. More long-term follow-up studies that assess the incidence of rebound growth after removal of the 8-plate are necessary in order to best evaluate its long-term efficacy.

CONTRAINDICATIONS, APPROPRIATE AGES

IMGG harnesses the patient's growing bones to correct the angular deformity, either reversibly or irreversibly, depending on the technique. As such, IMGG is contraindicated in patients with a physeal bone bar,[10] patients with closed physes,

TABLE 40.1 Age of Application

Author	*Age of Application*
Ballal et al.[12]	Mean: 11.6 y Range: 5.5–14.9 y
Boero et al.[14]	Mean: 10.10 y Range: 2.3–14.1 y
Burghardt and Herzenberg[5]	Mean: 9.6 y Range: 4–14.3 y
Guzman et al.[15]	Mean: 12.5 y Range: 10–16 y
Jelinek et al.[8]	Mean: 12.3 y Range: 2.9–16.0 y
Schroerlucke et al.[27]	Mean: 11 y Range: 7–14 y
Stevens[4]	Mean: 10.5 y Range: 1.7–17 y

or patients who are within 6 to 12 months of physeal closure (14 years bone age for females, 16 years bone age for males).[11] Historically, surgical treatment of lower limb angular deformities was contraindicated in children younger than the age of 8 years.[1] But more recently, children as young as 1.7 years of age are being reported,[4] and the trend toward treating younger children is becoming more widely accepted. Table 40.1 summarizes the most recent reported ages of patients treated with IMGG for lower limb angular deformities.

A bone age determination, made by analyzing the patient's hand radiograph, should be made in order to identify whether or not the patient has reached skeletal maturity.[12] This determination can now be made efficiently with the use of a shorthand method developed by researchers at the Hospital for Special Surgery that uses a single written criterion for each age rather than a single radiograph and multiple criteria (Fig. 40.1).[13] For more detailed information on growth assessment in pediatric patients, see Chapter 38.

For patients with genu valgum who still have immature growth plates, IMGG is the preferred temporary corrective strategy because it permits subsequent growth upon implant removal. This technique is effective for patients who have at least 6 to 12 more months of growth remaining.[4]

HOW MUCH CORRECTION TO EXPECT PER MONTH

When deciding to initiate IMGG therapy, it is important to consider the implant's rate of correction in order to avoid over- or undercorrection and appropriately monitor the patient's treatment trajectory. Ballal et al.[12] recently examined the rate at which the 8-plate corrected a cohort of 25 skeletally immature patients with either pathologic genu valgus or genu varus. The authors reported a mean correction rate of 0.7 degrees per month in the distal femur, 0.5 degrees per month in the tibia, and 1.2 degrees per month if the femur and tibia were treated simultaneously. They also found that children younger than the age of 10 years corrected at a faster rate, on average, than the children older than the age of 10 years (1.4 degrees per month vs. 0.6 degrees). Additionally, Boero et al.[14] reported a mean correction rate of 0.93 degrees per month in the distal femurs of 58 patients treated with the 8-plate for either pathologic genu valgus or varus.

In a cohort of 25 patients with 47 valgus deformities treated with a tension band plate on the distal femoral physis, Guzman et al.[15] reported a mean correction rate of the anatomic lateral distal femoral angle (aLDFA) of 0.96 degrees every 3 months, or 3.8 degrees per year. Consistent with the age-stratified results by Ballal et al.,[12] Guzman et al.[15] found that girls younger than 11 years of age and boys younger than 13 years of age corrected at a faster rate than older children (4.5 degrees per year vs. 3.4 degrees). Table 40.2 summarizes the most recent reported

Radiographic Criteria for Bone Age Determination	**Bone age (years)**	
	Males	**Females**
Appearance of hook of hamate ossific nucleus	12.5	10
Appearance of thumb sesamoid ossific nucleus	13	11
Width of proximal aspect of distal radius epiphysis equals width of distal aspect of distal radius metaphysis but has not yet begun to cap	13.5	—
Capping[a] of distal radius epiphysis	14	12
Closure[b] of thumb distal phalanx physis	15	13
Closure[b] of index finger distal phalanx physis	15.5	13.5
Closure[b] of index finger proximal phalanx physis	16	14
Closure[b] of index finger distal metacarpal physis (not tested)	—	15
Closure[b] of distal ulna physis (not tested)	—	16
Closure[b] of distal radius physis (not tested)	—	17

[a]Capping indicated by rounded osseous peak oriented proximally (on ulnar side).
[b]Closure indicated by osseous bridging = 50% of the physis.

Figure 40.1. Radiographic criteria for bone age determination. (Adapted from Heyworth BE, Osei DA, Fabricant PD, et al. The shorthand bone age assessment: a simpler alternative to current methods. J Pediatr Orthop. 2013;33[5]:569–574.)

TABLE 40.2 Rates of Correction with Implant-Mediated Guided Growth

Author	*Rate of Correction (degrees/month)*
Ballal et al.[12]	Distal femur: 0.7 degrees Proximal tibia: 0.5 degrees Femur + tibia simultaneously: 1.2 degrees
Boero et al.[14]	Distal femur: 0.93 degrees
Guzman et al.[15]	aLDFA: 0.96 degrees every 3 mo, 3.8 degrees per year Girls younger than 11 y of age: 4.5 degrees per year Boys younger than 13 y of age: 3.4 degrees per year
Schroerlucke et al.[27]	Average correction for genu varum and genu valgum: 0.42 degrees
Sung et al.[28]	Young children[a], distal femur: 0.71 degrees Young children, proximal tibia: 0.40 degrees Young children, distal tibia: 0.48 degrees Old children, distal femur: 0.39 degrees Old children, proximal tibia: 0.29 degrees Old children, distal tibia: 0.48 degrees

[a]Boys age 14 years or younger, girls age 12 years or younger.

rates of correction in patients treated with IMGG for lower limb angular deformities.

OVERCORRECTION CAN OCCUR

As a temporary measure, IMGG inherently requires routine serial follow-ups to prevent overcorrection of the deformity and ensure that hardware removal occurs at the appropriate time. It is critical for the treating physician to educate the patient regarding the significance of follow-ups to monitor the treated knee, as overcorrection may demand compensatory IMGG in the contralateral side should the patient fail to follow up. Saran and Rathjen[16] recommend a follow-up approximately every 4 months. Additionally, Blount and Clarke[3] recommend not leaving the epiphyseal staples on the growth plate for more than 2 years in a growing child.

SURGICAL TECHNIQUE

The surgical technique for fixation of different tension band plates typically follows the same general protocol and thus will be generalized for most commonly used implants. Before tension band plates can be applied, preoperative planning and radiologic analysis must occur to ensure appropriate application of the hardware. Standing anteroposterior (AP) and lateral radiographs that include the hip and the ankles should be analyzed to locate the patient's center of rotation of angulation (CORA), which will indicate the precise site and magnitude of the deformity to be corrected. Blunt dissection will reveal the periosteal surface, which should be carefully exposed to prevent injury to this layer. Periosteal stripping should be avoided, as it may lead to growth arrest or asymmetrical growth.

The following technical steps have been adapted from the technique manual published by Pega Medical for fixation of the Hinge Plate. Although this surgical protocol is relatively standard, innovation in tension band plates has resulted in a variety of plate designs, with more technical details specific to each plate type. A list of these guided growth constructs can be found in Table 40.3.

Under fluoroscopic imaging, a K-wire is introduced near the patient's growth plate to ensure proper implant alignment over the physis. If a template is being used, the template is centered over the physis on the lateral surface of the bone using the K-wire as a guide. If a template is not being used, then the tension band plate will be directly applied over the K-wire. Next, a second K-wire is introduced through one of the two main screw holes of the template (or tension band plate) at an angle away from the growth plate with the aid of a wire guide. After verification of the K-wire's position under fluoroscopy, a screw hole is drilled into the bone using a cannulated drill bit that matches the predetermined screw length. If a template is being used, then the template is removed at this point and

TABLE 40.3 Guided Growth Constructs

	Manufacturer	*Image*
eight-Plate	Orthofix (McKinney, TX)	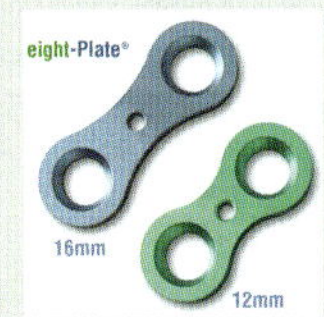 [a]
Hinge Plate	Pega Medical (Quebec, Canada)	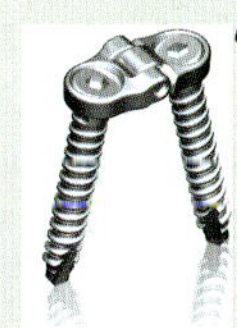 [b]
Peanut plate	Biomet (Warsaw, IN)	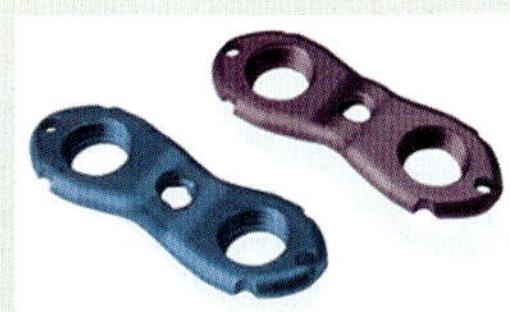 [c]
PediPlates	OrthoPediatrics (Warsaw, IN)	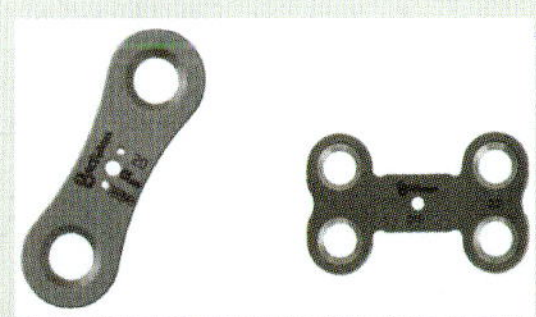 [d]

[a]From http://web.orthofix.com/Products/Products/Guided%20Growth%20System/Guided_Growth-Brochure_1304.pdf
[b]From Pega Medical. The Hinge Plate. http://www.pegamedical.com/en/products/Hinge-Plate-the-hinge-pediatric-plating-system.html. Accessed June 20, 2014.
[c]From Biomet. Peanut Growth Control Plating System. http://www.biomet.com/trauma/products.cfm?pdid=4&majcid=28&prodid=234. Accessed June 20, 2014.
[d]From OrthoPediatrics. PediPlates®. http://www.orthopediatrics.com/medical/product/PediPlates. Accessed June 20, 2014.

the tension band plate is directed over the guiding K-wire to ensure proper placement. The guiding K-wire is removed, and a cannulated screw is introduced into the bone surface so that it is perfectly center within the plate's first hole. Once the first screw is applied, proceed with the same method for drilling and screwing the second screw. It is important for the plate to be flush against the bone surface to prevent periosteal damage.

TECHNICAL CAUTIONS

If performing a medial distal femur epiphysiodesis, it is critical to minimize damage to the medial patellofemoral ligament (MPFL), which inserts just distal to the femoral growth plate on the surface of the medial epicondyle.[17] A recent experiment found that partial or complete transection of the MPFL occurred in 6 of 8 cadaveric knees after temporary mechanical hemiepiphysiodesis using a plate and two screws.[18] Therefore, we recommend placing the plate in the posterior one-third of the femur and avoiding transection of the MPFL when applying a growth modulating implant to this area. Current literature has illuminated cases of postoperative pain and decreased range of motion following temporary mechanical hemiepiphysiodesis,[8] and damage to the MPFL may be a significant contributing factor to these outcomes.

It is also critical to ensure that each of the screws is screwed directly into the center of the plate's two holes. Incorrect placement of the screws near the edge of the plate's holes can result in faulty plate fixation and ultimately implant failure. Figure 40.2 illustrates proper and improper screw position within the plate.

Finally, it is important to screw in the first screw prior to drilling the second hole. Following this recommendation will ensure that the second drill hole sits perfectly centered within the plate's second screw hole, thus optimizing the subsequent screw's positioning. A summary of the technical cautions for IMGG can be found in Table 40.4.

TABLE 40.4 Implant-Mediated Guided Growth Technical Principles

Technique	*Reasoning*
1. Avoid the periosteum.	Periosteal stripping may lead to growth arrest or asymmetrical growth.
2. Avoid the MPFL.	Damage to the MPFL may lead to postoperative pain and decreased range of motion.
3. Position each screw at the center of the plate's screw holes.	Improper positioning of the screws may result in faulty plate fixation and implant failure.
4. Screw the first screw before drilling the second hole.	This ensures proper positioning of the second screw.

IMPLANT-MEDIATED GUIDED GROWTH AND PATELLAR DISLOCATION

Children with pathologic genu valgum have an increased susceptibility to patellar instability and often present with a history of lateral patella dislocations. The MPFL has been identified as the major constraint against lateral patellar translation,[19] and genu valgum may contribute to the tendency toward patellar instability. Therefore, it is important to evaluate pediatric patients with recurrent patellar dislocations for genu valgum. Radiographic

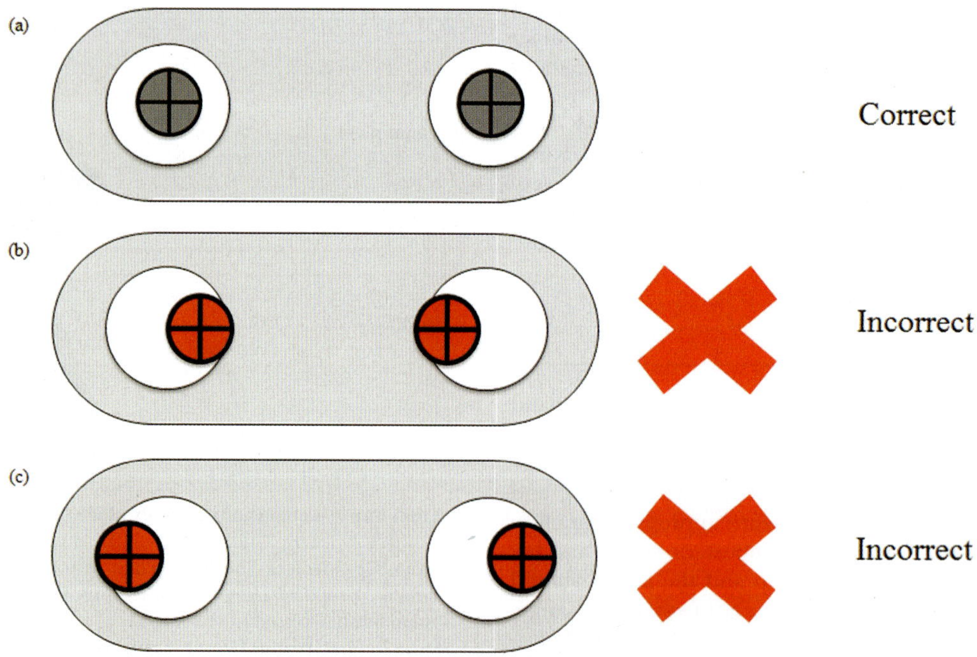

Figure 40.2. Surgical technique for application of an IMGG implant. Each screw should be applied in the precise center of each hole of the plate, as depicted in image *a*. Improper fixation of the screw near the edge of the hole of the plate can result in implant breakage and/or failure of therapy, as depicted in images *b* and *c*.

evaluation with a standing AP radiograph including the hip and the ankle is indicated if the space between the patient's ankles exceeds 10 cm while his or her knees are touching.[20]

To correct genu valgum angular deformities in young patients with concurrent recurrent patellar dislocations, we endorse IMGG. This technique prevents growth on one side of the growth plate while allowing unhindered growth on the opposite side until full angular correction is achieved, at which point the implant is removed and symmetrical linear growth resumes. Treatment of skeletally immature patients with genu valgum demands special attention because the implant is placed over the medial physis of the distal femur. IMGG is a less invasive, safer alternative to the more extensive surgical approaches such as corrective osteotomy.

CASES IN IMPLANT-MEDIATED GUIDED GROWTH

Genu Valgum Secondary to a Tibial Spine Avulsion Fracture

Recently, Fabricant et al.[21] identified one case in which IMGG effectively treated a lower limb angular deformity that manifested in a 13-year-old male after open reduction and internal fixation of a tibial spine avulsion fracture, the first reported complication of its type from this procedure. The patient presented 19 months after his original surgery with 19 degrees of genu valgum in the treated limb. In this patient, the screw that was introduced to achieve fixation for the previous avulsion fracture had crossed the lateral tibial physis, temporarily arresting growth on this side of the proximal tibia (Fig. 40.3). To correct the valgus deformity that developed, the authors of the case report removed the tibial spine screw and applied an 8-plate to the medial surface of the proximal tibia, as seen in the attached radiographs. After 11 months, radiographic and clinical examination revealed that the patient's lower extremity had attained neutral anatomic and mechanical axes, and the implant was removed.

Genu Valgum Secondary to Meniscal Insufficiency

IMGG has also been performed in the context of meniscal insufficiency in certain pediatric patients. Our institution reports the case of an 11-year-old female who underwent near-complete lateral meniscectomy at an outside hospital to treat her complex discoid lateral meniscus in her right knee followed by a meniscal transplant. She subsequently presented to our institution with osteoarthritic changes in her lateral compartment due to meniscal insufficiency as well as bilateral right greater

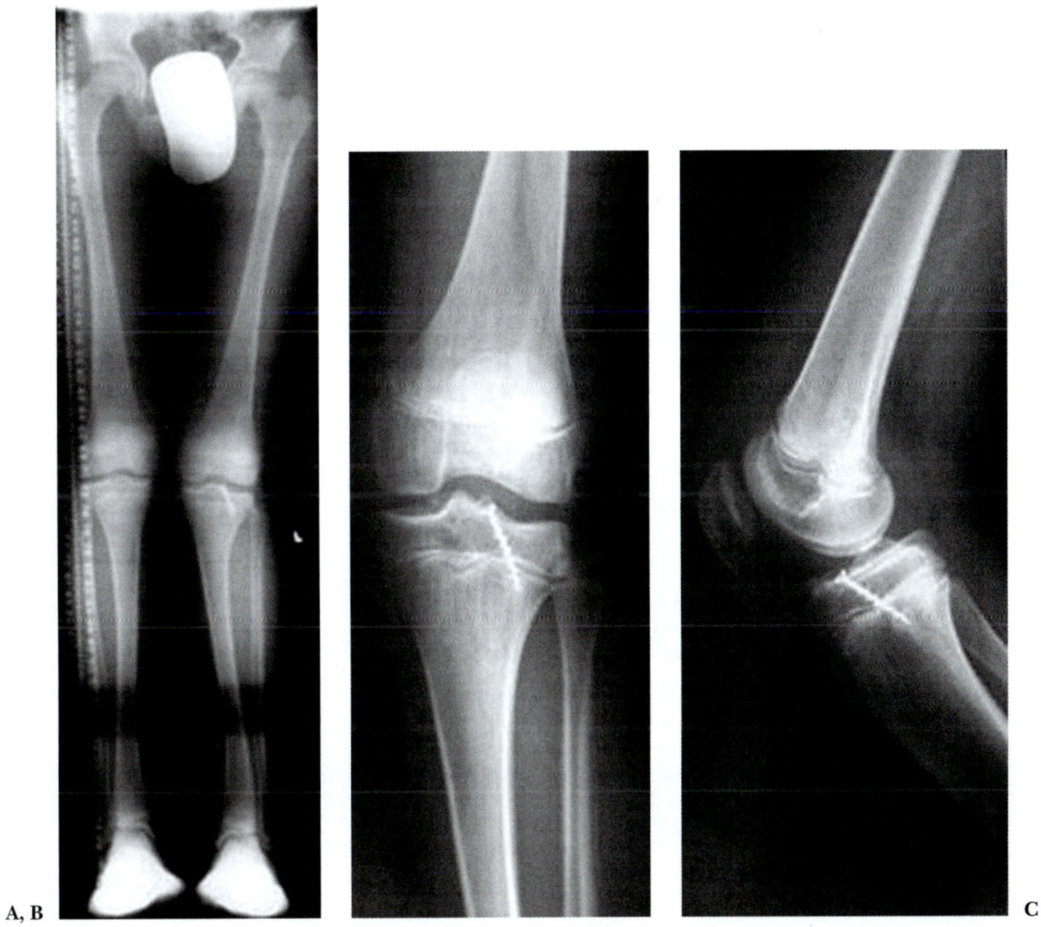

Figure 40.3. Unilateral genu valgum caused by the application of a transphyseal screw for the treatment of a tibial spine fracture in a 13-year-old male. **A.** Preoperative full-length standing film depicts 19 degrees of genu valgum in the left lower limb. **B,C.** Preoperative AP and lateral plain radiographs depict the orientation of the tibial spine screw. *(continued)*

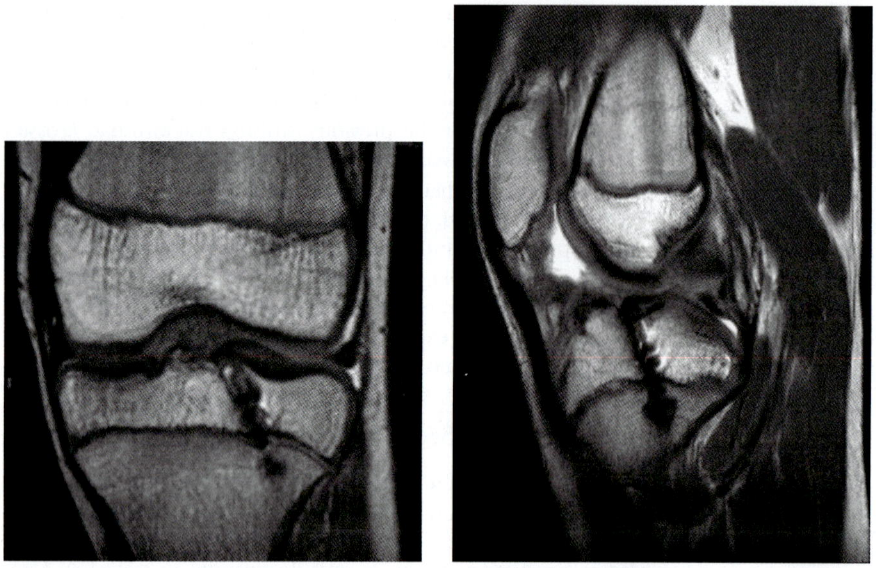

D, E

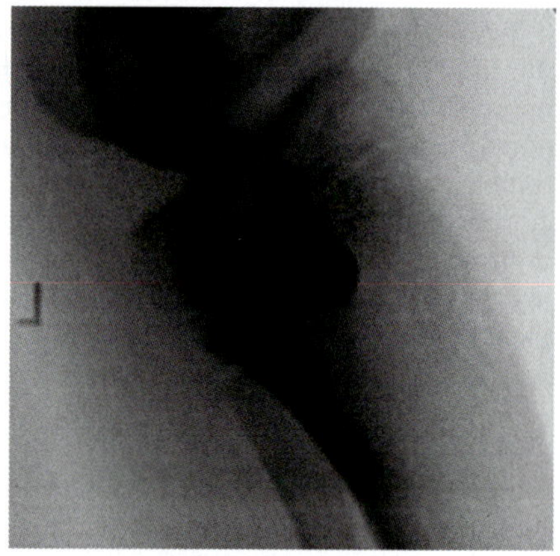

F

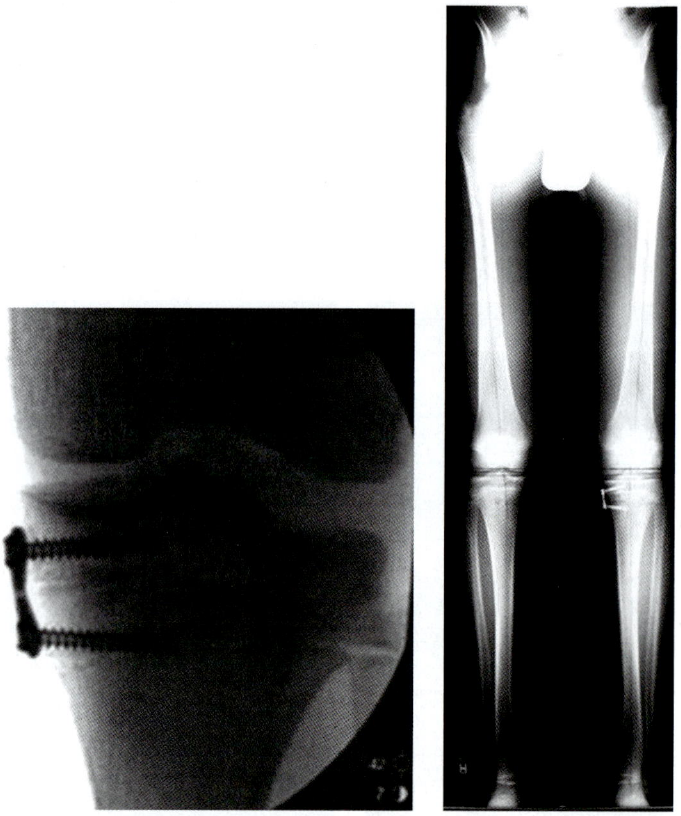

G, H

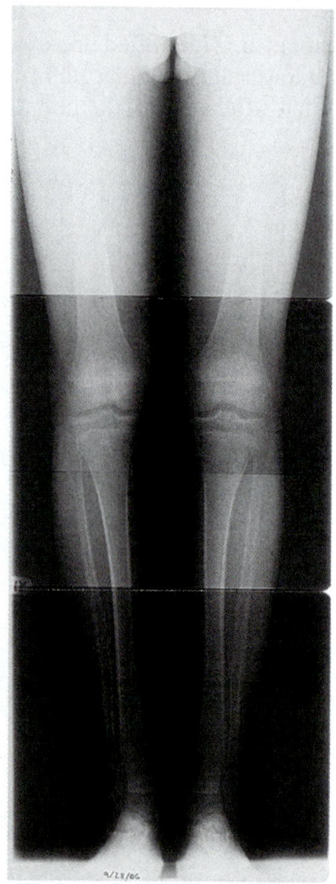

I

Figure 40.3. *(continued)* **D,E.** Preoperative coronal and sagittal magnetic resonance images depict screw fixation that extends through the proximal tibial physis. **F,G.** Intraoperative AP and lateral fluoroscopic images demonstrate correct application of the 8-plate to the medial surface of the proximal tibia. **H.** After 11 months of IMGG therapy, full-length standing AP radiographs reveal normal limb alignment. **I.** This full-length standing AP radiograph depicts the patient 4 months after removal of hardware with full correction of the varus deformity and normal angular alignment.

than left genu valgum. To treat these lower limb angular deformities, we performed mechanical hemiepiphysiodesis by applying 8-plates to the medial surfaces of the patient's right distal femur, right proximal tibia, and left distal femur. We removed the patient's hardware once she exhibited slight overcorrection and complete fusion of her growth plates, which occurred after 29 months of guided growth therapy. Her outcome was especially successful, as she was able to resume activity in lacrosse, volleyball, and snowboarding. Figure 40.4 demonstrates radiographs of this patient's correction from significant bilateral genu valgum to normal position.

Genu Varum and a Posterolateral Corner Injury

The use of IMGG is also indicated in patients who present with a history of posterolateral corner injury and concurrent genu varum. Repairing the posterolateral corner injury without first correcting the genu varum deformity can result in excess tension in the graft across the malaligned knee, which often results in graft failure.[22,23] As such, it has become common practice to correct the anatomic and mechanical axes of the lower limb in patients with angular deformities prior to performing any soft tissue reconstruction.[24]

A 15-year-old male patient presented at our institution with mild genu varum in the right distal femur with concurrent injuries to the posterolateral corner, posterior cruciate ligament (PCL), and lateral collateral ligament (LCL) as a result of a football injury. Figure 40.5 illustrates the patient after successful correction of his angular deformity with application of a Hinge Plate 11 months prior. The patient will next undergo reconstructive repair of his posterolateral corner, PCL, and LCL once he reaches skeletal maturity.

Genu Varum Secondary to Hypophosphatemic Rickets

Patients who are diagnosed with hypophosphatemic rickets often present with a combination of renal phosphate wasting, abnormal mineralization of bone, short stature, and/or progressive lower limb deformities.[25] The management of such patients often involves phosphate and 1,25-dihydroxyvitamin D supplementation; however, there is often a delay between the onset of therapy and the expected physiologic response. This delay can facilitate progression of the deformity. As such, early intervention to correct the mechanical axis can improve the efficacy of medical management by reducing pathologic loading.[26] Here, we present the use of IMGG to successfully correct bilateral genu valgum secondary to hypophosphatemic rickets in a patient at our institution.

The 10-year-old female initially presented with 16 degrees of genu valgum in her right knee and 13 degrees of genu valgum in her left knee. Sixteen months after bilateral application of 8-plates over the medial surfaces of her distal femoral physes, the right 8-plate was removed, and the patient underwent staged MPFL reconstruction, lateral releases, and quadriceps lengthening to treat her obligatory patellar dislocations. Figure 40.6 demonstrates correction of the patient's bilateral genu valgum after application of 8-plates.

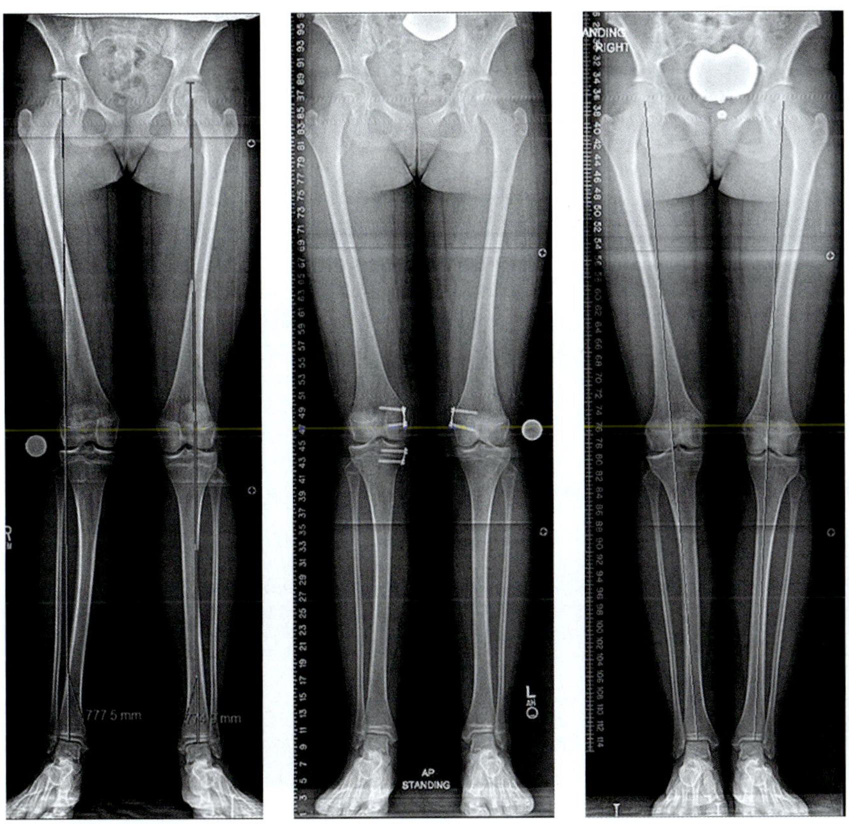

A, B C

Figure 40.4. Treatment of bilateral genu valgum in conjunction with meniscal insufficiency in a 13-year-old female. **A.** Full-length standing radiograph shows bilateral right greater than left genu valgum just prior to application of 8-plates for IMGG therapy. Mechanical axes of the lower limb depict the deformity. **B.** Full-length standing film portrays mild correction of the bilateral genu valgum 5 months after application of 8-plates on the right distal femur, right proximal tibia, and left proximal tibia. **C.** Three months post removal of hardware illustrates normal knee alignment, as indicated by the mechanical axes. Her outcome was especially successful, as she was able to return to competitive sports.

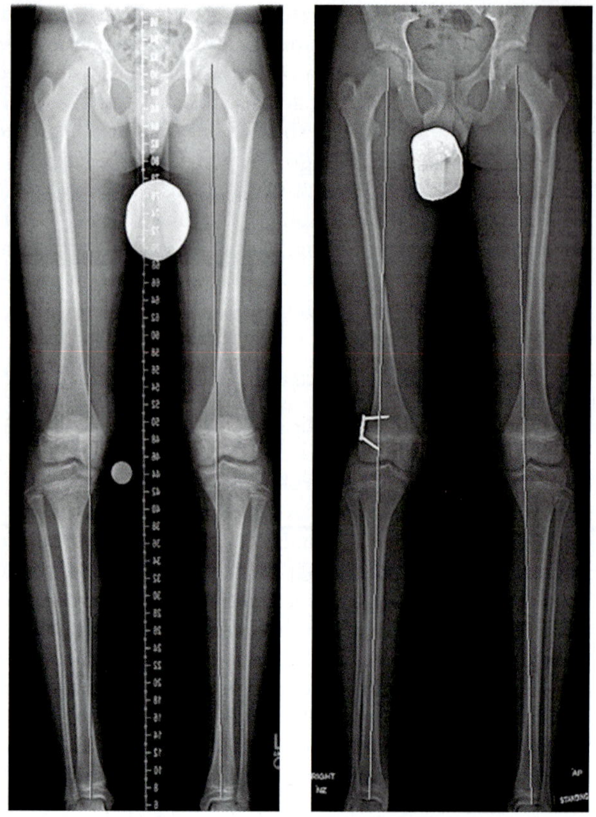

A B

Figure 40.5. Treatment of unilateral genu varum in conjunction with a posterolateral corner injury in a 15-year-old male. **A.** Full-length standing radiograph shows genu varum in the right lower limb 3 months prior to the application of an IMGG implant. The patient's lower limb angular deformity was corrected, and he will next undergo reconstructive repair of his posterolateral corner, PCL, and LCL once he reaches skeletal maturity. **B.** Full-length standing radiograph shows correction of the angular deformity after 11 months of IMGG therapy.

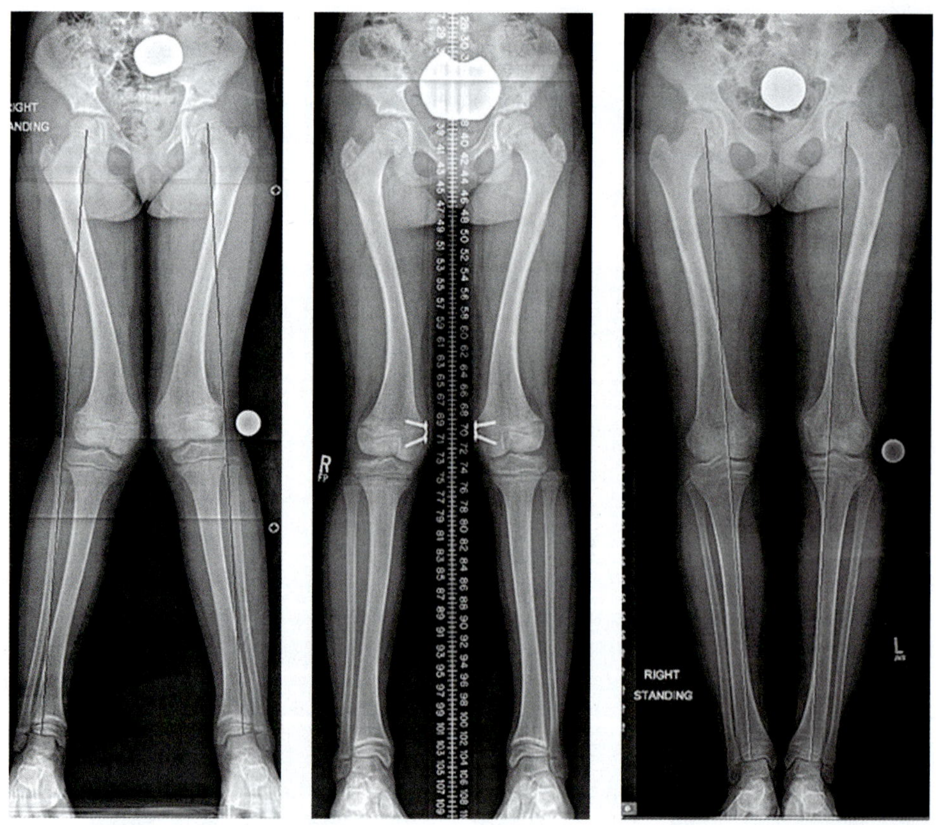

A, B C

Figure 40.6. Treatment of bilateral genu valgum secondary to hypophosphatemic rickets in a 10-year-old female. **A.** Full-length standing radiograph shows bilateral right greater than left genu valgum 3 months prior to application of 8-plates for IMGG therapy. Mechanical axes depict this deformity. **B.** Full-length standing radiograph 9 months after initial application of bilateral 8-plates. **C.** Full-length standing radiograph 9 months after removal of hardware on the left leg and 13 months after removal of hardware on the right leg. Mechanical axes indicate complete correction of the angular deformity. After correction of the genu valgum, patella reconstruction including MPFL reconstruction was performed.

REFERENCES

1. Salenius P, Vankka E. The development of the tibiofemoral angle in children. *J Bone Joint Surg Am.* 1975;57(2):259–261.
2. Tanamas S, Hanna FS, Cicuttini FM, et al. Does knee malalignment increase the risk of development and progression of knee osteoarthritis? A systematic review. *Arthritis Rheum.* 2009;61(4):459–467.
3. Blount WP, Clarke GR. Control of bone growth by epiphyseal stapling; a preliminary report. *J Bone Joint Surg Am.* 1949;31A(3):464–478.
4. Stevens PM. Guided growth for angular correction: a preliminary series using a tension band plate. *J Pediatr Orthop.* 2007;27(3):253–259.
5. Burghardt RD, Herzenberg JE. Temporary hemiepiphysiodesis with the eight-Plate for angular deformities: mid-term results. *J Orthop Sci.* 2010;15(5):699–704.
6. Wiemann JM IV, Tryon C, Szalay EA. Physeal stapling versus 8-plate hemiepiphysiodesis for guided correction of angular deformity about the knee. *J Pediatr Orthop.* 2009;29(5):481–485.
7. Niethard M, Deja M, Rogalski M. Correction of angular deformity of the knee in growing children by temporary hemiepiphyseodesis using the eight-plate [in German]. *Z Orthop Unfall.* 2010;148(2):215–221.
8. Jelinek EM, Bittersohl B, Martiny F, et al. The 8-plate versus physeal stapling for temporary hemiepiphyseodesis correcting genu valgum and genu varum: a retrospective analysis of thirty five patients. *Int Orthop.* 2012;36(3):599–605.
9. Gottliebsen M, Rahbek O, Hvid I, et al. Hemiepiphysiodesis: similar treatment time for tension-band plating and for stapling: a randomized clinical trial on guided growth for idiopathic genu valgum. *Acta Orthop.* 2013;84(2):202–206.
10. Goldman V, Green DW. Advances in growth plate modulation for lower extremity malalignment (knock knees and bow legs). *Curr Opin Pediatr.* 2010;22(1):47–53.
11. Anderson M, Green WT, Messner MB. Growth and predictions of growth in the lower extremities. *J Bone Joint Surg Am.* 1963;45-A:1–14.
12. Ballal MS, Bruce CE, Nayagam S. Correcting genu varum and genu valgum in children by guided growth: temporary hemiepiphysiodesis using tension band plates. *J Bone Joint Surg Br.* 2010;92(2):273–276.
13. Heyworth BE, Osei DA, Fabricant PD, et al. The shorthand bone age assessment: a simpler alternative to current methods. *J Pediatr Orthop.* 2013;33(5):569–574.
14. Boero S, Michelis MB, Riganti S. Use of the eight-Plate for angular correction of knee deformities due to idiopathic and pathologic physis: initiating treatment according to etiology. *J Child Orthop.* 2011;5(3):209–216.
15. Guzman H, Yaszay B, Scott VP, et al. Early experience with medial femoral tension band plating in idiopathic genu valgum. *J Child Orthop.* 2011;5(1):11–17.
16. Saran N, Rathjen KE. Guided growth for the correction of pediatric lower limb angular deformity. *J Am Acad Orthop Surg.* 2010;18(9):528–536.
17. Kepler CK, Bogner EA, Hammoud S, et al. Zone of injury of the medial patellofemoral ligament after acute patellar dislocation in children and adolescents. *Am J Sports Med.* 2011;39(7):1444–1449.
18. Bachmann M, Rutz E, Brunner R, et al. Temporary hemiepiphysiodesis of the distal medial femur: MPFL in danger. *Arch Orthop Trauma Surg.* 2014;134(8):1059–1064.
19. Rhee SJ, Pavlou G, Oakley J, et al. Modern management of patellar instability. *Int Orthop.* 2012;36(12):2447–2456.
20. Weeks KD III, Fabricant PD, Ladenhauf HN, et al. Surgical options for patellar stabilization in the skeletally immature patient. *Sports Med Arthrosc.* 2012;20(3):194–202.
21. Fabricant PD, Osbahr DC, Green DW. Management of a rare complication after screw fixation of a pediatric tibial spine avulsion fracture: a case report with follow-up to skeletal maturity. *J Orthop Trauma.* 2011;25(12):e115–e119.
22. Harner CD, Vogrin TM, Höher J, et al. Biomechanical analysis of a posterior cruciate ligament reconstruction. Deficiency of the posterolateral structures as a cause of graft failure. *Am J Sports Med.* 2000;28(1):32–39.
23. LaPrade RF, Resig S, Wentorf F, et al. The effects of grade III posterolateral knee complex injuries on anterior cruciate ligament graft force. A biomechanical analysis. *Am J Sports Med.* 1999;27(4):469–475.
24. Noyes FR, Barber-Westin SD. Anterior cruciate ligament revision reconstruction: results using a quadriceps tendon-patellar bone autograft. *Am J Sports Med.* 2006;34(4):553–564.
25. Petje G, Meizer R, Radler C, et al. Deformity correction in children with hereditary hypophosphatemic rickets. *Clin Orthop Relat Res.* 2008;466(12):3078–3085.
26. Eastwood DM, Sanghrajka AP. Guided growth: recent advances in a deep-rooted concept. *J Bone Joint Surg Br.* 2011;93(1):12–18.
27. Schroerlucke S, Bertrand S, Clapp J, et al. Failure of Orthofix eight Plate for the treatment of Blount disease. *J Pediatr Orthop.* 2009;29(1):57–60.
28. Sung KH, Ahn S, Chung CY, et al. Rate of correction after asymmetrical physeal suppression in valgus deformity: analysis using a linear mixed model application. *J Pediatr Orthop.* 2012;32(8):805–814.

CHAPTER

41

Alec A. Macaulay
Benton E. Heyworth

Surgical Treatment for Symptomatic Osgood-Schlatter Disease

INTRODUCTION

In 1903, Robert Osgood and Carl Schlatter independently published reports describing the clinical entity that now bears their surnames.[1,2] Osgood-Schlatter disease (OSD), also referred to as *Osgood-Schlatter syndrome*, is the eponym applied to tibial tubercle apophysitis, a common cause of knee pain in the adolescent athlete. It is characterized by activity-related painful inflammation in the cartilage of the tibial tubercle apophysis. Swelling and prominence of the tubercle can occur as well (Fig. 41.1) but are not necessarily or consistently present in the condition. Symptoms are generally worsened with physical activities, usually those that involve running, jumping, landing, cutting, or pivoting, but may instead simply be due to direct pressure on the tubercle, such as with kneeling. The symptoms of OSD typically resolve spontaneously around the time of skeletal maturity but may be present before this time to varying degrees for months, or even years, in some adolescents or preadolescents. A subset of patients with OSD experience persistent symptoms and disability *beyond* the time of skeletal maturity despite an appropriate course of conservative management. Surgical intervention to provide pain relief may be an option in these refractory cases.

ANATOMY

The tibial tubercle is the site of an apophysis, a chondro-osseous prominence or protuberance that experiences repetitive traction forces from a tendinous attachment. Prior to skeletal maturity, these tensile forces make the cartilaginous plate of the apophysis structurally different than the adjacent proximal tibial physis, which is subjected to compressive forces. The tibial tubercle apophysis has a large fibrocartilaginous component, helping it to withstand the strong tensile forces produced by the patellar tendon.[3]

The tibial tubercle has been described as developing through four stages during childhood and adolescence (Fig. 41.2).[4] The four stages have been named the *cartilaginous stage*, the *apophyseal stage*, the *epiphyseal stage*, and the *bony stage*. In the cartilaginous stage, the tubercle is entirely made of cartilage and not evident on x-ray. In the apophyseal stage, the secondary ossification center of the tubercle appears as a discrete entity. In the epiphyseal stage, the tubercle ossification center unites with the proximal tibia ossification center, but cartilage remains, deep to this bony portion of the apophysis. In the bony stage, the physis and apophysis ossify completely, or "close."[3]

ETIOLOGY

Multiple theories on the etiology of OSD have been proposed. These include mechanical avulsion, patellar tendon degeneration, avascular necrosis, and infection. However, the majority of research supports the mechanical theory that OSD is caused by repetitive traction-based microtrauma to the cartilaginous portion of the apophysis. There may also be one or more discreet episodes of new or increased tibial tubercle pain during the late cartilaginous or apophyseal stage, which can serve as inciting events for the more chronic, inflammatory condition.[3,5–8] However, OSD should be differentiated from a true tibial tubercle fracture, which generally requires a higher energy traumatic event and is distinct from the overuse phenomenon. In OSD, the aforementioned adaptive changes of the apophysis lead to the tubercle being vulnerable to traction forces. A tiny fragment or fragments of chondral tissue can be pulled proximally, away from the rest of the tubercle, and may generate small ossicles or fragments of bone. Discrete ossicles can form that are not confluent with the rest of the tibial tubercle[9] and may lead to pain, tenderness, local edema, and inflammation of the distal patellar tendon (patellar tendonitis).[5,9]

EPIDEMIOLOGY

OSD is a remarkably common cause of knee pain in adolescents of both sexes, with a higher incidence in boys than girls.[10] One study suggested that OSD affects 13% of adolescents.[11] However, it is almost twice as common (21%) in adolescents who are involved in sports and less than half as common (5%) in adolescents not involved in sports.[11] The apophyseal stage

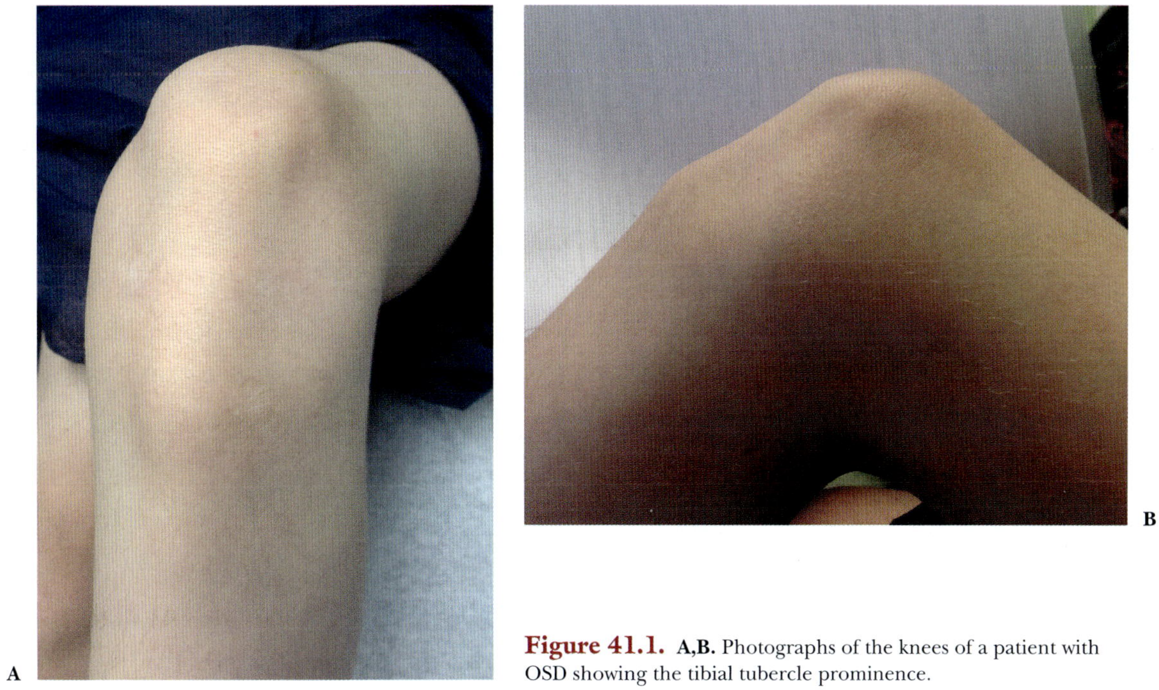

Figure 41.1. **A,B.** Photographs of the knees of a patient with OSD showing the tibial tubercle prominence.

of tibial tubercle development, which occurs roughly between the ages of 10 and 15 years, is the stage during which OSD most commonly arises. Studies have demonstrated the average age of symptom onset to be 12 to 15 years old.[11–13] A third to a half of afflicted adolescents have bilateral knee involvement.[10,11,14] When unilateral, OSD usually affects the knee of the jumping or "take-off" leg.[11]

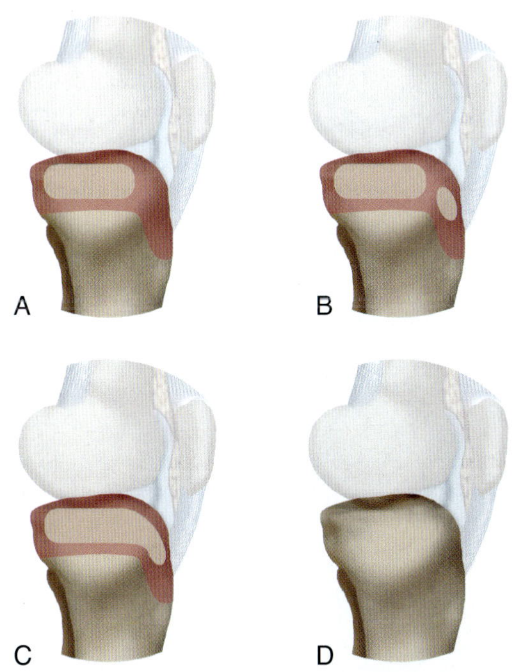

Figure 41.2. **A–D.** The four stages of tibial tubercle development.

EVALUATION

History and Physical Examination

The diagnosis of OSD is typically made based on history and physical examination findings rather than imaging findings. Patients will often complain of knee pain localized to the "front" of the knee or a "bump just below the knee." The duration of symptoms can vary from weeks to years. The pain experienced and degree of limitation can range from a mild, dull, achy discomfort to a severe limp, sometimes even requiring crutches.

Physical examination is critical for distinguishing OSD from other similar knee disorders that can affect adolescents or preadolescents. Tenderness in OSD is at the distal patellar tendon and tibial tubercle. A prominent tibial tubercle may be visible and tender free ossicles may be palpable.

The differential diagnosis of knee disorders similar to OSD includes two other overuse injuries of the knee extensor mechanism, namely patellar tendonitis and Sinding-Larsen-Johansson syndrome. However, these entities are generally distinguishable from OSD on physical exam because the pain and tenderness are at the proximal patellar tendon and distal pole of the patella rather than at the distal patellar tendon and tibial tubercle. Although rare, it is possible to have a combination of these overuse injuries at the same time.

Imaging

Radiographic findings in patients with active OSD will most commonly be absent, with no difference from normal knee x-rays in asymptomatic children. However, radiographs can, in some cases, support the diagnosis if one or more ossicles are seen on the lateral view. Moreover, x-rays are important for ruling out other pathology if knee symptoms are grossly

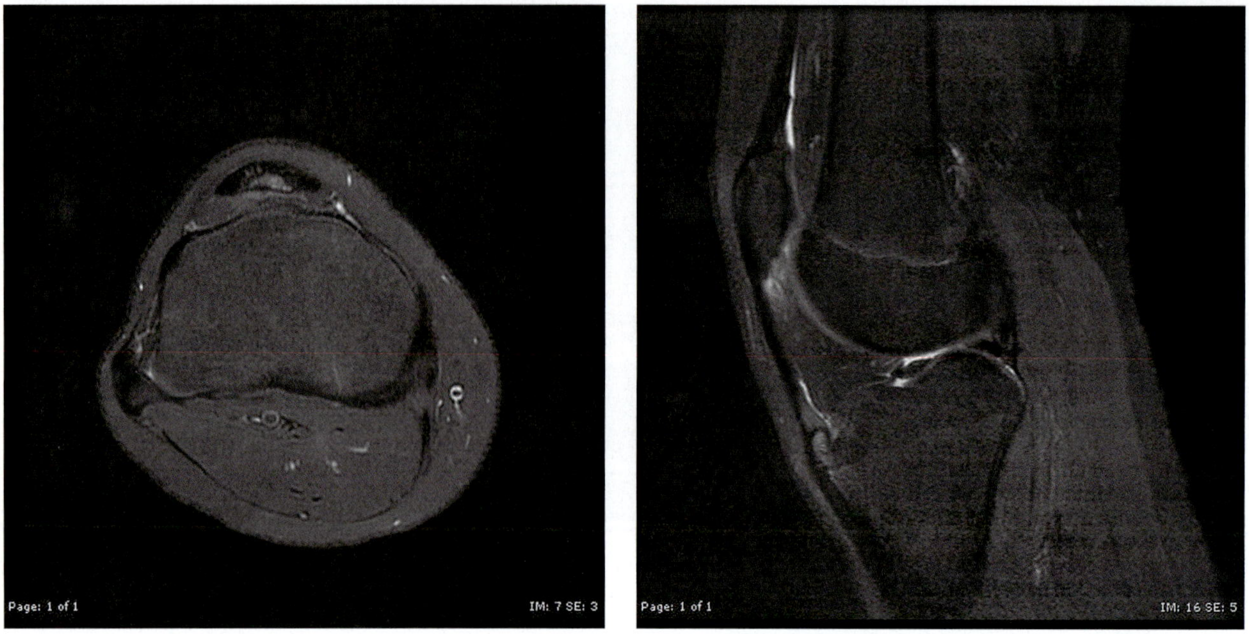

A B

Figure 41.3. Axial **(A)** and sagittal **(B)** T2 MRI in a skeletally mature patient with persistent OSD. The images show the free ossicle with increased signal as well as inflammation in the surrounding patellar tendon.

asymmetrical or are not limited to the region of the tubercle. Radiographs are recommended if surgery is being considered for a skeletally mature patient complaining of tibial tubercle pain. Standard anteroposterior (AP) and lateral views are generally sufficient when radiographs are obtained, although one study has suggested that a lateral view with 10 to 20 degrees of internal rotation allows for better visualization of the profile of the tibial tubercle.[10] Further imaging modalities, such as ultrasound and magnetic resonance imaging (MRI), have been shown to be effective at diagnosing OSD but are rarely needed (Fig. 41.3).[9,15,16]

The radiographic finding characteristic of OSD is a prominent tibial tubercle, with or without discrete ossicles anterior to the tibial tubercle (Fig. 41.4). Even in long-standing OSD, the involved tubercle may remain cartilaginous and not appear on x-rays.[17] MRI may have some value in these cases.

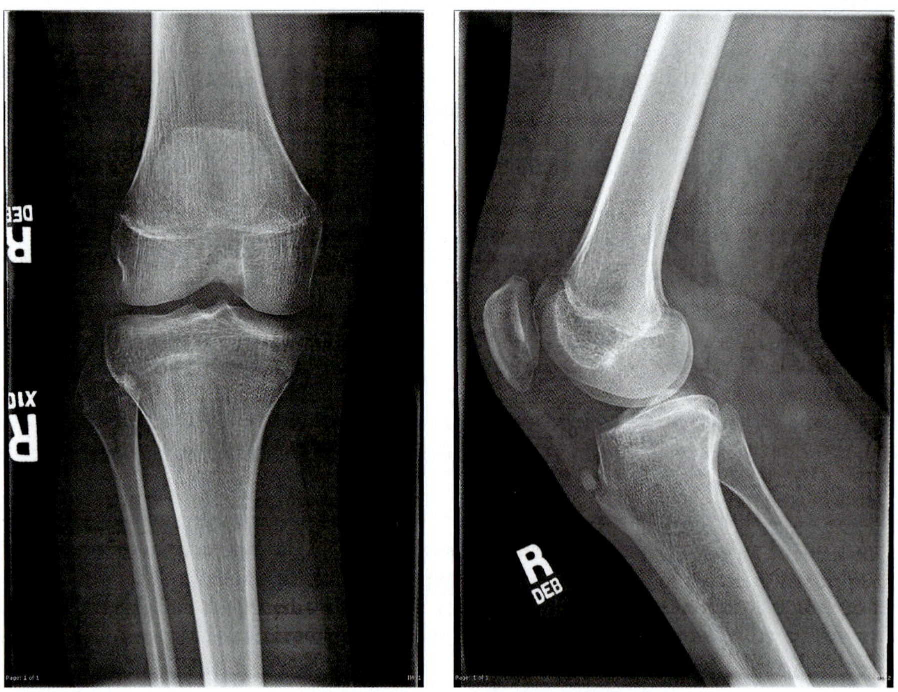

A B

Figure 41.4. AP **(A)** and lateral **(B)** x-rays of a skeletally mature patient with persistent OSD and the classic findings on the lateral x-ray of a prominent tibial tubercle and a free ossicle.

There has also been debate whether visible ossicles on x-ray are a prerequisite to surgical intervention in patients with recalcitrant OSD.[17,18]

TREATMENT

Natural History and Nonoperative Treatment

The mainstay of treatment for OSD is relative rest and activity modification. Other options include icing, oral anti-inflammatory medications, and physical therapy focusing on quadriceps and hamstrings strength and flexibility. Athletes may continue with their sports if these modalities give them relief, but increasing or unremitting pain may warrant complete rest for a period of weeks to allow the pain-inciting inflammation to resolve. Using a treatment dose regimen of around-the-clock oral anti-inflammatory medications for 2 to 4 weeks may be more effective in symptom resolution than using them on an as-needed basis. Some authors have suggested that even with significant improvement during such a hiatus, most adolescents will experience persistent limitations due to symptoms for approximately 6 months.[11]

The symptoms of OSD have classically been thought to improve with conservative measures and fully resolve with skeletal maturation of the tibial tubercle. Although this may be the case for the majority of adolescents, there is a subset of patients with OSD who have symptoms that persist after skeletal maturity. Importantly, Krause et al.[14] assessed 50 patients seen at an average of 9 years after the onset of OSD and found kneeling pain in 60% and other limitations in 24% of subjects. Similarly, Ross and Villard[19] found higher disability levels on knee outcome scores in 25 college athletes at an average of 7.6 years from the onset of OSD, when compared with age-matched controls that had not suffered from OSD.

OPERATIVE TREATMENT FOR OSGOOD-SCHLATTER DISEASE

The vast majority of patients with OSD will not require surgical intervention. Initial conservative measures and progression to skeletal maturity will result in symptom resolution and full return to function in most patients. In one study, less than 2% of patients treated for OSD ended up needing surgery, and even this may be an overestimate of the need for surgery given the selection bias present in the study.[20] However, as previously mentioned, there is a small subset of patients with persistent symptoms that do not respond to extensive conservative measures, even after skeletal maturity. The indications most authors describe for surgical intervention are a skeletally mature patient, failure of prolonged conservative treatment measures, continued knee pain, and functional limitations secondary to the knee pain. Kneeling pain alone is generally not a good indication for surgery, as a significant percentage of patients may still have this problem after surgery.[13]

Previously described surgical techniques used to treat recalcitrant OSD included tibial tubercle drilling and patellar tendon débridement. However, these have not been shown to provide reliable pain relief.[14,17] When indicated, free ossicle excision is currently the preferred surgical intervention for persistent OSD and has been shown in a number of studies to provide good pain relief.[5,13,17,18,20–22] Tibial tubercleplasty, in which a prominent tibial tubercle is smoothed down with a burr or osteotome, can be performed in addition to os excision if a prominent tibial tubercle is felt to be playing a role in kneeling pain. However, the results of tubercleplasty are less reliable than simple ossicle excision. More recently, reports of ossicle excision via an arthroscopic technique have emerged with favorable results.[23,24] However, the open technique remains more common and has a longer track record of consistent results.

AUTHORS' PREFERRED SURGICAL TECHNIQUE

The patient is positioned on a radiolucent operating room table, with a C-arm fluoroscopy unit brought in from the contralateral side. Tourniquet use is based on surgeon preference but optimizes visualization and identification of chondroosseous fragments within the patellar tendon. A longitudinal midline incision is made over the proximal tibial tubercle and distal patellar tendon. Dissection is performed down to the level of the paratenon, which should be divided sharply with meticulous elevation for later closure. Fluoroscopy should be used to identify the exact position of any ossicles or fragments, which are typically embedded in the posterior aspect of the distal patellar tendon. The overlying tendon is split in line with its fibers to minimize the effects on its structural integrity and to optimize postoperative healing. Alternatively, with the knee in maximum extension, the patellar tendon can be retracted to one side and ossicles identified from the backside, although this approach may be difficult without elevation of tendon fibers off of the bony tubercle. Ossicles can be excised with a scalpel or rongeur (Fig. 41.5). Care should be taken to look for all fragments not attached to the tibial tubercle, as some may be cartilaginous, thus not showing up on preoperative x-rays or intraoperative fluoroscopy. Following ossicle resection, tibial tubercleplasty may be performed in cases of a prominent or misshapen tibial tubercle, particularly if any sharp or irregular superficial margins exist. Again it is important not to disrupt the insertion of the patellar tendon. After thorough irrigation is performed to minimize any heterotopic bone formation within the tendon, one or more side-to-side absorbable sutures may be placed in the tendon split to optimize healing, followed by routine skin closure.

Postoperative rehabilitation involves weight bearing as tolerated with crutches for comfort. A knee immobilizer or hinged knee brace locked in extension may be used during ambulation for 4 to 6 weeks. Early range of motion from 0 to 90 degrees should be encouraged when not weight bearing, with straight-leg raises and quad sets encouraged. After 6 weeks, weight-bearing strengthening exercises should be performed, with an emphasis on eccentric exercises and other patellofemoral protocols and a progression to running and agility exercises. Return to sports is generally allowed within 3 to 4 months, provided symmetrical strength and stability are seen with dynamic, sports-specific exercises.

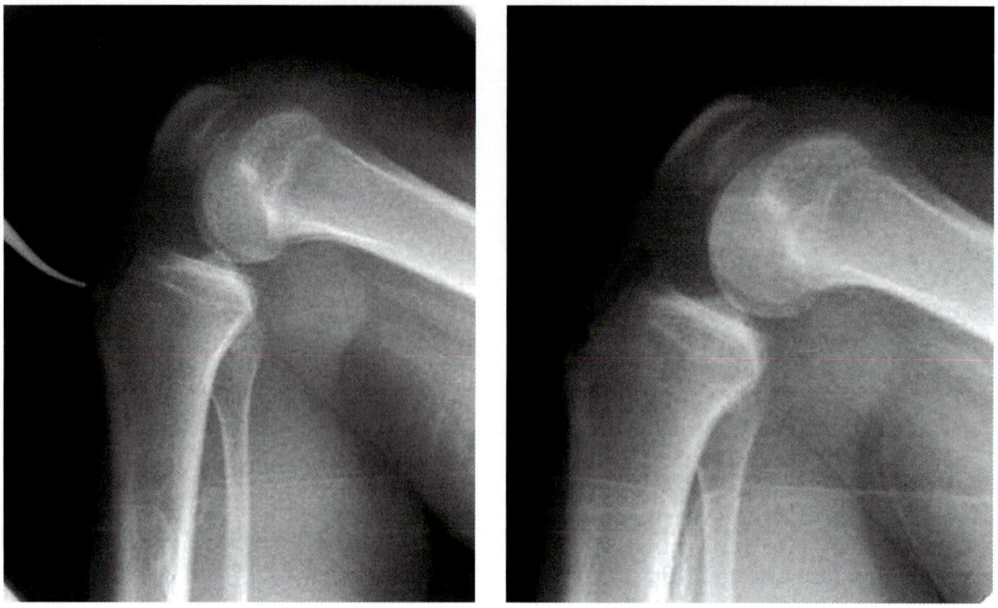

A B

Figure 41.5. Intraoperative fluoroscopy images before **(A)** and after **(B)** free ossicle excision.

REFERENCES

1. Osgood RB. Lesions of the tibial tubercle occurring during adolescence. 1903. *Clin Orthop Relat Res.* 1993;(286):4–9.
2. Schlatter C. Verletzungen des schnabelformigen Forstatzes der oberen Tibiaepiphyse. *Beitr Klin Chir.* 1903;38:874–887.
3. Ogden JA, Southwick WO. Osgood-Schlatter's disease and tibial tuberosity development. *Clin Orthop Relat Res.* 1976;(116):180–189.
4. Ehrenborg G, Engfeldt B. The insertion of the ligamentum patellae on the tibial tuberosity. Some views in connection with the Osgood-Schlatter lesion. *Acta Chir Scand.* 1961;121:491–499.
5. Mital MA, Matza RA, Cohen J. The so-called unresolved Osgood-Schlatter lesion: a concept based on fifteen surgically treated lesions. *J Bone Joint Surg Am.* 1980;62(5):732–739.
6. Ehrenborg G. The Osgood-Schlatter lesion. A clinical study of 170 cases. *Acta Chir Scand.* 1962;124:89–105.
7. Ogden JA. Radiology of postnatal skeletal development. X. Patella and tibial tuberosity. *Skeletal Radiol.* 1984;11(4):246–257.
8. Yashar A, Loder RT, Hensinger RN. Determination of skeletal age in children with Osgood-Schlatter disease by using radiographs of the knee. *J Pediatr Orthop.* 1995;15(3):298–301.
9. Hirano A, Fukubayashi T, Ishii T, et al. Magnetic resonance imaging of Osgood-Schlatter disease: the course of the disease. *Skeletal Radiol.* 2002;31(6):334–342.
10. Gholve PA, Scher DM, Khakharia S, et al. Osgood Schlatter syndrome. *Curr Opin Pediatr.* 2007;19(1):44–50.
11. Kujala UM, Kvist M, Heinonen O. Osgood-Schlatter's disease in adolescent athletes. Retrospective study of incidence and duration. *Am J Sports Med.* 1985;13(4):236–241.
12. Hanada M, Koyama H, Takahashi M, et al. Relationship between the clinical findings and radiographic severity in Osgood-Schlatter disease. *Open Access J Sports Med.* 2012;3:17–20.
13. Pihlajamaki HK, Mattila VM, Parviainen M, et al. Long-term outcome after surgical treatment of unresolved Osgood-Schlatter disease in young men. *J Bone Joint Surg Am.* 2009;91(10):2350–2358.
14. Krause BL, Williams JP, Catterall A. Natural history of Osgood-Schlatter disease. *J Pediatr Orthop.* 1990;10(1):65–68.
15. Lanning P, Heikkinen E. Ultrasonic features of the Osgood-Schlatter lesion. *J Pediatr Orthop.* 1991;11(4):538–540.
16. Blankstein A, Cohen I, Heim M, et al. Ultrasonography as a diagnostic modality in Osgood-Schlatter disease. A clinical study and review of the literature. *Arch Orthop Trauma Surg.* 2001;121(9):536–539.
17. Glynn MK, Regan BF. Surgical treatment of Osgood-Schlatter's disease. *J Pediatr Orthop.* 1983;3(2):216–219.
18. Nierenberg G, Falah M, Keren Y, et al. Surgical treatment of residual Osgood-Schlatter disease in young adults: role of the mobile osseous fragment. *Orthopedics.* 2011;34(3):176.
19. Ross MD, Villard D. Disability levels of college-aged men with a history of Osgood-Schlatter disease. *J Strength Cond Res.* 2003;17(4):659–663.
20. Weiss JM, Jordan SS, Andersen JS, et al. Surgical treatment of unresolved Osgood-Schlatter disease: ossicle resection with tibial tubercleplasty. *J Pediatr Orthop.* 2007;27(7):844–847.
21. Orava S, Malinen L, Karpakka J, et al. Results of surgical treatment of unresolved Osgood-Schlatter lesion. *Ann Chir Gynaecol.* 2000;89(4):298–302.
22. El-Husseini TF, Abdelgawad AA. Results of surgical treatment of unresolved Osgood-Schlatter disease in adults. *J Knee Surg.* 2010; 23(2):103–107.
23. Beyzadeoglu T, Inan M, Bekler H, et al. Arthroscopic excision of an ununited ossicle due to Osgood-Schlatter disease. *Arthroscopy.* 2008;24(9):1081–1083.
24. DeBerardino TM, Branstetter JG, Owens BD. Arthroscopic treatment of unresolved Osgood-Schlatter lesions. *Arthroscopy.* 2007; 23(10):1127.e1–1127.e3.

Index